Thieme

Manual of Functional and Aesthetic Rhinoplasty

Illustrated Stepwise Instructions with Videos

Alexander Berghaus, MD
Professor
Former Director, Department of Otorhinolaryngology
University Hospital, Campus Großhadern
Ludwig Maximilian University of Munich;
Private Practice
Munich, Germany

1026 Illustrations

Thieme
Stuttgart • New York • Delhi • Rio de Janeiro

Library of Congress Cataloging-in-Publication Data is available from the publisher.

Important note: Medicine is an ever-changing science undergoing continual development. Research and clinical experience are continually expanding our knowledge, in particular our knowledge of proper treatment and drug therapy. Insofar as this book mentions any dosage or application, readers may rest assured that the authors, editors, and publishers have made every effort to ensure that such references are in accordance with **the state of knowledge at the time of production of the book.**

Nevertheless, this does not involve, imply, or express any guarantee or responsibility on the part of the publishers in respect to any dosage instructions and forms of applications stated in the book. **Every user is requested to examine carefully** the manufacturers' leaflets accompanying each drug and to check, if necessary, in consultation with a physician or specialist, whether the dosage schedules mentioned therein or the contraindications stated by the manufacturers differ from the statements made in the present book. Such examination is particularly important with drugs that are either rarely used or have been newly released on the market. Every dosage schedule or every form of application used is entirely at the user's own risk and responsibility. The authors and publishers request every user to report to the publishers any discrepancies or inaccuracies noticed. If errors in this work are found after publication, errata will be posted at www.thieme.com on the product description page.

Some of the product names, patents, and registered designs referred to in this book are in fact registered trademarks or proprietary names even though specific reference to this fact is not always made in the text. Therefore, the appearance of a name without designation as proprietary is not to be construed as a representation by the publisher that it is in the public domain.

Thieme addresses people of all gender identities equally. We encourage our authors to use gender-neutral or gender-equal expressions wherever the context allows.

Georg Thieme Verlag KG
Oswald-Hesse-Straße 50
70469 Stuttgart, Germany
www.thieme.com

Translation: Renee Kulkarni, MD
Illustrations: Katja Dalkowski, MD
Cover design: © Thieme
Cover image source: © Thieme/Alexander Berghaus, Katja Dalkowski
Artwork on page ii: Horst Antes, 2024 (for Alexander)
Typesetting by TNQ Tech Private Limited, India

Printed in Germany by Westermann Druck Zwickau GmbH

5 4 3 2 1

ISBN: 978-3-13-241278-1

DOI: 10.1055/b000000272

Also available as an e-book:
eISBN (PDF): 978-3-13-241433-4
eISBN (epub): 978-3-13-258234-7

Contents

List of Videos

Preface

When I first started learning rhinoplasty more than 40 years ago, I immediately became engrossed in the subject. I didn't realize then that I was embarking on a very long journey that would take me through many ups and downs and through a maze of different methods, and that going astray would be a natural part of my progress.

The masters in the field at that time, from whom we used to learn with rapt attention, defended their views with conviction, and it seemed like it would just be a matter of imitating everything they did in the same way in order to become a good, successful nose surgeon oneself for ever after. Although they have the same level of commitment, today's teachers present very different content and convictions than were current 40 years ago, and some methods that were then regarded as forgotten have now become very up-to-date again. The reasons for these continuing changes – which also affect surgical ideas in fields other than rhinoplasty – lie in the constant expansion of empirical and statistical knowledge, and also in incessant technical advances in the field of surgery.

Over the decades, my professional pathway has consequently led through the narrow channels of closed endonasal procedures toward unlocking the gateway to open access. The path has led away from structured rhinoplasty toward surface procedures and foundational principles. Hammer, chisel, and rasp have been exchanged for electrical instruments and piezo technology. Sutures that used to be left in forever gave way to long-term dissolvable and eventually even quickly absorbable threads. The classic cast was superseded by plastic and ultimately aluminum splints, which were no longer left on the nose for weeks, but only for a few days. Patients were finally freed from the obligatory packing with nasal strips that I had first been taught was indispensable. And the strips were replaced with – nothing. Originally, surgical planning consisted of making a few unaided pencil strokes on a patient's photo. It has now become a simulation process involving computer-aided high technology, the perfection of which presents surgeons with even greater challenges.

Has it all been good – and if so, for whom? Of course, good and even very good results were also achieved with methods that may be regarded as outdated today – otherwise such methods would have been abandoned fairly quickly. However, there was a constant desire for greater reliability, predictability, safety, and precision in the methods used, and it is precisely in these areas that progress over the years has led to the benefits that patients and surgeons enjoy today. At the same time, none of the "old" traditional knowledge has been lost. When the opportunity arises, experienced surgeons are always happy to fall back on methods that no longer feature in the modern toolbox.

The aim of this book is to provide a coherent and comprehensible presentation of the full range of surgical techniques that I have found to be useful and helpful. In the best case, readers may find supportive and stimulating guidance on their way through the world of rhinoplasty – a path that may be different for each individual, and is rarely straightforward, but which in the end promises so much success and fulfillment for doctors and patients alike.

Alexander Berghaus
Munich, Spring 2025

Acknowledgments

My thanks are due to all those who have helped me with this book, and also to all who have provided encouragement, support, and companionship during my career in nose surgery.

Work on the book would have been inconceivable without the support provided by the publishing house's staff. Special thanks are due to Executive Editor Stephan Konnry, who supported me from the very first contact throughout the long development process with expertise, good advice, humor, and a great deal of patience. I am also grateful to Angelika M. Findgott, Snehil Sharma at Thieme Delhi, and Renee Kulkarni who translated part of the text into English. Michael Robertson did an excellent job as copy editor; but without the consistent support of Editor and Project Manager Anne Lamparter, I would hardly have managed the final stage of completion - many thanks to her!

With tireless commitment and artistic skill, Katja Dalkowski has translated my ideas into graphic representations. For almost all of the photos, the professional production and editing is owed to Andreas Steeger.

Dietmar Zühlke, Michael Handrock, Irene Flemming, Ronald Matthias, Ernst Kastenbauer, Rudolf Stellmach, and Hans Scherer provided me with support and encouragement in my career from a young age. Influential early teachers for me were Rodolphe Meyer and Eugene Tardy – already celebrated worldwide at that time as icons in the field of rhinoplasty. They taught me certain basic principles of nose surgery that I still take for granted today, and it was through their influence that rhinoplasty became the focus of my professional interest.

Important companions in the field of rhinoplasty with whom I have exchanged many suggestions and shared experience on our favorite topic, with friendly links often developing beyond nasal surgery, include in particular Hossam Foda – a good friend and partner, and not only in the countless rhinoplasty surgery courses we took part in together. Others also include Thomas Romo III, Stephen S. Park, Ira Papel, Wolfgang Gubisch, Gerhard Rettinger, Yves Saban, Enrico Robotti, Olivier Gerbault, Richard Davis, Charles East, Norman Pastorek, Peter Adamson, Julian Rowe-Jones, Fazil Apaydin, Roxana Cobo, Brian Wong, Richard Gentile, Jonathan Sykes, as well as Santdeep Paun, Milos Kovacevic, Jochen Wurm, Werner Heppt, Eckart Buttler, Holger Gassner, Sameer Ali Bafaqeeh, Mahmoud Elbestar, and Johan Reyneke. It was from Gary Burget that I learned that nasal reconstruction and rhinoplasty have a common denominator. Sometimes even short conversations have led to a valuable exchange of ideas, such as with Sam Most or Dean Toriumi.

Many thanks also to Chrisanthi Karapantzou for her spontaneous willingness to critically review chapter 22. Not to be forgotten are the medical staff members with a strong interest in the subject of rhinoplasty who, while still learners, asked me very shrewd questions – and by doing so also gave me more in return than they probably realized. In the meantime, they have successfully shaped their own careers, not always in the field of nose surgery: Stephan von Rothkirch, Sergije Jovanovic, Marc Bloching, Marion San Nicolò, Vanessa von Holzschuher, Klaus Stelter, Sven Becker, Christian Jacobi, Sebastian Strieth, Hjalmar "Charly" Hagedorn, Uli Harréus, and Christian "Sergeant" Pfeffer. Special thanks go to Martin Canis and Kariem Sharaf, who supported me in obtaining patient images from my previous post at the University of Munich's Grosshadern Hospital. I would also like to thank Alessandro Ferrario and Andrea Reho, Milan, for the nice opportunities to perform my surgery in beautiful Italy. Thanks also to Eva Wimmer, who has been an invaluable help in the postoperative aftercare of my patients since my time in private practice.

In the operating theaters in which I have worked, the support of the nursing staff always made a significant contribution to the success of procedures. The nursing teams headed by Gertrud Kreutz in Steglitz Hospital at the Free University of Berlin, Kerstin Deutschmann in the ENT Department at Martin Luther University of Halle-Wittenberg, Sofie Wohlgeschaffen at the University of Munich's Grosshadern Hospital, and Claudia Meyer in the ENT Department at the Helios Clinic in Dachau are all deserving of mention. I am also most recently grateful to Ruth Gröschel at Bernhard Wilhelm's clinic in Wolfratshausen and to her colleague Ginka Tatschkova, who, at 80 years old, still did a perfect job at the operating table.

I would also like to thank the patients who have placed their trust in me and often given me valuable feedback. Special thanks go to those who have allowed their photos to be used here.

Special thanks also go to Horst Antes, long-time friend and companion outside the operating room, for the beautiful frontispiece he created just for this book.

And, last but not least: Lisa, Frizzi, and Viko, who patiently endured the fact that the planned 2 years for creating this book ended up being 7 – thanks to you for your constant encouragement!

Technical Notes for Readers

The **photos** used in this volume are from a variety of sources. Almost all of the images were converted into a CMYK format and made available as .tif files by Andreas Steeger, professional photographer and long-time member of staff at Munich University Hospital.

Photographs of instruments and equipment were primarily taken by Andreas Steeger. Some of these images were also made available with the consent of manufacturers with whom we have been collaborating for many years. Only equipment and materials that the author has repeatedly tested are shown and described. Some companies have provided financial support for the production of this book – for example, to help cover translation costs. These contributions were gratefully received and had no influence on the content or design of the book.

Intraoperative photos were taken with various cameras (with the camera integrated into the surgical light, attached to the headband, or on a tripod; smartphone cameras). The image quality of these recordings naturally varies; occasionally, postprocessing was carried out by Andreas Steeger to improve the visibility of details, e.g., with increased contrast and revision of the coloring. Wherever it seemed useful, markings and arrows have been added.

Recognizable patient pictures are only shown if the individuals concerned provided written consent. Many of the photos were taken in the studio at Munich University Hospital, others in my office or clinic, in the latter case usually with a smartphone. Andreas Steeger standardized the image sections for the preoperative and postoperative images in order to improve comparability. Widely differing image colors were adjusted for the same reason.

Postoperative images taken at least 1 year after the operation have been used as far as possible. The depiction of minors was avoided as far as possible, even if the parents had given consent.

Videos were in part created with the same cameras as the photos, with the additional use of an endoscope if necessary. I edited the films with the Apple program iMovie and added spoken text. Video clips from medical device manufacturers have been used where indicated. All videos can be accessed by scanning the QR-code placed in each video-still in the book.

Almost all of the video clips show short segments of procedures or surgical steps that only illustrate the content of the corresponding chapter. An exception to this is Video 6.1, "Full-length preservation rhinoplasty," in which the complete process of a nose correction – in this case a preservation technique – can be followed almost unabridged.

The graphics were professionally created by Katja Dalkowski in accordance with my specifications. Together we have made every effort to present the often complicated surgical anatomy as accurately as possible. In the interests of better comprehensibility, less important details have occasionally been omitted. If existing graphics have been modified and revised in individual cases, this is marked accordingly.

1 Anatomy of the Nose

Successful outcomes in rhinoplasty require a thorough knowledge of anatomy, as in every field of surgery. Any knowledge gaps relating to anatomical structures and relationships should be filled by training on suitable specimens in anatomical or forensic institutes, or in specialized training centers. After years of experience in various training institutions, I can particularly recommend the courses offered by the European College of Aesthetic Medicine and Surgery (ECAMS; https://www.ecamedicine.com/). In these courses, rhinoplasty is learned step by step, theoretically and practically, using excellent material in a relatively small group with a very good ratio of lecturers to learners; the training situation is very similar to an intraoperative setting (▶ Video 1.1).

> Surgical courses that offer practical exercises on specimens and observation of live operations, as well as imparting theoretical knowledge, are particularly valuable.

1.1 The Bony Framework

The external skeleton of the nose consists of the **nasal bones** and the **frontal process of the maxilla** on either side (▶ Fig. 1.1). The internasal suture runs between the nasal bones, separated from the frontal process of the maxilla by the nasomaxillary suture. The inferior borders of these bones form the piriform aperture.

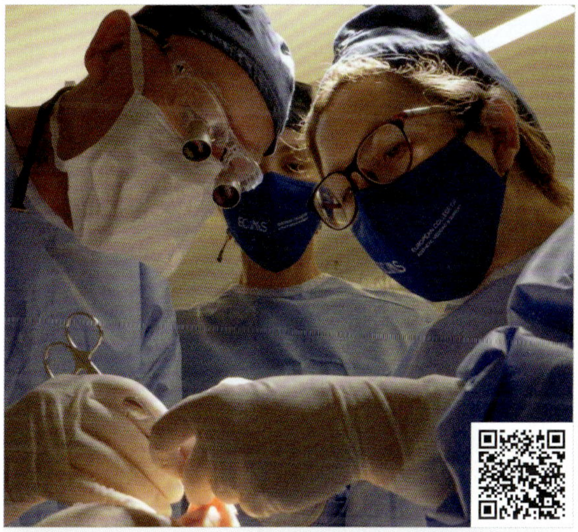

Video 1.1 The European College of Aesthetic Medicine and Surgery (ECAMS) rhinoplasty course.

> The "K-area" is the transitional zone between the cartilaginous and bony framework of the nose — i.e., at the rhinion — where the edges of these structures overlap.

The posterior aspect of the nasal septum comprises two bones, namely the perpendicular plate of the ethmoid and the vomer (▶ Fig. 1.2).

The nasal septum sits on the maxillary crest of the palate, which merges into the premaxilla, with its anteriormost part being the anterior nasal spine. The posterior edge of the vomer forms part of the choanae, the posterior nasal apertures. The nasal cavities and paranasal sinuses (frontal, sphenoidal, and maxillary sinuses, and ethmoid air cells) are closely related and interconnected. Ostial patency and optimal aeration of the paranasal sinuses is paramount for ensuring healthy upper airways (▶ Fig. 1.3).

The turbinates (superior, middle, and inferior nasal conchae) also have a bony framework. The inferior turbinate is the largest of these and the most important for regulating nasal airflow.

> Pathological processes may involve both the nasal septum and the inferior and middle turbinates. Nasal septal deviation may frequently be present, while the inferior turbinate is susceptible to hypertrophy. Surgical diminution of the turbinates is thus often needed in order to relieve nasal obstruction (▶ Fig. 1.3, ▶ Fig. 1.4)

Most of the inferior turbinate consists of vascularized soft tissue, covered with mucous membranes, and not of bone (▶ Fig. 1.5, ▶ Fig. 1.6). Persistent nasal congestion is therefore most commonly due to inferior turbinate hypertrophy and may require surgical diminution of the soft tissues overlying the turbinate.

The inferior turbinates and the floor of the nasal cavity form the boundaries of the inferior meatus, while the middle meatus lies between the middle and lower turbinates. The maxillary sinus opens into the middle meatus, and the nasolacrimal duct into the inferior meatus (see ▶ Fig. 1.3, ▶ Fig. 1.5).

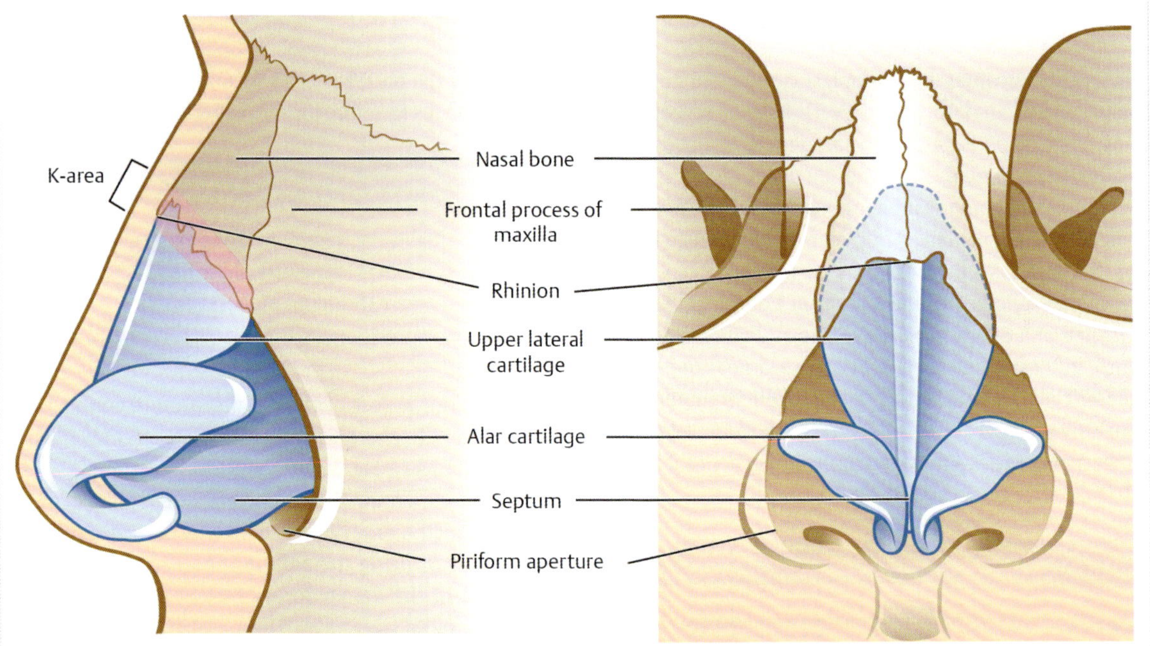

Fig. 1.1 Bony nasal framework. The nasal bones form the bony framework of the outer nose together with the frontal processes of the maxilla.

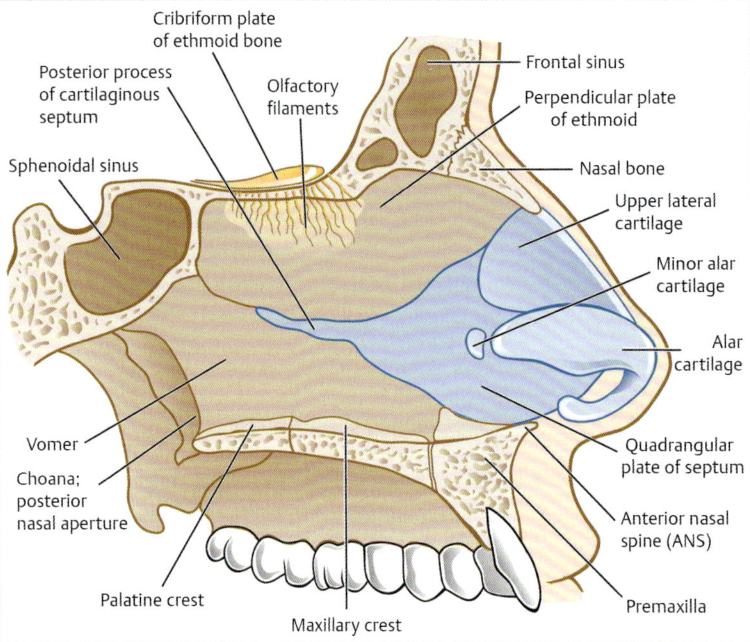

Fig. 1.2 Inner nose, sagittal; view of the septum. The cartilaginous quadrangular plate and the bony perpendicular plate, together with the vomer, are the supporting elements of the nasal septum.

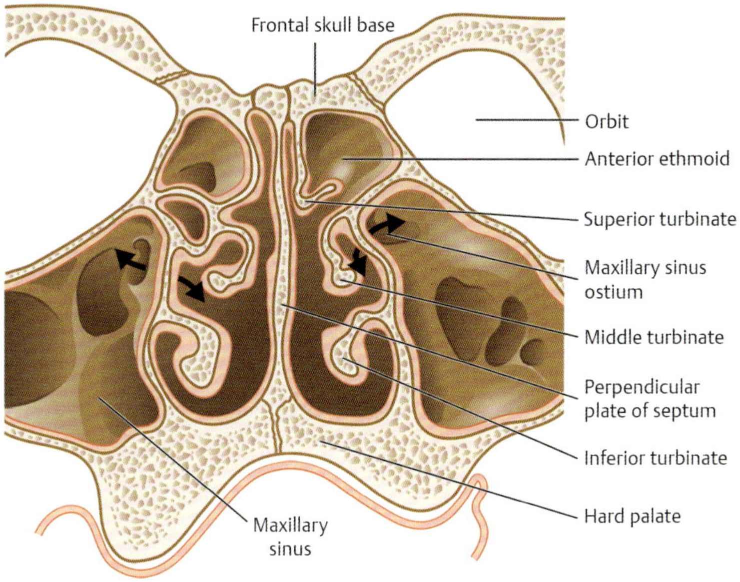

Fig. 1.3 Inner nose, deep cross-section at the level of the maxillary sinuses. The cross-section shows the close relationship of the nasal cavities to the paranasal sinuses.

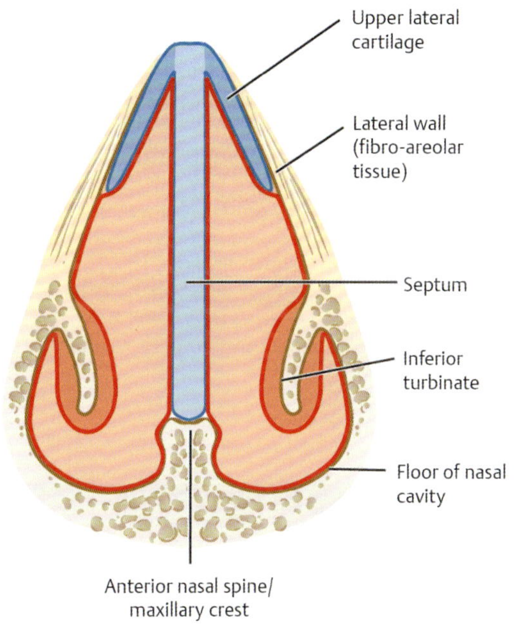

Fig. 1.4 Inner nose, cross-section. The septum and the inferior turbinates are most commonly involved in functional disorders of the nose.

1.2 The Cartilaginous Framework

The anterior two-thirds of the nasal framework consists of cartilage, which provides the mobility and flexibility needed in view of the frequent movement of the nose and repeated touching of the nasal tip. The septum, to which the upper lateral cartilages (ULC) are fused, and the alar cartilages are the most important cartilaginous structures of the nose, both from a functional and a surgical point of view (▶ Fig. 1.7).

> ✔
>
> A variable portion of the cranial aspect of the cartilaginous septum and the upper lateral cartilages in the "K-area" is virtually buried beneath the nasal bones and is directly accessible only after removal of the overlying bone (e.g., during correction of a nasal hump). This anatomical detail is of the utmost importance from the surgical viewpoint (▶ Fig. 1.1, ▶ Fig. 1.7).

A small triangular region of the lateral nasal wall between the upper lateral cartilage, the lateral crus of the alar cartilage (i.e., the lower lateral cartilage, LLC), and the piriform aperture consists only of fibrous tissue, unsupported by stable structural elements (see ▶ Fig. 1.1).

The caudal end of the upper lateral cartilage articulates with the cranial (i.e., cephalic) rim of the lateral crus of the alar cartilage as an "alar scroll," with the edge of the upper lateral cartilage curling outward and that of the lower lateral cartilage curling inward. This cartilaginous articulation may be either loose or rigid (▶ Fig. 1.8).

This area is of particular functional importance for nasal breathing. Here, the lateral nasal wall and the septum form what is known as the **(inner) nasal valve** at the level of the caudal rim of the upper lateral cartilage.

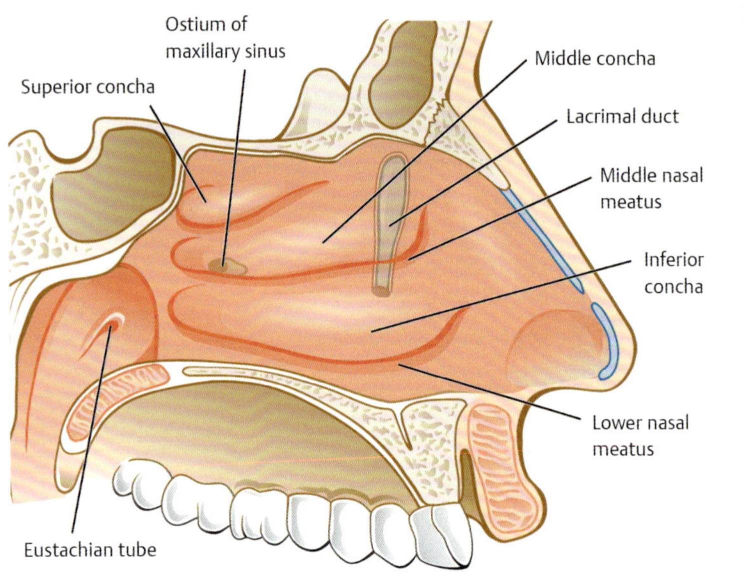

Fig. 1.5 Inner nose, view of the lateral wall. The three turbinates divide the nasal cavity into three meatus. The ostium of the maxillary sinus opens into the middle meatus, while the lacrimal duct opens into the inferior meatus.

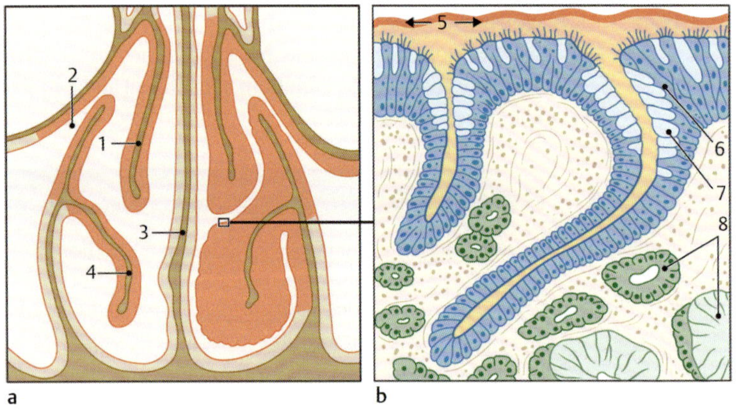

Fig. 1.6 Nasal turbinates and mucosa. **(a)** Frontal section through the nose. The nasal mucosa is unswollen on the left side and swollen on the right. 1, Middle turbinate; 2, maxillary sinus, ostium; 3, nasal septum; 4, inferior turbinate. **(b)** Respiratory mucosa. 5, Mucus layer; 6, respiratory epithelium with cilia; 7, goblet cells; 8, mucosal glands.

> The angle of opening of this valve plays a crucial role in regulating nasal airflow (▶ Fig. 1.9) and should be at least 15° to allow smooth nasal breathing.

A smaller angle may result in obstruction of nasal breathing despite a stable cartilaginous framework. This is typically seen in the "tension nose," characterized by a high, narrow nasal bridge with a high anterior septal angle (see case study, ▶ Fig. 10.13). If the cartilage is weak or compromised by prior rhinoplasty, it may result in collapse of the internal nasal valve despite a normal angle.

> The importance of the counterpart, the **external nasal valve**, must also not be underestimated. This valve is represented by the nostril, bounded medially by the caudal septum and laterally by the caudal edge of the alar cartilage, which may also be floppy and weak. Preoperative evaluation should focus on precise localization of the vulnerable area if a functional disorder is present. Alar rim grafts can be used to reinforce weak external nasal valves (see section 10.3).

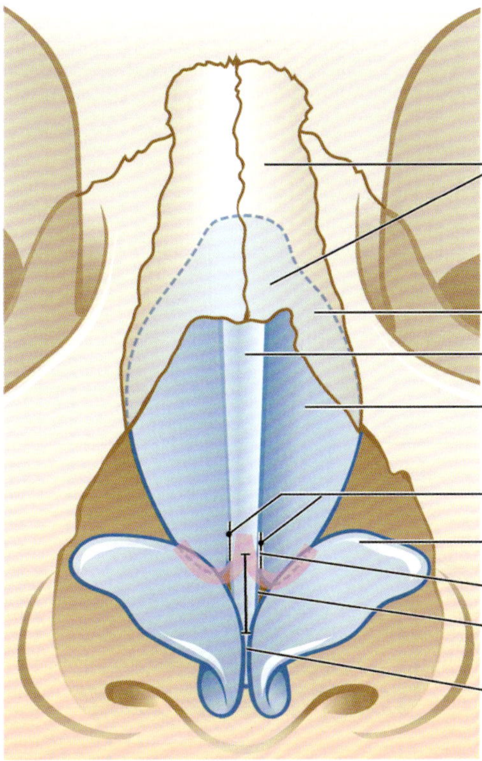

Fig. 1.7 Bony and cartilaginous framework of the nose. The nasal cartilage is partly covered by bone at its cranial aspect.

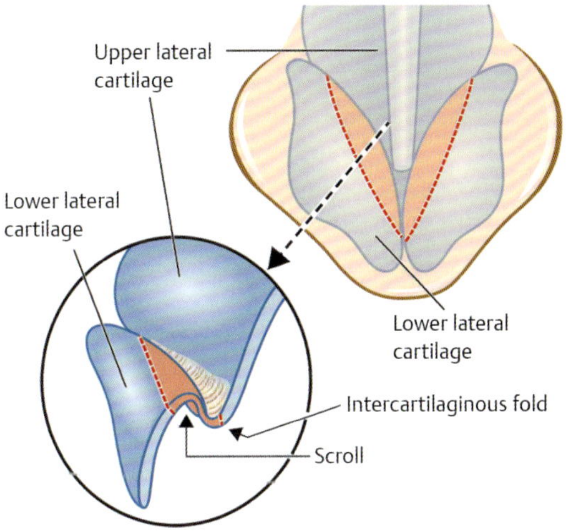

Fig. 1.8 Intercartilaginous fold with "scroll." The upper and lower lateral cartilages (ULC, LLC) are connected at the intercartilaginous fold by an undulating segment of cartilage (scroll).

1.2.1 The Alar Cartilages

The alar cartilages constitute a structural cornerstone of the tip of the nose, and knowledge of their anatomy is essential for the surgeon, particularly for mastering nasal tip surgery.

The configuration of the alar cartilages, with their medial and lateral crura, determines key features of the nasal tip, such as the height and width of the nasal domes, the opening angle of the nares, and also the width and prominence of the columella. Medial stabilization of the alar cartilages by connective and fibrous tissue connecting it to the caudal septum, which in turn rests firmly on the anterior nasal spine, is equally important (▶ Fig. 1.10).

Loss of stability between the anterior nasal spine, the caudal septum, and the medial and lateral crura of the alar cartilages may result in sagging of the nasal tip, with consequent development of functional disorders and nasal deformities. The surgeon must therefore pay special attention to the stability of this complex.

Jack Anderson developed the concept of a three-legged frame (tripod) in this context, on which the equilibrium of a stable anterior nose is based (▶ Fig. 1.11). The central, anterior limb of this "tripod" consists of the columella, with the medial crura of the alar cartilages and the caudal

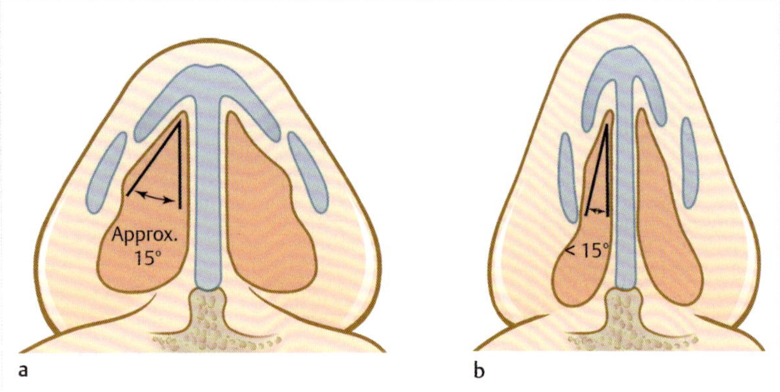

Fig. 1.9 The nasal valve. (a) Normal opening angle of the nasal valve. **(b)** Narrow opening angle, with so-called tension nose.

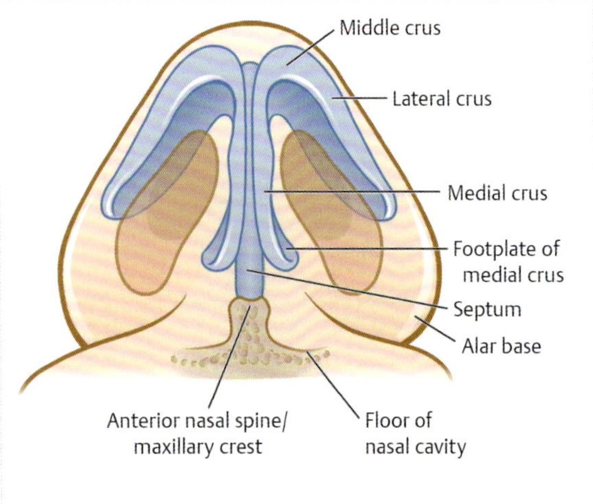

Fig. 1.10 Base of the nose. The medial crura, with the caudal rim of the septum supporting the nasal tip, while the lateral crura help to keep the nostrils open.

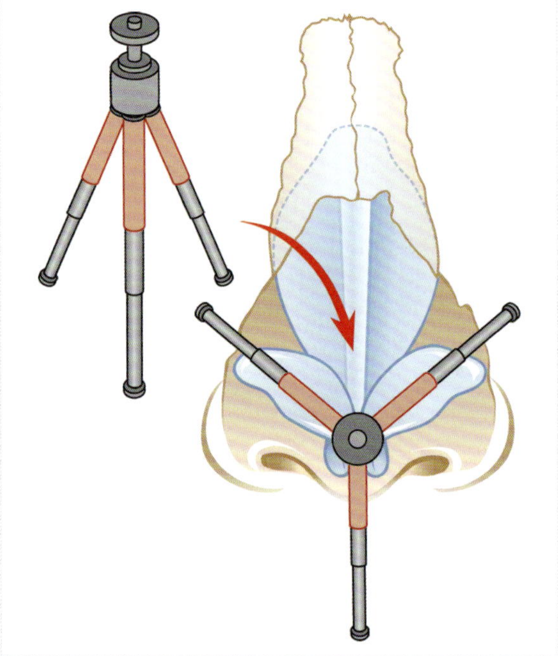

Fig. 1.11 The anterior nose as a tripod (model by Jack Anderson). The notion that the tip of the nose rests on three defined, stable "legs" is a valuable contribution to understanding the "construction" of the nose for successful functional outcomes in rhinoplasty.

edge of the cartilaginous septum, while the lateral crura of the alar cartilages form its lateral supports.

> ✓
>
> The anatomy of the nasal entrance also shows that the width of the base of the nose is only marginally influenced by the alar cartilages (▶ Fig. 1.10). Surgical corrections of the alar base therefore usually require direct interventions on the skin and soft tissue of the alar base.

The **medial** crus of the alar cartilage can be subdivided into the footplate and columella segments. Distinct from it is the **middle** crus, which in turn is further subdivided into lobular and domal segments (▶ Fig. 1.12).

The middle and lateral crura meet at the alar dome, which defines the nasal tip. The dome may also be referred to as the lateral genu, analogous to the medial genu between the middle and medial crus.

The middle crura form an angle of about 30–45° with one another (**angle of divergence**), while the columellar and lobular segments of the medial crura also form an angle of 30–45° on the lateral view (**angle of rotation**; columella–lobular angle).

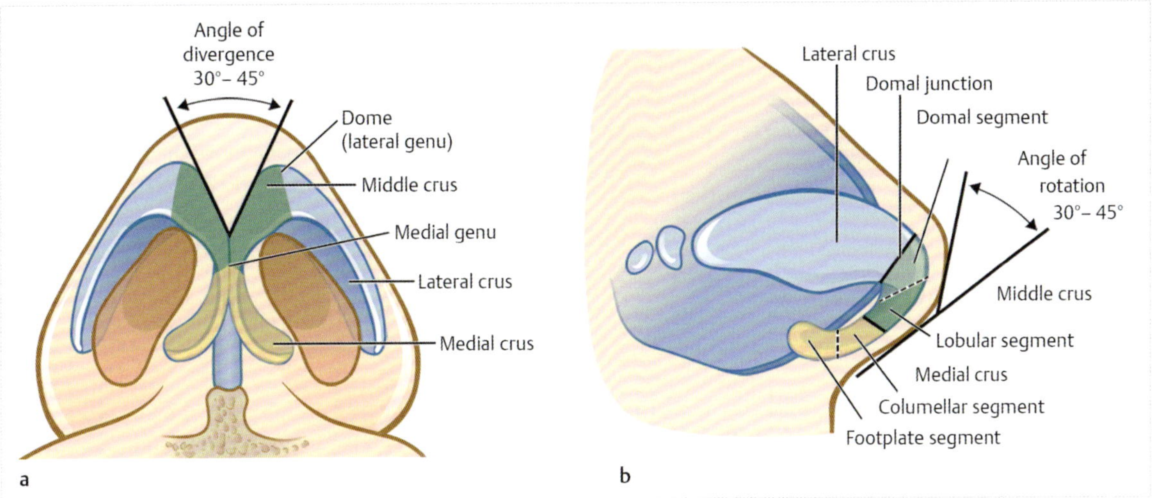

Fig. 1.12 Anatomy of the alar cartilages. (a) A middle crus is visualized in addition to the medial and lateral crura; note the "angle of divergence." **(b)** Subdivision of the medial crus; note the "angle of rotation."

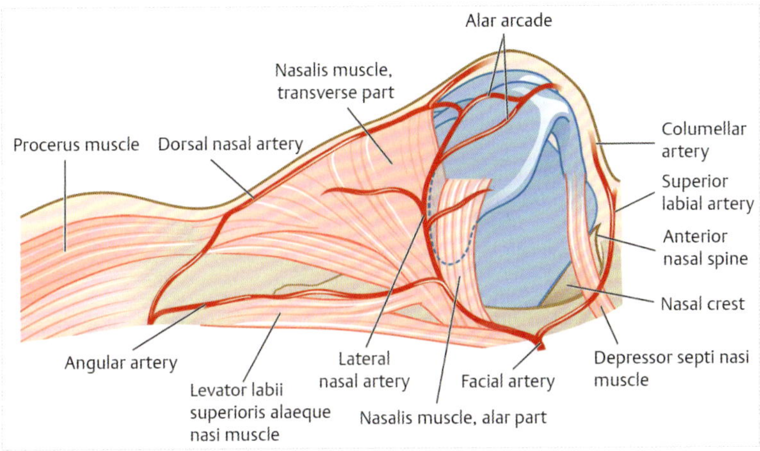

Fig. 1.13 Muscles and arteries of the outer nose. The angular artery and vein connect the vessels of the nose to the ophthalmic circulation.

> ✔
>
> It is the dense connective tissue of the nasal ala, rather than the cartilage, that provides stability to the inferolateral circumference of the nostrils.

1.3 Muscles of the Nose

The muscles of the nose contribute to facial expression and play a minor functional role. The nasalis muscle is present at the lateral aspect, while the depressor septi nasi lies caudally between the cartilaginous structures of the columella and the premaxilla (▶ Fig. 1.13). The latter may give rise to a troublesome lowering of the nasal tip in some individuals during laughing or other oral movements, which can be treated by severing this muscle. A similar, although transient, effect can be achieved by eliminating muscle pull using botulinum toxin (e.g., Botox), a neurotoxin.

The procerus muscle attaches to the nasion (see ▶ Fig. 1.13), and its fibers extend vertically to the forehead; this muscle may be bulky enough to influence the shape of the nasofrontal angle. Repetitive action of the procerus gives rise to glabellar furrows, and resection of its fibers occasionally becomes part of a rhinoplasty.

1.3.1 SMAS

The superficial musculoaponeurotic system (SMAS), which plays an important role in facelifts, can also be seen as a separate preparation layer between the skin and the framework of the nose. Occasionally, this layer may be used to cover bone and cartilage at the end of a rhinoplasty.

1.4 Vascular Supply

The outer nose is mainly supplied by branches of the facial artery and vein (▶ Fig. 1.13). These vessels are connected to the ophthalmic circulation via the angular artery and vein. Injections into the nose may therefore rarely cause ocular complications. Blindness is a feared risk. Although it is extremely rare, according to literature reports it is by no means an isolated occurrence, especially after filler injections (see Chapter 22).

In the columella, nasal surgeons regularly encounter two small but quite well-developed arteries during open surgery. These branches arise from the superior labial artery at the level of the columella and connect to the dorsal nasal artery on the nasal bridge and the lateral nasal artery over the lateral walls via a vascular network over the nasal domes ("alar arcade"; ▶ Fig. 1.13, ▶ Fig. 1.14).

Obliteration of arterial vessels that supply the nasal skin can rapidly lead to skin necrosis and requires prompt intervention (see Chapter 22).

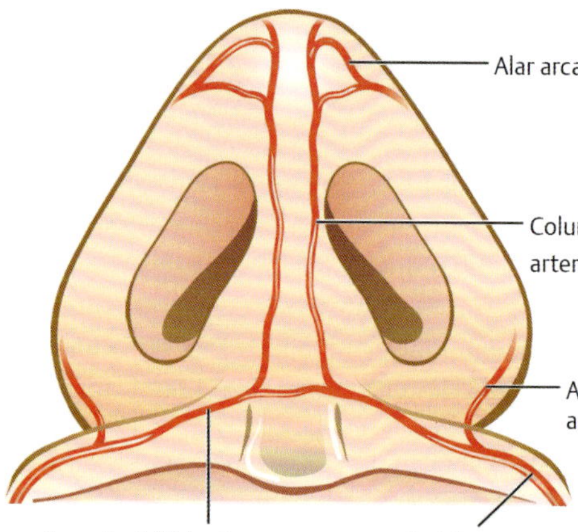

Fig. 1.14 Arteries of the nasal base. Columellar vessels are inevitably exposed during the transverse skin incision for the "open approach."

> ✔
>
> Injection of an epinephrine-containing local anesthetic occasionally gives rise to a rapidly evolving, circumscribed, white discoloration of the skin due to epinephrine-induced vascular constriction. This phenomenon is generally transient and not worrisome. However, one should carefully consider the need for injection of vasoconstrictors in patients with irradiated or otherwise severely diseased skin.

Intraoperative bleeding can be minimized by precise preoperative injection of vasoconstrictors and dissection in anatomical layers. However, the rich blood supply to the nose may occasionally give rise to recurrent heavy bleeding during rhinoplasty. Intraoperative hemostasis using bipolar coagulation is usually necessary in such cases.

> ✔
>
> Surgeons should select the lowest effective power setting for bipolar coagulation in order to prevent unintentional tissue burns, especially when treating bleeding points in subcutaneous tissue.

1.5 Nerve Supply

For sensitivity, the skin of the nose is supplied by the first and second branches of the trigeminal nerve. In the inner nose, the fibers of the olfactory nerve are of major importance. They originate in the receptors of the olfactory epithelium at the posterosuperior aspect of the septum and pass through the olfactory foramina in the cribriform plate of the ethmoid bone, ending at the olfactory bulbs (see ▶ Fig. 1.2). Dissection in this region should therefore be avoided or reduced to an absolute minimum in order to prevent lesions of the skull base, with olfactory disorders.

The nasopalatine nerve, which supplies sensory innervation to the upper incisors and parts of the central upper lip, runs close to the maxillary crest and the inferior edge of the septum. Careful handling of the maxillary crest during septoplasty may help avoid injury to the nerve and subsequent sensory disorders. Such sequelae are of particular importance for musicians who play wind instruments, for instance; preoperative history-taking and explanation therefore also need to take the occupational risk for the patient into account.

1.6 Skin

The skin of the nose just at its tip is typically thin. The skin is firmer above the tip and not infrequently has thick fibroadipose subcutaneous tissue. The skin over the bony nasal bridge is thinner, only to become more voluminous at the nasion (▶ Fig. 1.15).

It is in the interest of every rhinoplasty surgeon and patient to avoid injuries to the skin. Unavoidable incisions for surgical access (at the columella during the open technique, at the base of the nose for nasal base corrections) are placed in predefined furrows and folds and thus rendered "invisible" as far as possible by appropriate localization and incision lines.

The anatomy of the skin over the nose does not differ significantly from that of other areas of the face (▶ Fig. 1.16). It is essential to bear in mind that the thickness of the skin over different regions of the nose may have significant intraindividual and interindividual variability, which in turn may decide the outcome of rhinoplasty. Both excessively thick and thin skin may be problematic during rhinoplasty. Thick skin may obscure delicate structures, especially at the tip of the nose, so that rhinoplasty may result in little more than a rounded, plump appearance. Extremely thin skin, on the other hand, reveals every edge in the cartilage, and with it the smallest asymmetries and irregularities.

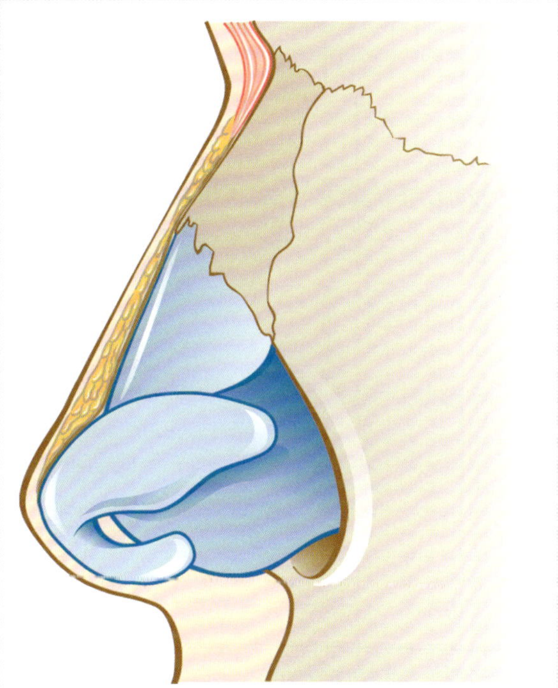

Fig. 1.15 Skin thickness over the nasal bridge. Subcutaneous tissue is thickest above the tip of the nose (supratip area) due to the presence of a layer of fibroadipose tissue. Muscles contribute to the volume of subcutaneous tissue in the region of the nasofrontal angle.

In connection with "thick skin," not every layer of skin is necessarily particularly strong. Patients with epidermis and dermis of normal thickness may be found to have particularly well-developed subcutaneous tissue, which essentially consists of connective and adipose tissue, as well as some vessels. This fibroadipose subcutaneous tissue can be carefully thinned out, while avoiding injury to the dermis and the vessels running within it parallel to the surface.

The view that an excellent postoperative outcome cannot be achieved in rhinoplasty patients who have this type of thick skin is not generally correct. Modest, careful thinning of subcutaneous tissue frequently enables the delicate contours of the cartilaginous framework to define the shape of the nose. In other cases, building somewhat stronger cartilaginous structures at the tip may overcome the disadvantages of thick skin. Patience is vital in the postoperative period until the new nasal contours become apparent over weeks and months as swelling diminishes.

1.7 Ligaments

What are called "ligaments" are bundles of fibrous connective tissue between the perichondrium and the subcutaneous layer on the nose, or connecting cartilage and bone structures or cartilage structures with each other. These ligaments appear to be important for tip stability. In surgery, they may be severed, or spared, or severed and restored at the end (▶ Fig. 1.17).

Laterally, the "scroll ligaments" are found along the intercartilaginous fold between the upper and lower lateral cartilages. A distinction can be made between a **vertical** and a **horizontal (longitudinal) scroll ligament**: the vertical ligament connects the scroll area with the hypodermis, while the horizontal band connects the upper and lower lateral cartilages together.

Medially, the dermocartilaginous **Pitanguy ligament, with its superficial portion** (inserting into the orbicularis oris muscle) **and deep portion** (inserting into the depressor septi nasi muscle, DSN), stretches over the edge of the anterior septum. These fiber bundles can either be protected in a targeted manner or, after they have been cut through using the open technique, they may be sutured again at the end in order to improve the attachment of the skin to the nasal skeleton.

Other such ligaments are the **vertical piriform attachment** and **piriform ligaments, the interdomal and the intercrural (suspension) ligaments** (▶ Fig. 1.17). If these ligaments are severed during surgery and cannot be restored, stability is reduced, especially in the tip of the nose, and it needs to be reestablished using appropriate sutures.

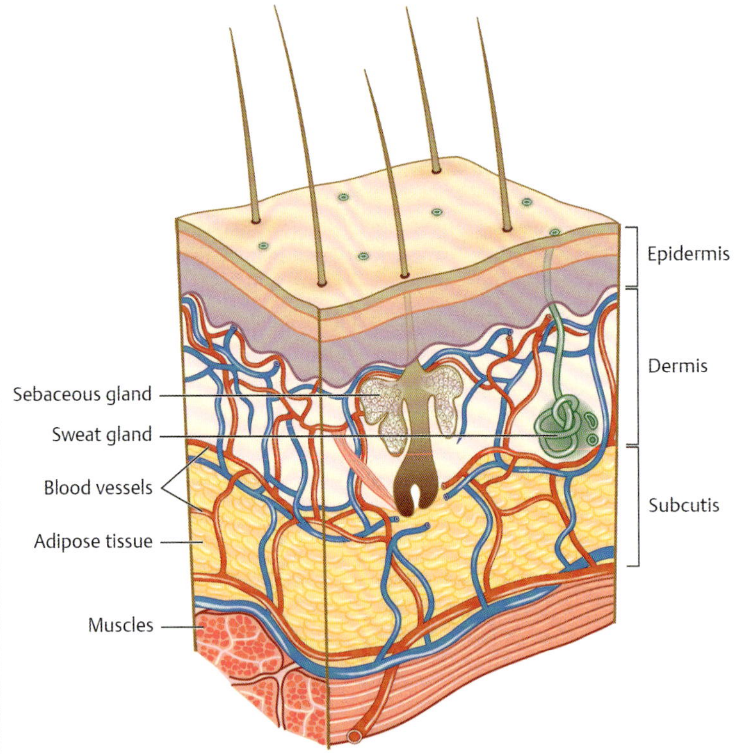

Fig. 1.16 Skin layers. The layers of skin over the nose are essentially no different from those over other parts of the body. Hair is sparse; the amount of subcutaneous fat may be relevant for the external shape of the nose.

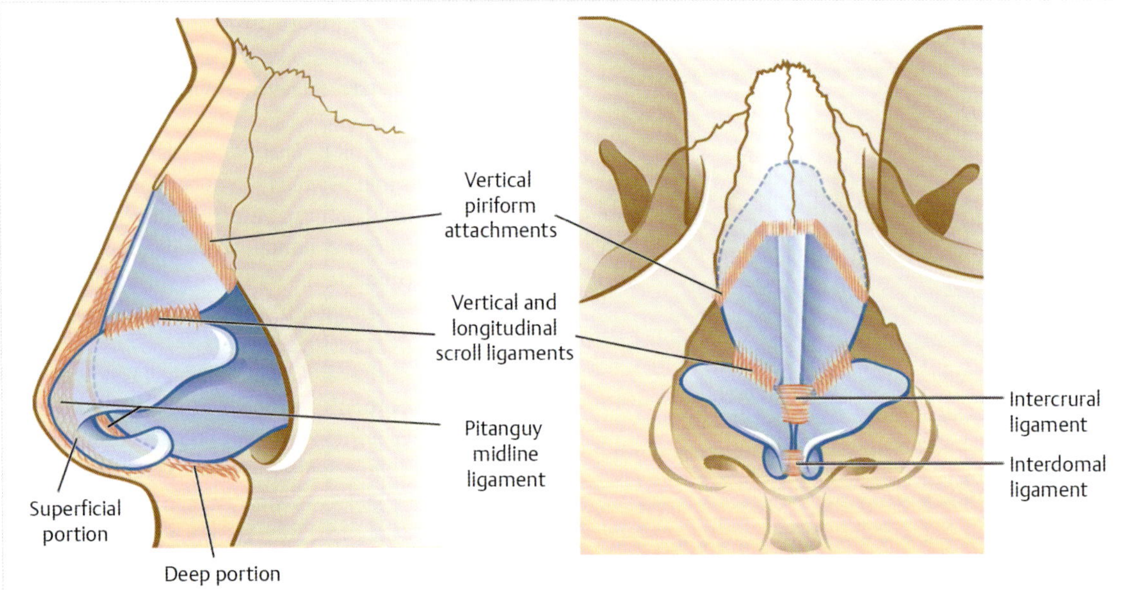

Fig. 1.17 Nasal ligaments. Vertical piriform attachments, interdomal (see also ▶ **Fig. 7.4 a,b**) and intercrural ligaments, scroll ligaments, and the Pitanguy midline ligament (see also ▶ **Fig. 8.58a,b**, ▶ **Fig. 8.59**).

Bibliography

Anderson JR. A new approach to rhinoplasty. Trans Am Acad Ophthalmol Otolaryngol. 1966; 70(2):183–192

Anderson JR. A reasoned approach to nasal base surgery. Arch Otolaryngol. 1984; 110(6):349–358

Daniel RK. The nasal tip: anatomy and aesthetics. Plast Reconstr Surg. 1992; 89:216–224

Daniel RK, Palhazi P. The nasal ligaments and tip support in rhinoplasty: an anatomical study. Aesthet Surg J. 2018; 38(4):357–368

Han SK, Jeong SH, Lee BI, Kim WK. Updated anatomy of the dermocartilaginous ligament of the nose. Ann Plast Surg. 2007; 59(4): 393–397

Patel RG. Nasal anatomy and function. Facial Plast Surg. 2017; 33(1):3–8

Pitanguy I. Revisiting the dermocartilaginous ligament. Plast Reconstr Surg. 2001; 107(1):264–266

Pitanguy I, Salgado F, Radwanski HN, Bushkin SC. The surgical importance of the dermocartilaginous ligament of the nose. Plast Reconstr Surg. 1995; 95(5):790–794

Saban Y, Andretto Amodeo C, Hammou JC, Polselli R. An anatomical study of the nasal superficial musculoaponeurotic system: surgical applications in rhinoplasty. Arch Facial Plast Surg. 2008; 10(2):109–115

Saban Y, Andretto Amodeo C, Bouaziz D, Polselli R. Nasal arterial vasculature: medical and surgical applications. Arch Facial Plast Surg. 2012; 14(6):429–436

San Nicoló M, Berghaus A, Jacobi C, Kisser U, Haack M, Flatz W. The nasal valve: new insights on the static and dynamic NV with MR-imaging. Eur Arch Otorhinolaryngol. 2020; 277(2):463–467

2 Proportions of the Nose

A nose that is considered "normal" or "aesthetically pleasing" meets specific criteria relative to the face regarding size, length, width, and other details. Artists were already working on standard values as a measure of beauty in ancient Rome and in Greek antiquity. Most rules of proportion that were developed in ancient times still apply today; others have been added more recently through investigations in anthropology and plastic surgery.

Thorough knowledge of the nasofacial proportions that contribute to a normal or "beautiful" appearance is thus crucial for successful rhinoplasty. Although nasal surgeons may be familiar with basic aesthetic facial proportions, in-depth knowledge helps in decision-making on modifying the nasal contours to create an aesthetically pleasing appearance. The following sections therefore highlight essential aspects of nasal proportions.

Intensive study by artists such as Leonardo da Vinci and Albrecht Dürer revealed that strict rules of mathematical proportion by no means automatically created a "beautiful" image of the human body when applied to works of art. The same also applies to facial cosmetic surgery: beauty is concealed in countless details, and ultimately lies in the eye of the beholder. This is why faces are often perceived as beautiful even when significant deviations from the ideal values for beautiful proportions are found on closer examination.

✓

An awareness of the rules of proportion is therefore vital and useful for the facial cosmetic surgeon, but it cannot be regarded as the sole yardstick for every operative decision.

Research has shown that a desire for nose correction may also conceal an unconscious desire to make the nose appear less conspicuous. The eyes and mouth appear to count most from the beauty point of view, and a hooked or long, pointed nose is problematic, as it evidently distracts the viewer from other facial details. On the other hand, a public personality who is regarded as an "idol" may also be perceived as attractive despite having a less than aesthetically ideal nose; the nose is then considered "striking" rather than "ugly." The proportions of a White (light-skinned) face are generally used as a standard, and not only in the Western world.

2.1 Horizontal Trisection of the Face

A face with proportions that are perceived as balanced can be divided into three roughly equal segments using four horizontal dividing lines (▶ Fig. 2.1). A line passing through the trichion (at the hairline), another through the glabella, a third through the subnasale, and finally a line passing through the menton under the chin divide the face into upper, middle, and lower thirds. The nose occupies approximately the middle third of the face.

The hairline recedes with age, while tooth loss and bone atrophy result in shrinking of the lower third of the face. The ears and the nose grow throughout life, resulting in a shift in the proportions of the three horizontal divisions of the face. Older individuals may thus have a relatively large nose, with drooping of the nasal tip. A desire for nose correction in such cases may result from an unconscious yearning for a more youthful appearance.

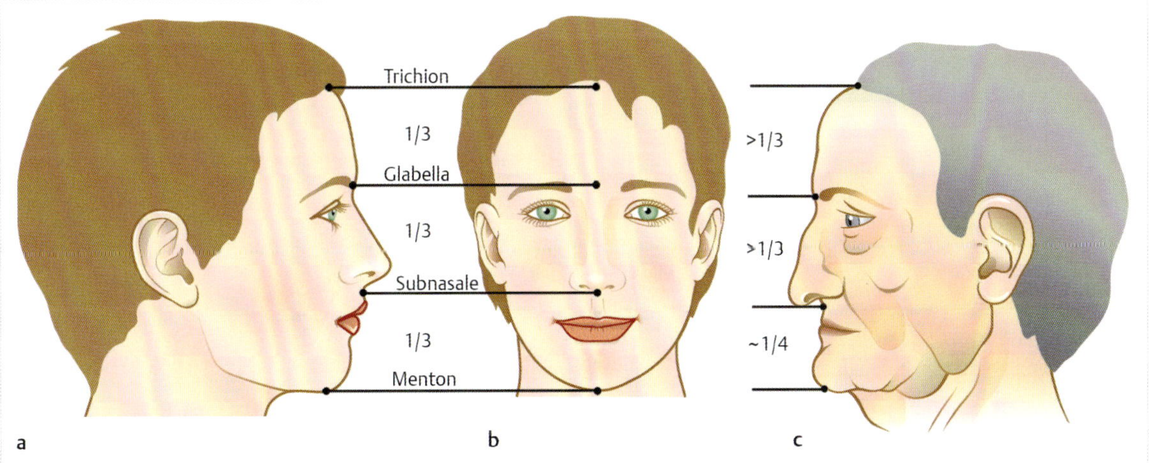

Fig. 2.1 Horizontal trisection of the face. (a, b) In young individuals. **(c)** In the elderly.

2

> Successful nose reduction surgery with elevation of the nasal tip does in fact frequently impart a fresher, more youthful expression to the face (see ▶ Fig. 2.14).

2.2 Vertical Division of the Face into Fifths

Vertical lines divide a well-proportioned face into five segments. The nose occupies the center, while each eye occupies another fifth, and the lateral segments extend to the helix of the ears (▶ Fig. 2.2).

In practice, however, the nasal ala are often seen projecting slightly beyond the boundary lines of the middle fifth in aesthetically appealing faces (corresponding to a vertical line drawn through the medial canthus), without the nasal base appearing too broad. Significant widening of the nasal base, with considerable lateral crossing of these lines, may call for narrowing of the alar base using alar wedge excisions (see section 14.1).

2.3 Nasal Length to Width Ratio

If segment A between the nasion (attachment of the nasal root to the forehead) and the nasal tip (pronasale; tip-defining point; tip) defines the length of the nose, and segment B between the alar furrows defines its width, then A should be greater than B (▶ Fig. 2.3). If this is not the case, surgical narrowing of the nasal base or lengthening of the nose may be considered.

2.4 Midline and Dorsal Aesthetic Line (DAL; Eyebrow–Nasal Tip Line)

Not every detail of the face needs to be symmetrical for an aesthetically pleasing appearance. On the contrary: mild asymmetry enhances attractiveness and gives the face an individual character. However, the nose, which occupies the center of the face, should be largely symmetrical, and all significant points of measurement should lie exactly on the center line (▶ Fig. 2.4). Patients often closely examine such details after a rhinoplasty. It is therefore important for the surgeon to draw the patient's attention to existing asymmetries preoperatively, so that preexisting deviations are not later interpreted as the result of the operation.

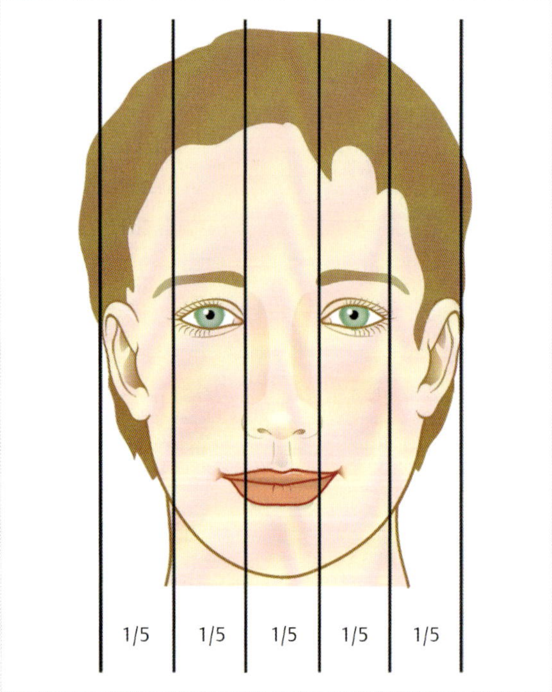

Fig. 2.2 Division of the face into vertical fifths. The width of the nose occupies approximately the middle fifth of the face.

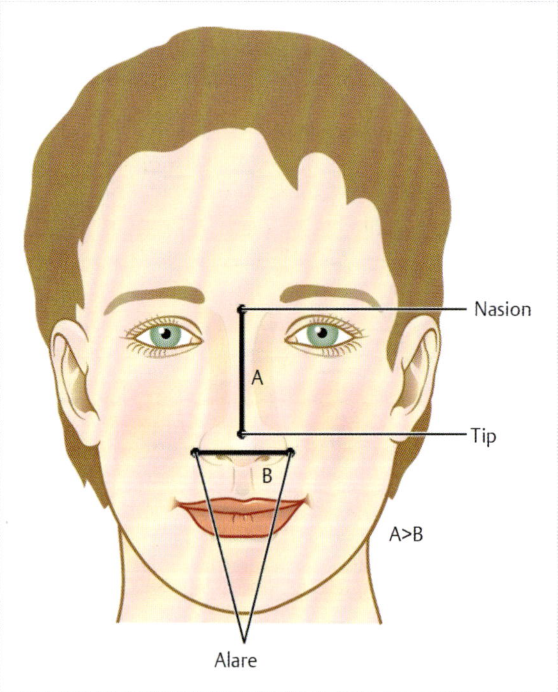

Fig. 2.3 Length–width ratio of the nose. The length of the nose in White people **(A)** exceeds its width **(B)**.

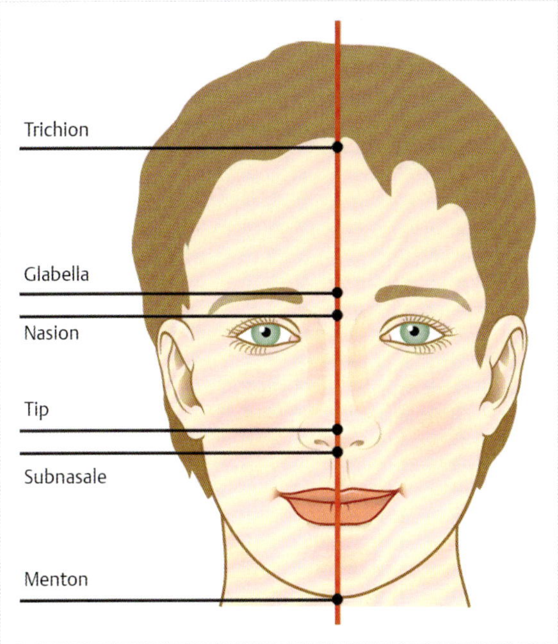

Fig. 2.4 Midline symmetry. All critical points of measurement of the nose (trichion, glabella, nasion, tip, subnasale, menton) ideally lie on the central axis of the face. The alar points (Fig. 2.3) are symmetrically positioned.

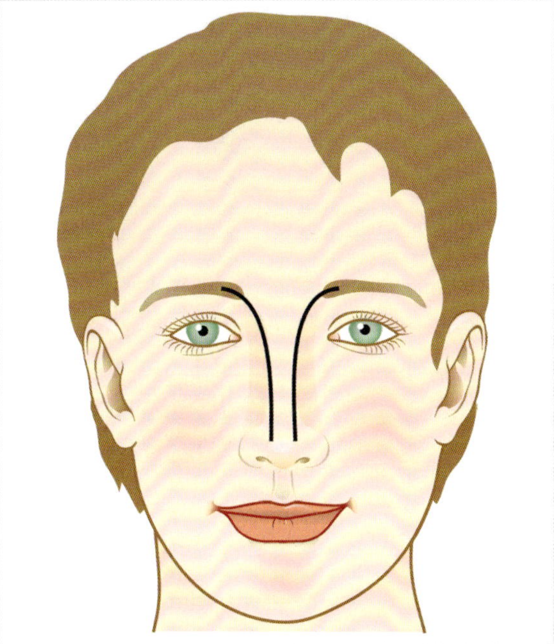

Fig. 2.5 Dorsal aesthetic lines (DALs). The dorsal aesthetic line extends in a slightly curved arc symmetrically on both sides from the eyebrow to the nasal tip (brow–tip aesthetic line).

A proportionate and well-balanced nose allows symmetrical, harmoniously curved lines to be drawn on either side from the medial end of the eyebrows to the two nasal tip points; these dorsal aesthetic lines (DALs) are oriented along the midline, are continuous, and do not show any irregularities (▶ Fig. 2.5).

Noses with asymmetry of such measuring points and lines have to undergo detailed analysis to identify the causative deformity, which must then be corrected accordingly (▶ Fig. 2.6a, b).

2.5 Profile Angles of the Nose and Face

Some angles that can be measured in the profile of a face are of particular importance for the analysis of nasal proportions.

The **nasolabial angle** (▶ Fig. 2.7b) between the columella and the upper lip measures about 95° in males and 105° in females. The slightly larger angle in females is associated with a mildly pronounced upward rotation of the nasal tip.

The **nasofrontal angle** between the nasal dorsum and forehead is approximately 125°, similar to the **nasomental angle** between the nasal dorsal line and the tip of the chin (approximately 124°; ▶ Fig. 2.7c).

The **nasofacial angle** is formed between a vertical line passing through the nasal radix and the chin, and the nasal dorsal line, and optimally measures 35° (▶ Fig. 2.7a, ▶ Fig. 2.8a, b).

2.6 Projection

The **projection** of the nose is also determined by the nasofacial angle. This is the distance between the nasal tip and the face. The nasal tip is said to be overprojected if this distance is too large. The female nose is slightly less projected than the male nose; the nasofacial angle may thus be 34° in females and closer to 36° or more in males (▶ Fig. 2.9, ▶ Fig. 2.10, ▶ Fig. 2.11a–d, ▶ Fig. 2.12a, b).

The importance of the nasofacial angle for nasal projection is illustrated in ▶ Fig. 2.10: the larger this angle, the greater the projection of the nose.

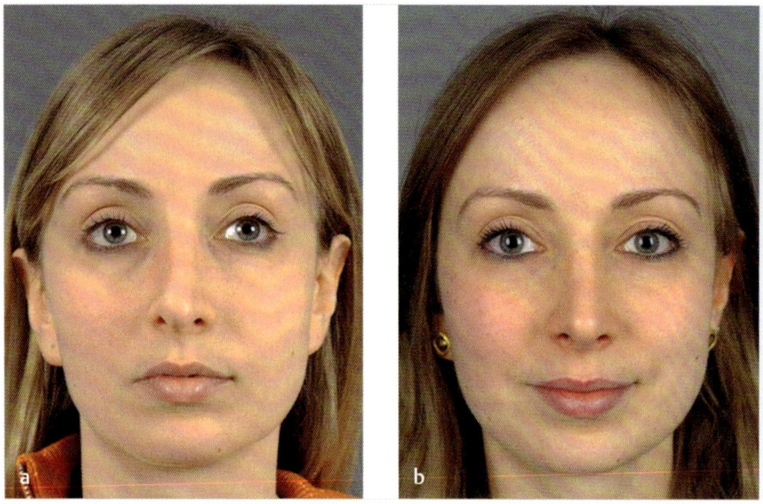

Fig. 2.6 Asymmetry of the nose; case study. (a) Asymmetry of the nose is often perceived as particularly annoying. Here, the tip in particular deviates from the midline, and the dorsal aesthetic lines are asymmetrical. **(b)** Condition after rhinoplasty. In addition to the deviation, the asymmetry of the tip-defining points has also been corrected.

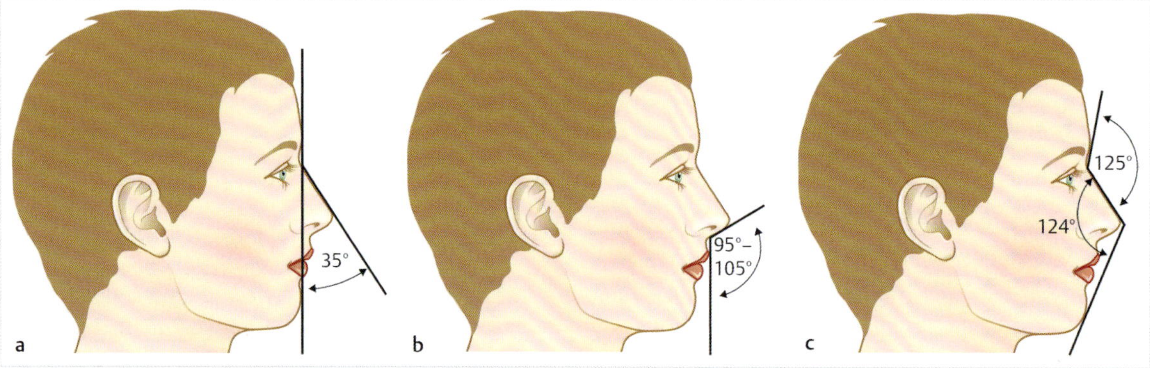

Fig. 2.7 Nasal and facial angles in profile. (a) Nasofacial angle. **(b)** Nasolabial angle. **(c)** Nasofrontal and nasomental angles.

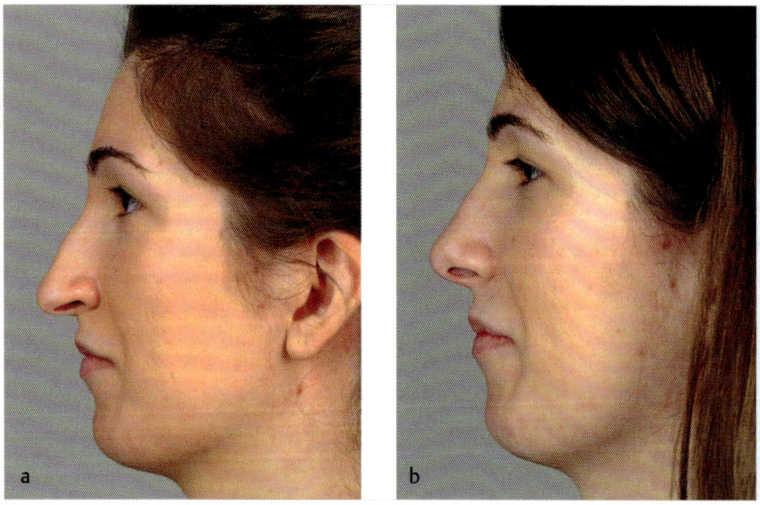

Fig. 2.8 Nasofacial and nasolabial angles; case study. (a) Narrow nasofacial and nasolabial angles. **(b)** Post correction.

2.7 Rotation

While projection describes the distance of the nasal tip from the face, rotation expresses the extent to which the tip of the nose is raised or lowered. Increasing rotation implies that the nasal tip moves upward on the lateral view on a circular arc, the center of which lies approximately above the external auditory meatus (▶ Fig. 2.13).

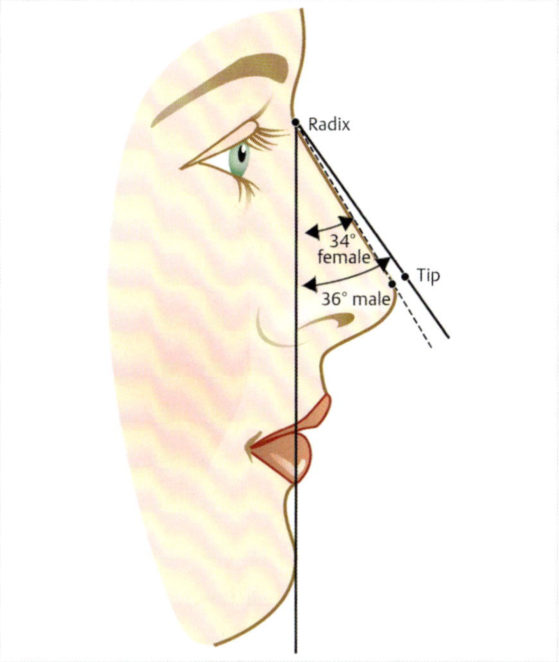

Fig. 2.9 Nasofacial angle. The nasofacial angle and nasal projection are slightly larger in men than in women.

> ✔
>
> The angle of rotation is of considerable importance for the appearance of a nose. Elevation of a "droopy" nasal tip (underrotation) is very often part of, or even the main objective of, a rhinoplasty (▶ Fig. 2.14; see also ▶ Fig. 2.8a, b).

2.8 Hump, Saddle, and Supratip Break

The profile of the nasal dorsum is defined by the nasal dorsal line extending between the nasion and the nasal tip. Elevations above this line on the lateral view are referred to as "**humps**" (▶ Fig. 2.15a, ▶ Fig. 2.16, ▶ Fig. 2.17a, b, ▶ Fig. 2.18a, b).

Any irritating lowering below this line is a **saddle** (▶ Fig. 2.15b, ▶ Fig. 2.20).

A slight depression of the supratip region may be desired or tolerated as a "**supratip break**," especially in women (▶ Fig. 2.15c).

Men sometimes tolerate, or even desire, a minimally raised or curved nasal dorsum, which still cannot be referred to as a hump, rather than a completely straight dorsum. Arab patients, among others, occasionally insist that such an elevation or even a distinct hump should be

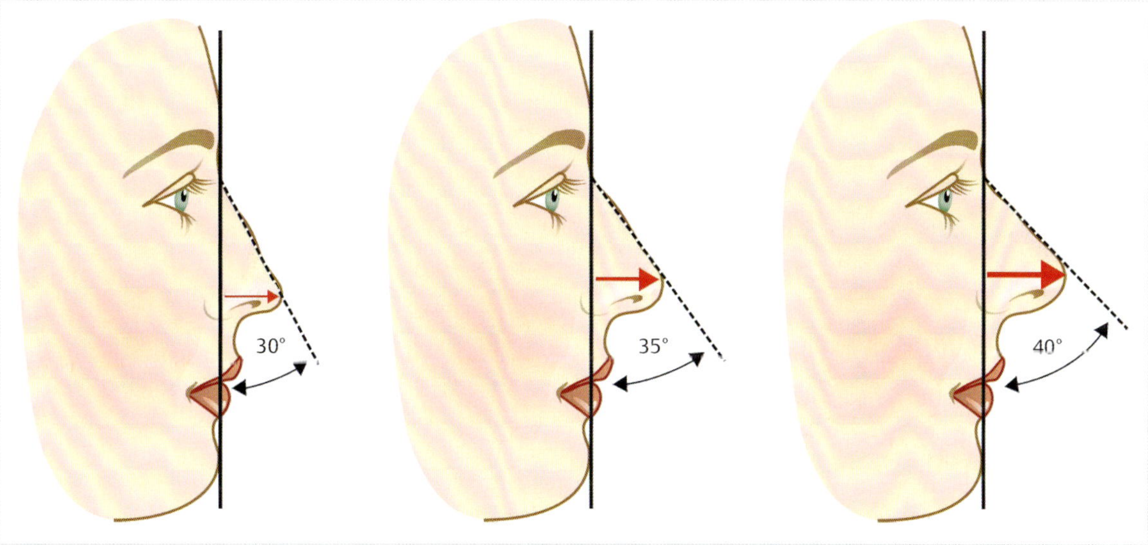

Fig. 2.10 Nasal projection and nasofacial angle. The larger the nasofacial angle, the greater the projection of the nose.

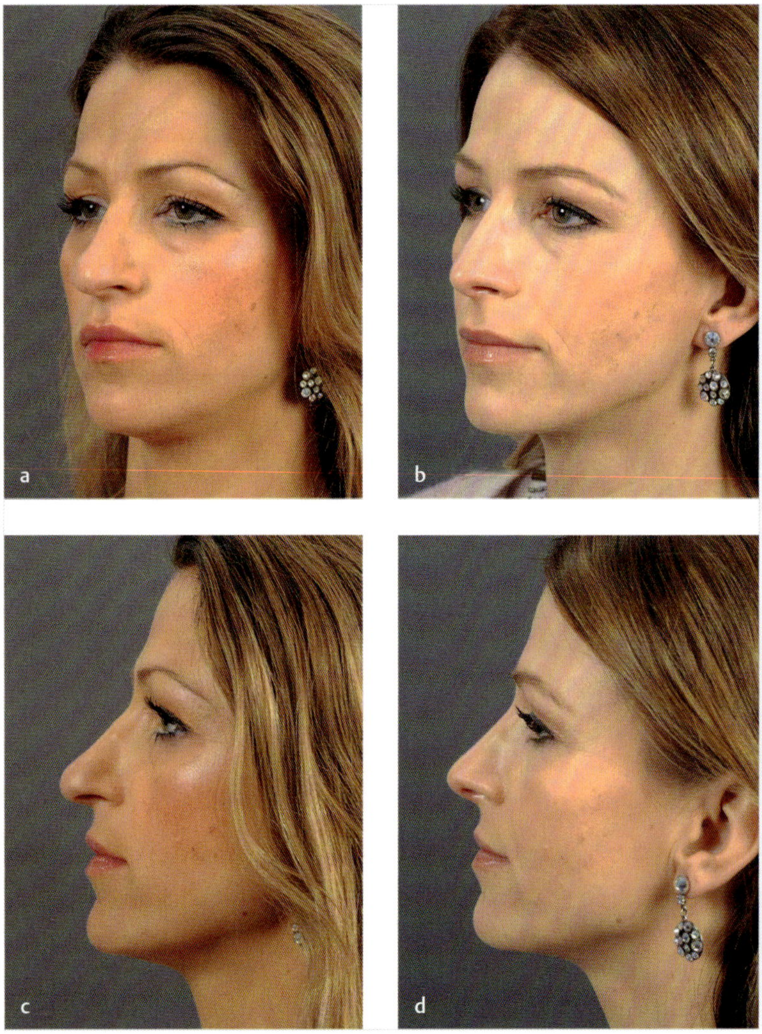

Fig. 2.11 Projection; case study. (a, c) Overprojection of the nose, mainly due to an oversized tip. **(b, d)** Condition after rhinoplasty, with reduced projection and a slight increase in rotation.

retained during rhinoplasty to preserve this typical feature of their nose (▶ Fig. 2.19). Patients are very appreciative when such details are successfully implemented during surgery.

> ✔
>
> An exaggerated supratip break, especially in combination with a markedly elevated nasal tip, may create the impression of an aesthetically unappealing **snub nose**.

2.9 Position of the Nasal Radix

The nasal length, the position of the nasal radix, and nasal tip projection are ideally proportional to one another. Radix projection is defined as the distance between the medial canthus of the eye and the nasion on the lateral view. This distance is about 0.33 times the distance between the nasion and the nasal tip (radix tip, RT); its absolute value fluctuates around 10 mm (▶ Fig. 2.21, ▶ Fig. 2.22a,b, ▶ Fig. 2.23a).

Analogous to the above, the nasal tip projection, measured from the alar crease to the nasal tip, should be 0.67 of the nasal dorsal length.

A high or low nasion is determined by its position relative to the upper eyelid (▶ Fig. 2.23a–c).

The radix normally lies approximately at the level of the center of the upper eyelid or the edge of the eyelashes (▶ Fig. 2.23a). A "low radix" is present if it lies significantly below that level (▶ Fig. 2.23b, ▶ Fig. 2.24a, b), whereas a "high radix" lies higher than the crease of the upper eyelid (▶ Fig. 2.23c).

The ideal position of the nasion relative to the forehead in side view can also be described: it lies at a distance of 4–6 mm behind the glabella (▶ Fig. 2.23a).

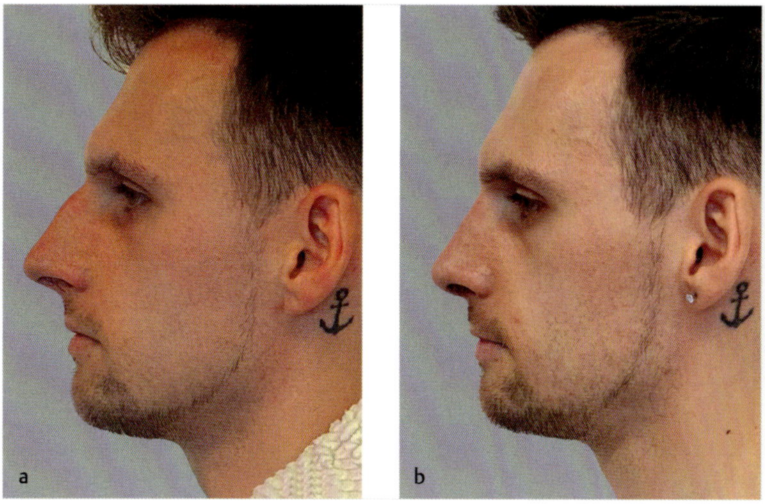

Fig. 2.12 Projection and nasolabial angle; case study. In the male patient with a large nose, the reduction must not be exaggerated during correction. The male nose remains larger than a female nose. **(a)** Pronounced projection, with a wide open nasolabial angle. **(b)** Condition after rhinoplasty.

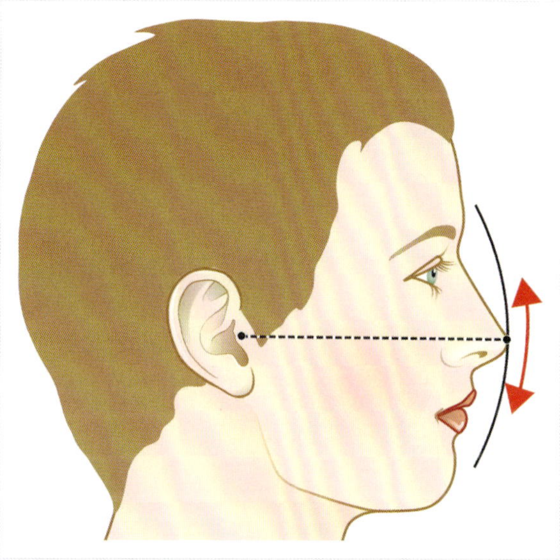

Fig. 2.13 Rotation. "More rotation" means raising the nasal tip; "less rotation" means lowering the tip.

2.10 Nostril Dimensions on the Lateral View

> A good-looking nostril is **comma-shaped** in the side view.

The distance from a line drawn through the longitudinal axis of the nostril to the nasal alar rim on the lateral view is ideally no more than 2 mm (▸ Fig. 2.25a).

Alar retraction is said to be present if this distance is greater (▸ Fig. 2.25c; see case study in ▸ Fig. 10.22).

Shortening of the distance between the nasal alar rim and the columella results in the columella being pulled up behind the ala on the lateral view, an appearance known as "**hidden columella**" (▸ Fig. 2.25b, ▸ Fig. 2.26a, b).

The distance from the central axis of the nostril to the edge of the columella is approximately 2 mm; a **hanging columella** is said to be present if this distance is longer (▸ Fig. 2.25d).

The nasal alar rim, which defines the upper edge of the nostril, can be further subdivided into anterior and posterior segments, with the posterior segment comprising approximately two-thirds of the arcuate contour. Its maximum convexity lies at the transition to its anterior third. A line drawn through the posterior aspect of the nasal alar rim forms an angle of about 45° with its anterior third (▸ Fig. 2.27). The upper edge of the nostril runs in a harmonious curve. A visible angle at this point is undesirable (known as a "Chinese hat" deformity; see ▸ Fig. 9.7, ▸ Fig. 10.22c, ▸ Fig. 10.43).

The distance from the anterior edge of the nostril to the nasal tip ("inner tip"; infratip lobule) corresponds to about 70% of the length of the nostril in individuals with well-proportioned nasal tips (▸ Fig. 2.28).

2.11 The Nasal Base

Rules of proportionality also apply to the base of the nose. The lobule comprises about one-third of the height, while the columella contributes about two-thirds when viewed from below. The nasal tip angle is formed by the ala of the nose, and measures approximately 60° in White people, about 90° in Asians, and about 120° in Black people when viewed from below (▸ Fig. 2.29, ▸ Fig. 2.30a–c). Ethnic widening of the nasal base results in movement of the axis of the nostril from a more vertical to a more horizontal plane.

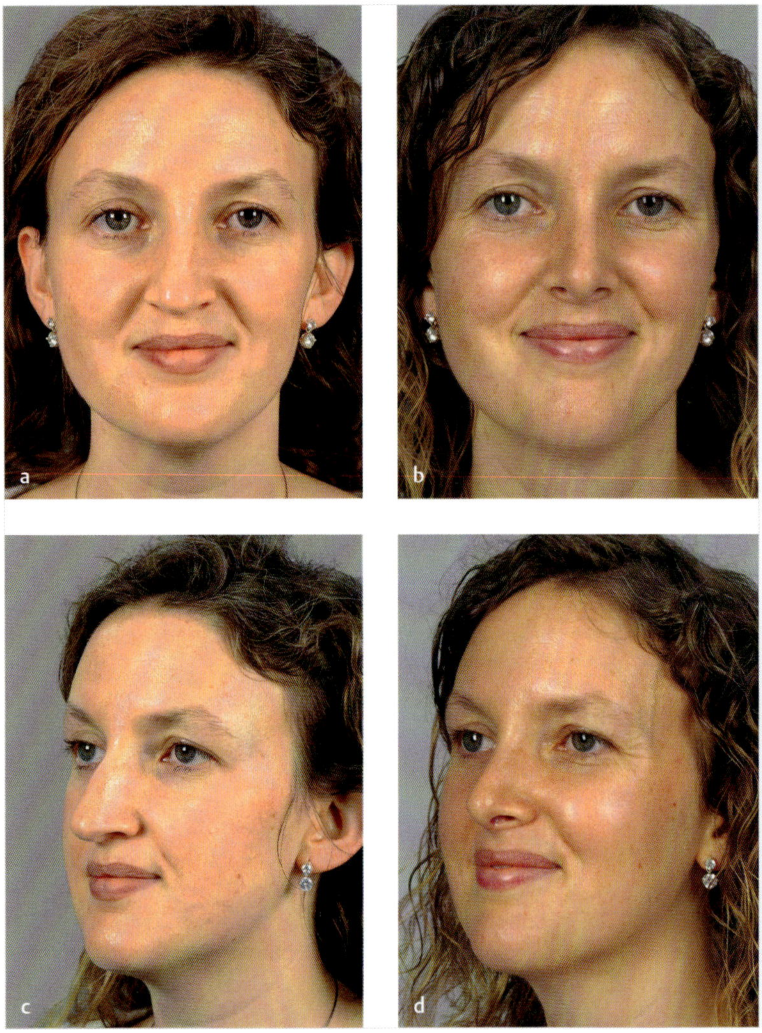

Fig. 2.14 Rotation; case study (a, c) An underrotated, “droopy” nasal tip – especially in combination with a hump – is characteristically seen in the elderly. **(b, d)** Rhinoplasty thus also has a rejuvenating effect. The nasal asymmetry corrected by the procedure should also be noted.

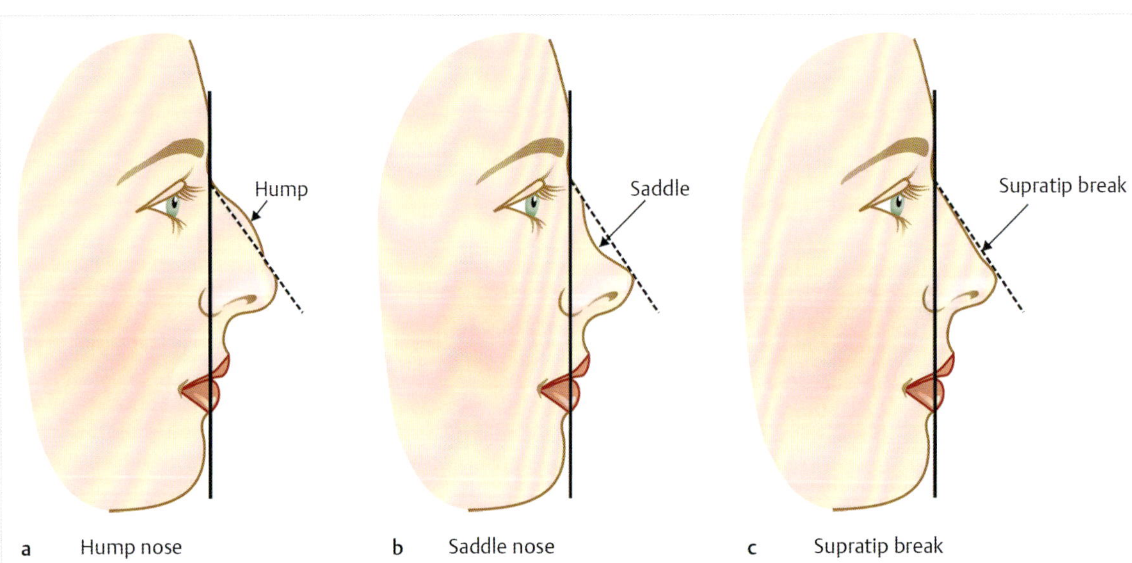

Fig. 2.15 Variations of the nasal dorsal profile. (a) Hump. **(b)** Saddle. **(c)** Supratip break, and nasal dorsal line (nasion–tip).

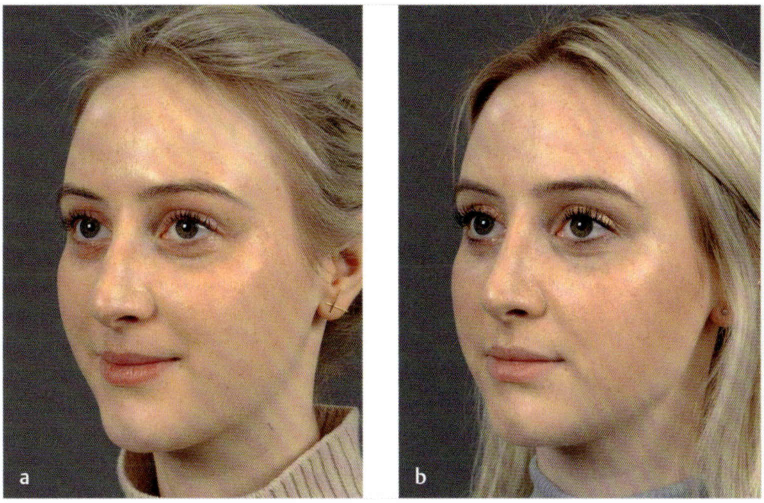

Fig. 2.16 Nasal hump; case study 1. **(a)** Nasal hump. **(b)** After rhinoplasty.

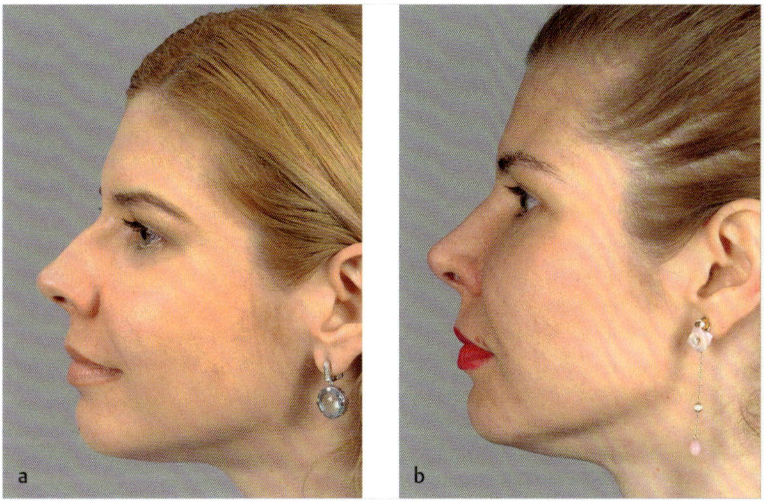

Fig. 2.17 Nasal hump; case study 2. **(a)** Even correcting a small hump can give the nose an attractive profile. **(b)** Postoperative result.

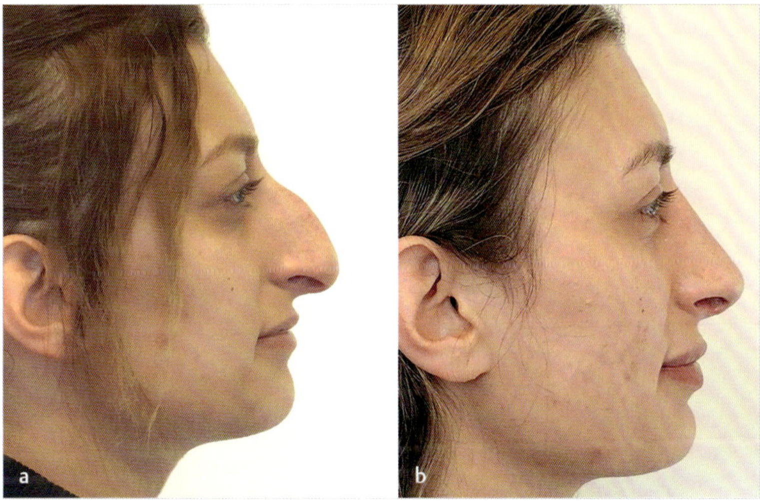

Fig. 2.18 Large hump on a large nose. **(a)** A large nose with a large hump has a significant influence on the physiognomy of a young woman's face. **(b)** Note that rhinoplasty correction does not result in an extremely tiny nose. But in addition to the hump, the angle of rotation and the hanging tip are also corrected.

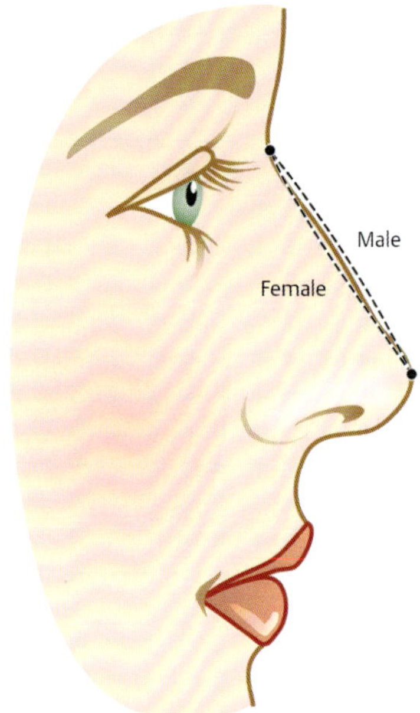

Fig. 2.19 Nasal dorsum in men and women. The nasal dorsal line runs slightly below the nasion–tip line in women, while it may lie slightly above this in men.

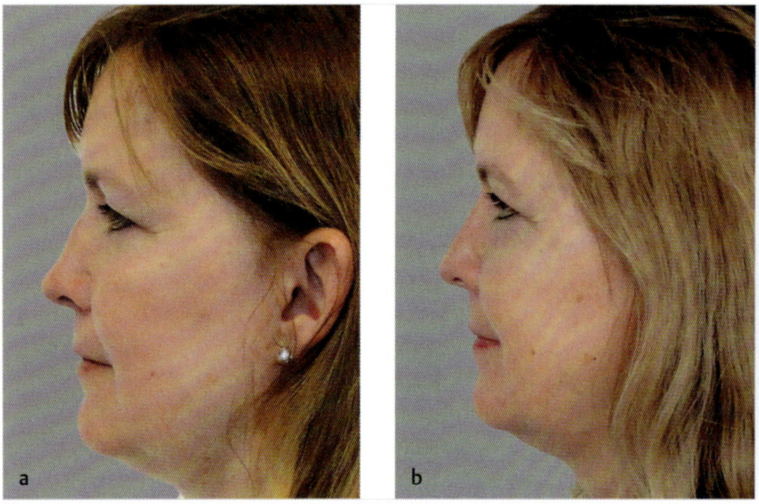

Fig. 2.20 Saddle nose; case study. **(a)** Saddle nose after a septoplasty operation carried out elsewhere. **(b)** After corrective surgery using conchal cartilage graft. The patient did not want correction of the accompanying small hump.

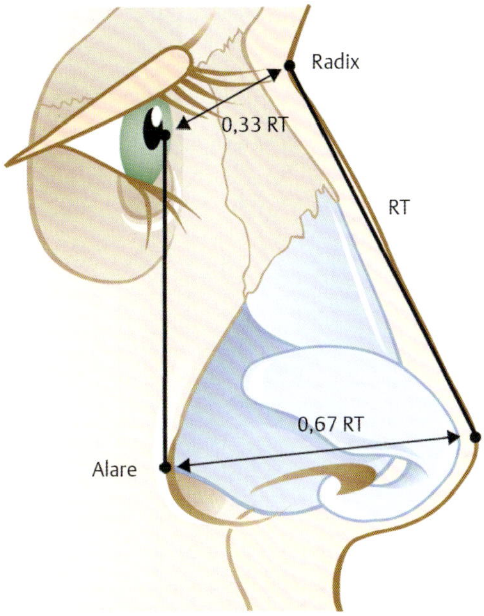

Fig. 2.21 Position of the nasal radix and the nasal tip. The nasal dorsal length (RT) is related to the height of the nasal radix (× 0.33) as well as to the projection of its tip (× 0.67) (adapted from TD Wang, 2010).

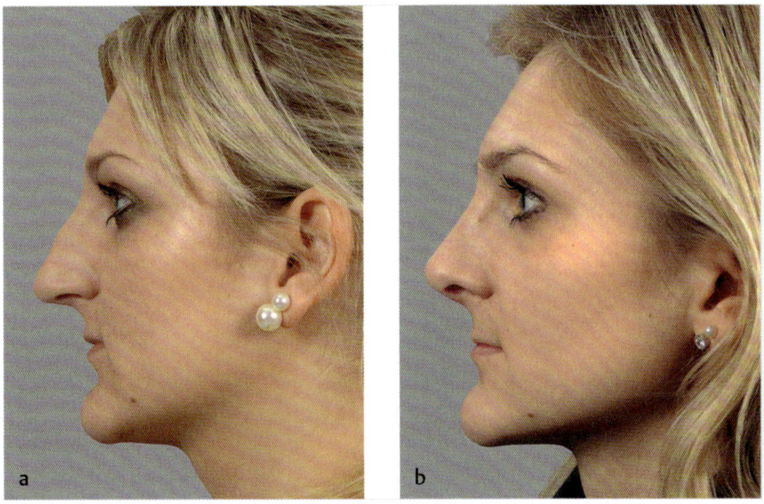

Fig. 2.22 Overprojected radix with an overall large nose; case study. (a) An overprojected radix, with a large distance to the medial canthus. **(b)** After structure rhinoplasty with reduction of the radix projection.

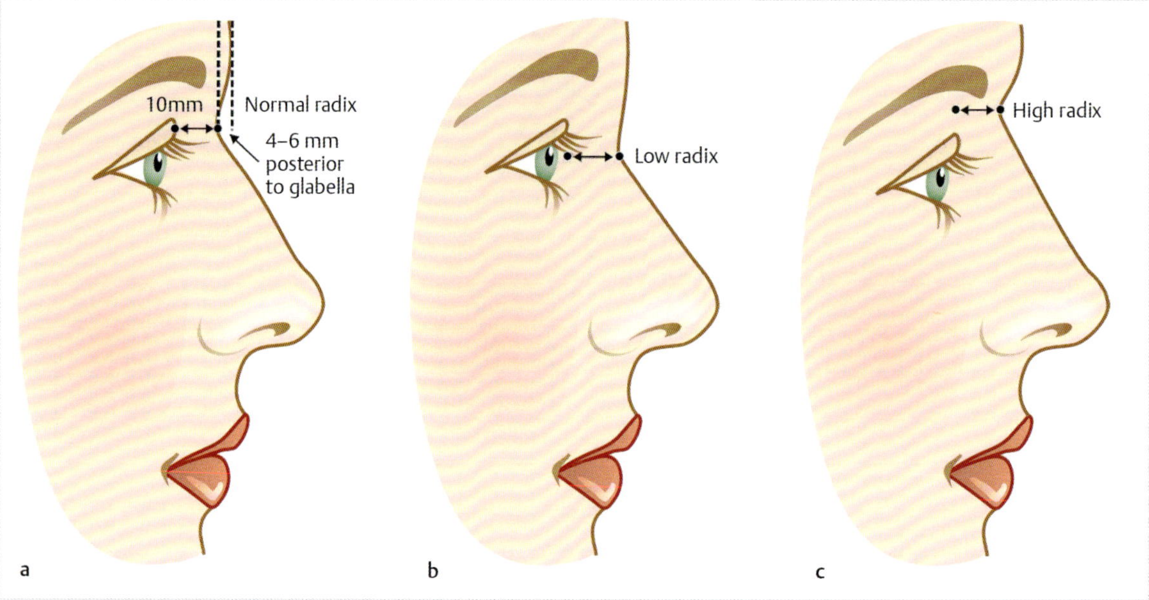

Fig. 2.23 Position of the nasal radix relative to the upper eyelid and the glabella. (a) The radix typically lies at the level of the lower half of the upper eyelid, about 10 mm from the medial canthus and 4–6 mm posterior to the glabella. **(b)** Low radix. **(c)** High radix.

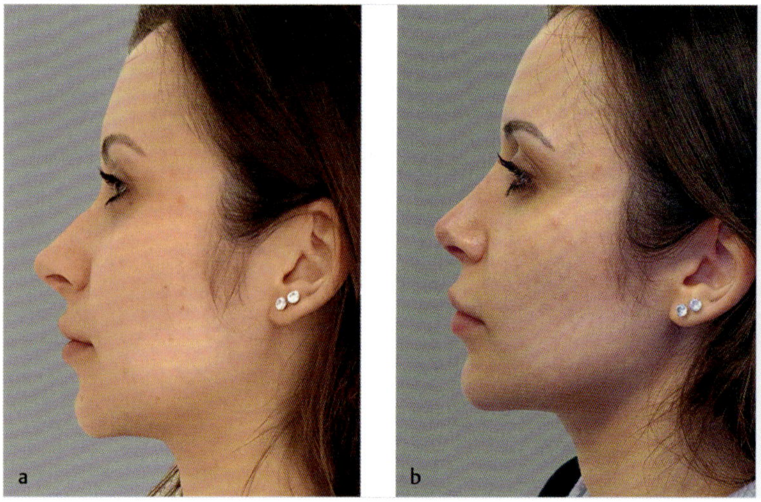

Fig. 2.24 Deep-seated radix; case study. (a) Excessively deep radix (low radix) following a rhinoplasty carried out elsewhere. **(b)** After revision rhinoplasty with a radix graft (see section 17.2.2); the nasolabial angle has also been revised.

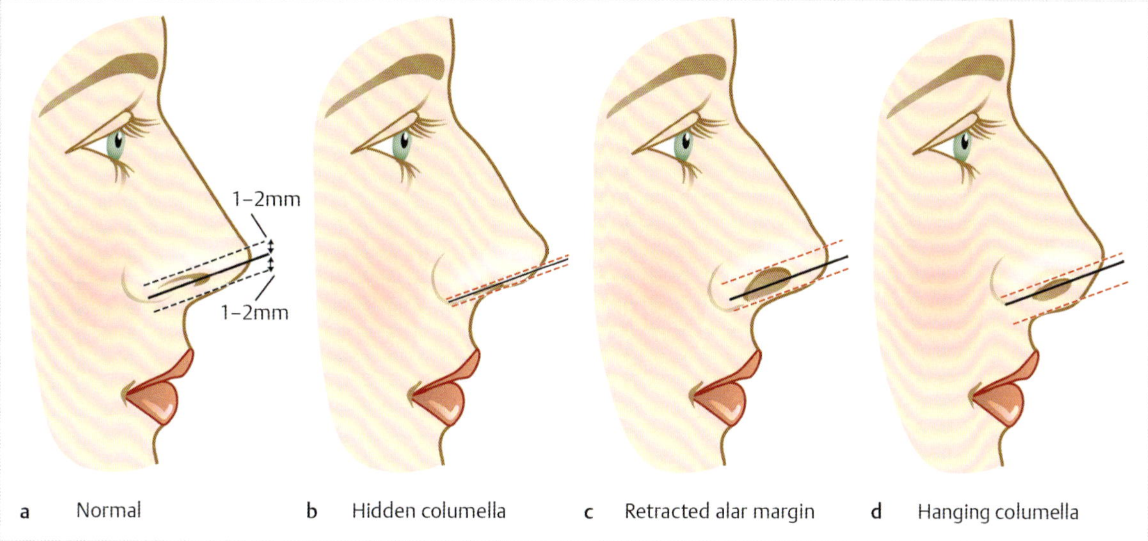

Fig. 2.25 Lateral view of the nostril – relationship of the nasal alar rim to the columella. **(a)** Normal appearance; the alar rim and columella lie at a distance of 1–2 mm from a central axis passing through the nostril. **(b)** Hidden columella. **(c)** Retracted alar rim (see ▶ **Fig. 10.22a–d**). **(d)** Hanging columella.

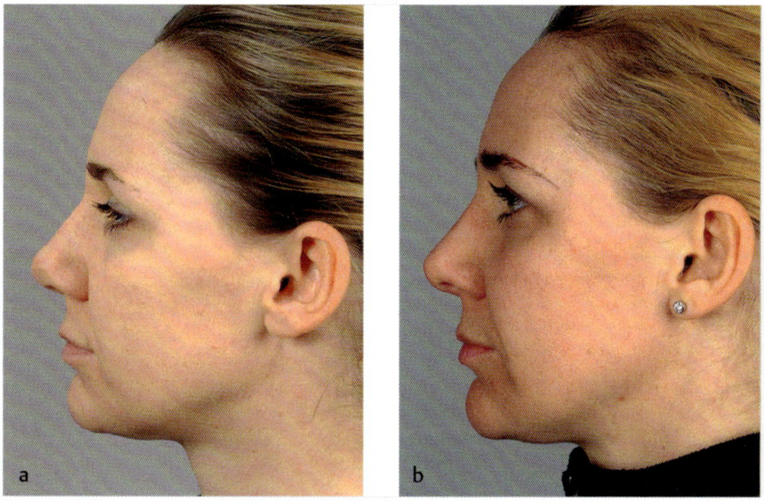

Fig. 2.26 Hidden columella; case study. **(a)** Hidden columella. **(b)** Surgical outcome after rhinoplasty, with correction of the hidden columella using an extended columella strut graft and elevation of the nasal alar rim with lateral suspension sutures.

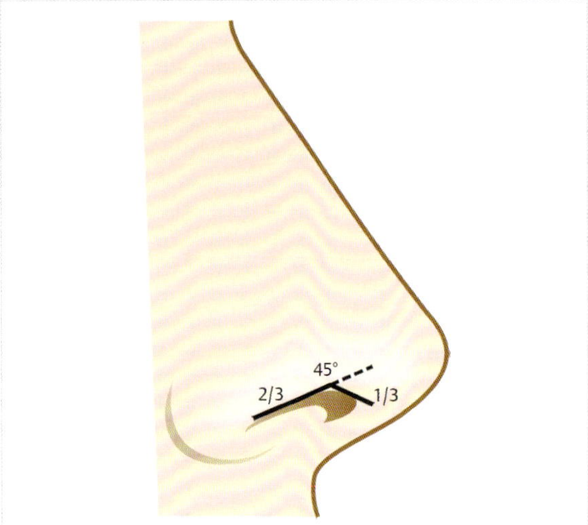

Fig. 2.27 Contour of the nasal alar rim. The anterior third of the nasal alar rim inclines caudally.

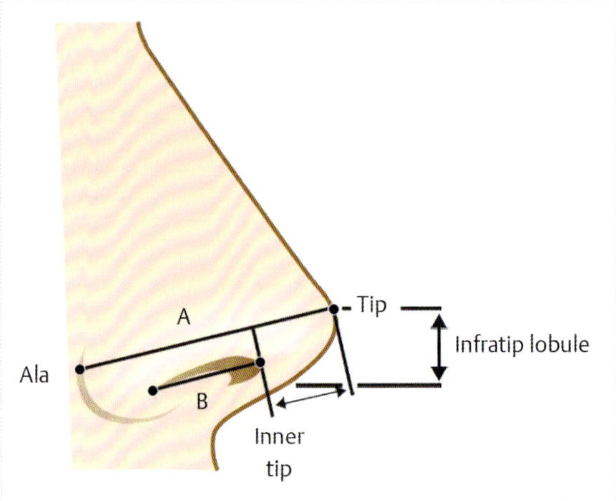

Fig. 2.28 Dimensions of the nostril and lobule (inner tip). Ala–tip = A; nostril length = B. The length of the inner tip (infratip lobule) corresponds to approximately 0.3 × A or approximately 0.7 × B.

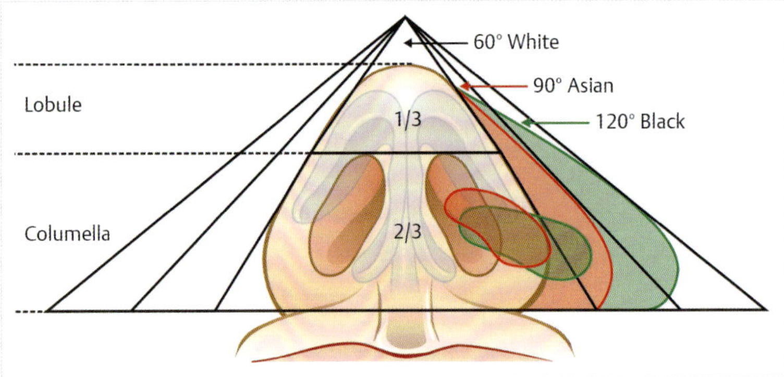

Fig. 2.29 Dimensions of the nasal base with ethnic differences. The angle between the nasal ala is larger in Asian and especially Black noses than in White ones. The axis of the nostril moves from a vertical to a more horizontal position.

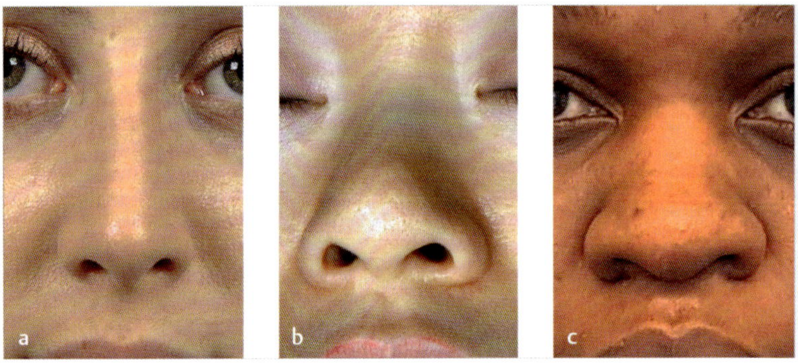

Fig. 2.30 Different configurations of the nasal base. (a) White patient. **(b)** Asian patient. **(c)** Black patient.

Bibliography

Braunfels S. Der "vermessene" Mensch. Anthropometrie in Kunst und Wissenschaft. Munich-Graefelfing: Heinz Moos; 1973

Farkas LG, Munro JR. Anthropometric facial proportions in medicine. Springfield: Thomas; 1987

Naini FB, Cobourne MT, Garagiola U, McDonald F, Wertheim D. Nasofrontal angle and nasal dorsal aesthetics: a quantitative investigation of idealized and normative values. Facial Plast Surg. 2016; 32(4):444–451

Patel PN, Most SP. Concepts of facial aesthetics when considering ethnic rhinoplasty. Otolaryngol Clin North Am. 2020; 53(2):195–208

Powell N, Humphreys B. Proportions of the aesthetic face. New York: Thieme Stratton; 1984

Wang TD. [Nasal dorsal augmentation]. HNO. 2010; 58(9):907–911

3 Preoperative Assessment and Preparation

The preparation phase is extremely important for the success of the operation.

> ✔
>
> It is important for both doctor and patient to be prepared to approach the surgical treatment as a joint action in good agreement and with positive expectations, in which they have the same goal in mind regarding the surgical result and at the same time are both aware of the risks that are present in the procedure. This agreement first needs to be established, and it is not always possible right away.

The surgeon contributes to successful preoperative planning by following a systematic approach.

3.1 Case Analysis

Case analysis includes careful history-taking (▶ Table 3.1). Awareness of the patient's living conditions is essential, as it provides crucial information about exposure to certain stressful situations in the postoperative period that may jeopardize the surgical result (sports; dust and dirt in the workplace; wearing glasses; dealing with small children or pets, etc.). These conditions have to be discussed with the patient preoperatively for appropriate planning of the postoperative phase and include planned trips, sports activities and exercise, appearances in public or in front of a camera, and so on (see Chapter 24).

Table 3.1 Patient history

General history
• Gender
• Age
• Occupation/social situation
• Marital status
• Nationality
Medical history
• Health status, incl. conditions of heart, circulation, lungs, blood coagulation, nervous system, psyche, and others
• Previous or concomitant operations or illnesses
• Allergies
• Medications
Specific medical history related to the nose
• Symptoms
• Nasal breathing status
• Diseases / operations / trauma to the nose and paranasal sinuses
• Self-assessment of the cosmetic abnormality

Computed tomography (CT) or magnetic resonance imaging (MRI) may be indicated in patients with preexisting disease, previous operations, or trauma to the nose and/or paranasal sinuses. Occasionally, a patient may require surgery on the paranasal sinuses together with a rhinoplasty (for example, patients with chronic sinusitis).

Any anticoagulant medication must be discontinued or changed, if necessary. The patient's general history and medication history also have to be discussed with the anesthesiologist in advance.

> ✔
>
> The indication for rhinoplasty is debatable in patients who are in poor general health, have severe comorbidities, acute illnesses, or alcohol or drug addiction. Heavy smoking may also be added to the list, given the risk of impaired wound healing.

These restrictions mainly apply to cosmetic nasal correction; the severity of symptoms has to be taken into account when weighing up the benefits and risks of functional nasal surgery.

Surgical reports from any prior operations on the nose should be obtained – e.g., to determine whether certain implants or transplants may have been used. However, such information is frequently lacking, as surgical reports are not available and patients are poorly informed about the details of previous operations. One must therefore be prepared for an element of surprise during revision surgery.

3.2 Impaired Nasal Breathing

Preoperative assessment of nasal breathing is crucial before rhinoplasty. Any planned operation must include relief of nasal obstruction in patients with impaired nasal breathing, and this may directly affect the surgical approach. This is often linked to the question of whether and to what extent a health-insurance company will bear the cost of functional correction. The surgeon must explicitly clarify this aspect preoperatively with the patient and/or the insurance provider; a written declaration of cost coverage from the body concerned should be obtained in advance, if necessary. The same also applies to concomitantly planned sinus surgery.

Preoperative diagnosis and documentation of nasal obstruction may also be relevant from a forensic point of view.

3.2.1 Septal Deviation, Inferior Turbinate Hypertrophy, Nasal Valve Incompetence

A carefully elicited history may already reveal the cause of obstructed nasal breathing. **Constantly** obstructed unilateral or – less frequently – bilateral nasal breathing suggests a diagnosis of **septal deviation** (▶ Fig. 3.1b). Nasal congestion that fluctuates and alternates between the two sides is usually attributable to **hypertrophy of the inferior turbinates**, particularly if it becomes worse when recumbent (on lying down to sleep, for instance) (▶ Fig. 3.1a). This can be explained by the greater fluid content in the soft tissues of the head region in the horizontal body position.

Turbinate hypertrophy is the most common cause of nasal obstruction that requires treatment. It may be due to an allergy, and can be excluded by an allergy test in suspected cases. The disorder is also observed relatively frequently even in the absence of allergies, and is then due to a nonallergic response to nonspecific stimuli (vasomotor rhinitis). The condition is due to hypertrophy of the soft tissues overlying the turbinates (▶ Fig. 3.1a, on the right) and rarely to enlargement of the bony turbinate itself (▶ Fig. 3.1a, on the left). Both findings may occasionally be present in combination.

Turbinate hyperplasia is also commonly seen in combination with septal deviation.

Nasal valve incompetence or weakness of the lateral nasal wall usually presents as nasal obstruction on deep inspiration, or even on inspiration at rest in severe cases (▶ Fig. 3.1c).

Lateral nasal wall collapse occasionally occurs after aggressive surgical procedures on the upper or lower lateral cartilages during rhinoplasty (▶ Fig. 3.1c). Collapse of the lateral cartilages is frequently evident as a visible retraction of the lateral nasal wall on inspiration, while at the same time patients complain of nasal obstruction.

Adhesions or **synechiae** between the septum and the lateral nasal wall or the middle or inferior turbinate after prior surgery or previous illness may give rise to constant nasal obstruction on the affected side. The degree of obstruction depends on the extent of the adhesions. Fine synechiae may remain asymptomatic and may go unnoticed, while denser adhesions may cause near-complete obstruction of the nasal airway (▶ Fig. 3.2a).

High septal deviation under the roof of the nose deserves special mention (▶ Fig. 3.2b). It may be missed on a cursory examination and can give rise to symptoms of nasal valve incompetence in the intercartilaginous region.

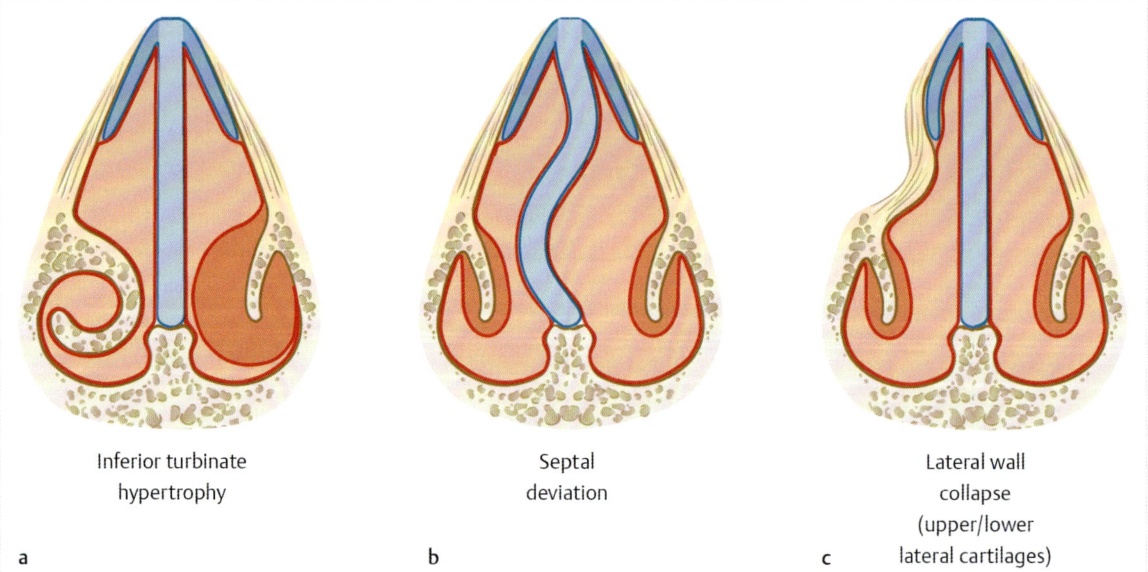

Fig. 3.1 Causes of nasal obstruction (1). Pathological conditions in the lateral nasal wall and turbinates. **(a)** Turbinate hyperplasia. **(b)** Septal deviation. **(c)** Lateral wall collapse.

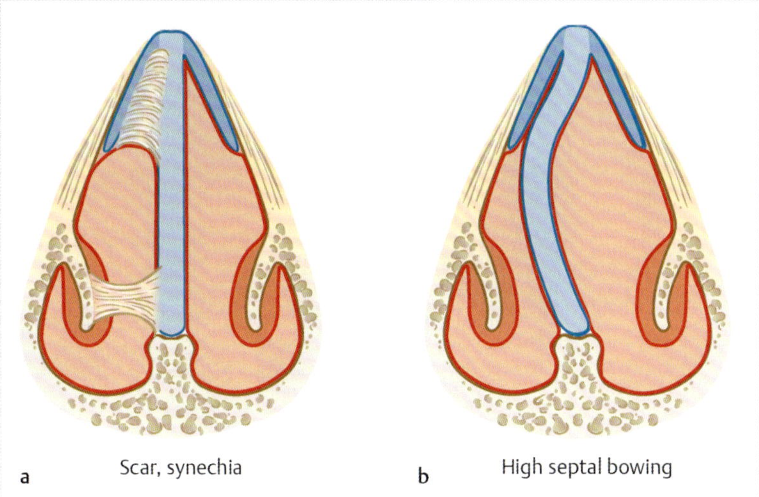

Fig. 3.2 Causes of nasal obstruction (2). Causes of narrowing under the roof of the nose, such as cicatricial postoperative or traumatic adhesions (synechiae) **(a)** and high septal deviation **(b)**, are frequently identified using only a 0° or 30° nasal endoscope.

Other causes of nasal obstruction include **polyps,** such as those due to chronic sinusitis, benign and malignant **tumors**, pneumatized middle turbinate (**concha bullosa**), **choanal stenosis**, etc. A detailed description of these and other entities is beyond the scope of this book. Referral to an ear, nose, and throat (ENT) surgeon is indicated for optimal clinical evaluation if any of these conditions are suspected or the findings are unclear, and the nose surgeon does not treat the findings himself.

3.2.2 Diagnostic Investigations

Clinical Examination of the Nose

Examination of the nose mainly involves external and internal inspection. Additional special procedures are required for evaluation of nasal airway obstruction.

The shape and dimensions of the nose are evaluated during **inspection.** A crooked nose, narrow nostrils, or retraction of the lateral wall, worsening on inspiration, may indicate the presence of a functional disorder.

From a cosmetic surgical perspective, the surgeon has to evaluate the extent to which the nasal proportions deviate from the standard dimensions. It is also important to document the presence of scars due to previous surgery or trauma, and dynamic changes, such as the frequently troublesome drooping of the nasal tip when laughing.

Palpation is needed to assess the bony and cartilaginous framework, as well as cartilaginous consistency and stability (▶ Fig. 3.3). Palpation is especially important for identifying the presence of mobile bone fragments, as well as step deformity, if any, in patients with a history of recent trauma. Any visible scars should be palpated to determine whether they are fixed or mobile. Troublesome abnormalities of the nasal framework are occasionally better felt than seen.

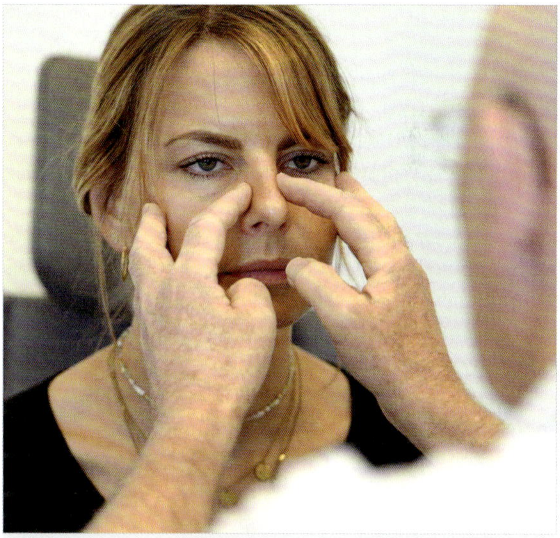

Fig. 3.3 Palpation of the nose. Both sides of the nose are palpated for comparison.

Examination of the Inner Nose

Examining the nasal cavities using a **speculum** is still the most important method for rapidly assessing the interior of the nose. A powerful, well-focused head lamp and a slim speculum, usually held in the left hand, are used, while the right hand maneuvers the position of the patient's head in order to visualize the superior or inferior meatus (▶ Fig. 3.4).

Touching the septum may be uncomfortable or even painful, and should be avoided in all endonasal examinations. However, it may be unavoidable during palpation with a fine instrument, which may be necessary after septoplasty to determine the adequacy of residual septal

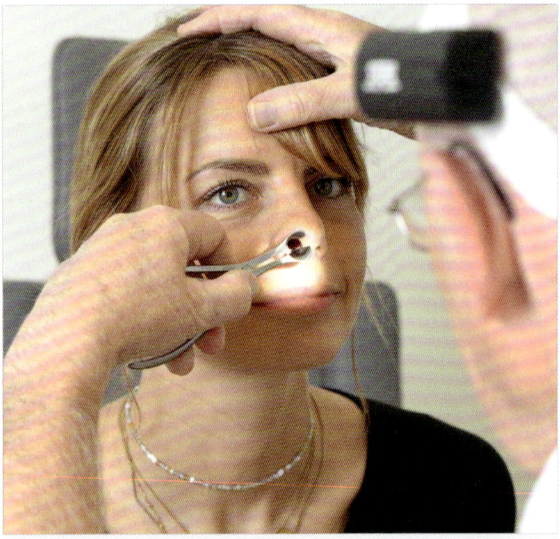

Fig. 3.4 Speculum examination of the inner nose. A head lamp is usually employed for speculum examinations.

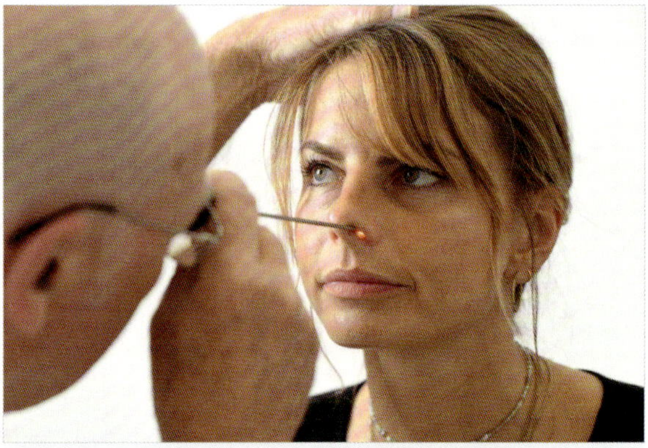

Fig. 3.5 Examination with a nasal endoscope. Examining the nose using a slim telescope with a light source allows the most accurate evaluation of the interior of the nose.

cartilage as graft material for a planned rhinoplasty. Palpation of the septum is a crucial diagnostic test in such cases.

Also important is the assessment of the size and appearance of the inferior turbinates, the state of the mucous membranes, alignment of the septum, and any visible pathology. One should not fail to examine the region under the roof of the nasal cavity, to avoid overlooking the presence of high septal deviation.

The nasal cavity can be examined more precisely using a fine **endoscope** (▶ Fig. 3.5). These rigid endoscopes, with a viewing angle of 0–30°, should not exceed a diameter of 3 mm for nasal endoscopy to prevent unpleasant contact with the walls of the nasal cavity. In conjunction with a camera, the endoscopic image can be conveniently viewed on a monitor and, for example, endoscopic images can also be taken.

A good light source allows excellent anatomical visualization right down to the nasopharynx. Tubal openings can be visualized, and the maxillary ostia in the middle meatus are usually also visible. Prior application of a decongestant spray (naphazoline) facilitates examination in patients with nasal mucosal congestion by inducing transient vasoconstriction and relieving congestion. Applying a local anesthetic spray (lidocaine) reduces mucosal sensitivity to touch in both children and sensitive adults.

Cottle Test and Similar Procedures

The Cottle maneuver helps improve nasal obstruction due to **incompetence or narrowing of the nasal valve.**

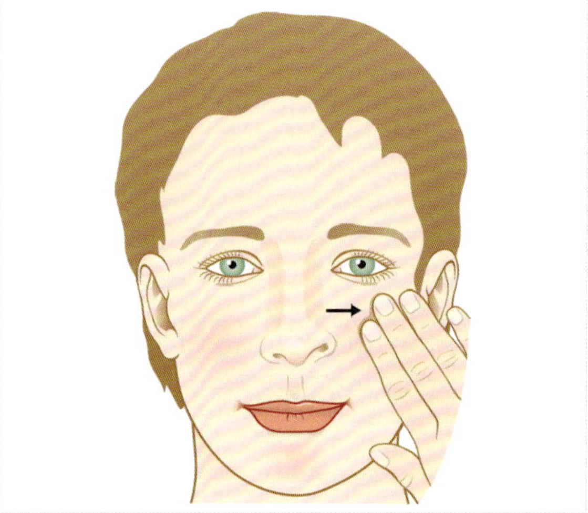

Fig. 3.6 Cottle test. The cheek on the side to be evaluated is gently pulled laterally with one or two fingers to open the nasal valve. This leads to improved inspiratory flow in patients who have weakness or narrowing of the valve.

The cheek on the side to be evaluated is gently pulled laterally with one or two fingers to open the valve (▶ Fig. 3.6, ▶ Fig. 3.7).

An elevator can also be used to lift the nasal ala from within and thus relieve nasal obstruction (▶ Fig. 3.8, ▶ Fig. 3.9). These maneuvers are helpful for locating the site of obstruction precisely.

Relief of nasal obstruction during inspiration by lifting the nasal tip also indicates nasal valve incompetence (▶ Fig. 3.10). The central pillar of Anderson's "tripod" – i.e., the entire anterior nose with the columella and the caudal septum – is usually weak in such cases.

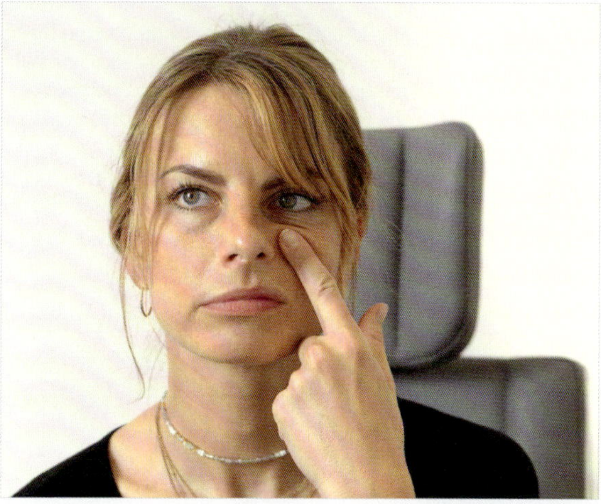

Fig. 3.7 Cottle test. Patients with incompetent or narrow nasal valves often experience relief of nasal obstruction when they apply the Cottle maneuver themselves.

Evaluation of Transnasal Airflow (Rhinomanometry)

Application of decongestant nasal spray (naphazoline) is a relatively simple clinical method for identifying the effect of mucosal congestion and turbinate hypertrophy on nasal breathing. Symptomatic patients with nasal obstruction who are found to have enlarged turbinates and narrow nasal passages on a speculum or endoscopic examination typically have a significant reduction in turbinate size and dilation of the nasal airways, with notable relief from nasal obstruction, within 5–10 minutes of application of the decongestant spray. In contrast, decongestion of the nasal mucosa does not provide any perceptible relief from nasal obstruction due to nasal septal deviation or nasal valve incompetence.

Rhinomanometry is a diagnostic tool for objective evaluation of the respiratory function of the nose by measuring transnasal airflow. Each nostril is evaluated

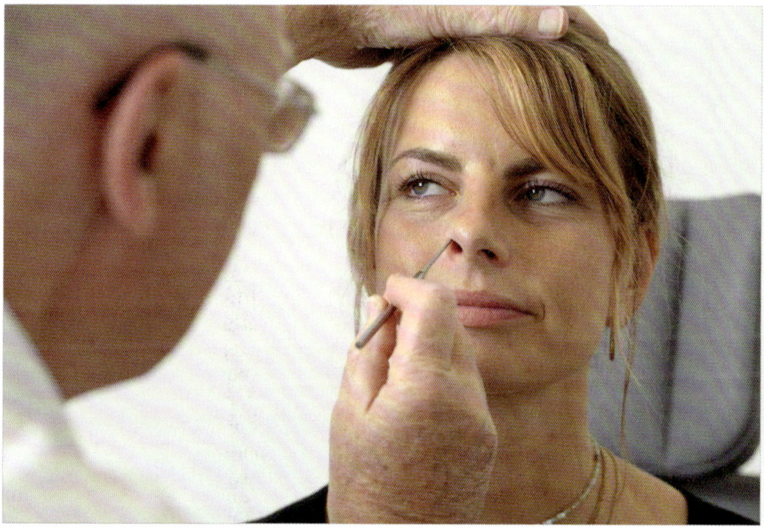

Fig. 3.8 Instrumental opening of the nasal valve. Lifting of the nasal ala with a fine elevator improves breathing in patients with valvular incompetence.

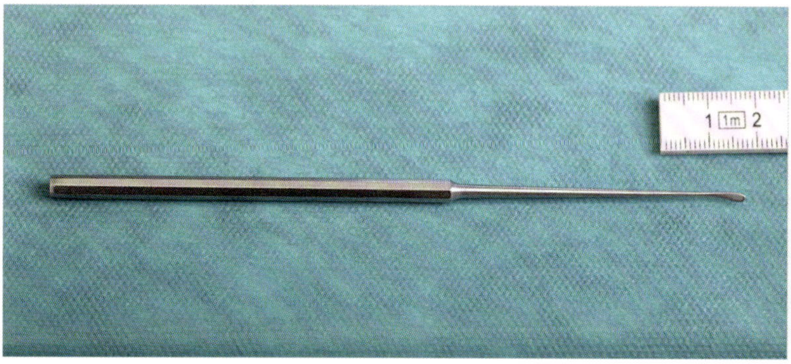

Fig. 3.9 Fine elevator. The instrument for this examination must not be too bulky, so as not to hinder breathing.

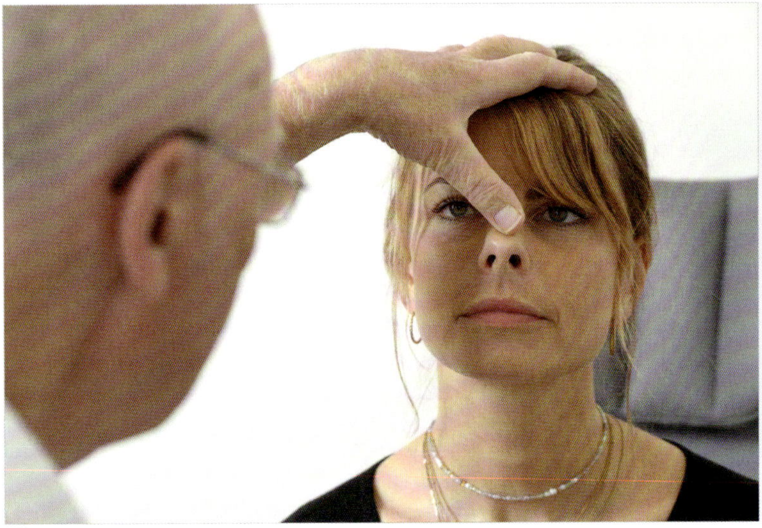

Fig. 3.10 Lifting the nasal tip. Raising the nasal tip often restores the patency of nasal passages in patients with incompetence of the nasal valves and anterior nose.

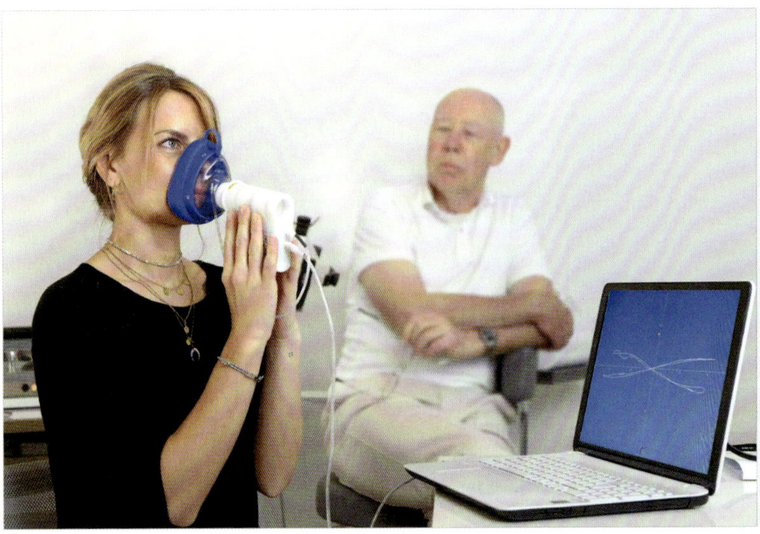

Fig. 3.11 Rhinomanometry. A pressure tube is attached to the nostril under the mask.

separately. The procedure is carried out both before and after the application of a decongestant nasal spray (naphazoline) (▶ Fig. 3.11). The objective findings obtained include absolute values and a typical curve from which nasal flow or the extent of obstruction may be derived (▶ Fig. 3.12). Inspiratory values are depicted in the image on the right, while expiratory values are seen on the left. The steeper the curve, the better the nasal air flow, and the lesser the degree of nasal obstruction.

However, rhinomanometric measurements may be misleading, resulting in unreliable assessment of nasal airflow; both false-negative and false-positive findings have been observed. Rhinomanometry is technically unfeasible when the nasal cavities are completely occluded, with no readings being obtained. Data obtained in patients with a septal perforation are likewise unreliable.

✓

Rhinomanometry cannot be used for objective assessment of disorders that are due to an incompetent nasal valve or collapsed nostril; placement of a nasal "olive" in the nostril precludes measurement of nasal airflow in this area.

A detailed medical history is therefore of the utmost importance in such cases. Together with clinical and endoscopic examination of the nose, the patient's medical history often provides a clearer picture of the type, extent, and cause of the disorder than the findings obtained with these technical procedures.

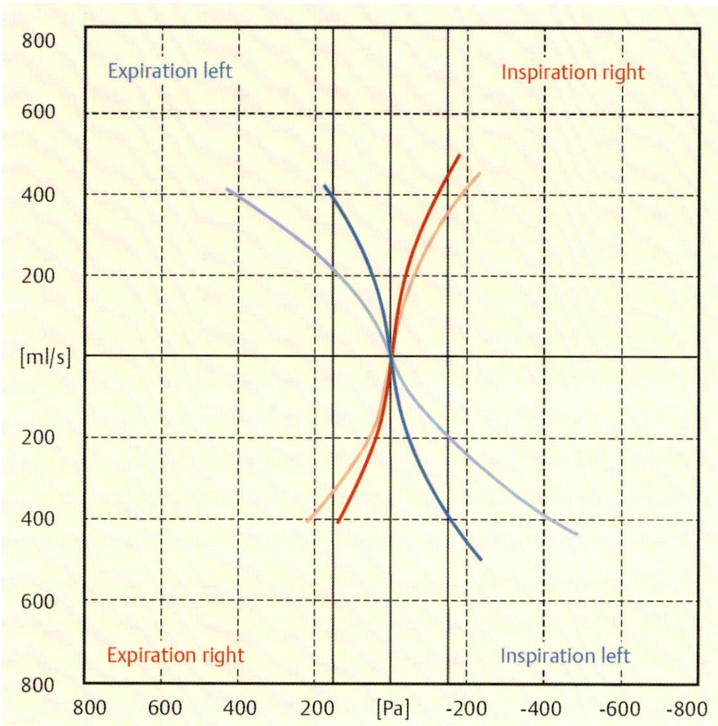

Red: right side of nose
Blue: left side of nose
Pale colored: before decongestion
Brightly colored: after decongestion

Fig. 3.12 Rhinomanometry curve. Graphic representation of a rhinomanometry measurement result. Typical rhinomanometry curves before and after the application of decongestant spray, leading to a moderate improvement in nasal patency (from Mlynski and Pirsig, 2018).

Also worth mentioning here is *acoustic rhinometry*, an objective technique used to assess the geometry of the nasal cavity based on the analysis of reflected sound waves. However, this method is not widely used in ENT facilities and is unfortunately also error-prone.

Czermak Plate

Czermak's test is a fairly simple method for rapid detection of abnormal nasal airflow (▶ Fig. 3.13). Czermak's plate is a smooth metallic plate that is held directly under the patient's nostrils, with an arched recess facilitating close contact with the upper lip. Exhalation of air through the nose fogs the plate, which gives an idea of the volume of air exhaled. The semicircular markings on the plate surface roughly quantify the degree of fogging caused by the expired air (none, mild or severe), and comparison of the two sides is possible.

It should be pointed out that this plate can only be used to assess expiratory nasal flow. Obstruction of inspiratory nasal airflow, as in nasal valve disorders, cannot be detected using this method. The Czermak plate is primarily used in phoniatrics, specifically to document the nasality of certain sounds, as in patients with cleft lip and palate.

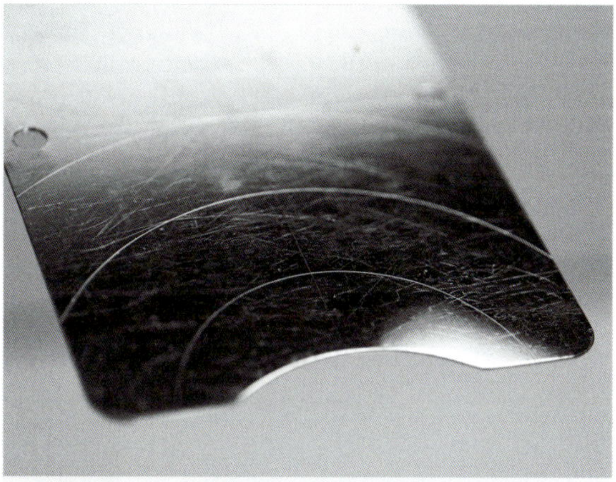

Fig. 3.13 Czermak plate. The inscribed rings are helpful for quantitative assessment of fogging caused by expired nasal air (KARL STORZ SE & Co. KG, Tuttlingen, Germany).

Imaging

Detailed preoperative evaluation of the bony framework and soft tissues of the nose and paranasal sinuses may be useful from both a functional and cosmetic standpoint.

3

High-resolution **computed tomography** (CT) or **digital volume tomography** (DVT) of the nose and paranasal sinuses optimally depict the regional anatomy, as well as pathological states such as diseased sinuses, fracture lines following trauma or previous operations, deviation of the bony framework and septum, and the bony component of a nasal hump, as well as pneumatized middle turbinates (concha bullosa, not uncommon when there is an obstruction in nasal breathing) (▶ Fig. 3.14a–c).

Magnetic resonance imaging (MRI) is advantageous, as it does not involve any exposure to radiation, in contrast to CT; however, bony structures are not directly visualized.

> ✓
>
> Although analyzing imaging findings is a job for the radiologist, surgeons can also benefit from learning image interpretation themselves.

Other causes of nasal obstruction include chronic inflammation or tumors of the nose and/or paranasal sinuses. The diagnosis and treatment of these diseases are beyond the scope of this book. Reference may be made to ENT textbooks for more information.

3.3 Desire for Cosmetic Correction

Many patients have had a long-standing desire for cosmetic correction of the nose, ever since childhood or adolescence, before they seek the services of a skilled surgeon. Others may wish to undergo surgical correction because someone has made them feel insecure by pointing out a nasal abnormality; however, short-term decision-making regarding surgery should be avoided. Rhinoplasty cannot be undertaken on a whim and needs to be strongly indicated; the patient alone should decide for or against the operation, rather than their family or partner — and not the doctor either.

> ✓
>
> A second or even a third consultation should be recommended if the necessity for the operation or the timing of surgery is ambiguous or in doubt. This gives patients sufficient time to rethink their decision.

3.3.1 Interviewing the Patient

It is advisable to first have patients describe in their own words what bothers them most about their nose and the corrections they believe are most important to them, before discussing the surgeon's ideas about possible changes to the nose. I then outline my assessment and decide whether I initially agree with the patient or find it difficult to understand the patient's wishes. If I note discrepancies or distinctly unrealistic patient expectations, I am happy to suggest a computer simulation of the expected postoperative outcome using professionally produced photos.

At this relatively early stage in communication with the patient, it often becomes apparent whether difficulties are likely to arise along the way or whether patients feel they have met the "right" surgeon.

One should not be put off by patients who want to be in control of the situation right from the outset, saying they "by no means" want any change in the appearance of a hooked nose or a (hanging) tip during correction of other abnormalities, or that the surgeon should "only use a closed technique" or "by no means osteotomies." Patients like this should be thoroughly examined, the findings should be analyzed, and it should then be calmly explained to them why, for instance, the open technique is more suitable in the given case, that the nose will look aesthetically more appealing without a hump or with a

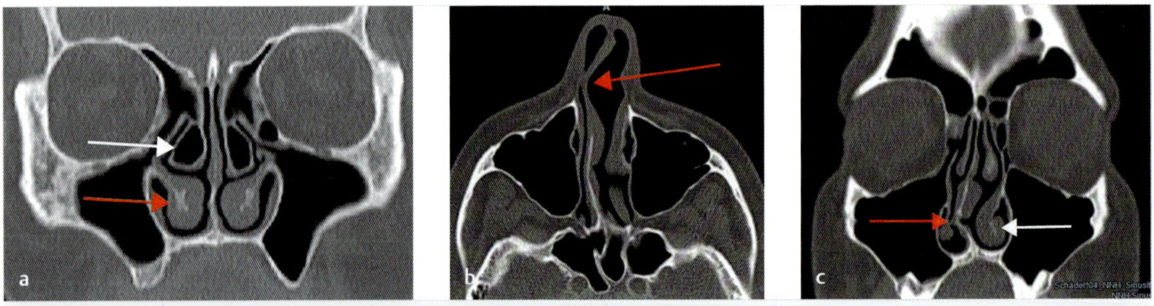

Fig. 3.14 Computed tomography (CT) of the paranasal sinuses, showing bilateral concha bullosa (white arrow in **a**), septal deviation (red arrow in **b** and **c**), and inferior turbinate hypertrophy (red arrow in **a**, bilateral; white arrow in **c**).

rotated tip, or that a good outcome cannot be expected without osteotomies, etc. The patients are laypeople in this field, and sensible individuals can usually be convinced if good computer-simulation images support the professional recommendations.

Surgeons should not hesitate to refuse surgery in a given case if they and the patient disagree about the objectives of the operation. The same applies to extreme expectations of the surgical outcome, such as wanting to have a nose similar to Michael Jackson's in his later years – a star whose nose allegedly underwent more than 30 operative interventions in all (one patient actually expressed this desire to me). Such patients do better if referred to a specialist for psychosomatic disorders.

3.3.2 Photography

Preoperative and postoperative photographic documentation of the findings is an indispensable part of rhinoplasty. Photos of the entire face are taken, with close-ups of the nose only being required in exceptional cases, such as for the documentation of scars. Frontal, both lateral, and two oblique views are the most important, and a perspective view of the nose is obtained from below (▶ Fig. 3.15a–l).

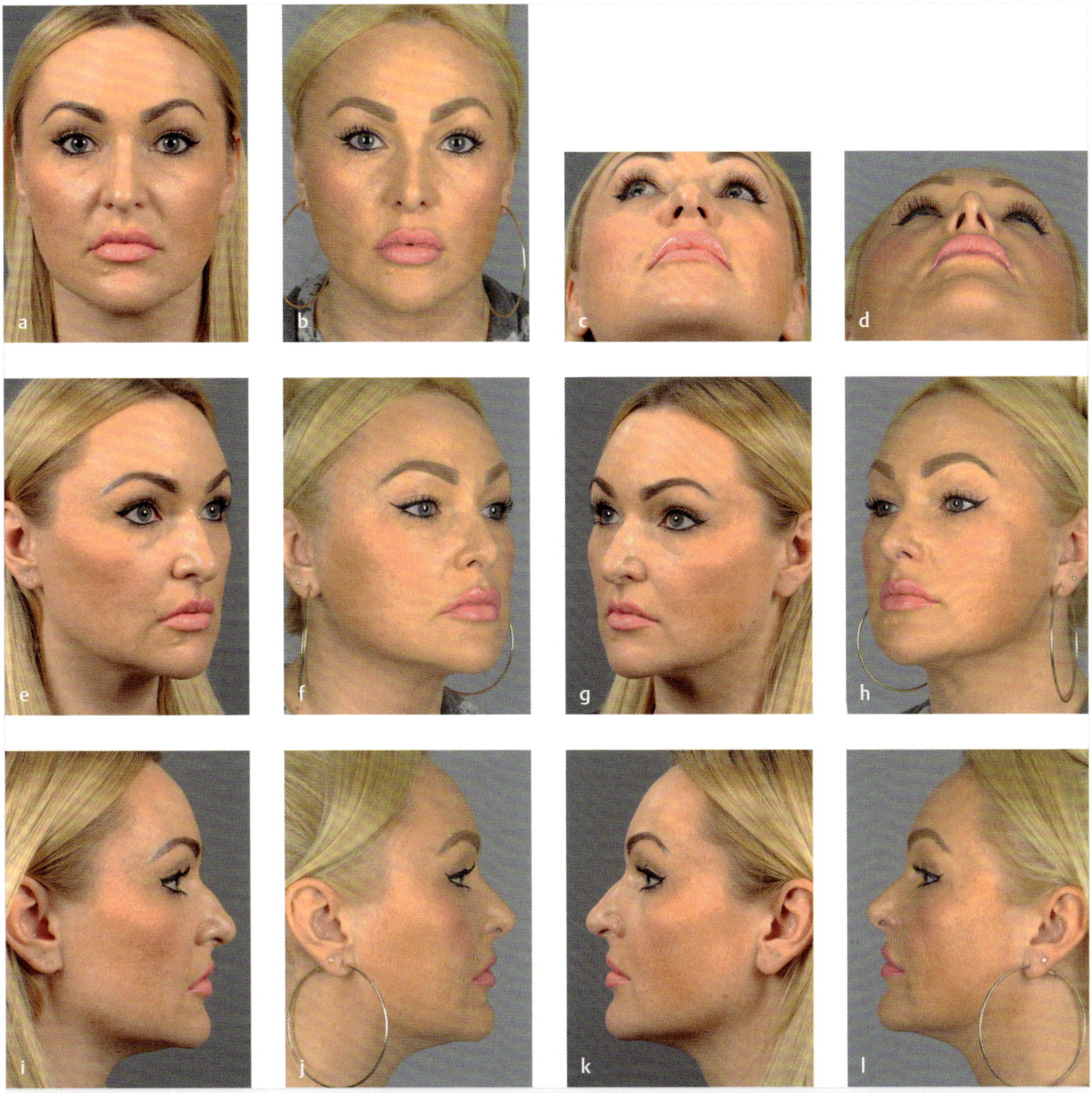

Fig. 3.15 Preoperative and postoperative photography: case study. The patient's nose has a hump and a slightly drooping tip (**a, c, e, g, i, k**). Postoperative images (**b, d, f, h, j, l**). Frontal (**a, b**), base view (**c, d**), two oblique views (**e, f, g, h**), bilateral side views (**i, j, k, l**); preoperative images (left) and postoperative images (right).

A complete series of standardized images ensures a clear depiction of the nasal deformity, while allowing optimal comparison of the preoperative and postoperative states.

When appropriate, photos are taken from below (see ▶ Fig. 7.1a,b, ▶ Fig. 11.12a, b, ▶ Fig. 19.4c,d), from above (the "helicopter view"), and with the patient smiling. A modified "helicopter view," with the image plane parallel to the nasal dorsum, may also clearly delineate a crooked nose (▶ Fig. 3.16).

A lateral view obtained while the patient is smiling may demonstrate a reduction in the nasolabial angle – i.e., sinking of the nasal tip.

The photos are taken with a neutral, monochrome, light background; care must be taken to avoid casting a drop shadow. It is therefore best not to use a flash, unless professional photo studio equipment is available. Smartphone photos can also be used, although cell-phone cameras are equipped with a powerful wide-angle lens. The nose may appear unnaturally large and voluminous, as it is located further anteriorly in the image when taken from a short distance – as in a "selfie" (▶ Fig. 3.17a, b). It is best to hold the cell-phone camera at an appropriate distance from the face (approximately 1.5 m) to avoid this type of distortion; the required sections of the image may be digitally enlarged later, if necessary.

It must be ensured that the preoperative and postoperative photographs are taken from exactly the same angle. This may be difficult to achieve, especially for oblique views. It requires precise alignment of the face, and can be accomplished, for instance, by asking the patient to look at a defined point in space for the oblique views. Alternatively, the head can be rotated sideways in such a way that the nasal tip barely touches the contour of the cheek when the face is viewed from the front.

All images are stored digitally and can therefore be electronically processed. This is particularly important for computer simulation of a possible surgical outcome – an

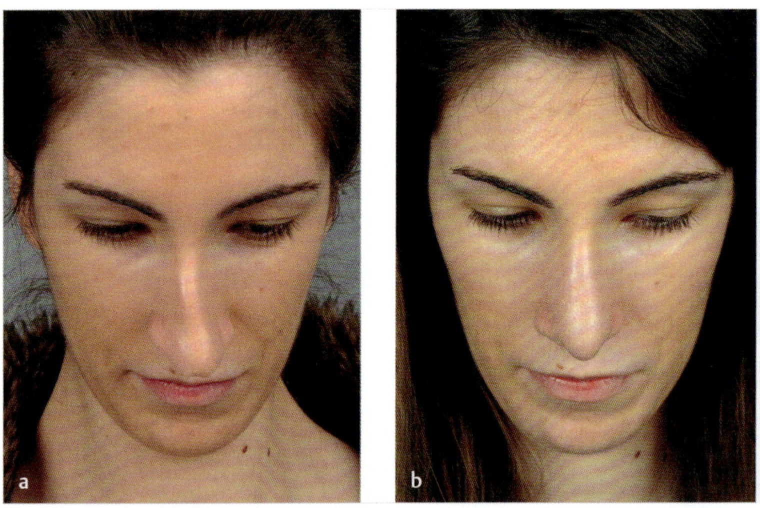

Fig. 3.16 Modified "helicopter view." (a) A modified "helicopter view" of the nasal dorsum from above clearly depicts a nasal deviation preoperatively. **(b)** Status post rhinoplasty for comparison.

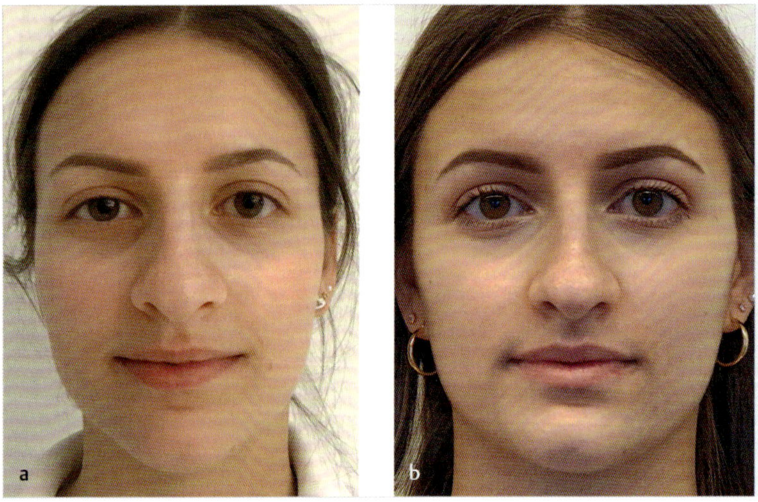

Fig. 3.17 Comparison of a selfie shot with distance photography. (a) Selfie of a patient before rhinoplasty, showing distorted nasal and facial proportions. The nose is disproportionately large, and the ears seem to merge into the background. **(b)** Distance photograph of the same patient, with real proportions for comparison (compare with ▶ Fig. 13.5 for the postoperative outcome).

essential component of preoperative planning for both the patient and physician.

Three-dimensional preoperative and postoperative comparisons are possible using **video recordings** (▸ Video 3.1). For videos, it is best to have patients slowly turn the head from side to side while they are sitting on a chair in front of the camera, which faces the face (▸ Video 3.2).

3.3.3 Computer Simulation

I use the software program AlterImage (Seattle Software Design, Seattle, Washington, USA) to simulate possible results after rhinoplasty on the basis of digital photos (▸ Video 3.3).

Image processing requires a powerful PC or laptop with a high-quality monitor and a comfortable, good-quality computer mouse. The images can be edited using an electronic pen or keyboard, but editing is far more challenging without a mouse. This image editing program is easy to use and is largely self-explanatory. However, the user must either already have or must acquire expertise in relation to nasal and facial proportions and skill in optimizing the shape of the nose (▸ Fig. 3.18a–d).

High-quality prints of the simulation should be obtained, as they serve as valuable guides during surgery (compare with ▸ Fig. 4.4.). Some patients prefer to take printed simulation images with them after the consultation so that they can discuss them with family or friends (▸ Fig. 3.19).

Expensive photo paper is preferable, but is not a must if a high-quality color printer is available that also allows high-resolution printing on plain paper.

It must be made amply clear to the patient that the simulation does not guarantee a specific postoperative outcome and should be regarded as an aid to preoperative planning. Every printout of a simulated postoperative result should therefore clearly state the following: "This simulated computer image only serves to help plan corrective surgery of the nose. The simulation images do not show a guaranteed result, and the surgical result will differ from that depicted in the image." This message is reinforced during the preoperative information discussion, both verbally and in writing, and is acknowledged and signed by the patient.

The doctor's simulation images of the suggested outcome should not be regarded as a "dictate" to which the patient has to submit. On the contrary, mutual discussion of a simulated outcome should encourage patients to formulate their ideas and desires regarding the postoperative result. Both doctor and patient must finally agree on the surgical objectives, including details such as the width of the tip, nostril size, and nasal dorsal height, to mention only a few.

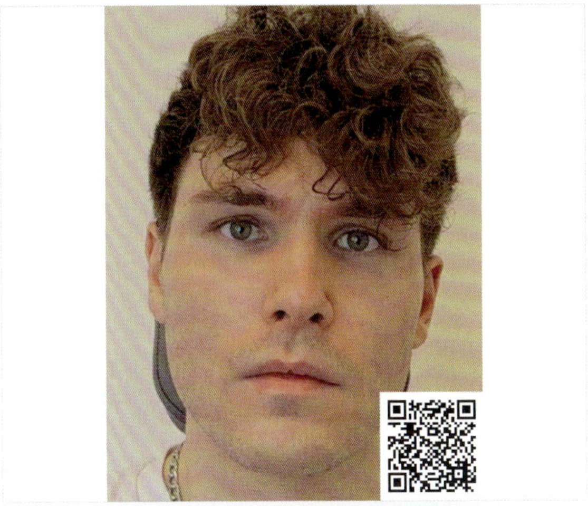

Video 3.1 Three-dimensional preoperative and postoperative comparisons, photo and video documentation.

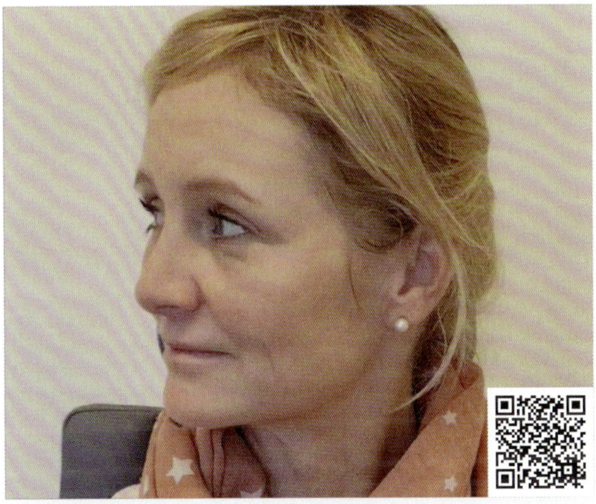

Video 3.2 Photo and video documentation of a patient slowly turning her head from side to side while sitting on a chair in front of the camera.

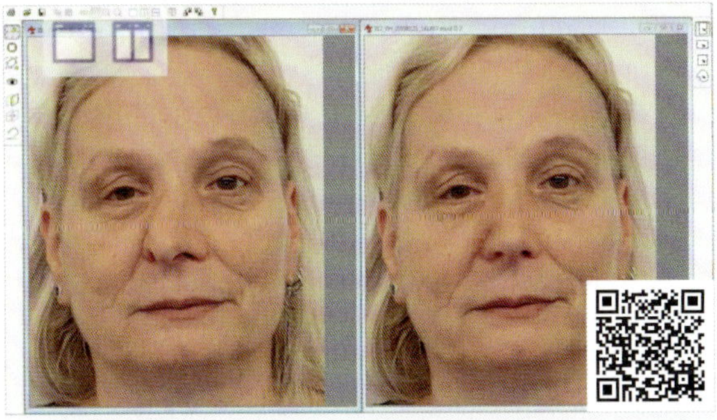

Video 3.3 Computer simulation of possible results on the basis of digital photos.

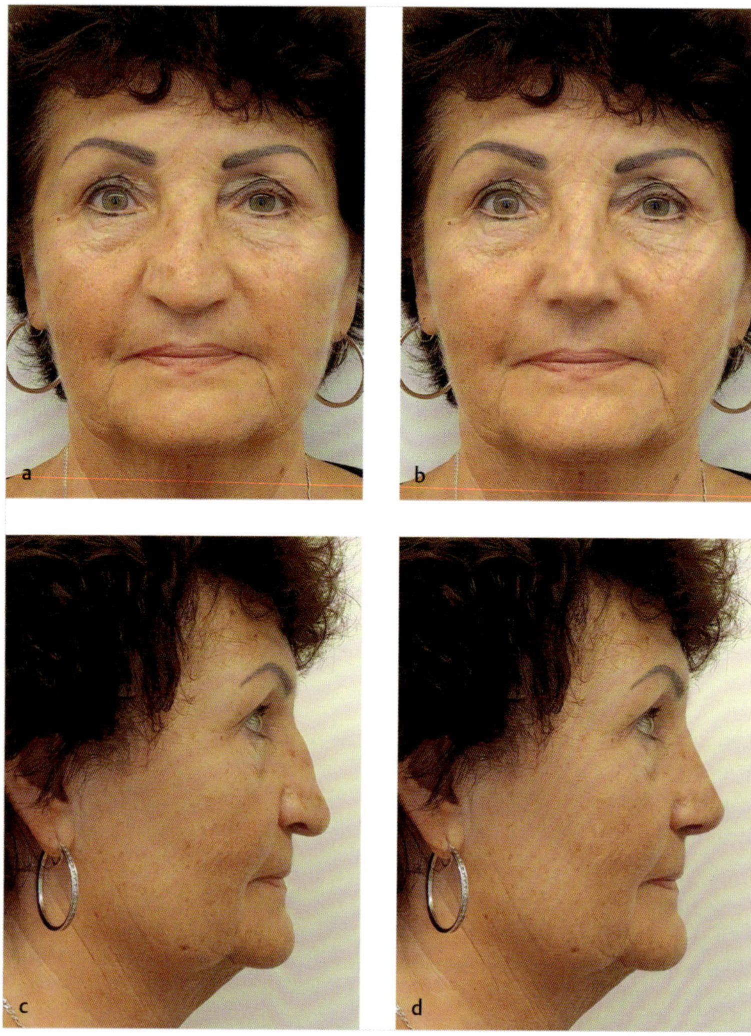

Fig. 3.18 Frontal and lateral simulation. Original and simulated frontal **(a, b)** and lateral images **(c, d)** using the AlterImage software program, before rhinoplasty (compare with ▶ Fig. 17.5 for the actual postoperative result).

In my routine practice, it is extremely rare for patients to decline the offer of a simulation. I always offer simulated images of the frontal *and* lateral views, and patients are highly appreciative of this. However, good frontal simulation requires some additional practice. I mostly edit images on my PC on my own, without being pressured for time; I then share the high-resolution paper printouts with the patient, keeping the original and simulation side by side (▶ Fig. 3.19). Image processing or modification can also be carried out in the presence of the patient.

Patients may occasionally ask for the simulated images to be e-mailed to them; while I do not decline this request, I prefer to discuss the simulated result in person.

This type of joint preoperative planning thus provides an excellent opportunity to identify in good time whether the doctor and patient are on the same page with regard to the desired outcome, or whether there are significant differences that first need to be addressed.

✓

Simulation is thus very helpful for avoiding interventions in which the goals of the doctor and patient are widely different. For this reason, I produce a simulation before every rhinoplasty and discuss it with the patient, even if this has not been requested.

For intraoperative use, I prefer to see the profile of the patient's nose with the simulated image set over the preoperative original one. This is possible with the PowerPoint program, which makes it possible to position the two pictures precisely one over the other and give each nasal profile a specific "artistic effect" and transparency (▶ Fig. 3.20). These superimposed images make it possible to see exactly the areas in which the profile is to be changed, and to what extent (▶ Video 3.4).

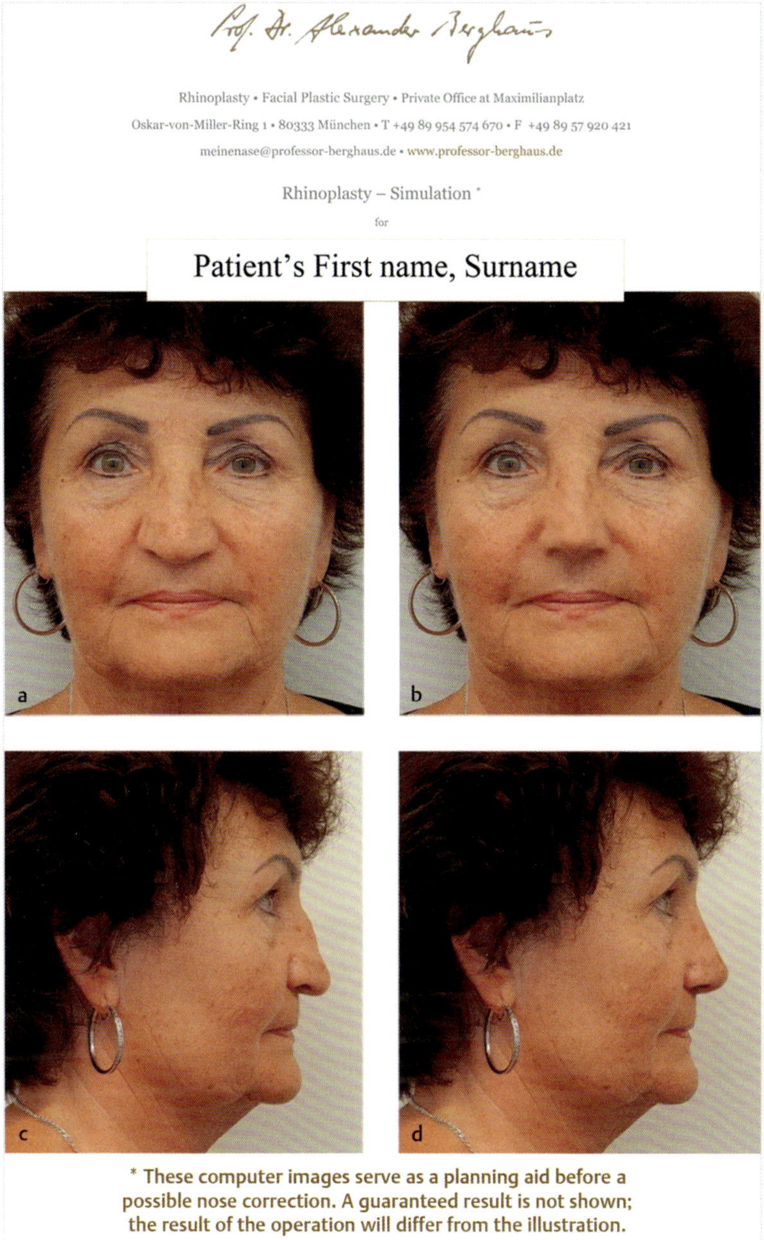

Fig. 3.19 Paper printout of simulated images. The text under every printout of simulated images emphasizes the fact that they do not guarantee an identical postoperative outcome.

3.3.4 Patient Information and Declaration of Consent

A written and documented preoperative informative discussion must be held between the doctor and the patient once all doubts regarding the surgical objectives have been clarified and the costs have been settled by mutual agreement. The details of the operation are explained to the patient, who is provided with a written list of possible risks and postoperative complications.

Professionally prepared printed forms for this purpose are available on the market and are widely used in Germany for rhinoplasty, as for most other medical interventions. They are prepared by a panel of medical and legal experts (▶ Fig. 3.21).

> ✔
>
> However, this does not absolve the physician from the obligation to personally discuss all surgical risks with the patient – simply handing out a printed form for signature does not do justice to the situation, particularly in cosmetic surgery, and is not acceptable.

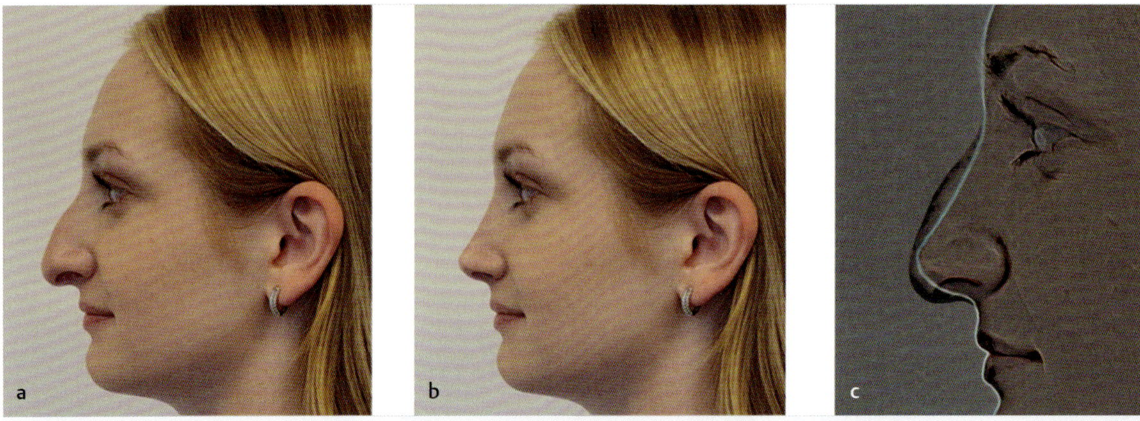

Fig. 3.20 Superimposed images (c) of the original (a) and simulation (b). Presenting the original and the simulation as superimposed images makes it possible to see exactly in which areas the profile should be changed, and to what amount.

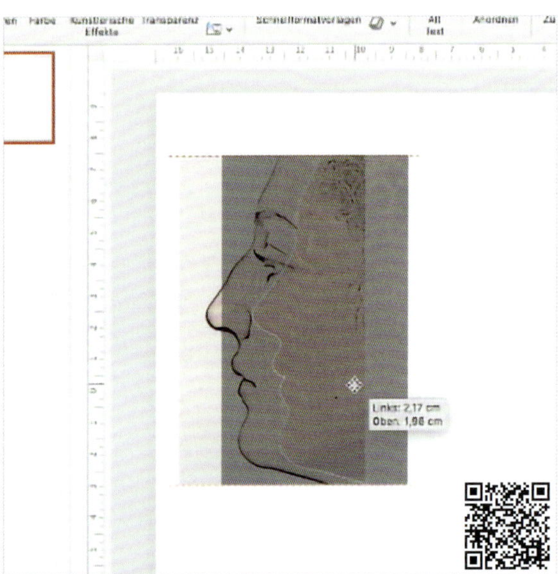

Video 3.4 How to overlay the original and the simulation in PowerPoint.

In Germany, in the event of a dispute, the courts appreciate when handwritten, individual entries on the form show that a detailed personal conversation actually took place between doctor and patient.

The patient must be informed about the typical **medical** risks of nasal surgery and must also be aware that the procedure also carries a risk regarding the **cosmetic** outcome. The **patient information sheet** (▶ Fig. 3.21) mentions all aspects that are relevant to the planned intervention, and these also have to be discussed verbally.

The patient is also apprised that health-insurance companies do not generally cover the costs of aesthetic operations and that follow-up cost insurance cover is available for cosmetic interventions (see section 24.10).

The type of anesthesia and the choice of the incision are also mentioned, and the operative procedure is outlined in brief. The patients declare their consent for an extension of the operative procedure, as well as blood transfusion or the use of blood plasma products, provided these are absolutely necessary during the operation. They must be informed about possible placements of internal and external nasal splints and swelling of the nose in the early postoperative phase, and should be aware that complete postoperative assessment is only possible after roughly 12 months and that any decision on revision surgery can only be taken after that.

Possible **general complications** such as injury to the skin or nerves, allergies, or intolerance to the materials used, bleeding or secondary hemorrhage, infections and their potential consequences, thromboses, and embolism are described in detail.

Specific risks of nasal surgery are likewise explained in detail, including injuries to the lacrimal duct or the base of the skull, visual impairment including blindness, loss of smell, sensory disorders of the nose and upper lip, obstructed nasal breathing, septal defect, unattractive scars, pain, dryness of the nose, and more.

It is noted that a specific result cannot be guaranteed, not even an outcome based on simulated images. The patient information sheet also contains behavioral recommendations following the procedure, such as position-

GB01600040601

Clinic/Practice

Thieme Compliance PO 4 *GB*

Surgical Correction of the Nose

(Septorhinoplasty)

Patient name and address

Hello,

The purpose of this informed consent leaflet is to help you prepare for the patient-doctor discussion. Please read it carefully before the discussion and complete the questionnaire carefully and completely. For better readability, we use male pronouns but are addressing all genders with them.

Why is the procedure recommended?

The shape, the size and the position of the nose (fig. 1) can impair the harmony of the face significantly (e.g. crooked nose). A change in the shape of the external nose but also a deviated septum (the wall dividing the nasal cavity into halves), a constricted internal nasal valve or enlargement of the turbinates (hypertrophy of the erectile tissue) inside the nose can obstruct nasal breathing. Disorders of both shape and function of the nose can be remedied or at least improved surgically. In particular in the case of noses already treated surgically or of very marked deformities of the nose, a satisfying result can frequently be achieved after several operations only, however. This also applies to nose deformities in patients with cleft lip and palate/jaw deformity.

Assumption of costs

If the procedure is performed purely for aesthetic reasons, public/private health insurance does not usually cover the cost of the procedure or any follow-up treatment in the case of complications. It is therefore recommended that you discuss the question of costs with the doctor/health insurance provider in advance. Furthermore, you should also consider taking out insurance which will cover treatment of any possible complications arising as a result of elective plastic surgery.

The procedure

The operation is usually performed under general anaesthesia; you will be informed about this procedure and the associated risks in a separate patient-doctor discussion.

The nose is accessed either by an external (open) approach after making an incision across the columella (the bridge of tissue between the nostrils) to open the nose and lifting the tissue or through the nostrils (fig. 3). External incisions causing almost invisible scars can be required across the columella, the base of the nasal wings, behind the tip of the nose, at the root of the nose, or the sidewalls (fig. 2).

During rhinoplasty, excessive cartilage and bone are removed and/or straightened if they are crooked. The skin then adjusts to the newly created nose shape.

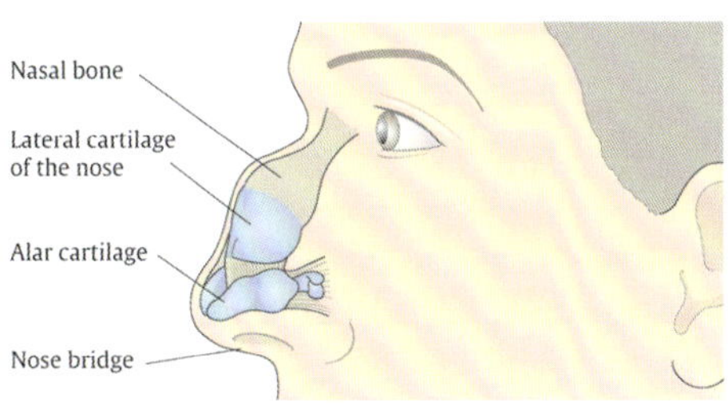

Fig. 1: Structure of the nose

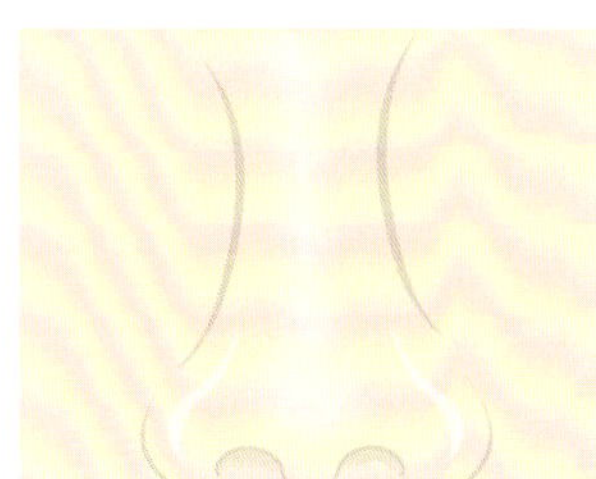

Fig. 2: Sketch for the doctor to mark the incision lines

PO 4/GB · 08/2023 · 06/2024ez · 08/2024 · Seite 1/6

Informed Consent Documentation · Publisher: R.-W. Bock (Medizinrecht) · Empfohlen vom Expertenrat Deutscher Nasenchirurgen e.V. · Founding Publisher: Prof. W. Weißauer · Medical Speciality Editor: Prof. W. Gubisch · Authors: Prof. W. Gubisch, Dr. S. Allert

Edition 08/2023
Transl. 06/2024ez
PDF 08/2024
Order Number: GB016004

Fig. 3.21 Informed consent form for patients. The first and last page of a patient information sheet: The handwritten and typewritten notes and the signatures of the patient and surgeon document the fact that the patient has been personally briefed during a preoperative information discussion. The complete form consists of 7 pages, of which only 2 are shown here. (Informed consent form PO04 from the Thieme-Compliance-System. Published by Thieme Compliance GmbH, Erlangen, Germany. http://www.thieme-compliance.de)

(Continued)

3

Doctor's comments

I have informed the patient about the procedure using the informed consent leaflet at hand, focusing on the following aspects and individual unusual circumstances (e.g. risk profile; underlying diseases; alternative treatment methods; medications; additional treatment methods; chances of success; instructions; follow-up care; special urgency or demands on the body; duration of the discussion; determination of the patient's ability to comprehend; minors; patient has a legal surrogate decision-maker/a legal guardian; patient has appointed a legal representative/provided a medical power of attorney; information provided in response to the patient's questions, etc.):

A **surgical correction of the nose** is planned for you.

Proposed date for the operation: ____________________

Date

Only in case of refusal to consent

I was informed about the planned measure. I do **not** consent to its implementation. I was emphatically informed that my refusal might result in health consequences if an operation is indicated.

Place, date, time

Patient

Patient's guardian*

Witness (if applicable)

Doctor

Statement of Consent

I have read the informed consent leaflet, and I understand it. The above-named measure, its nature and significance, alternatives, the risks and possible associated complications, chances of success, possible necessary changes, extensions as well as additional/subsequent procedures have been fully explained to me in a patient-doctor discussion with

doctor ____________________.

My questions have been answered completely and clearly.

I have **no further questions**, feel that the **counselling was satisfactory**, do **not need any further time for consideration** and **consent** to the proposed measure and any medically necessary, including unforeseeable, changes, extensions, additional and subsequent procedures.

I will follow the doctor's **instructions**.

Place, date, time

Patient

Patient's guardian*

Doctor

* Only if the patient is a minor: If only one of the patient's guardians signs, with this signature, they confirm that they have sole custody of the child or that they are acting in agreement with the other of the patient's guardians. As a rule, both of the patient's guardians should sign for major procedures. Minor patients who are able to comprehend should also always sign.

PO 4/GB · 08/2023 · 06/2024ez · 08/2024 · Seite 6/6

Fig. 3.21 (*Continued*)

ing in bed, driving restrictions, care of the nose, response to sneezing, wearing glasses, treatment of the skin, and precautions during exercise and sports activities.

All other planned measures are mentioned along with their individual risks, including removal of ear cartilage (inflammation, deformity of the ear) or costal cartilage (scarring of the chest, pneumothorax, inflammation, absorption, and deformation of the cartilage transplant).

This list is by no means exhaustive or applicable to all cases; its contents must be personalized for each patient, depending on the planned operation. "Off-label" use of pharmaceutical preparations, if any, must also be mentioned.

Finally, the patient information sheet contains several questions for the patient relating to information about themselves, their state of health and any known illnesses, allergies, or intolerance. The name of the physician who is obtaining informed consent is mentioned. Patients then sign the document, stating that they have no further questions, are well-informed, and have had enough time to think over the procedure once again. The date and time of signature are documented. This information sheet is usually provided about 2–10 days before the operation and not on the day of surgery itself, to give the patient adequate time to think the procedure over or ask any questions.

I have become accustomed to clearly mentioning the cosmetic risk during the preoperative discussion and I take pains to describe dealing with the postoperative outcome if it fails to meet expectations (see section 24.20). This relieves the patient of the fear that they may be stranded with an unacceptable postoperative outcome. When talking about possible revision surgery, I also discuss the approximate costs the patient is likely to incur for the procedure.

3.3.5 Rhinoplasty in Children and Adolescents

The surgeon bears a special responsibility while operating on minors, and the indication must be considered very carefully in such cases. Surgical correction is indicated in children and adolescents if the problem is primarily *functional*. Rejecting an operation that is essential to restore unobstructed nasal breathing in this age group – with the argument that the nose is "not yet fully grown" – is incomprehensible. The nose grows throughout life, and it is therefore difficult to define a particular age at which this growth has been completed.

In addition, young people suffer as much as adults from severely obstructed nasal breathing and associated mouth breathing; persistent nasal obstruction, especially in this age group, may result in chronic sinusitis. Correction is therefore indicated in children when there is an unmistakable functional disorder due to nasal septal deviation – including, for instance, straightening of a crooked nose if the functional disorder cannot be corrected by other means. ▶ Fig. 3.22a–f, as well as ▶ Fig. 3.23a–d and ▶ Video 3.5 show an example of a crooked nose with deviated septum and hump in an adolescent.

Cosmetic rhinoplasty in children is a rare exception, but may also be indicated. I have encountered a few children and adolescents with marked external abnormalities of the nose and severe psychological problems, even to the point of social withdrawal and isolation from friends and schoolmates ("I don't go outside any more, because everyone looks at my nose and makes fun of me"). The remarkable change in the demeanor of these young individuals following a successful rhinoplasty was notable. They appeared cheerful, outgoing, and reintegrated into their peer groups, with significant improvement in school grades.

My conversations with pediatric psychiatrists have revealed that many of these specialists are also in favor of a surgical solution to problems of this type in some circumstances. Referring affected youngsters for psychotherapy may lead to increasing stigmatization and further isolation ("Paul can't come to the birthday party because he has an appointment with his psychotherapist"). In addition, well-qualified specialists are not always available and long waiting times for psychotherapeutic treatment are standard.

All of these aspects need to be carefully examined in each case, and preferably in consultation with pediatric psychiatrists. Both parents or legal guardians are required to sign the informed consent form if a decision is taken to operate. The physician must also document that they have made sure that the child does have an abnormal finding and is suffering from an identifiable self-awareness disorder.

> ✔
>
> In some countries, the surgeon may also be required to comply with legal requirements regarding cosmetic surgery on minors.

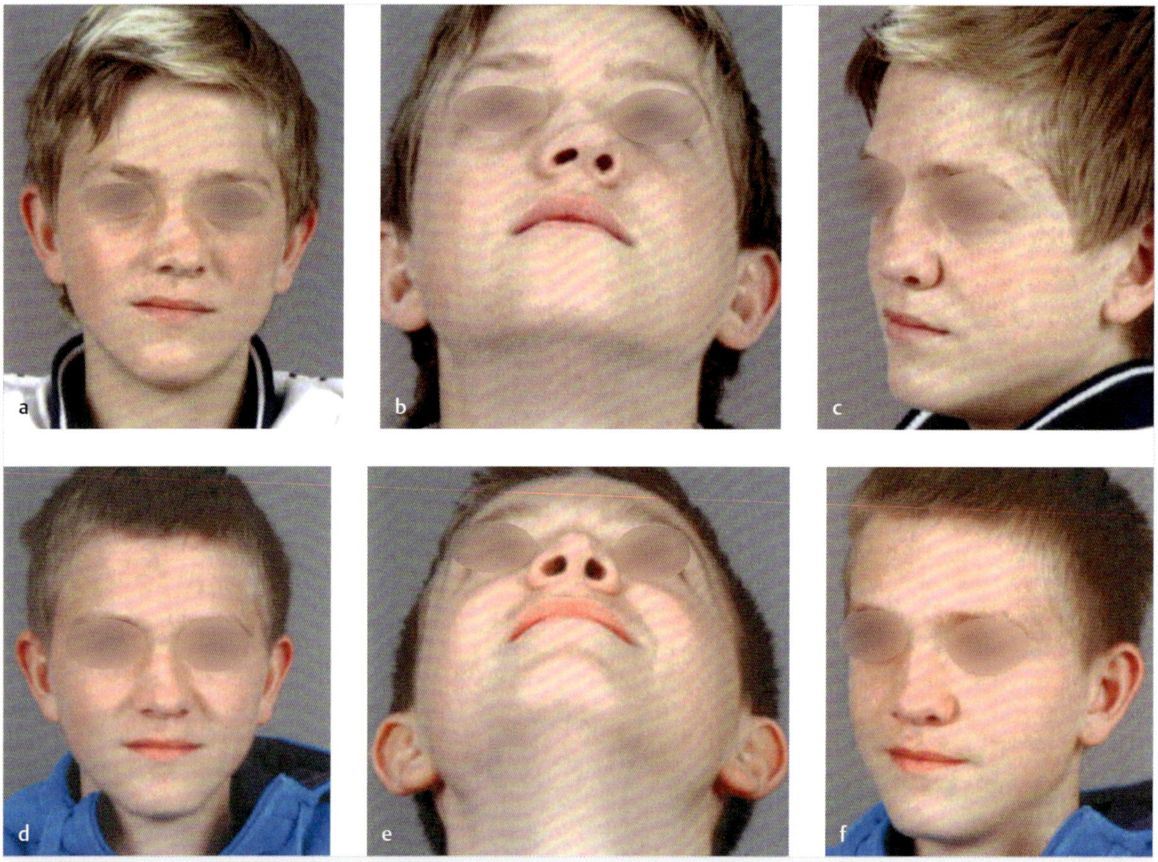

Fig. 3.22 Functional and cosmetic rhinoplasty in an adolescent.
Noticeable nasal deformity with significant nasal breathing obstruction after childhood nasal trauma in a 15-year-old teenager **(a-c)**. Significant functional and cosmetic improvement after septorhinoplasty **(d-f)**.

3.3.6 International Patients

A qualified interpreter must be present during the preoperative informative discussion with international patients who speak a foreign language and are not able to communicate with the physician. This discussion must be as detailed as in all other cases, even though it may take longer than usual. In Germany, the fact that a preoperative informative discussion was conducted with the help of an interpreter must be documented, as must the quality of the translation.

Surgery on international patients should be deferred if the interpreter's linguistic skills seem to be inadequate and the translation does not convey essential facets of the informative discussion to the patient.

3.3.7 The "Difficult" Patient

The surgeon may face a "difficult case" when operative correction in the patient concerned is likely to be a surgical challenge. This needs to be distinguished from dealing with difficult patients per se, irrespective of the findings. Physicians may be particularly challenged if they are confronted with both situations in a given patient.

Regardless of the above, preoperative red flags may indicate that a patient may not be a suitable candidate for a given cosmetic procedure. In general, a patient with realistic expectations despite a marked, troublesome deformity will eventually be satisfied if there is an unremarkable clinical course and an acceptable outcome ("green flag patient"; ► Fig. 3.24). The situation is even more difficult if a patient with a barely visible cosmetic nasal deformity has exceptionally high expectations of a perfect outcome ("red flag patient"; ► Fig. 3.24). Patients with a barely noticeable nasal deformity who think "It can't get any worse than this!" need to have the limitations, risks, and dangers of such an operative procedure clearly explained to them.

The surgeon must also avoid raising unreasonable expectations of the postoperative outcome. This situation can be illustrated with the example of a staircase with five steps, with a very unsightly appearance at the first

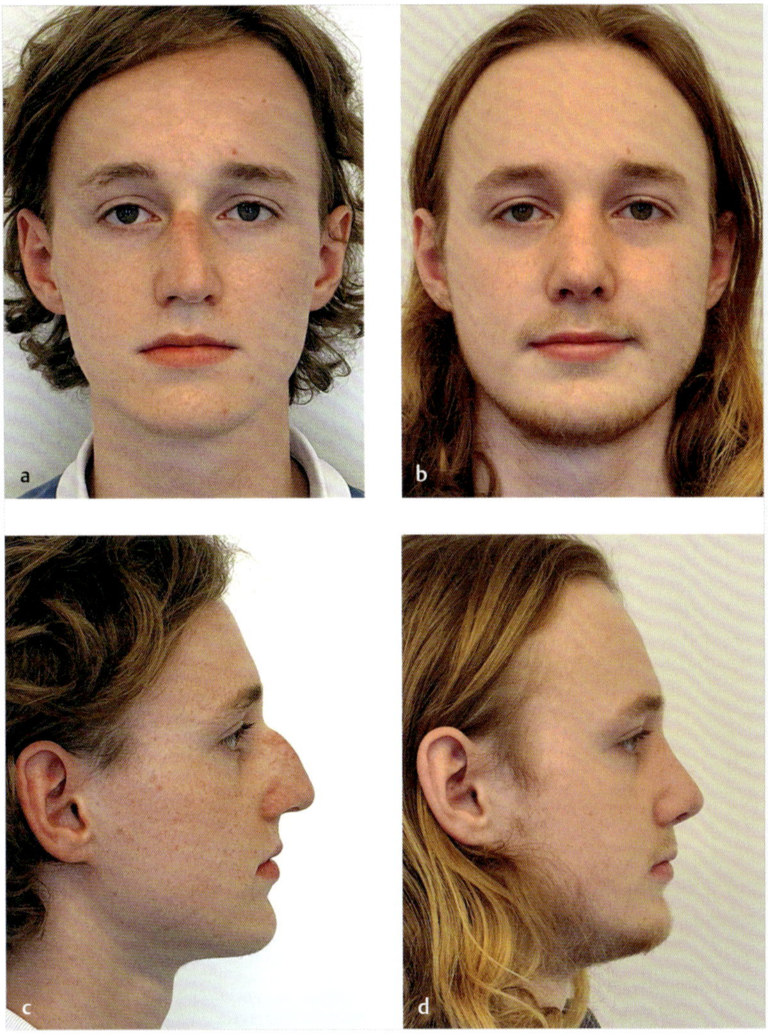

Fig. 3.23 Crooked nose with deviated septum and hump in an adolescent. (a, c) Preoperative frontal and side views. **(b, d)** The result after septoplasty, with correction of the nasal deviation and hump removal.

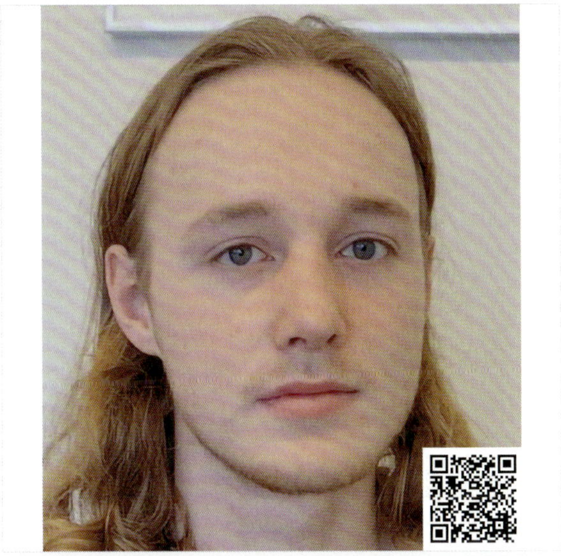

Video 3.5 Crooked nose, with deviated septum and hump in an adolescent (video documentation).

step and an aesthetically perfect fifth step. Both the doctor and patient should understand that surgical intervention may improve the appearance by one, two, or at best three steps. A surgeon can scarcely achieve the transformation of an extreme deformity into a flawless nose (▶ Fig. 3.25), and both parties have to reach this consensus during a detailed preoperative discussion. Surgeons should not hesitate to refuse the intervention if their objectives differ very widely from those of the patient; this is especially true if patients desire atypical nose shapes that are not encouraged by the surgeon. The patient should consult an appropriately qualified psychiatrist or psychosomatic therapist if a severe psychiatric disorder is suspected in a given case.

A rare special case are patients with **Body Dysmorphic Disorder** (BDD).

BDD is a mental disorder in which the affected person has an extreme focus on certain aspects of their appearance that they find disfiguring or unattractive, even

3

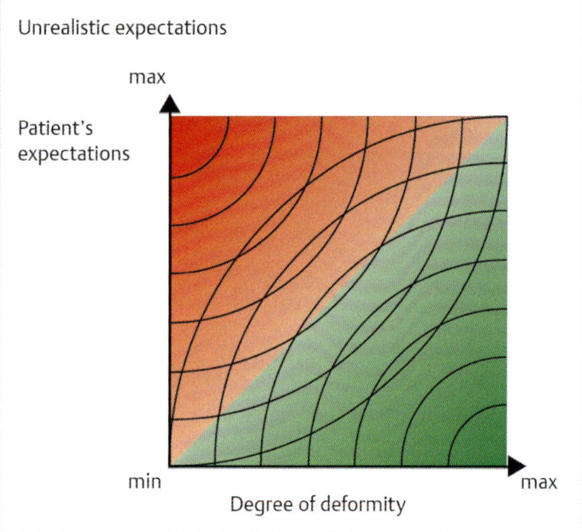

Fig. 3.24 Green flag and red flag patients (adapted from Gorney, 1993). Patients with minor deformities and high expectations of the postoperative outcome may be extremely difficult to please ("red flag" patients). Conversely, this is generally easier in patients with marked nasal deformities and fewer expectations ("green flag" patients).

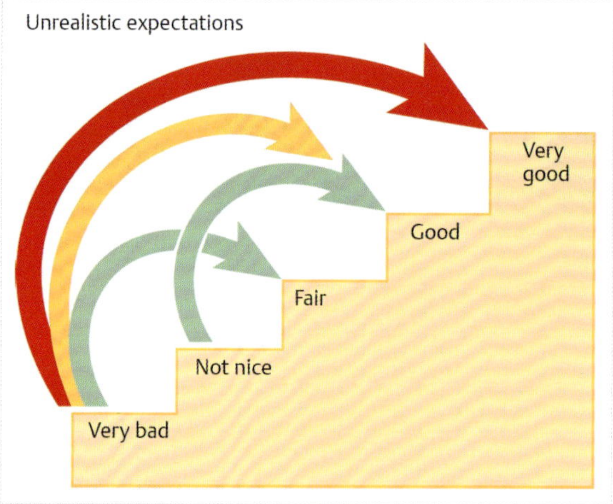

Fig. 3.25 Postoperative expectations. In a single operation, it is difficult to improve the appearance of a nose by more than two steps on the staircase shown.

though these features are objectively not perceived or only slightly perceived by others. The perception of one's own body is distorted, which can lead to intense worry, shame and often to repeated alterations of appearance, e.g. through excessive use of cosmetics, frequent cosmetic procedures or severe overweight or underweight.

This diagnosis is suggested by a medical history of numerous plastic surgeries, although the deformities complained of are often difficult to understand objectively. Those affected do not belong on the operating table, but in the care of a psychiatrist or psychologist; treatment consists primarily of psychotherapy after specialist diagnosis.

It cannot be predicted with any certainty before the operation whether or not dealing with a patient will be difficult *postoperatively*. The patient's attitude after the intervention also depends on whether and to what extent the surgical outcome meets expectations. Rarely, however, patients may be dissatisfied with their new appearance despite an aesthetically pleasing result being achieved.

Bibliography

Berghaus A. Pediatric cosmetic rhinoplasty. Paper presented at a miniseminar on "Rhinoplasty Pearls & Pitfalls" at the Annual Meeting of the American Academy of Otolaryngology–Head and Neck Surgery (AAO-HNS), San Diego, CA, USA, 2009

Clappier M, Tanna N. Preoperative evaluation of the rhinoplasty patient. Clin Plast Surg. 2022; 49(1):1–11

Gorney M. Patient selection in rhinoplasty: practical guidelines. In: Daniel RK, ed. Aesthetic plastic surgery: rhinoplasty. Boston: Little, Brown; 1993

Harounian J, Tham T, Dodhia S, Pearlman S. Accuracy of surgeon predictions in rhinoplasty outcomes using computer imaging: a quantitative analysis of dorsal height. Facial Plast Surg Aesthet Med. 2023; 25(2):186–188

Heilbronn C, Cragun D, Wong BJF. Complications in rhinoplasty: a literature review and comparison with a survey of consent forms. Facial Plast Surg Aesthet Med. 2020; 22(1):50–56. DOI: 10.1089/fpsam.2019.29007.won

Johnson MD. Management of pediatric nasal surgery (rhinoplasty). Facial Plast Surg Clin North Am. 2017; 25(2):211–221

Mlynski G, Pirsig W. Funktionell-ästhetische Rhinochirurgie. Stuttgart: Thieme; 2018

Tripathi PB, Elghobashi S, Wong BJF. The myth of the internal nasal valve. JAMA Facial Plast Surg. 2017; 19(4):253–254

Ward B, Ward M, Fried O, Paskhover B. Nasal distortion in short-distance photographs: the selfie effect. [Letter] JAMA Facial Plast Surg. 2018; 20(4):333–335

4 Arrangement of the Patient, Instruments, Equipment, and Staff in the Operating Room

4.1 Preparing the Patient and Operating Room for Surgery

Rhinoplasty is usually performed with the patient under general anesthesia in an operating room that meets the legal standards for sterility and hospital hygiene. Minor corrective surgery on the nose is often performed under local anesthesia, with or without sedation.

> ✔
>
> The surgeon must ensure that all necessary equipment such as drills, piezoelectric and suction devices, and appropriate instruments, suture materials, etc., required for the operation are available before the procedure starts.

The surgeon, anesthetist, and scrub nurse confirm the identity of the patient and details of the planned surgery one last time (in a "team time-out") while ensuring that the patient is appropriately positioned for the procedure. The operation may last 2–3 hours, or significantly longer in patients who are undergoing interventions such as revision surgery with rib cartilage transplantation.

An antibiotic (such as a cephalosporin, ampicillin, or sultamicillin) should be administered perioperatively, bearing in mind the duration of the operation. Intravenous administration of an adjusted dose of prednisolone in the perioperative period can help to counter postoperative pain and swelling, but this is individually tailored.

In the orally intubated patient, the tube runs in a caudal direction over the lower lip across the midline and is adequately secured with an adhesive plaster. A tube extension ("goose throat") prevents interference with the surgeon's hand, so that the airway connectors and filters come to rest over the sternum. The nasopharynx is occluded transorally using a commercially available soft-foam (Brusis type) tampon secured with two threads, which prevents blood and irrigation fluid from draining into the deeper airways and esophagus without inducing mucosal lesions in the palate or throat (▶ Fig. 4.1).

The patient is placed in the supine position, while the head may be raised slightly on a head rest. The face is disinfected preoperatively, and the nasal cavities are cleaned with pointed tip swabs. Brief insertion of naphazoline swabs (e.g., Privin) decongests the mucosa and turbinates, which are likewise disinfected. For this preparation process, a small separate instrument set should be available to the surgeon, containing a nasal speculum (▶ Fig. 4.2), bayonet forceps (▶ Fig. 4.3), pointed tip

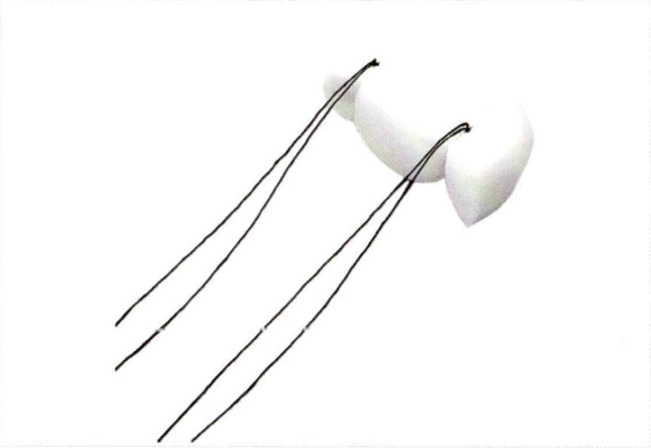

Fig. 4.1 The Brusis nasopharyngeal tampon consists of soft foam packing, secured by two threads. (Copyright SPIGGLE & THEIS Medizintechnik GmbH, Overath, Germany. Reprinted with permission.)

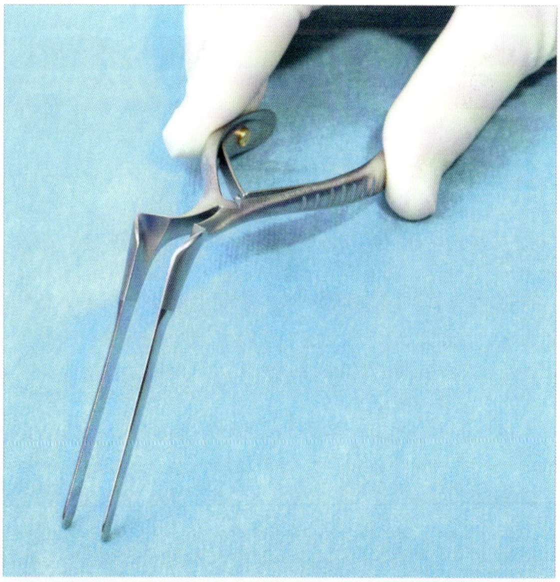

Fig. 4.2 Nasal speculum. The slender blades of the speculum allow optimal visualization of the nasal cavity (KARL STORZ SE & Co. KG, Tuttlingen, Germany).

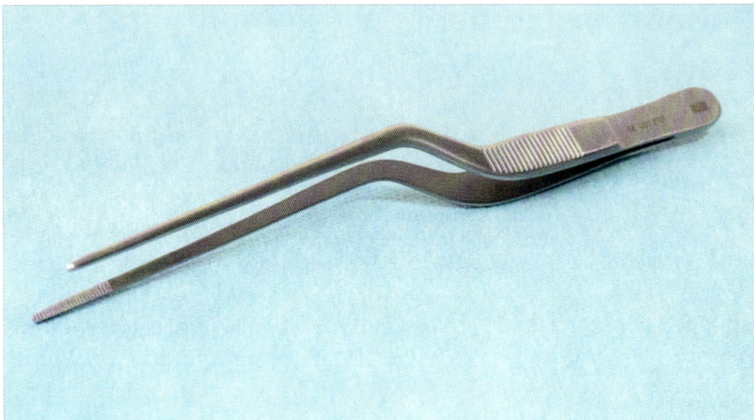

Fig. 4.3 Bayonet forceps. The bayonet forceps allows optimal visualization when swabs are being inserted into the nose (KARL STORZ SE & Co. KG, Tuttlingen, Germany).

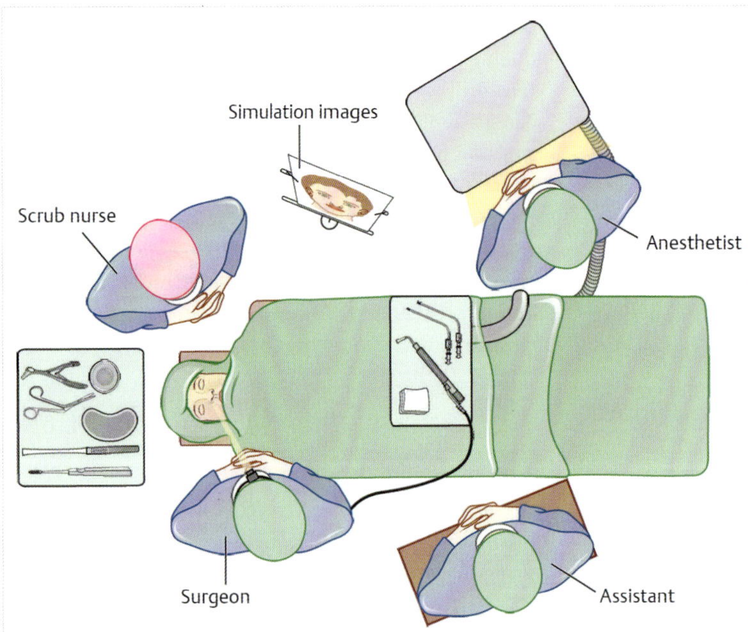

Fig. 4.4 Arrangement at the operating table. The scrub nurse or an assistant stands at the head end opposite to the surgeon, while the anesthetist is at the foot end. For teaching purposes, one observer may stand to the surgeon's right. The surgeon has an unobstructed view of the patient's photos and simulated images.

swabs, compresses, disinfectant solution, and local anesthetic. Surgical drapes around the operative field leave uncovered the forehead up to the hairline, the eyes, cheeks, mouth with upper lip, and upper row of teeth, to allow intraoperative assessment of nasal proportions in context with the face.

The auricle should also be disinfected and infiltrated with local anesthetic in case auricular cartilage is required. One half of the thorax should also be prepared if costal cartilage harvesting is necessary. Preparation of the left chest wall is recommended if a separate team is available for rib graft harvesting, which enables the surgeon to operate simultaneously on the nose while standing to the right of the head.

> ✔
>
> Infiltration of the operating field with the local anesthetic lidocaine (Xylocaine) and epinephrine (Suprarenin) is carried out before sterile draping and surgical hand disinfection. This extends the time for which the local anesthetic takes effect and increases its efficacy. The actual procedure starts once the surgeon has donned a surgical gown and gloves.

The scrub nurse stands with the instrument table at the head end, while the anesthetist is positioned with his or her equipment at the foot end (▶ Fig. 4.4). The assistant, if present, stands to the opposite side of the patient. For teaching purposes, one observer may stand to the surgeon's right on the same side of the patient. The observer can also use a small footstool to look over the surgeon's shoulder. Only the surgeon may wear a head lamp for optimal illumination; this may be required in addition to the operating light during surgery on the inner nose.

> A head lamp worn by the assistant does not improve lighting conditions further, and is often disturbing; the two head lights and cones of light may collide and thus give rise to confusion.

The scrub nurse assists from the opposite (left) side of the patient in the absence of an assistant, and can readily pass surgical instruments to the surgeon.

The patient's face is cleaned with sterile octenidine dihydrochloride and phenoxyethanol (e.g., Octenisept) and draped as described above before the start of the surgical procedure.

> The advantage of using octenidine dihydrochloride and phenoxyethanol (e.g., Octenisept) is its lack of irritation, especially of the conjunctiva.

Everyone involved, including spectators, must wear protective goggles in addition to a surgical mask in the vicinity of the operating field, especially when aerosol-generating piezoelectric devices or burrs are being used, with possible splashes of rinsing water.

I prefer using an adjustable metallic mirror, if possible, attached to the operating table across from me during rhinoplasty, allowing visualization of the nasal and facial profile in a strictly lateral view (▶ Video 4.1, ▶ Fig. 4.5a–c). The mirror makes it possible to constantly visualize the profile of the nose not only from the right side, where I stand, but also from the opposite (left) side, and this greatly improves surgical precision and symmetry.

The nurse may hand the surgeon a sterile mirror during the procedure, if necessary, if the mirror cannot be assembled for technical reasons.

Paper printouts of the patient's preoperative frontal and lateral images are also arranged at eye level across from me and to the left of the patient, together with the simulated images and handwritten notes, if necessary, highlighting the intended objectives of the operation (see ▶ Fig. 3.20).

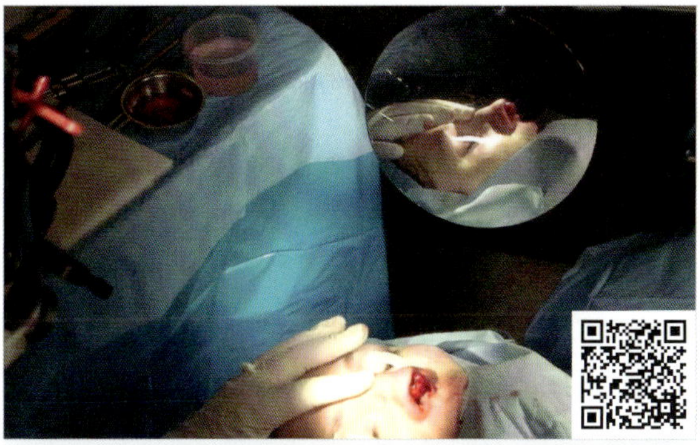

Video 4.1 The rhinoplasty mirror.

> The operating field is mainly illuminated by the beam of the head lamp, with a particularly strong light source for adequate illumination even of the depths of the nasal cavity. Additional lighting is suitable for open surgery, and the surgeon should not forgo the use of the ceiling operating theater light.

Together with the head lamp, magnifying glasses with high magnification ensure surgical precision (▶ Fig. 4.6).

4.2 Intraoperative Photo and Video Documentation

A monitor within the surgeon's field of view shows an image of the surgical site captured by a camera while the procedure is being documented using photography or video recordings, or for the benefit of observers in the operating room.

The camera can be integrated into the operating lamp or its handle, or fixed to a separate articulated arm. The Karl Storz company offers professional solutions for this purpose in the form of the Vitom camera with integrated fiberoptics, which also allows three-dimensional visualization with appropriate equipment. Most of the video clips for this book were documented using this excellent system.

The starCam camera supplied by the starMed company, a head-mounted camera that can also be attached to a tripod, is also well-suited for use in the operating room (▶ Fig. 4.7).

Viewers may find a head-mounted camera for video sequences of lengthy surgical procedures troublesome, as they inevitably follow every head movement and change in the direction of the surgeon's line of sight.

Both preoperative and postoperative images, as well as digital photos and video recordings of the intraoperative procedure and findings, are archived. These images allow

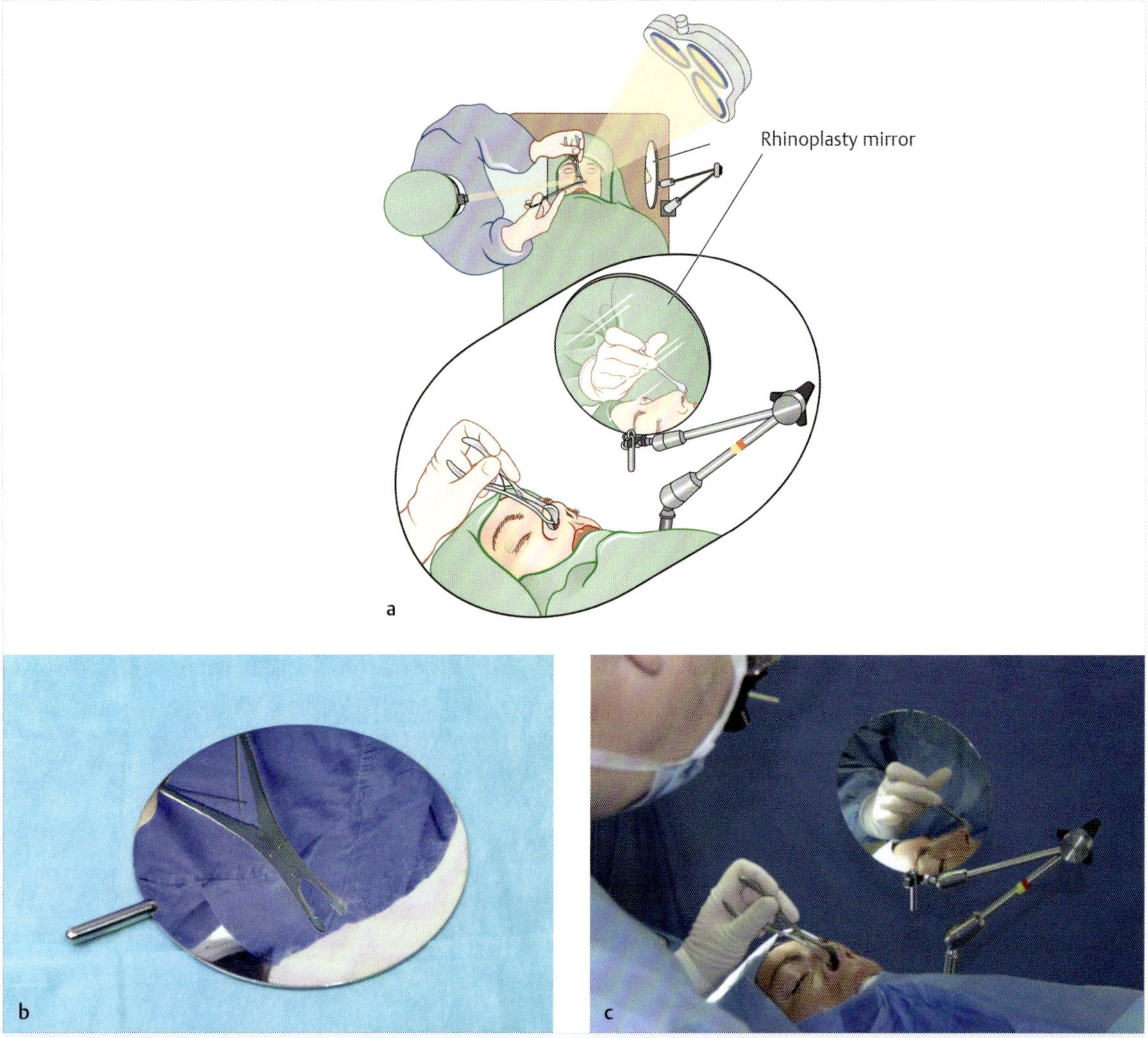

Fig. 4.5 Arrangement at the operating table with a rhinoplasty mirror. (a) The mirror allows the surgeon to view real-time changes in the nasal profile while operating. **(b)** A metallic rhinoplasty mirror (KARL STORZ SE & Co. KG, Tuttlingen, Germany). **(c)** The intraoperative situation.

the surgeon to retrospectively analyze surgical maneuvers during an intervention and relate them to the surgical outcome. This documentation is essential if the operative procedure is to be presented in lectures and publications. It is advisable to set up a reliable archive system, with clearly labeled files and folders for a large number of patients, so that various images of an individual case or of a thematically sorted group can be easily found and classified. The digital camera software provided by starMed comprises an integrated archiving program that is a handy tool for image classification.

Intraoperative image documentation may theoretically also be relevant from a forensic point of view in a given case, although I have as yet to encounter such a situation. Intraoperative images can also be taken by an assistant using a smartphone, in the absence of other technology. Patients are rarely interested in seeing intraoperative images of the procedure.

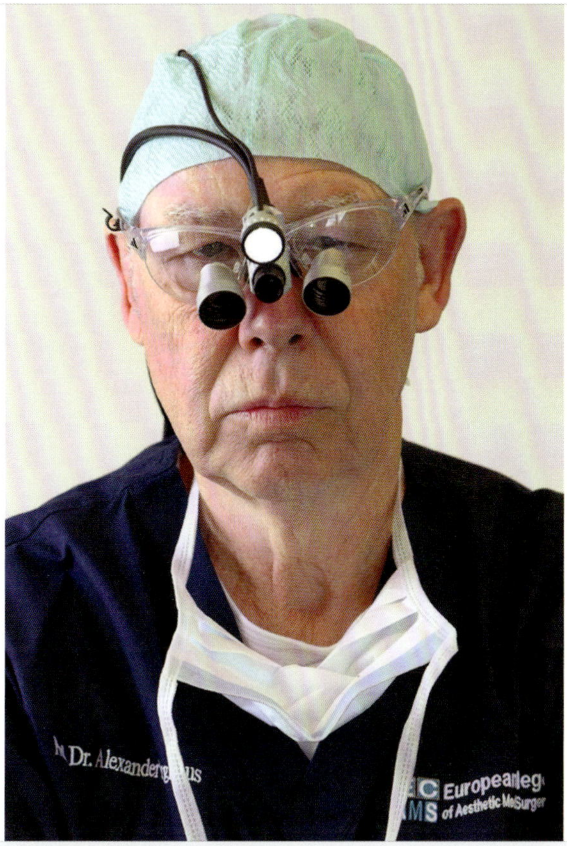

Fig. 4.6 Head lamp, magnifying glasses, safety goggles. The head lamp is battery-operated; the magnifying glasses and protective glasses are adjusted precisely to the surgeon's working distance during surgery. In the example shown, the optionally available head camera is also mounted with the magnifying glasses.

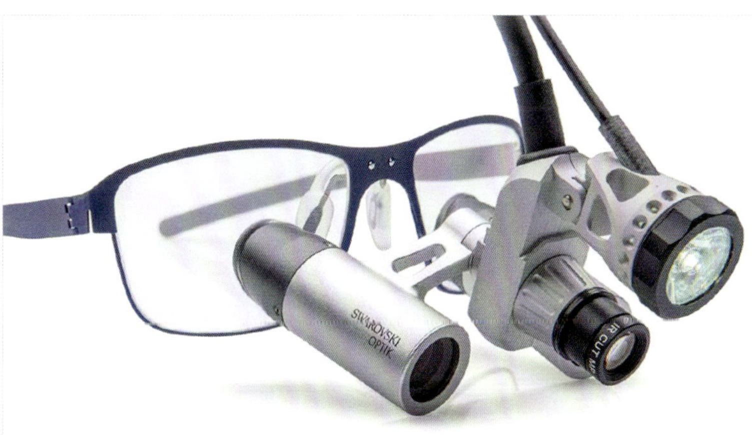

Fig. 4.7 The starCam camera. The fully high-definition photo/video starCam camera (shown here with magnifying glasses and head lamp) can also be used without glasses on the tripod. (Copyright starMed GmbH & Co. KG, Grafing, Germany. Reprinted with permission.)

5 Turbinate Surgery

Inferior turbinate reduction does not form an integral part of rhinoplasty and is therefore addressed separately. Inferior turbinate (or inferior concha) hypertrophy is an extremely common condition, and turbinate reduction (usually with modest radiofrequency treatment, with or without lateralization) is therefore frequently recommended in conjunction with rhinoplasty. If indicated, this minor procedure is performed after disinfection and local infiltration, but before the skin incision for rhinoplasty. It regularly helps improve nasal congestion once the postoperative healing process is completed. Rhinoplasty patients who suffer from nasal obstruction preoperatively due to hypertrophic turbinates are grateful for the long-term functional relief that is obtained after appropriate turbinate reduction in a low-risk and easy way.

The inferior turbinates therefore have to be examined beforehand during nasal endoscopy. Soft-tissue hypertrophy may involve the head, middle third of the body, or the posterior end of the turbinate, where it may be particularly marked and troublesome (▶ Fig. 5.1). The technique and extent of the selected therapeutic procedure depend on the site and extent of turbinate hypertrophy (▶ Fig. 5.1).

5.1 Radiofrequency Treatment

Targeted radiofrequency (RF) therapy is carried out in patients with moderate to marked turbinate hypertrophy by inserting and activating a **radiofrequency needle** once or twice into each of the hypertrophic regions of the turbinate – the anterior, middle, and posterior thirds (▶ Video 5.1, ▶ Fig. 5.1, ▶ Fig. 5.2a, b).

The posterior third of the turbinate frequently requires somewhat more intense application of RF. The mucosa should not be ablated and should at most exhibit slightly whitish discoloration during the procedure (▶ Fig. 5.3).

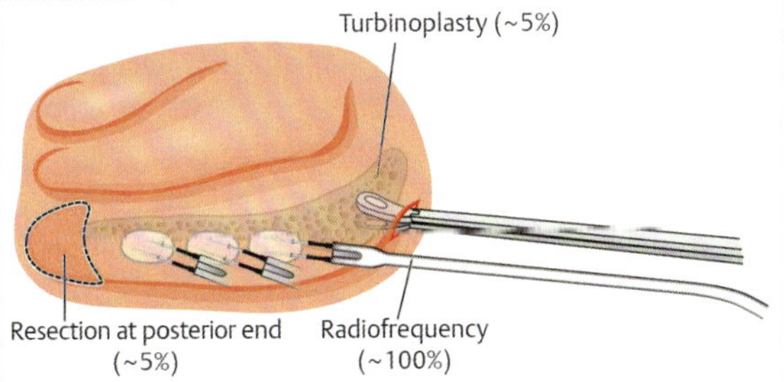

Fig. 5.1 Inferior turbinate surgery. The size of the hypertrophic inferior turbinates is reduced using radiofrequency therapy, turbinoplasty, and / or resection of their posterior ends. The approximate percentage of each method used in cases of turbinate hypertrophy is indicated in parentheses.

> ✔ Straight forward-viewing telescopes allow optimal visualization of the posterior third of the turbinate during radiofrequency application in narrow noses.

Radiofrequency treatment does not usually cause significant bleeding; the nasal cavity is aspirated after the procedure.

The soft tissues that have been treated heal by scarring and contraction, leading to turbinate reduction and improved nasal breathing. Patients should be informed beforehand that wound healing and subsequent long-term improvement in nasal breathing may take a few days to weeks, and regular suctioning and cleaning of the nose may be necessary until then.

Partial resection of the posterior third of the inferior turbinate may rarely be indicated if marked inferior turbinate hypertrophy leads to severe choanal obstruction (see ▶ Fig. 5.1). Radiofrequency application in this region should be undertaken beforehand to prevent bleeding, which occurs far more frequently after resection than following RF treatment alone.

> ✔ The classic conchotomy – i.e., removal of a large amount of soft tissue from the turbinate, typically using angled conchotomy scissors – should be rejected in favor of the procedures described above. Conchotomy is associated with a risk of excessive soft-tissue loss, resulting in a dry nose and the dreaded “empty nose syndrome,” which is resistant to treatment.

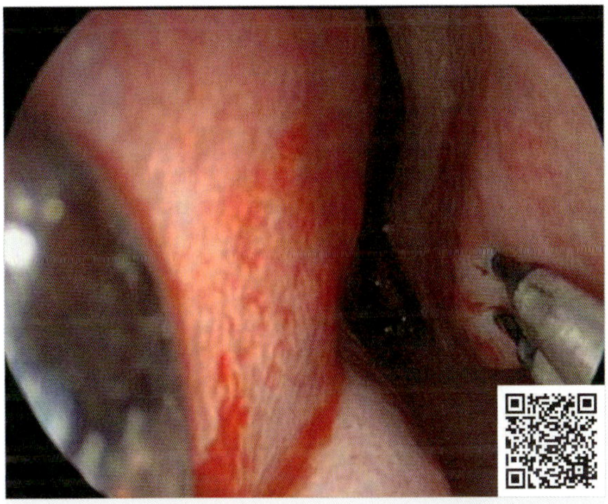

Video 5.1 Radiofrequency treatment of the inferior turbinates.

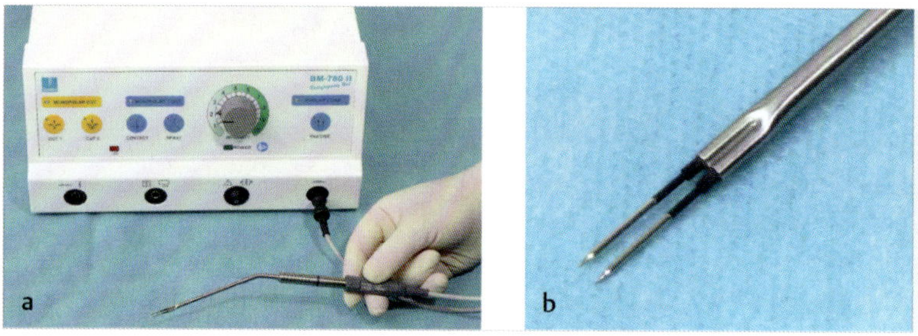

Fig. 5.2 Radiofrequency technique. (a) The intensity of the electric current is regulated using the radiofrequency control unit (Sutter Medizintechnik GmbH, Emmendingen, Germany). **(b)** The Sutter bipolar needle is suitable for radiofrequency application to the turbinate (Sutter Medizintechnik GmbH, Emmendingen, Germany).

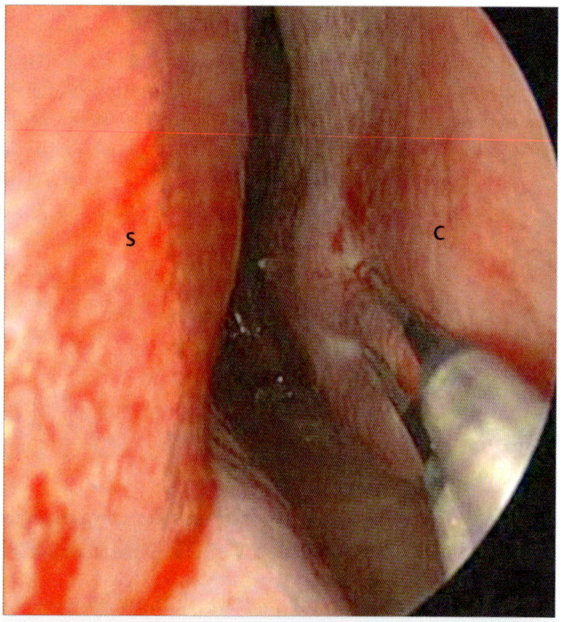

Fig. 5.3 Radiofrequency treatment of the inferior turbinate using a Sutter needle. S: septum; C: inferior turbinate.

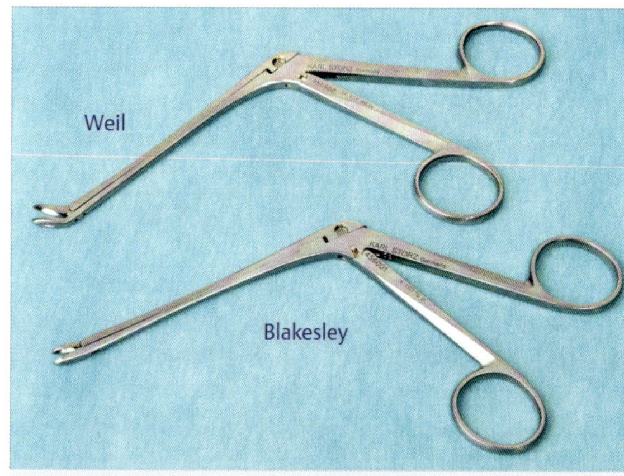

Fig. 5.4 The Weil and Blakesley instruments. Weil or Blakesley–Wilde (top: angled, KARL STORZ SE & Co. KG, Tuttlingen, Germany) and Blakesley instruments (bottom: straight, KARL STORZ SE & Co. KG, Tuttlingen, Germany).

5.2 Turbinoplasty and Lateralization

Inferior turbinate hypertrophy is not necessarily due to voluminous soft tissue; enlargement of the bony component (the os turbinale) may occasionally obstruct nasal airflow. Doubtful cases can be assessed with the patient under general anesthesia, using careful palpation of the turbinate. Soft-tissue reduction alone is not effective in such cases, and treatment consists of removing parts of the hypertrophic bone (turbinoplasty) or outfracture of the inferior turbinate.

Turbinoplasty is carried out for turbinate reduction in the area of the head of the turbinate. A small incision is made over the head of the turbinate (see ▶ Fig. 5.1), the bony framework is identified, and the intact overlying soft tissues are pushed aside. Excessive turbinate bone is then removed with an instrument such as the Weil or Blakesley nasal forceps (▶ Fig. 5.4) or a suitable bone punch, or by piezo surgery if available. The dislodged soft tissues are then repositioned, and the incision is closed with absorbable sutures.

"Outfracture" or lateropositioning of a bony outgrowth of the inferior turbinate, narrowing the lumen, is an elegant and relatively simple procedure. The technique involves lateral repositioning of the os turbinale, with an increase in airway patency. The procedure is performed either alone or in combination with radiofrequency treatment, and typically starts with placement of an elevator (e.g., a raspatory) medial to the inferior turbinate in the inferior meatus. Force is then directed toward the lateral nasal wall in order to fracture the os turbinale not at its stable base, but at the knee-shaped transition to the more delicate peripheral segment. The otherwise intact turbinate is then displaced laterally along with the overlying soft tissues (▶ Fig. 5.5).

In appropriate cases, this procedure typically has an impressive and immediate beneficial effect on the width of the inferior meatus, extending to the choanae.

In rare cases, when the bone of the turbinate is very hard, a predetermined breaking point can be marked in the bone using piezo technology or a chisel before lateralization.

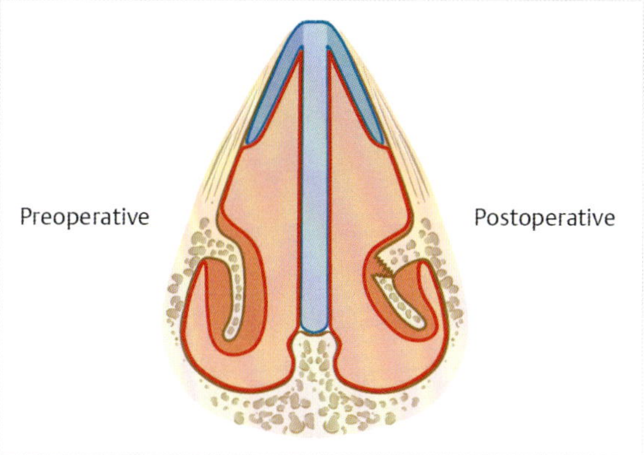

Fig. 5.5 Outfracture (lateropositioning) of the inferior turbinate. Lateralization of the inferior turbinate (on the right side in the illustration) results in significant widening of the airway. Fracturing of the lateral nasal wall must be avoided.

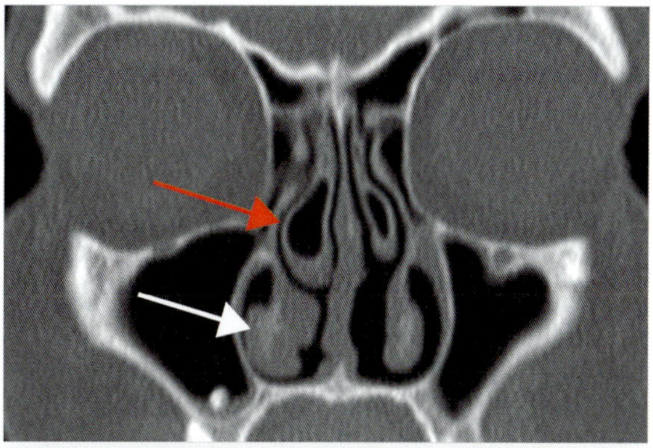

Fig. 5.6 Concha bullosa. Computed tomography of the paranasal sinuses optimally depicts bilateral concha bullosa (with the right side larger than the left, red arrow). A hypertrophic right inferior turbinate is also seen (white arrow). Both structures can be seen to obstruct the right nasal airway.

> ✓
>
> Fracturing of the lateral nasal wall must be avoided. Damage to the nasolacrimal duct with fracture of the medial maxillary sinus wall appears to be a potential, but very rare, risk with this maneuver. To avoid this complication, care is taken to ensure that the os turbinale does not fracture at its base with the medial maxillary sinus wall, but below its "shoulder," at the attachment of the thin peripheral bone element.

Marked septal deviation may be present in a given case, obscuring visualization of the middle and posterior aspects of the turbinate, and hindering access. These areas are addressed in the same session, once septoplasty is complete.

5.3 Concha Bullosa

Enlargement of the **middle turbinate** caused by pneumatization of its bony component (concha bullosa) may also contribute significantly to nasal obstruction. This abnormality may be overlooked in nasal endoscopy; it is best seen in a computed tomography scan (▶ Fig. 5.6). However, the middle turbinate forms part of the paranasal sinuses, specifically the ethmoid cells. Describing surgical interventions in this region is beyond the scope of this book. Basically, a concha bullosa abnormality should be corrected by lateral excision of the pneumatized middle turbinate and is primarily treated by ear, nose, and throat (ENT) specialists with experience in this field.

Bibliography

Bergmark RW, Gray ST. Surgical management of turbinate hypertrophy. Otolaryngol Clin North Am. 2018; 51(5):919–928

Cavaliere M, Mottola G, Iemma M. Comparison of the effectiveness and safety of radiofrequency turbinoplasty and traditional surgical technique in treatment of inferior turbinate hypertrophy. Otolaryngol Head Neck Surg. 2005; 133(6):972–978

Scheithauer MO. Surgery of the turbinates and "empty nose" syndrome. GMS Curr Top Otorhinolaryngol Head Neck Surg. 2010; 9:Doc03

Sommer F, Lindemann J, Scheithauer MO, Hoffmann TK, Veit JA. [Nasal turbinate surgery]. HNO. 2017; 65(5):443–456–German.

6 The Open Approach Technique in Rhinoplasty

Before starting the procedure, the surgeon has to decide on the appropriate surgical approach. Rhinoplasty can be performed using either a closed or an open approach.

> ✓
>
> The terms "open rhinoplasty" and "closed rhinoplasty" are often heard. Strictly speaking, they are misleading: "rhinoplasty" includes all measures required for nose surgery. The words "open" and "closed" only refer to the access route that is chosen for it.

6.1 Considerations on the Sequence of Surgical Steps

The open procedure will be described first here, as it is more important and is universally employed. I use this approach in about 90% of cases. The procedural sequence may vary; I usually prefer the following **workflow**:

1. **Cleaning, disinfection, local infiltration,** protection of the eyes
2. **Treatment of the inferior turbinates** (radiofrequency, lateroposition; see Chapter 5)
3. **Incision** for the open approach, dissection of the skin flap
4. Manipulation of the **bony framework**
   a) Removal of a bony hump (piezo technique / osteotome / rasp)
   b) Paramedian osteotomies (optional; piezo technique / osteotome)
   c) Lateral osteotomies (piezo technique / osteotome)
   d) Piezo **boreholes and suture fixation** of nasal bones
   Or:
   e) Preservation rhinoplasty (see section 8.4)
5. **Visualization of the upper lateral and alar cartilages** and the **caudal septum**
6. **Septoplasty / harvesting of septal cartilage** as graft material for rhinoplasty
7. Manipulation of the **middle third of the nasal framework** (correction of a cartilaginous hump / autospreader flaps / spreader grafts, if necessary)
8. Preparation and **correction of the shape of the alar cartilages**
9. Rotation and nasal tip projection (domal sutures; tongue-in-groove procedure, etc.)
10. Final manipulation of the **nasal dorsum**, correction of irregularities
11. Application of tip, rim, and other **grafts**
12. **Thinning of subcutaneous tissue** on the skin flap (optional)
13. **Lip lift** (rare; optional)
14. **Wound closure**
15. **Alar wedge, nostril sill resections**
16. Insertion of **Doyle splints** (optional)
17. **Dressing / splint**

> ✓
>
> The complete procedure for a nose correction (in this case a preservation rhinoplasty) can be followed in ▶ Video 6.1.

It goes without saying that individual steps may be omitted if unnecessary, and the operative sequence can be modified on the basis of individual needs – especially in patients undergoing revision surgery.

If necessary, I harvest conchal cartilage before starting surgery on the nose, and proceed in the same manner with harvesting of costal cartilage. However, rib harvesting should ideally be carried out in parallel by a second team, standing opposite the surgeon on the other side of the chest. This approach saves time, since the costal cartilage can then be harvested simultaneously during rhinoplasty, without the surgeons getting in each other's way.

> ✓
>
> The sequence of surgical steps above also applies to the description of these procedures in the following chapters. The basic steps are described to start with, and alternative and special measures and solutions for particular problems are explained in subsequent sections.

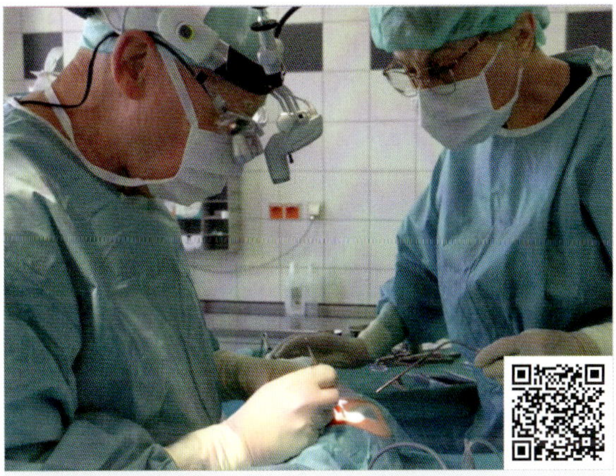

Video 6.1 Full-length preservation rhinoplasty.

6.2 Cleaning, Disinfection, Protection of the Eyes

The face is washed with disinfectant; alcoholic and other solutions that irritate the conjunctiva should be avoided. Octenidine dihydrochloride (Octenisept), a nonirritant, is preferable instead. As this agent reduces the adhesiveness of surgical drapes, the face has to be dried with a sterile compress after disinfection.

The nasal cavities are also cleaned and disinfected. Pointed swabs or tamponade strips impregnated with naphazoline (Privin) may be inserted for mucosal decongestion, if necessary.

The eyes are closed with suitable tape or Steri-Strips. This is necessary in particular for patients who have incomplete eyelid closure while anesthetized, such as those with a history of blepharoplasty or with endocrine orbitopathy.

6

6.3 Local Infiltration

The local anesthetic – lidocaine (Xylocaine) or articaine with epinephrine (Ultracaine with Suprarenin, 1 : 100,000 or 1 : 200,000) is usually infiltrated using a 5-mL syringe and a 25-G cannula (0.5 × 25 mm). The total volume injected usually ranges from 3 to 5 mL.

The following structures are infiltrated (▶ Video 6.2):

- The columella and membranous septum (▶ Fig. 6.1)
- The anterior third of the quadrangular plate of the septum (▶ Fig. 6.2), as well as the subperichondrial or subperiosteal regions of the septum further posteriorly if surgical dissection is required in these areas
- Subcutaneous tissue of the columella
- Subcutaneous tissue over the nasal tip and alar domes, starting from the "soft triangle" at the anterior circumference of the nostrils on either side (▶ Fig. 6.3)
- Subcutaneous tissue of the nasal dorsum, starting from the intercartilaginous fold on either side (▶ Fig. 6.4)
- Soft tissue over the lateral nasal slopes, extending from the piriform aperture at the level of the head of the inferior turbinate (▶ Fig. 6.5)

The nose is cleaned again with a disinfectant solution, followed by draping of the surgical field (see Chapter 4). The infiltration has time to take effect while the surgeon proceeds with hand disinfection, increasing the chances of a bloodless procedure.

6.4 Nasal Hair

Dense nasal hair that impedes visualization of the nostril has to be shortened with a pair of sharp scissors immediately before the incision, and suctioned off immediately (▶ Fig. 6.6, ▶ Video 6.2).

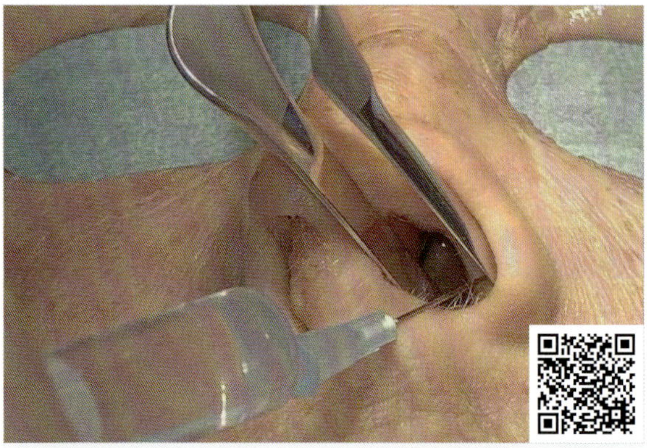

Video 6.2 Local anesthetic infiltration and shortening of nasal hair.

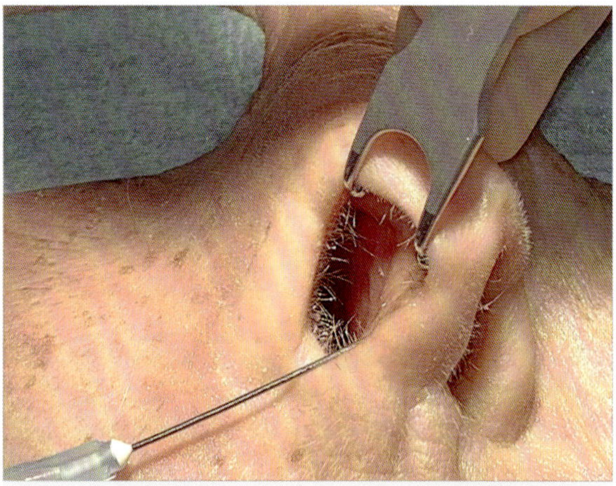

Fig. 6.1 Infiltration of the columella.

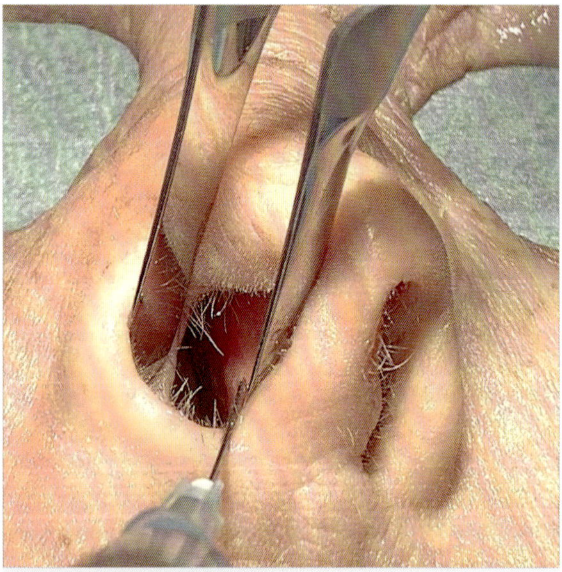

Fig. 6.2 Infiltration of the septum.

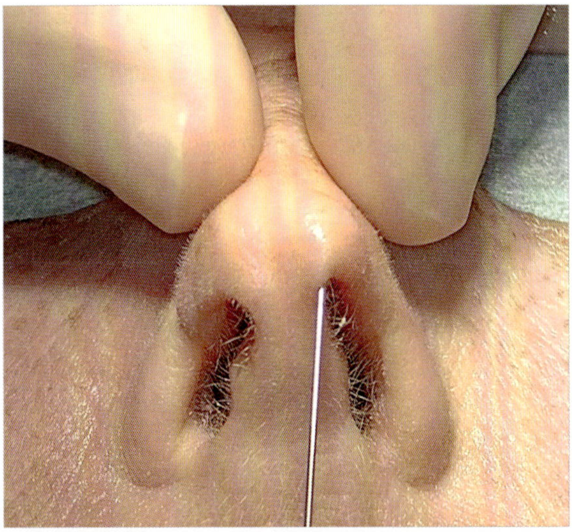

Fig. 6.3 Infiltration of the subcutaneous tissue of the nasal tip.

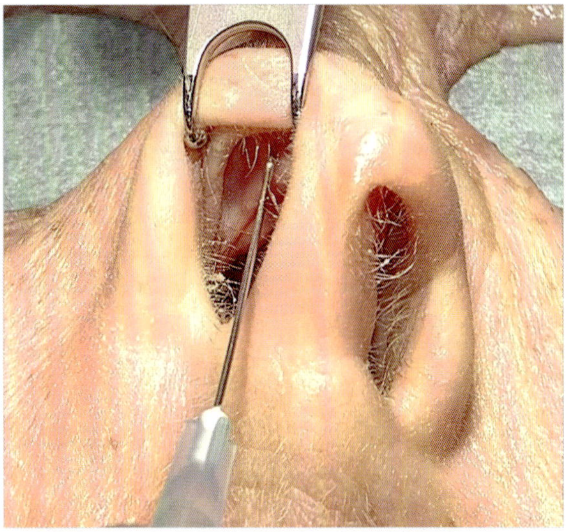

Fig. 6.4 Infiltration of the intercartilaginous fold and the nasal dorsum.

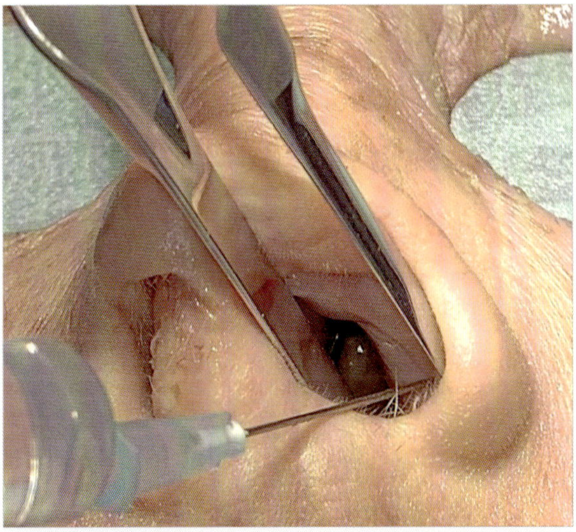

Fig. 6.5 Infiltration of the lateral nasal slope.

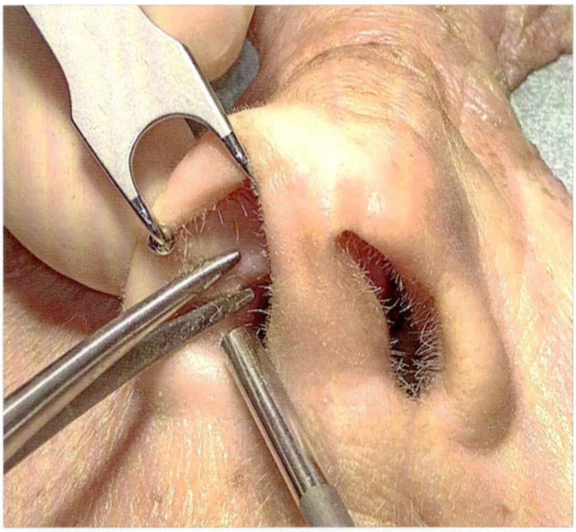

Fig. 6.6 Shortening and suctioning of nasal hair.

6.5 The Incision for the Open Approach

The incision for open rhinoplasty access (▸ Video 6.3) comprises a combination of bilateral incisions along the caudal margin of the alar cartilages (▸ Fig. 6.7), with a W-shaped incision at the columella (inverted V incision; see ▸ Fig. 6.14).

While a Kilner alar retractor with buttons (▸ Fig. 6.8) is being used to lift the edge of the nostril, the middle finger pushes the alar cartilage anteriorly against the scalpel. The vestibular skin at the caudal margin of the alar cartilage is then incised from lateral to medial using a no. 15 blade ("marginal incision"). If the cartilaginous rim is not palpable (this can be checked using the butt of the knife), the hairline along the nostril can be used as a rough, but inconsistently reliable, landmark (▸ Fig. 6.9).

A rim incision (an incision made along the rim of the nostril, ▶ Fig. 6.10) may be used as an alternative (not as a supplement) to the marginal incision (an incision along the caudal margin of the lower lateral cartilage).

The rim incision (▶ Fig. 6.10) may be used in exceptional cases – for example, in revision surgery in patients with marked scarring, if placement of a graft at the lower edge of the alar cartilage (rim graft) is required. The rim incision generally provides easy access to the lateral caudal area of the nasal ala. As a rule, however, a rim graft is introduced through a marginal incision into a pocket created at the edge of the nostril (see section 10.3).

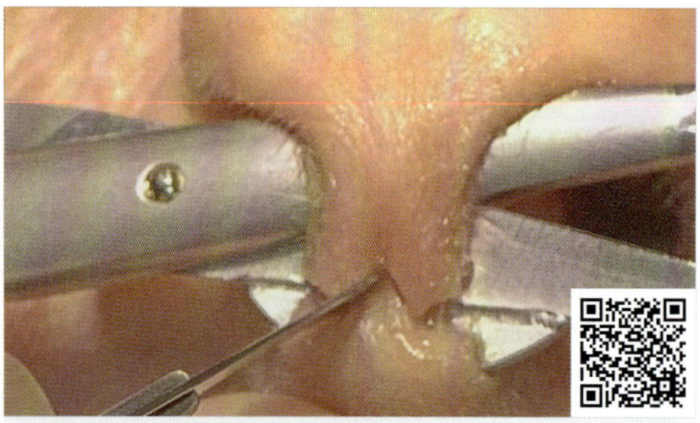

Video 6.3 Incision for open-access rhinoplasty.

Once these incisions are complete on each side, the columellar skin is undermined with a pair of fine, pointed scissors (▶ Fig. 6.11), starting at the right columellar incision and using a combination of cutting and spreading movements.

This preparation is carried out just anterior to the medial crura of the alar cartilages, and any injury to these needs to be painstakingly avoided. Dissection is continued with the scissors until the skin is sufficiently detached and the tip of the instrument emerges in the columellar incision on the opposite side. The scissors are advanced under the skin until the scissor blades are centered exactly at the narrowest part of the columella under the skin. It is an advantage if the scissors have a widening on the right branch, which can serve as a working plate for the knife (▶ Fig. 6.11). The scissors are then opened carefully, slightly stretching the skin over the lower blade of the scissors (or the "working plate," if present). This provides a stable supporting surface for the inverted V incision in the columellar skin (▶ Fig. 6.12).

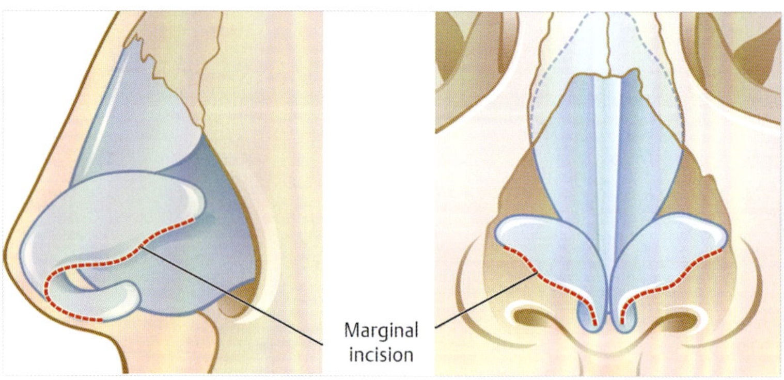

Fig. 6.7 Bilateral marginal incision. The marginal incision follows the caudal edge of the alar cartilage; it is continued as a columellar rim incision for the open approach (see also ▶ Fig. 6.14).

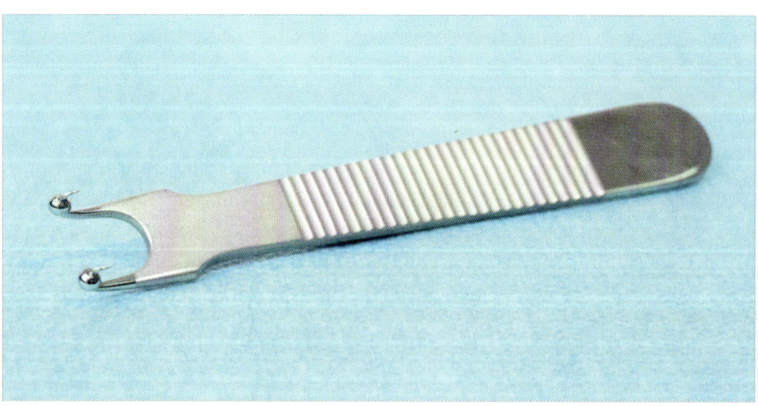

Fig. 6.8 The double-pronged retractor with buttons (Kilner hook). The retractor holds the alar rims securely; the small spherical buttons on the prongs prevent both deep penetration and tissue injury (KARL STORZ SE & Co. KG, Tuttlingen, Germany).

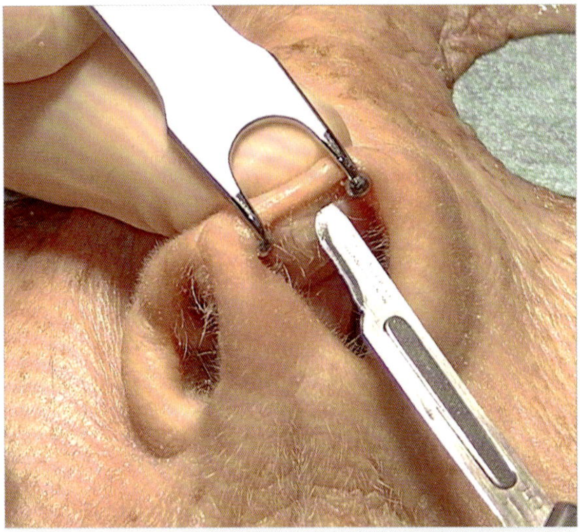

Fig. 6.9 Marginal incision. The incision follows the cartilage edge medially to about halfway along the rim of the columella, a little over the narrowest point of the columella toward its base.

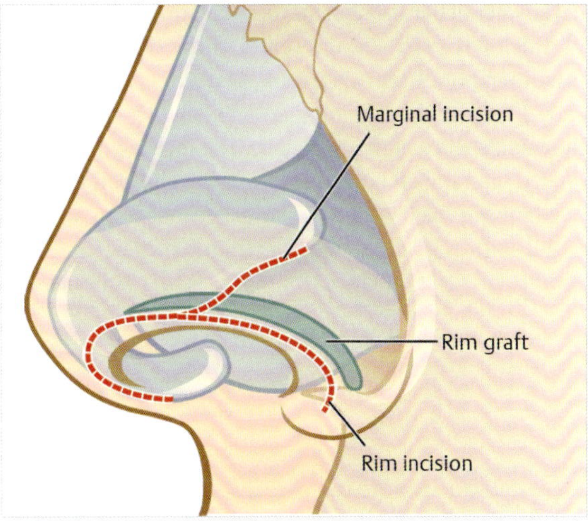

Fig. 6.10 Rim incision. The rim incision is made along the edge of the nostril and is an optional alternative to the marginal incision, e.g. in patients who require a rim graft.

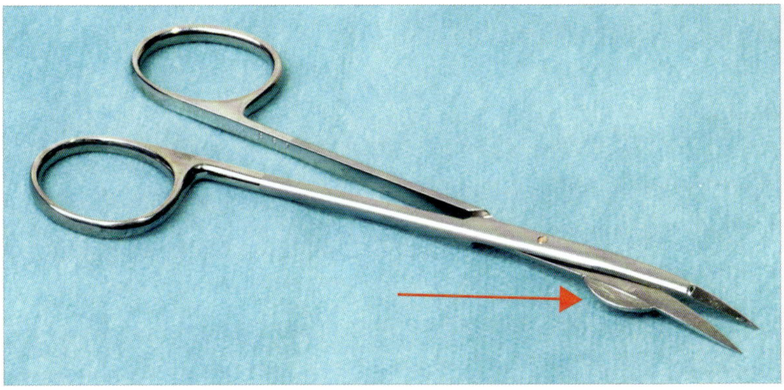

Fig. 6.11 Pointed scissors with a "working plate" attached to the lower (right) blade (red arrow) (KARL STORZ SE & Co. KG, Tuttlingen, Germany).

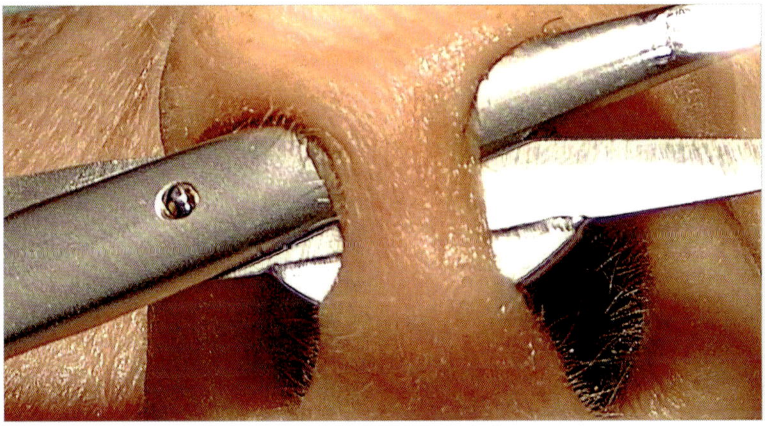

Fig. 6.12 Dissection of the skin over the columella. The skin is stretched slightly prior to the incision.

The columellar incision starts at the tip of the inverted V, which lies exactly at the center of the columella, at its narrowest point (see ▶ Fig. 6.14). The two limbs of the inverted V form an angle of approximately 45° and occupy the middle third of the columella. The incision is then extended laterally on both sides from the end points of the two limbs of the inverted V. These incisions form an angle of 90° with the lateral edge of the columella – i.e., perpendicular to it (▶ Fig. 6.13, ▶ Fig. 6.14). This incision meets the incisions on both sides at the columellar rim. Any residual fibers along the incision are severed with sharp scissors.

The edge of the columellar flap is raised with a fine double-pronged retractor once the incision for the open approach is complete (▶ Fig. 6.15).

Bleeding often occurs from two fine columellar arteries in the subcutaneous tissue running parallel to the medial crura of the alar cartilages, which are severed during the

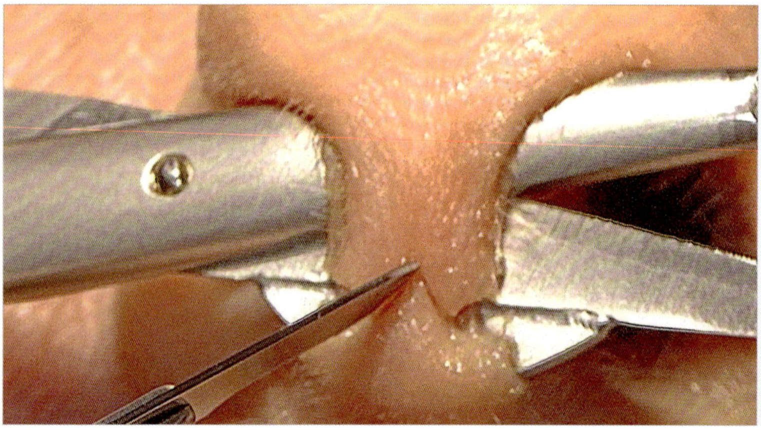

Fig. 6.13 The inverted V incision in the columella skin on the working plate of the slightly splayed scissors.

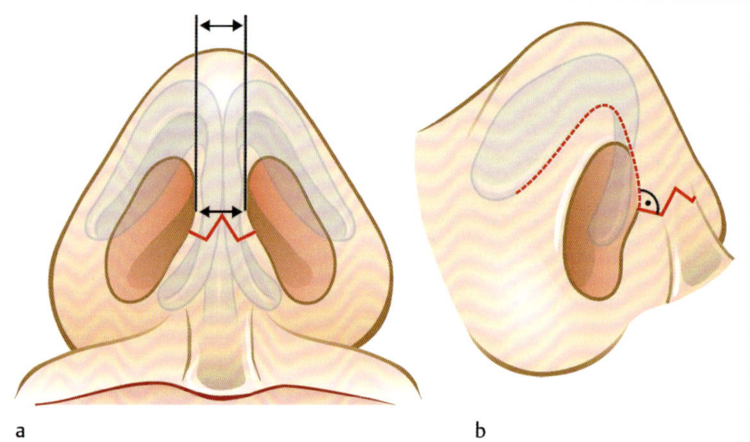

Fig. 6.14 Diagram of the inverted V incision on the columella for the open approach. **(a)** The tip of the inverted V lies exactly at the narrowest point of the columella. **(b)** The lateral incisions meet the edge of the columella at an angle of 90°.

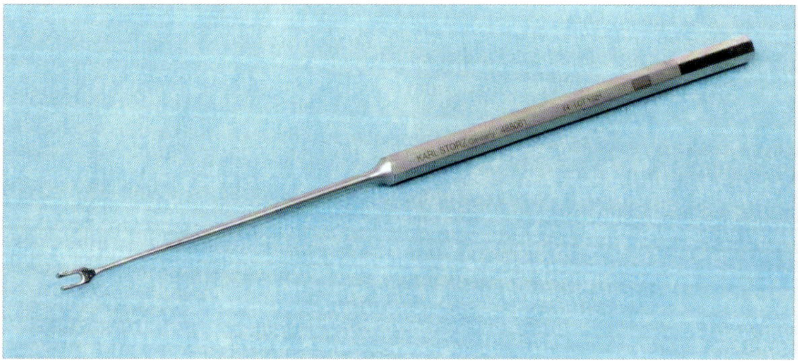

Fig. 6.15 Fine double hook. The double hook has to be narrow enough to lift the delicate skin of the columella with both prongs (KARL STORZ SE & Co. KG, Tuttlingen, Germany).

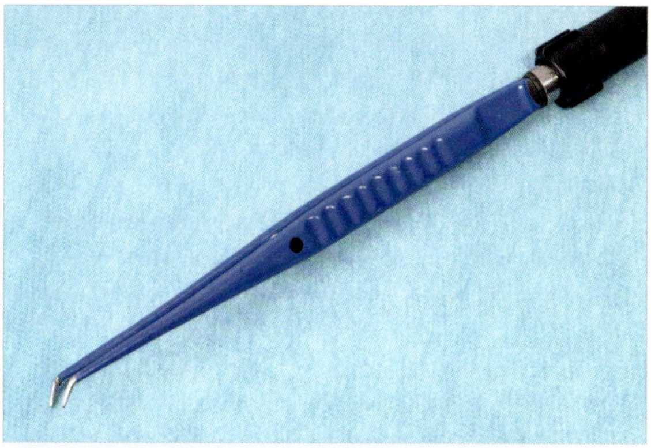

Fig. 6.16 Fine bipolar forceps (Erbe Elektromedizin GmbH, Tübingen, Germany).

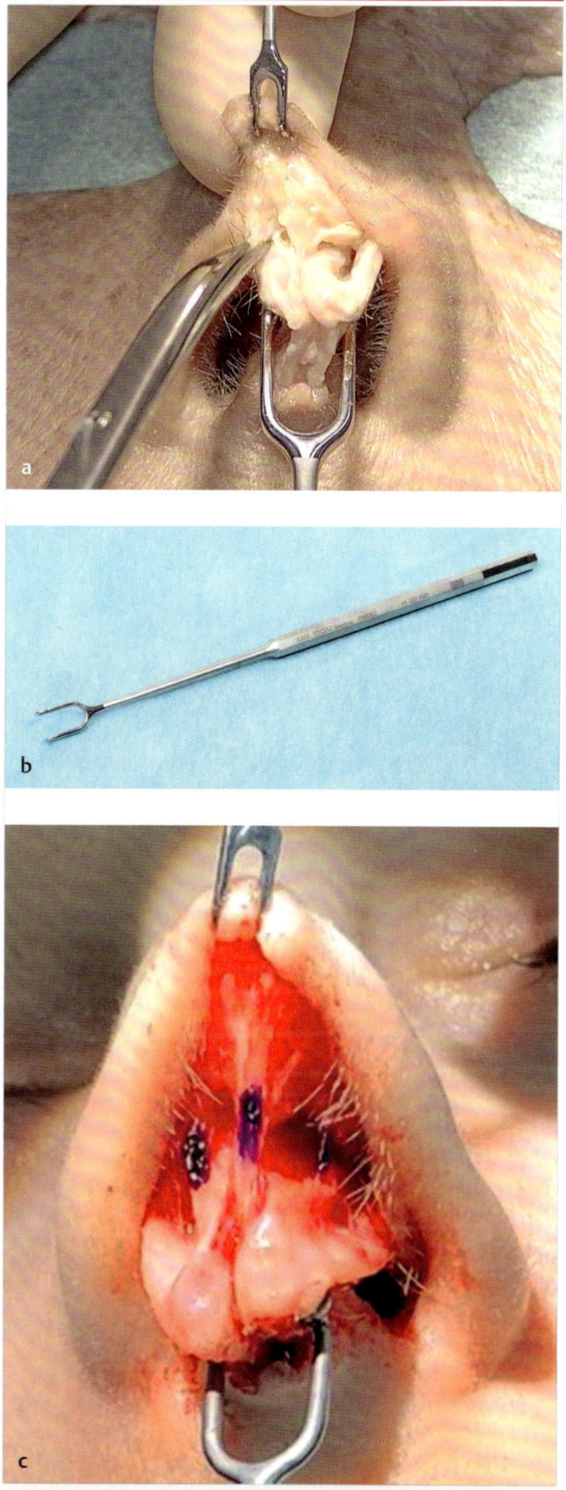

Fig. 6.17 Elevation of the skin flap over the nasal framework. Dissection of the skin flap. **(a)** Visualization of the alar domes. **(b)** The double hook inserted under the domes of the alar cartilages has to be sufficiently wide (KARL STORZ SE & Co. KG, Tuttlingen, Germany). **(c)** The Pitanguy and vertical scroll ligaments have been dissected free and marked in color.

transverse skin incision (see ▶ Fig. 1.13, ▶ Fig. 1.14). These vessels are coagulated with a fine bipolar forceps, slightly angled at the tip (▶ Fig. 6.16).

> Low bipolar power settings (approximately 10–15 W, depending on the device) and the penetration depth, if adjustable (e.g., level 1), are selected to prevent injury to the skin.

Hemostasis is achieved throughout the operation using these forceps and the same power setting.

6.6 Raising the Skin Flap

The skin flap is raised over the nasal framework, with the alar cartilages pulled caudally by an assistant or by the scrub nurse using a medium double-pronged retractor; this grasps the alar domes from below, with a prong on either side of the columella (▶ Fig. 6.17a, b).

While the skin flap is being raised using the fine double-pronged retractor, the skin and subcutaneous tissues are tightened against the pulling of the second double-pronged retractor under the alar domes to facilitate dissection (▶ Fig. 6.17a). Yaşargil's double-pronged spring hook with a bulldog clamp (for attachment to the surgical drape) comes in very handy during this phase of the operation, if an assistant is unavailable (▶ Video 6.4, ▶ Fig. 6.18).

The skin is then gradually detached from the cartilaginous framework using a pair of sharp scissors, mostly with cutting movements and occasionally with spreading movements (▶ Video 6.5; ▶ Fig. 6.17a). The tip of the scissors lies directly over the alar cartilages as far as possible, at least directly over the perichondrium, if not in a subperichondrial plane. The medial crura are then followed cranially to arrive at the alar domes as the next landmarks.

The lateral crura are traced, starting at the domes, and are visualized along their entire extent. Maintaining constant contact with the cartilaginous framework, one arrives at the complex of the middle third of the nasal framework – i.e., the nasal dorsum with the upper edge of the septum (W-ASA segment; see ▶ Fig. 1.7) and the attached upper lateral cartilages, lying between the cephalic margins of the alar cartilages. At this stage of the dissection, the surgeon can decide whether to expose the vertical scroll ligaments and the Pitanguy ligament when raising the skin flap (compare with ▶ Fig. 1.17, ▶ Fig. 8.58, ▶ Fig. 8.59). The ligaments can be dissected free, marked in color, then separated and later readapted with sutures to suit the anatomy when the wound is closed (▶ Fig. 6.17c).

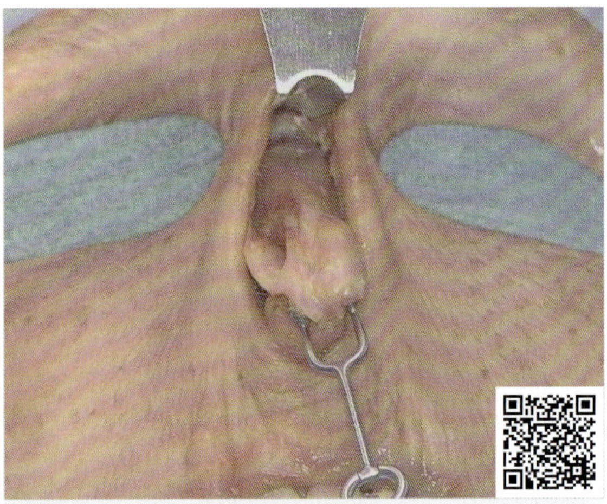

Video 6.4 Inserting and removing the spring hook.

The small double-pronged retractor on the skin flap is then exchanged for a "shortened Aufricht retractor" to improve visualization in this area (▶ Fig. 6.19).

Dissection of the skin flap can end there if manipulation of the alar cartilages alone is desired. However, it continues further during the typical rhinoplasty that is far more commonly performed, which also includes manipulation of the middle and upper (bony) nasal framework. The shortened Aufricht retractor (▶ Fig. 6.19) is then again replaced with the classic standard-length Aufricht retractor (▶ Fig. 6.20).

Cartilage dissection continues further with a pair of slightly larger scissors (▶ Fig. 6.21). Remaining directly over the cartilage of the middle third of the nasal dorsum, the bone is reached (▶ Fig. 6.22).

The skin is lifted with the superficial musculoaponeurotic system (SMAS) attached, but the perichondrium and periosteum may be primarily left intact over the nasal framework. These layers can later be mobilized separately as a perichondrium–periosteal flap, as a cover for the corrected nasal dorsum if needed.

To access the bone and work on it directly, its periosteum is elevated; the bone is completely exposed over the area of planned hump removal up to the nasal radix, or laterally somewhat beyond the intended lateral osteotomy, when surface surgery with piezo instruments is employed.

Mobilization of the skin must be continued even further in the direction of the glabella if the nasal radix is to be lowered (in order to deepen the nasofrontal angle).

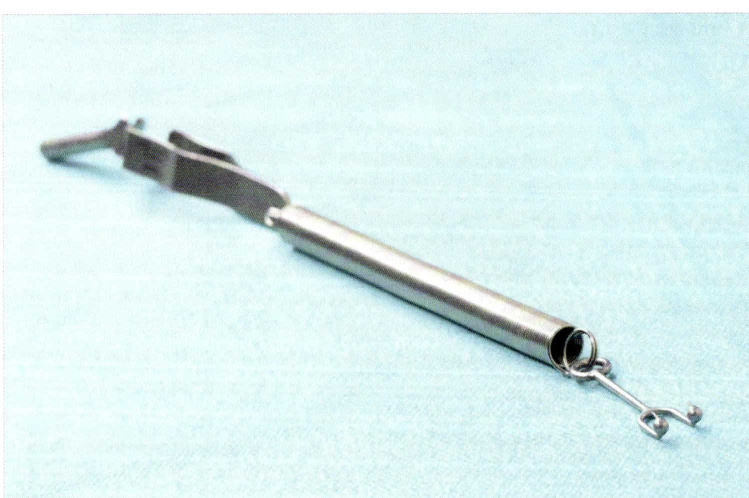

Fig. 6.18 The Yaşargil double-pronged spring hook with a bulldog clamp. The double-pronged retractor is inserted under the alar domes, as shown in ▶ Fig. 6.17a. The bulldog clamp is fixed to the drape under slight tension, avoiding the need for an assistant (KARL STORZ SE & Co. KG, Tuttlingen, Germany).

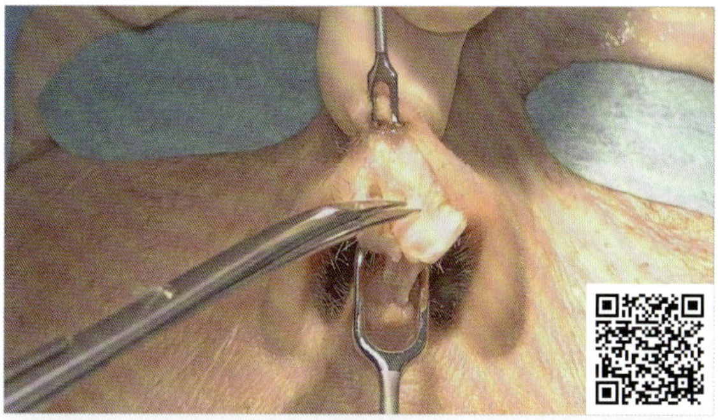

Video 6.5 Elevation of the skin flap.

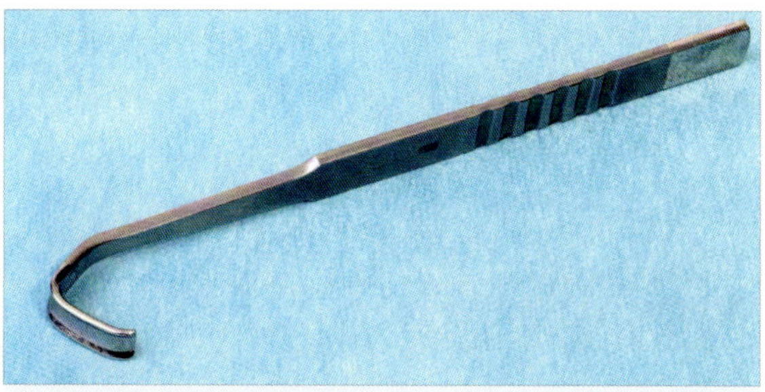

Fig. 6.19 The shortened Aufricht retractor (KARL STORZ SE & Co. KG, Tuttlingen, Germany).

> As explained in greater detail in Chapter 8, there are considerable differences between the surgical procedures used when working on the bone using the piezo technique and classic osteotomy using a chisel and osteotome. Exposure of the nasal bone during chisel osteotomies is required only for hump removal or for controlled paramedian osteotomies. Lateral osteotomies are usually carried out using a blind technique while palpating with a finger, as with the closed approach. In contrast, lateral piezo osteotomy requires extensive exposure of the nasal bones beyond the facial processes of the maxilla (in the so-called “extended open approach”).

The first phase of rhinoplasty thus concludes with complete dissection of the skin flap and visualization of the anatomical structures. The Aufricht retractor (see ▶ Fig. 6.20), which has been hand-held up to this point, is now replaced with the self-retaining nasal skin retractor with weight and chain (▶ Video 6.6; ▶ Fig. 6.23a-c). This allows the surgeon to use both hands during surgery,

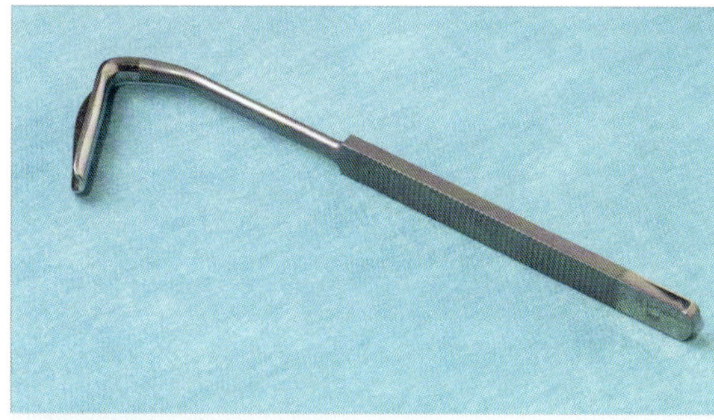

Fig. 6.20 The Aufricht retractor (KARL STORZ SE & Co. KG, Tuttlingen, Germany).

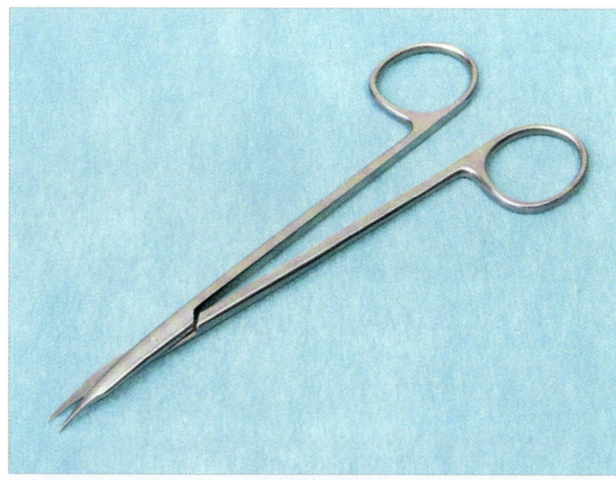

Fig. 6.21 Scissors for dissection at the nasal dorsum. For dissecting the dorsum, more robust scissors are suitable than those used on the columella and the alar cartilages (KARL STORZ SE & Co. KG, Tuttlingen, Germany).

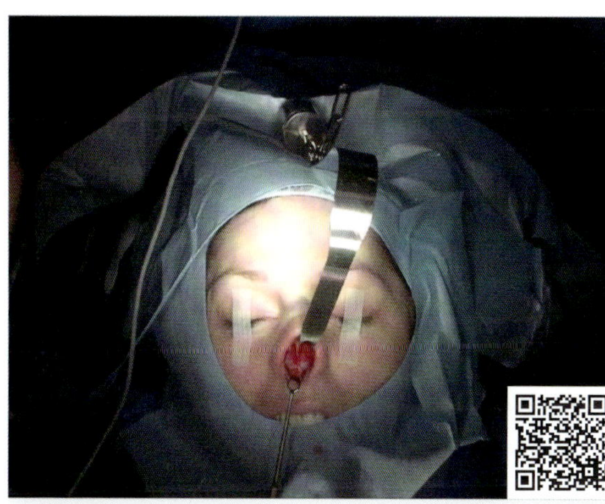

Video 6.6 Insertion and removal of the self-retaining Aufricht retractor.

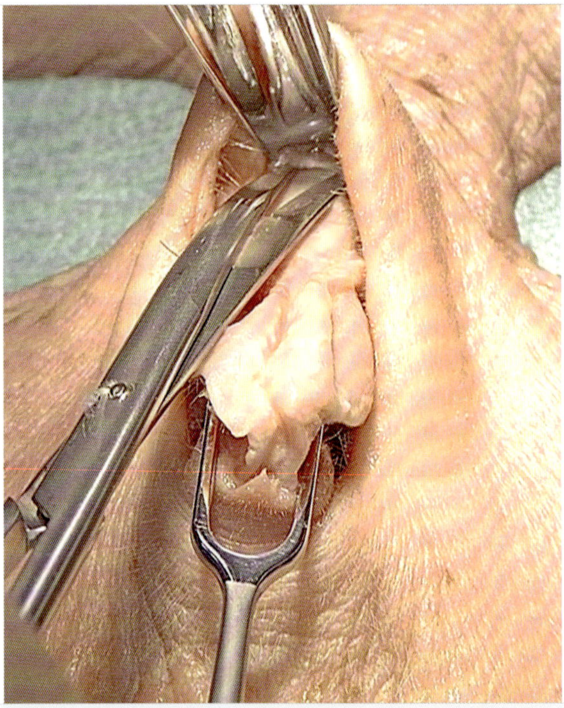

Fig. 6.22 Dissection of the skin flap on the nasal dorsum, with visualization of the cartilaginous and bony framework.

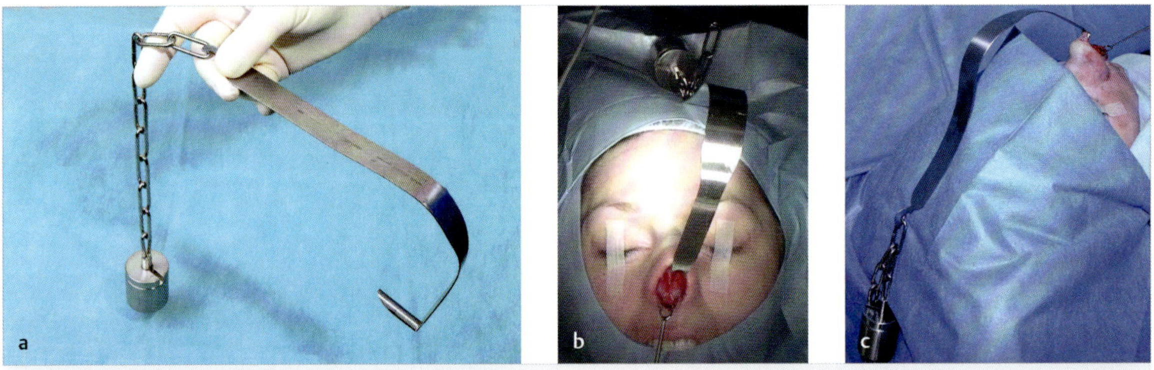

Fig. 6.23 The self-retaining Aufricht retractor with an added weight. (a) The chain and weight are attached to the retractor (KARL STORZ SE & Co. KG, Tuttlingen, Germany). **(b, c)** The curvature of the retractor can be adjusted by bending it to any situation as required. This is a self-retaining instrument.

especially while working on the middle and anterior thirds of the nose.

The entire surgical field is examined for any sources of bleeding before one proceeds further with manipulation of the bony and cartilaginous framework, and hemostasis is achieved using bipolar cauterization. Hemostasis of occasional diffuse bleeding is usually achieved by intermittent insertion of moistened compress strips. Epinephrine is required only in exceptional cases when there is heavy bleeding. The anesthetist should be consulted in case of persistent excessive bleeding, to assess whether hypotension may be induced to the extent permissible for the patient.

✔

Repeated washing and cleaning of the entire surgical field is recommended for reasons of hygiene and to ensure continued visualization.

Bibliography

Anderson JR, Ries WR. Rhinoplasty: emphasizing the external approach. New York: Thieme-Stratton; 1986

Berghaus A.. New rhinoplasty instruments: columella scissors and self-retaining Aufricht retractor. Plast Reconstr Surg Glob Open. 2016; 4: e789. DOI: 10.1097/GOX.0000000000000767

Daniel RK. Mastering rhinoplasty: a comprehensive atlas of surgical techniques with integrated video clips. Heidelberg: Springer; 2010

Gruber RP, Peck GC. Rhinoplasty: state of the art. St. Louis: Mosby-Year Book; 1993

Guyuron B. Rhinoplasty. Philadelphia: Elsevier; 2012

Johnson CM, Toriumi DM. Open structure rhinoplasty. Philadelphia; Saunders 1990

Peck GC. Techniques in aesthetic rhinoplasty. 2nd ed. Philadelphia: JB Lippincott; 1990

Sheen JH, Sheen A. Aesthetic rhinoplasty. 2nd ed. St. Louis: CV Mosby; 1987

Toriumi DM. Structure approach in rhinoplasty. Facial Plast Surg Clin North Am. 2005; 13(1):93–113

Toriumi DM. Structure rhinoplasty: lessons learned in 30 years. Chicago, IL: DMT Publishing; 2019

Totonchi A, Guyuron B. The external rhinoplasty approach. Clin Plast Surg. 2022; 49(1):49–59

7 Septoplasty

Septoplasty is often required together with a rhinoplasty to correct a deviated nasal septum ("septorhinoplasty"). ▶ Fig. 7.1 shows a typical case study. As explained earlier, septoplasty and harvesting of septal cartilage are performed after correction of the bony nasal framework, in connection with dissection of the alar cartilages and exposure of the caudal edge of the septum. Septoplasty is described at this point so that the following chapters can focus on the surgical steps involved in rhinoplasty.

The hemitransfixion incision – usually the incision of choice for septoplasty without rhinoplasty – can also be used to obtain access to the septum with an open rhinoplasty. In most cases, however, the caudal edge of the septum is exposed for corrective septal procedures during open rhinoplasty, allowing easy access to the septum and eliminating the need for a separate hemitransfixion incision.

7.1 Septoplasty via an Open Approach

Accessing the septum during **open rhinoplasty** is more laborious than with a closed procedure using a hemitransfixion incision, but it allows far better visualization and manipulation (▶ Video 7.1).

The alar cartilages are first separated in the midline. Dissection may be limited to the medial crura if required; however, the alar cartilages are usually completely separated from each other to expose the caudal edge of the septum and the anterior septal angle. The alar cartilages are first pulled aside with a fine double hook (see ▶ Fig. 6.15), and the septal edge is exposed by dissection with a pair of pointed scissors (see ▶ Fig. 6.21). Septoplasty is then continued with a slim, relatively long speculum (▶ Fig. 7.2; ▶ Fig. 7.3a, b). The interdomal ligaments connecting the medial crura can be left intact if the nasal tip does not require correction. Access to the septum is then obtained below these ligaments (▶ Fig. 7.4a, b).

7.2 Septoplasty via a Hemitransfixion Incision

Alternatively, septoplasty may be carried out before the incision for the open approach, or during any other stage of rhinoplasty, via a **hemitransfixion incision**, as is usual for septoplasty alone – i.e., using the closed approach (▶ Video 7.2; ▶ Fig. 7.5). This access route may be useful in isolated cases if the medial crura of the alar cartilages and the caudal septum do not require manipulation during open rhinoplasty.

Some surgeons place the hemitransfixion incision a few millimeters behind the caudal edge of the septum, but I prefer incising the vestibular skin strictly along the caudal edge of the septum and to its left side (▶ Fig. 7.5, ▶ Fig. 7.6a).

7.3 The Cartilaginous Septum

Regardless of the approach, the anterior 5–10 mm of the caudal septum is dissected using a pair of sharp scissors or a scalpel, since tough connective tissue and muscle fibers insert into cartilage in this region (see ▶ Fig. 7.3b). These tough connecting fibers have to be sharply separated to expose the subperichondrial plane in direct

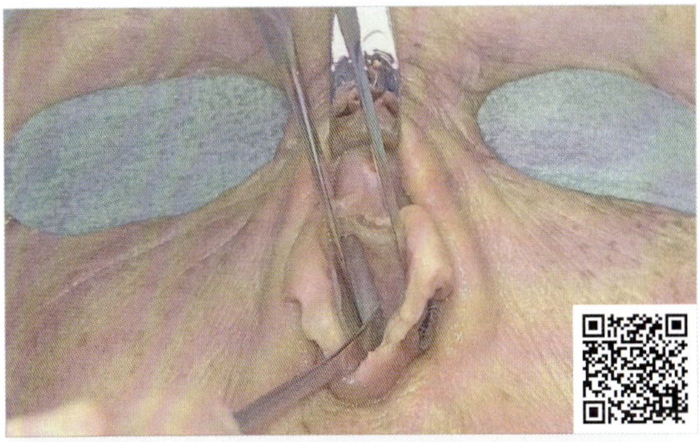

Video 7.1 Exposing the septum and anterior nasal spine.

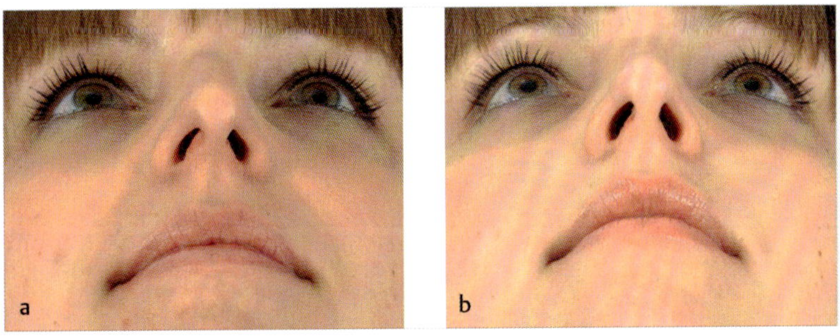

Fig. 7.1 Septal deviation with subluxation; case study. (a) The patient had obstructed nasal breathing, with septal deviation and subluxation of the caudal edge of the septum to the right. **(b)** Post septorhinoplasty.

7

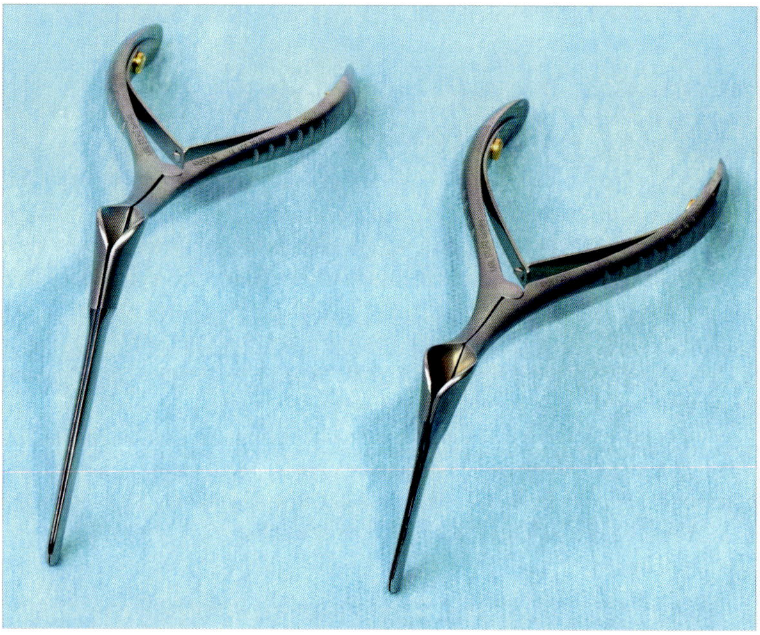

Fig. 7.2 Two long specula for septoplasty. The slim design facilitates visualization of narrow regions during treatment of the septum (KARL STORZ SE & Co. KG, Tuttlingen, Germany).

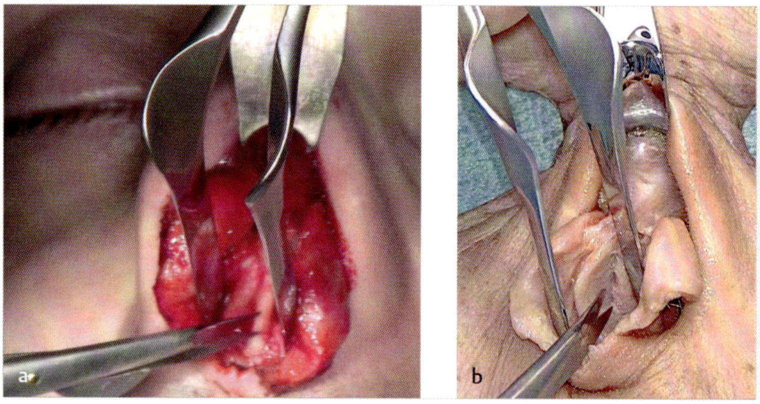

Fig. 7.3 Access to the septum via the open approach. (a) Separation of the alar cartilages, with visualization of the caudal edge of the septum. **(b)** Exposure of the cartilaginous septum (in a cadaver specimen).

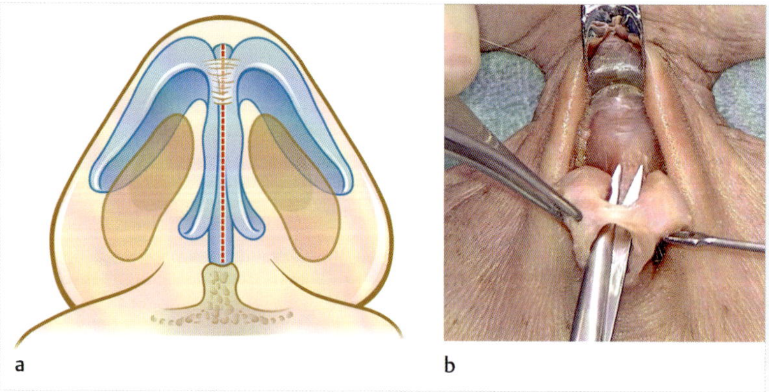

Fig. 7.4 Access to the septum via the open approach, with preserved domal ligaments. The interdomal ligaments can be left intact if corrective surgery of the alar domes is not required, but the caudal edge of the septum can still be exposed ("dome bridge"). **(a)** Schematic diagram. **(b)** As seen in a cadaver specimen.

contact with the cartilage a little further posteriorly. The sharp and then blunt edges of the Freer elevator (▶ Fig. 7.7) can then be advanced relatively easily in this plane with upward and downward movements to detach the mucoperichondrium (▶ Video 7.3; see ▶ Fig. 7.6b, ▶ Fig. 7.8). The septal cartilage appears with a bright

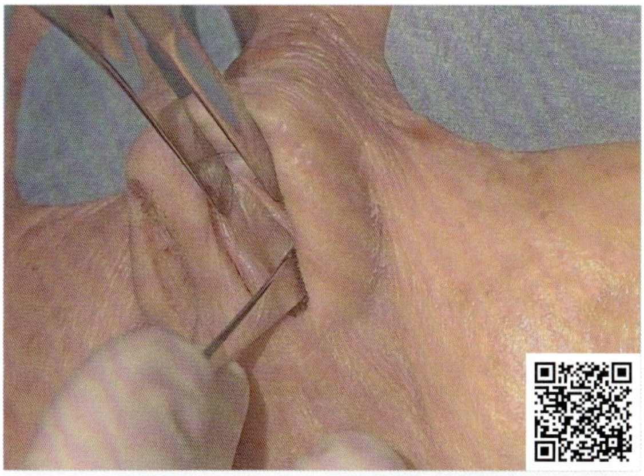

Video 7.2 Endonasal septoplasty via a hemitransfixion incision.

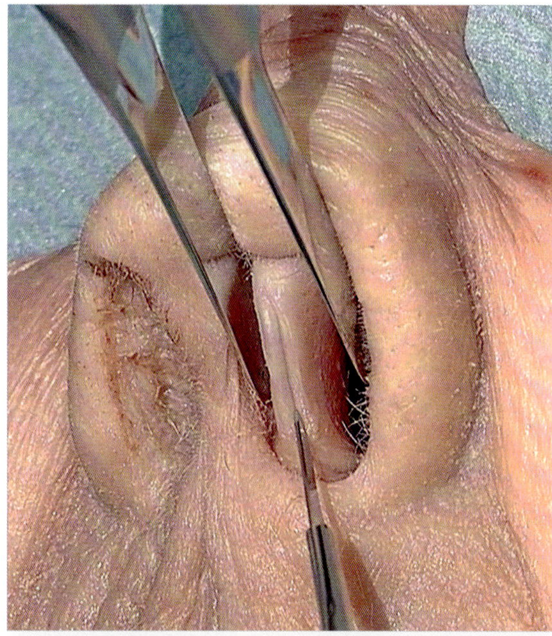

Fig. 7.5 Left hemitransfixion incision. Manipulation is easier with a left-sided hemitransfixion incision, precisely over the caudal edge of the septum (seen in a cadaver specimen).

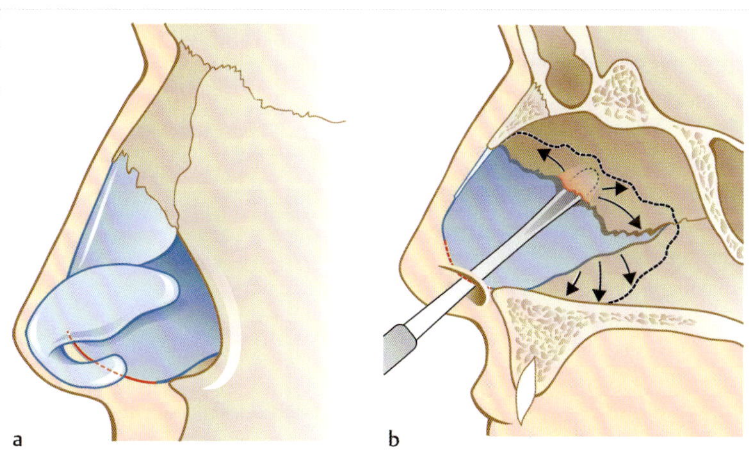

Fig. 7.6 Septoplasty. (a) Hemitransfixion incision (red line) over the caudal edge of the septum. **(b)** Dissection of the mucoperichondrium and mucoperiosteum of the cartilaginous and bony septum.

white to yellow and slightly bluish, shiny color below the mucoperichondrium. This appearance is lacking if there is an intervening layer of soft tissue obscuring the cartilage, no matter how delicate.

> "When it's blue (i.e., the cartilage) — you're through (i.e., the perichondrium)."

This dissection is performed **bilaterally**, if necessary, to make it possible to operate on the cartilage with an unobstructed view of the deviated septum. Unilateral elevation of the mucoperichondrium is sufficient if corrective surgery of a short segment or harvesting of a small piece of septal cartilage is required.

Dissection of the mucous membrane is continued beyond the osseocartilaginous junction. Long and thin specula are used for manipulation of further back segments of the septum (see ▸ Fig. 7.2).

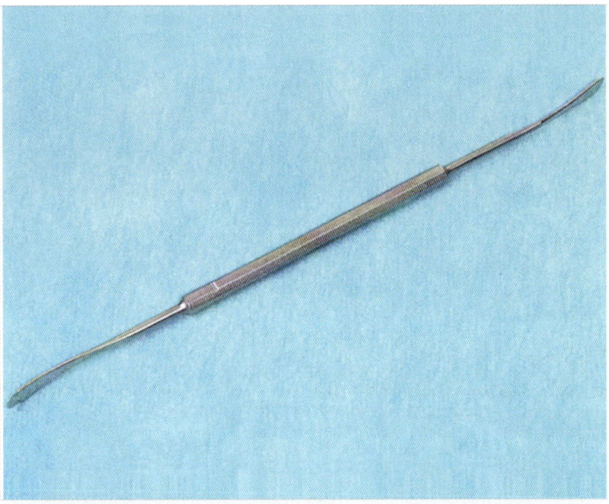

Fig. 7.7 Freer elevator. The double-ended Freer elevator is equipped with an extra sharp blade at one end (on the left in the image), while the opposite end is blunt (KARL STORZ SE & Co. KG, Tuttlingen, Germany).

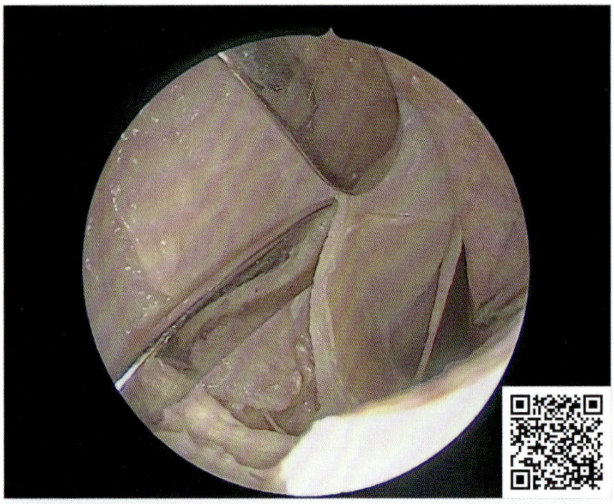

Video 7.3 Exposure of the maxillary crest and removal of septal cartilage.

The septum is completely exposed once the anterior nasal spine and the maxillary crest have been visualized. The perpendicular plate of the bony septum is exposed to the extent necessary for correction of septal deviation, and the insertion of the upper lateral cartilage is visualized under the nasal dorsum. If necessary, the dissection can be continued over the maxillary crest to the floor of the nasal cavity. This is useful for correcting deviations of the crest.

The subsequent steps depend on the nature of the septal deformity that requires correction. The inferior septal edge is frequently found to be dislocated out of the maxillary crest, or even with it, resulting in a deviated septum. The septum may alternatively bulge under tension between the nasal dorsum and the maxillary crest. Excision of a cartilaginous strip from the inferior edge of the septum, after separation of the cartilaginous septum from the maxillary crest, effectively corrects its dislocation from the crest or relieves tension in the cartilage in both these instances (known as "basal release") (▸ Fig. 7.9). However, this may result in loss of contact between the posterior septal angle and the anterior nasal spine, depriving the septum of its inferior support and allowing it to migrate inferiorly or posteriorly. This can be prevented by suture fixation of the posterior septal angle to the anterior nasal spine after correction of septal deviation. The suture is looped around the spine, or through a borehole drilled into the spine using the piezo technique, a drill, or a sturdy cannula (see ▸ Fig. 7.12).

The cartilaginous septum frequently deviates vertically from the midline together with the caudal edge of the perpendicular plate of the ethmoid bone. The quadrangular plate is corrected by first sharply separating it from the caudal bony rim of the perpendicular plate (▸ Fig. 7.10). After that, the cartilaginous plate can usually

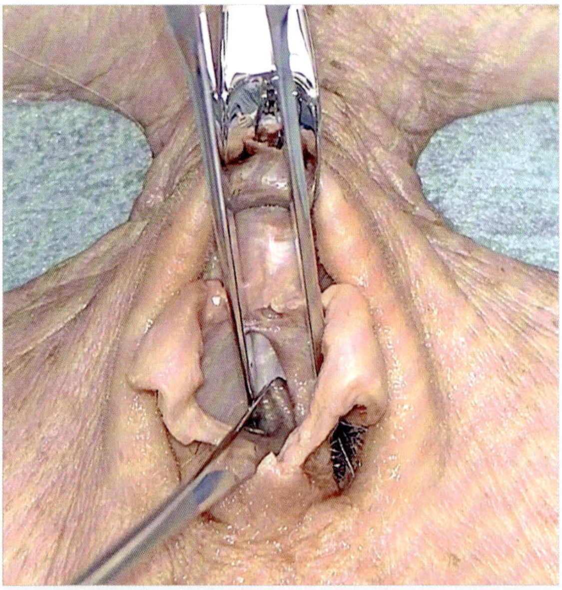

Fig. 7.8 Dissection of the mucoperichondrium using the Freer elevator with the open approach. Tough strands of tissue are first loosened with the sharp end of the instrument. In the subperichondrial layer, dissection with the blunt end is then easier and safer.

be repositioned to the midline only after resection of a narrow vertical strip of cartilage from the posterior edge of the cartilaginous septum. This requires a vertical cartilaginous incision, followed by dissection and removal of the cartilaginous strip (▸ Fig. 7.11a, b).

Marked convexity of the quadrangular plate may necessitate an arcuate cartilaginous incision extending from

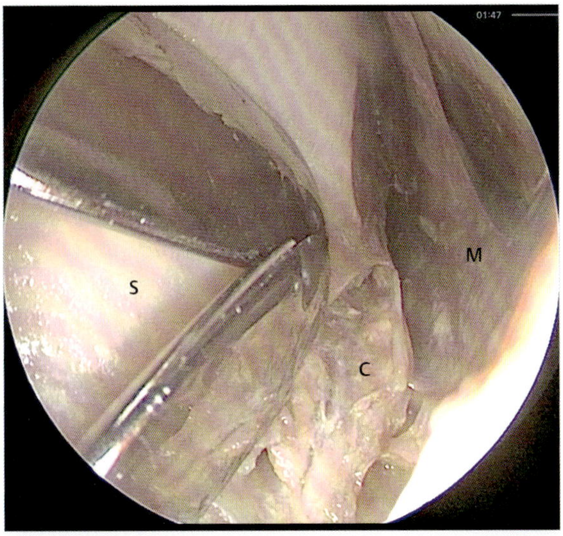

Fig. 7.9 **Dissection of the maxillary crest.** The cartilaginous septum (S) is separated from the maxillary crest (C) using the Freer elevator; the mucosa (M) is kept intact.

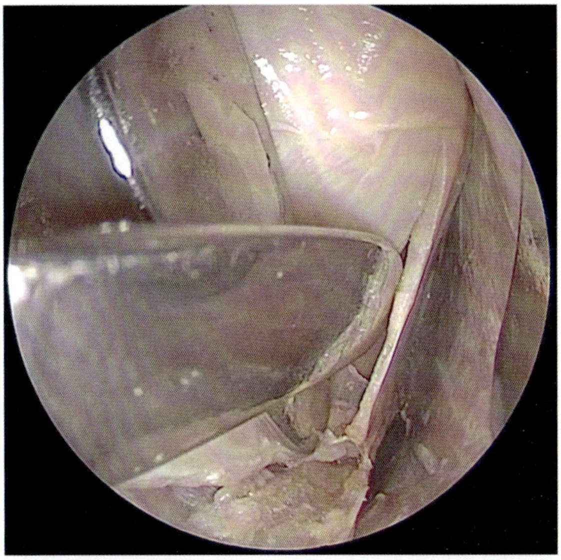

Fig. 7.10 **Separation of the cartilaginous septum from the perpendicular plate.**

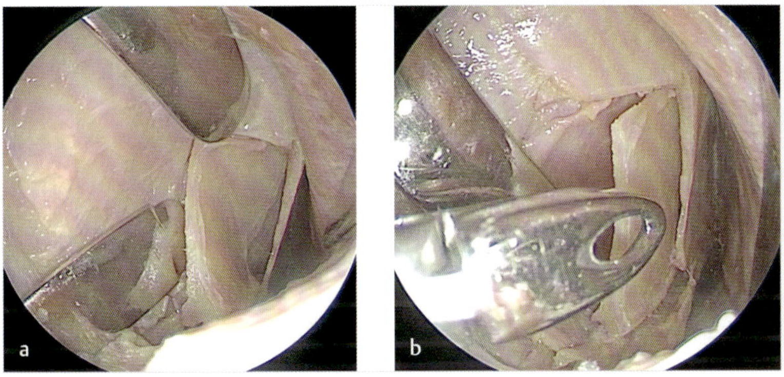

Fig. 7.11 **Resection of a vertical strip of cartilage. (a)** A vertical cartilage incision is made in front of the deviation. **(b)** Removal of deviated cartilage with the Blakesley nasal forceps (see ▶ Fig. 5.4).

a posteroinferior to an anterosuperior direction under the nasal roof, to facilitate easy repositioning of the cartilaginous septum into the midline.

> ✔
>
> All pieces of cartilage removed from the septum constitute invaluable graft material for subsequent rhinoplasty and are carefully preserved in saline solution.

7.4 The L-Strut

Contact between the septum and the anterior nasal spine must be preserved during resection of parts of the quadrangular plate (unless intentional lowering of the nasal tip is desired), and an intact, L-shaped cartilaginous strip ("L-strut"), 8–10 mm wide, must be preserved both under the nasal dorsum and also at the caudal edge of the septum (▶ Fig. 7.12). This angular strip of cartilage has to be stable and firmly attached to the anterior nasal spine and the nasal bone or perpendicular plate in the "keystone area" ("K-area"). Stability at these fixed points must be secured by drill holes and sutures if necessary.

The K-area is a zone of approximately 1 cm at the osseocartilaginous junction at the rhinion of the nasal dorsum (see ▶ Fig. 1.1). The stability of this zone is particularly important.

A kink in the L-strut is relevant from a functional point of view, and often results in an aesthetically unappealing nasal deviation. This buckled cartilaginous segment is corrected by division, usually followed by resection; stability has to be restored subsequently by splinting with so-called spreader grafts (▶ Fig. 7.13, ▶ Fig. 7.14, ▶ Fig. 7.15a, b; see also section 9.4).

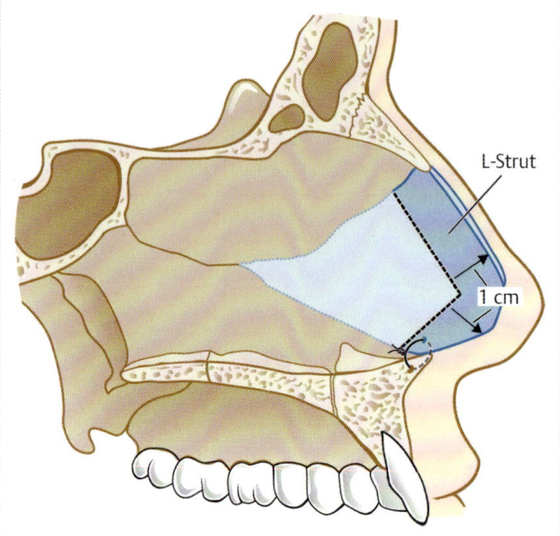

Fig. 7.12 L-strut. During septoplasty or harvesting of a septal cartilage graft, a contiguous strip of cartilage approximately 10 mm wide is preserved in the dorsal and caudal areas of the nasal septum (L-strut) to maintain structural stability and prevent external deformity. It is crucial that this angled piece of cartilage should rest firmly on the anterior nasal spine and that it is firmly connected to the nasal bone in the "keystone area" (K-area).

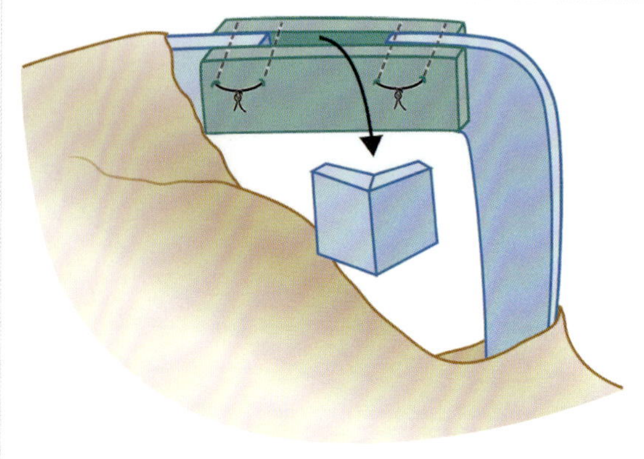

Fig. 7.13 L-strut and spreader grafts (lateral view). Surgical correction of a kink in the L-strut by resection and reconstruction with spreader grafts.

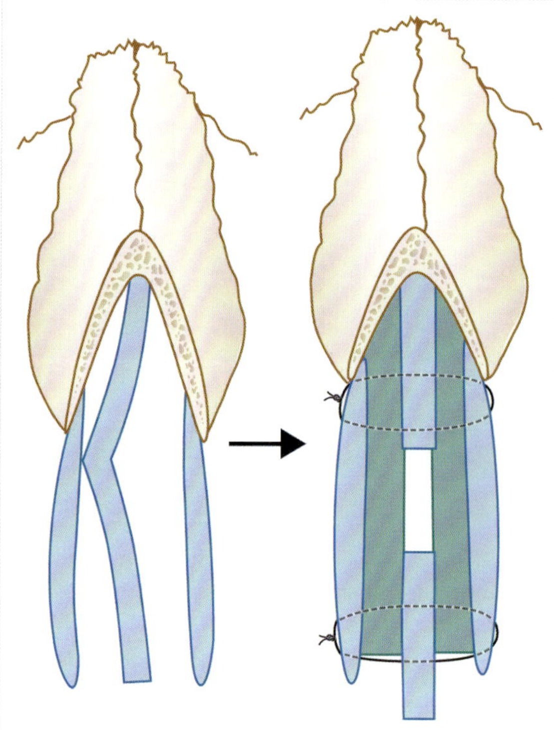

Fig. 7.14 L-strut and spreader graft (cranial view). Resection of a kink in the L-strut and reconstruction with spreader grafts. The reconstructed L-strut with spreader grafts is firmly sutured to the upper lateral cartilages, and to the nasal bones or the perpendicular plate of the septum if necessary.

7.5 Extracorporeal Septoplasty

Extracorporeal septoplasty is a valuable method for reconstructing a severely deviated septum that cannot be corrected in any other way and has been detached from its anchor points and removed as a whole or, more often, subtotally. The deformed septal cartilage is then reconstructed as a plane cartilage plate on the instrument table (extracorporeally) or remodeled to form a stable L-shaped cartilage graft, which is then repositioned and anchored in the nose to restore stability. Individual flat segments of the markedly deviated septum are joined together with several fine sutures to form a flat cartilaginous sheet (▸ Fig. 7.16a–c).

Other options for correcting a deviated septum include isolated resection of sharp kink formations or thinning of markedly thick nasal cartilage, especially at the level of narrow nasal valves.

7.6 The Bony Septum

Deviation of the quadrangular plate often continues as a bony deformity (such as kinking, deviation, or widening) of the perpendicular plate of the ethmoid bone. These abnormalities are well visualized on preoperative computed tomography (▸ Fig. 7.17). Functional deformities may extend posteriorly from the vomer into the anterior wall of the sphenoid sinus, or upward from the perpendicular plate into the lamina cribrosa (and thus to the olfactory fibers).

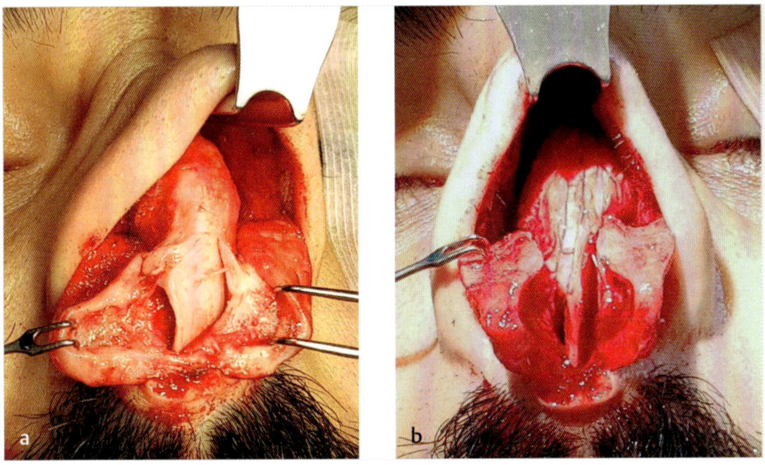

Fig. 7.15 Surgical correction of deviated L-strut, intraoperative. (a) Septal deviation with vertical posttraumatic kinking. **(b)** Resection of the kink and reconstruction with spreader grafts.

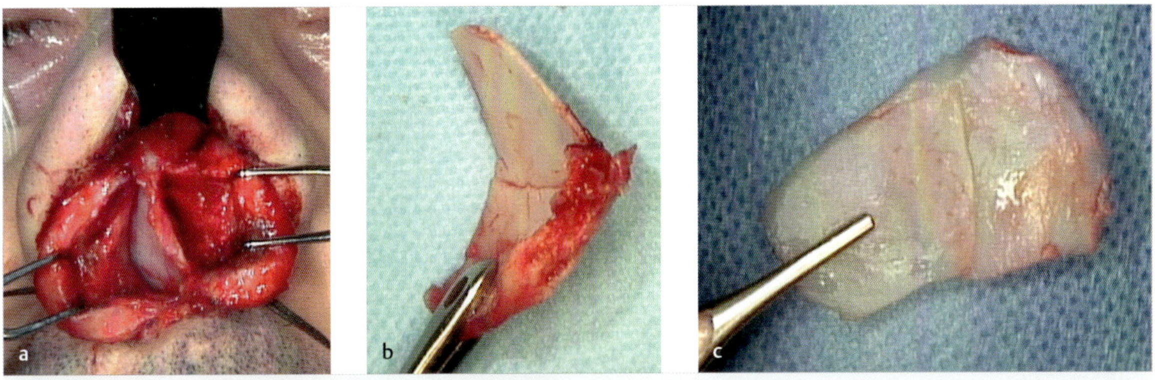

Fig. 7.16 Extracorporeal septoplasty. (a) Marked septal deviation. **(b)** Resected septum. **(c)** Correction with extracorporeal septoplasty.

> Uncontrolled fracturing of bone with bone forceps in these areas is therefore not recommended, since the fracture lines may extend into the lamina cribrosa at the base of the skull, with resultant injury to olfactory fibers or the skull base and dura, with loss of smell, cerebrospinal fluid rhinorrhea, and further complications.

It is safer to sever the bone below the base of the skull with a pair of sharp double-jointed bone scissors (Becker–Caplan septum scissors, ▶ Fig. 7.18) or the exceptionally safe piezo technique (see section 8.3). Deviated bone that has been cut around in this manner can be loosened and removed with little risk (▶ Video 7.4).

7.7 The Maxillary Crest

A deviated and functionally disturbing maxillary crest does not necessarily require complete resection. Fracturing of its base and subsequent rotation of it to the midline is often sufficient, while avoiding injury to the vessels and sensory nerves running in the crest. This spares the surgeon the sometimes laborious process of achieving hemostasis of spurting blood from the bone, while avoiding postoperative sensory disorders in the upper lip and teeth for the patient.

7.8 Cartilage Replantation after Septoplasty

Cartilage or bone obtained from the septum can be flattened or leveled and reimplanted between the layers of septal mucosa at the end of the procedure, unless it is required for reconstruction of the external nose. Reimplantation may be useful for possible revision surgery even if it is not necessary from the functional point of view in the presence of an intact L-strut. Reimplanting compact cartilaginous discs is therefore preferable to using crushed or fragmented material, which offers little stability and is also difficult to recover and reuse in a later operation.

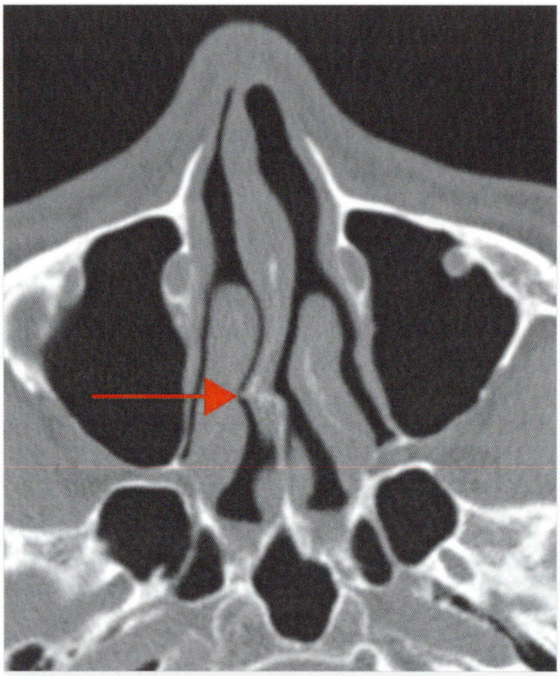

Fig. 7.17 **Deviation of the bony septum.** The axial computed tomography scan shows bone abnormalities best. Septal deviation in contact with the turbinate mucosa is seen (red arrow).

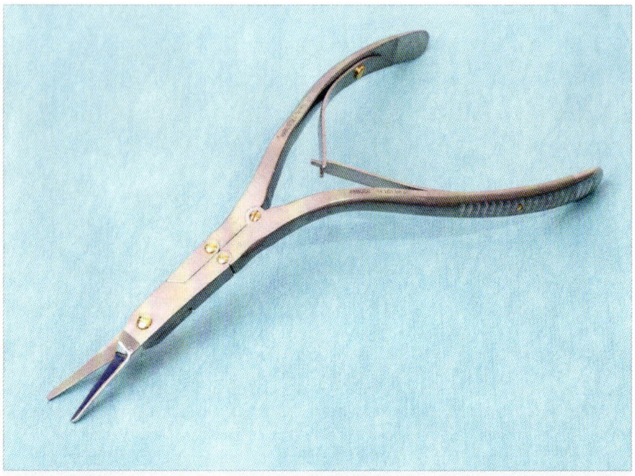

Fig. 7.18 Surgical double-joint bone scissors. These scissors cut even solid bone far back in the bony septum both precisely and efficiently (KARL STORZ SE & Co. KG, Tuttlingen, Germany).

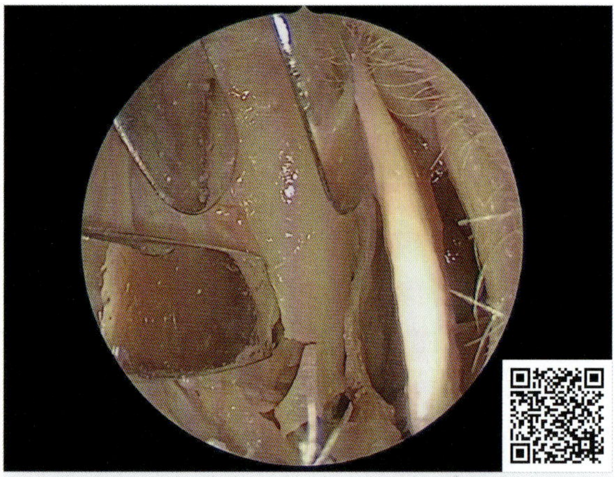

Video 7.4 Endonasal septoplasty.

7.9 Septal Perforation

Septal perforation (a hole in the nasal septum) is an undesirable consequence of surgical procedures on the nasal septum such as septoplasty, following trauma, or due to constant "nose picking." Cocaine abuse is a less common cause and may give rise to septal defects of considerable size.

Symptoms of this condition include a whistling sound during nasal breathing, obstructed nasal breathing, excessive nasal secretions and crusting, and recurrent minor nosebleeds. Large perforations can result in a loss of dorsal nasal support, leading to a saddle nose (sunken nasal dorsum; see section 19.2) and/or a retracted columella (see Chapter 11). Techniques for closing septal perforations are discussed in section 19.5.

7.10 Wound Closure after Septoplasty

The mucosa is readapted to the osseocartilaginous framework after completion of septoplasty, and any mucosal tears are repaired with rapidly absorbable sutures (e.g., 5-0 polyglactin 910, Vicryl Rapide). Triple-layer septal defects with bilaterally deficient mucosa and an absence of underlying cartilage have to be repaired, since there is a high risk of permanent septal perforations developing in such cases.

Suturing the mucosa to the septal cartilage using continuous, horizontal mattress sutures is worthwhile, with the needle passing through all three layers several times in a zigzag or starlike manner from one side of the septum to the other (▶ Fig. 7.19). All three layers of the septum are thus well apposed during the healing phase; the rapidly absorbable sutures dissolve on their own within 8–10 days.

The hemitransfixion incision (in the closed technique) is closed with three or four single interrupted sutures, also with rapidly absorbable suture material.

Doyle splints can also be inserted and sutured to the septum, especially after extensive surgical correction of a deviated septum (▶ Fig. 7.20). These tube-like silicone

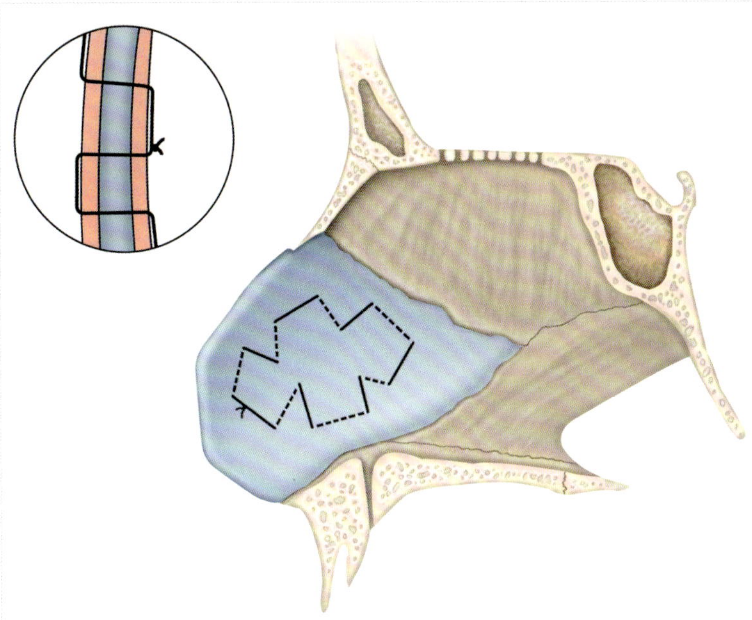

Fig. 7.19 Mattress suture after septoplasty. This zigzag suture closes the dead space between the cartilage and the mucosa, adapts the layers of mucosa to the cartilage, helps stabilize the septum, and often makes the use of splints superfluous. (From Behrbohm and Tardy, eds., *Essentials of septorhinoplasty*, 2nd ed., Stuttgart: Thieme, 2016.)

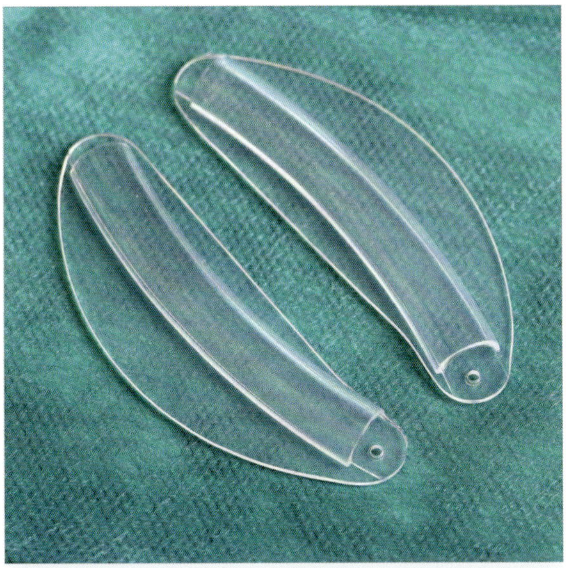

Fig. 7.20 Doyle splints. These silicone splints with tubes support the inner nose for a few days after extensive septoplasty and reconstruction. They are not troublesome for the patient, enable nasal breathing, and can be easily removed (SPIGGLE & THEIS Medizintechnik GmbH, Overath, Germany).

endonasal splints are removed 2–3 days later; they ensure patency of the nasal lumen (enabling nasal breathing), support the septum, and — together with mattress sutures — effectively prevent the development of a septal hematoma. These splints are not troublesome for the patient.

If Doyle splints are inserted, the patients should be given an antibiotic postoperatively. The splints block drainage from the paranasal sinuses and interfere with their ventilation, which may encourage the development of sinusitis.

In the open technique, the surgical wound is closed in a typical manner (see Chapter 15).

The **caudal** septum, together with the medial crura of the alar cartilages, is extremely important for the columellar and nasal tip profile. The important corrective measures in this region are therefore separately summarized in Chapter 11.

Bibliography

Davis RE. Rhinoplasty and septoplasty. In: Snow J, Wackym A, eds. Ballenger's otolaryngology head and neck surgery. 17th ed. Shelton: BC Decker/People's Medical Publishing House; 2009:633–639

Gomulinski L. The severely deviated septum—the way I solve the problem. Facial Plast Surg. 2006; 22(4):240–248

Gruber RP, Nahai F, Bogdan MA, Friedman GD. Changing the convexity and concavity of nasal cartilages and cartilage grafts with horizontal mattress sutures: part II. Clinical results. Plast Reconstr Surg. 2005; 115 (2):595–606, discussion 607–608

Gubisch W. The extracorporeal septum plasty: a technique to correct difficult nasal deformities. Plast Reconstr Surg. 1995; 95(4):672–682

Gubisch W. Twenty-five years experience with extracorporeal septoplasty. Facial Plast Surg. 2006; 22(4):230–239

Most SP, Rudy SF. Septoplasty: Basic and Advanced Techniques. Facial Plast Surg Clin North Am. 2017; 25(2):161–169

Sirinoglu H, Yesiloglu N, Ersoy B. A new perspective for spreader graft use in severely deviated septum: is septal continuity an obligation for a stable and straight nasal septum? Facial Plast Surg. 2016; 32(4):460–468

8 Reduction of the Bony Nasal Framework

Reduction of the bony nasal frame is often carried out during primary rhinoplasty. Augmentation, primarily necessary for revision surgery, is required much less often. The term "hump reduction" does not adequately describe the measures required here and is by no means always appropriate.

> It is important to understand that it is not just about lowering the height of the bridge of the nose, but that the surgeon must have an adequate command of the bony and cartilaginous framework of the nose as a whole (▶ Fig. 8.1a–d).

8.1 Overview of Techniques and General Considerations

Modern rhinoplasty offers the surgeon a selection of methods for reducing the bony bridge of the nose.

▶ **Structure rhinoplasty.** This is the classic traditional method of working in rhinoplasty. Each individual structural element (nasal dorsum, side walls, septum, etc.) is considered individually and is treated as an isolated item. Chisels and rasps are primarily used on bones with this methodology, which has predominated during the last few decades.

▶ **Surface rhinoplasty.** With this procedure, the surface of cartilage and bone is primarily processed in order to

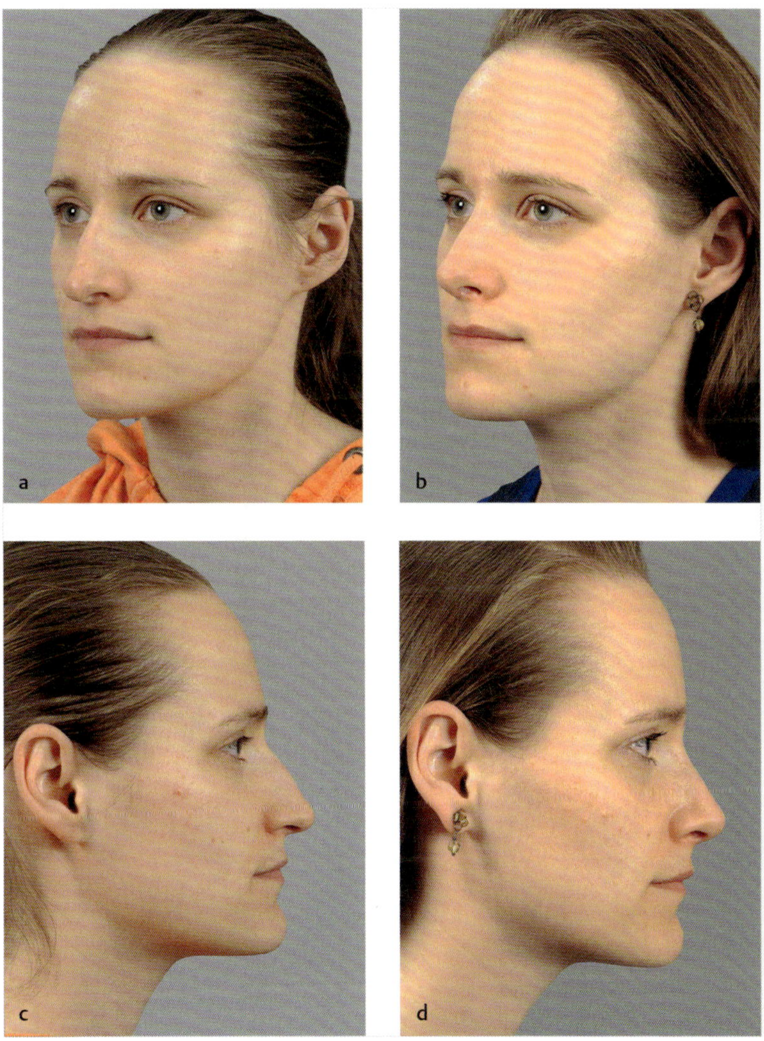

Fig. 8.1 Correction of a hump nose; case study. (a, c) Even a relatively small hump, especially in combination with a drooping nasal tip (tip drop), can significantly affect facial expression. **(b, d)** Status post corrective rhinoplasty with hump removal.

influence the shape of the nose. This way of working on the bony frame has become particularly important due to the advent of piezo technology in rhinoplasty ("osteoplasty").

▸ **Foundation rhinoplasty.** In this approach, the working principle is to mobilize the nose at the base and to change the position of the superstructure while maintaining its integrity. This procedure, which is basically well known from the early times of nose surgery, has become quite important again in recent years under the term "preservation rhinoplasty." This is where the terms "push down" and "let down" belong.

▸ **Hybrid rhinoplasty.** The surgeon should be aware that simply relying on just one procedure in the method used does not always lead to the best goal. Often, a combination of different techniques leads to the best result – especially, for example, a combination of foundation (preservation) techniques with surface procedures. This can then be called a hybrid rhinoplasty.

In this book, the principles of all these procedures are described. For the author, the use of piezo technology has become increasingly important. The advantages of piezo technology are also seen in preservation rhinoplasty, which has gained greater significance. At the same time, it is essential for the rhinoplasty surgeon to know how to use osteotomes, chisels, and rasps, which is why the use of these instruments has to be described with equal importance.

The surgeon must be aware that dorsal hump reduction alone (in the sense of resection) nearly always results in visual widening of the nose in the frontal view, unless additional measures are taken (▸ Fig. 8.2). These include lateral osteotomies or fracturing of the lateral nasal walls and thus the nasal bones during hump reduction, followed by medial repositioning or medialization to achieve a narrowing. This protocol, however, need not be strictly followed. The patient is evaluated preoperatively (e.g., during computer simulation), to assess whether narrowing of the nasal pyramid is required in addition to hump reduction (which is usually the case), or whether medialization of the nasal bones can be dispensed with, as in patients with a very narrow but high nasal pyramid and a small hump (▸ Fig. 8.3a–d). In addition, it should be checked whether the given case might be suitable for a preservation technique in which the nasal framework is lowered overall (see section 8.4).

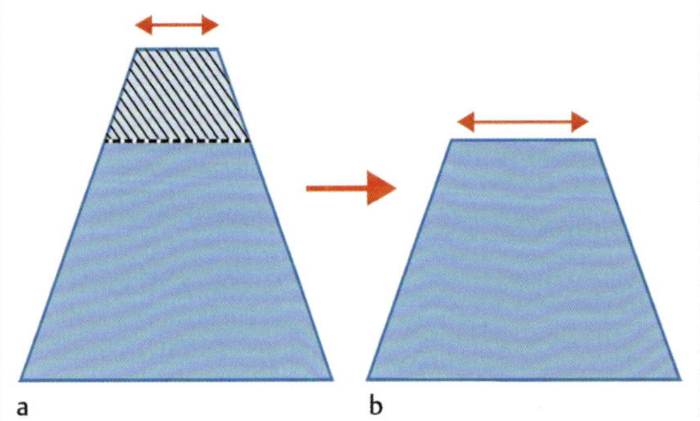

Fig. 8.2 Effect of hump removal on the visual width of the nasal dorsum (schematic cross-section of the nose). Hump removal **(a)** results in a wider appearance of the nasal dorsum, in the absence of other measures **(b)**.

> ✓
>
> I generally recommend that the patient should not be given any preoperative assurance that "the bone will not be fractured." Intraoperative findings may differ from those expected – the nose may appear too wide after hump reduction, and an osteotomy may be required to narrow the nose. Performing an osteotomy despite a promise to the contrary may result in unpleasant legal disputes between patients and physicians (regardless of the cosmetic outcome).

It is not uncommon for patients to come for revision surgery after hump removal without the desirable lateral osteotomies, as the surgeon had either failed to identify the need for this procedure or did not implement it. Such noses may appear excessively wide, and an **"open roof"** may be present. This refers to a condition in which the bony walls stand more or less wide open at the nasal dorsum after hump removal. In these cases, one can often feel the edges of the nasal bones on the bridge of the nose with one's finger under the skin, between which a depression can be felt.

Closure is usually achieved by medialization of the lateral walls of the nose after an osteotomy, failing which the nasal dorsum will lack a bony cover and is only covered by skin. This results in the unsightly palpable or visible "open roof" defect over time, with retraction of the skin into the gaps between the septum and the lateral walls. Such patients also complain of headaches, which only improve after revision surgery to correct this deformity.

The periosteum over the nasal dorsum has to be elevated before the bone in this region can be surgically corrected. The periosteum can be lifted off either together with the skin flap or separately from it. Sharply entering the subperiosteal plane over the bone to expose it while

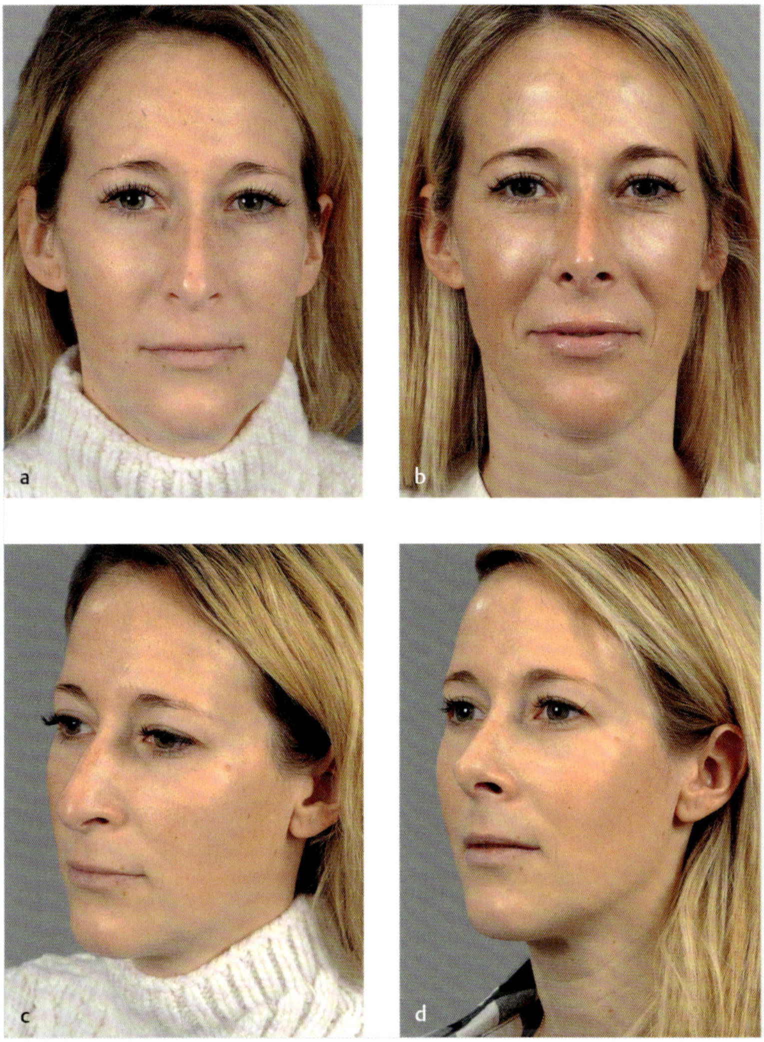

Fig. 8.3 Removal of a narrow hump. A narrow nasal framework that does not require further narrowing with lateral osteotomies after hump removal.
(a, c) Preoperative status. **(b, d)** Postoperative status; also note the improvement in nasal tip rotation after rhinoplasty.

dissecting the skin flap saves time and simplifies the preparation, but cannot be achieved in every case. The periosteum must occasionally be separately elevated, since it is firmly attached to the bone, as in patients with severe scarring who are undergoing revision surgery.

The Joseph raspatory is ideally suited for periosteal elevation (▶ Fig. 8.4, ▶ Fig. 8.5), but a piezoelectric device penetrates a little deeper into the bone for complete removal of the periosteum (see section 8.3).

A bony hump can be removed using an osteotome, a bone rasp, a drill, or a piezoelectric device. Chisels, saws, drills, or piezoelectric devices can be used for osteotomies. The piezoelectric technique described in this chapter has several advantages in comparison with other methods.

The push-down and let-down techniques are used for dorsal preservation, with the dorsal hump basically being lowered along with the nasal framework instead of being resected. This method is discussed separately below (see section 8.4).

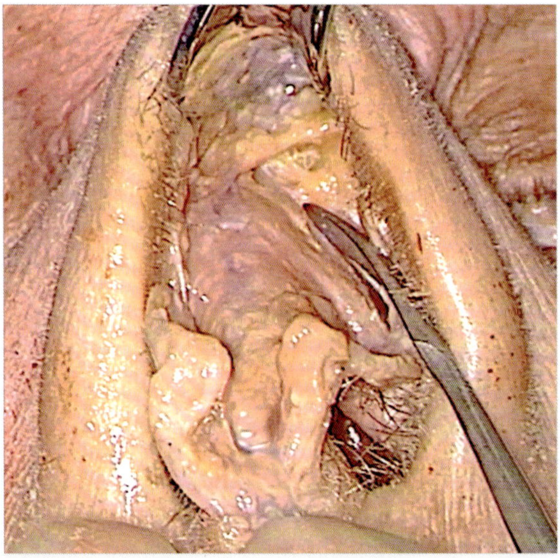

Fig. 8.4 Periosteal elevation using the Joseph raspatory. Open technique; demonstrated in a cadaver specimen.

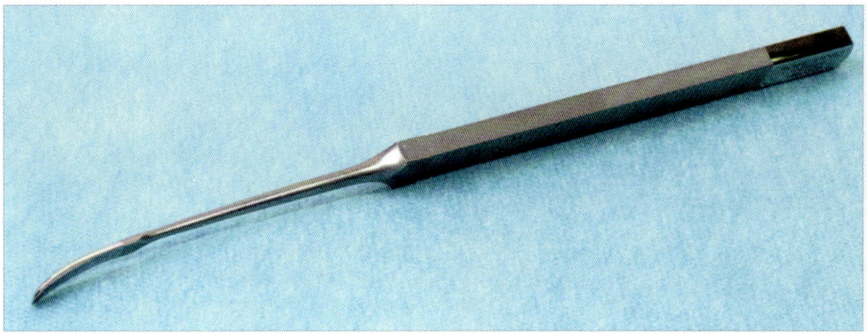

Fig. 8.5 Joseph raspatory (KARL STORZ SE & Co. KG, Tuttlingen, Germany).

8.2 Working with Osteotome, Rasp, and Chisel

> ✓
>
> Even if the piezo technology is preferred, it is strongly recommended that every nose surgeon should also be trained in the use of the classic surgical instruments. Like any other device, the piezo device can fail, and this could lead to problematic situations if the surgeon does not have a “plan B” available in the form of a hammer, chisel, and rasp.

Corrective surgery of the skeletal framework using conventional instruments can be performed using both closed and open access routes. An “extended” open approach is unnecessary and unfeasible.

8.2.1 Conventional Hump Removal Using an Osteotome and Rasp

> ✓
>
> Regardless of whether an open or closed approach is chosen, the handling of osteotome, rasp and chisel does not differ.

Among the conventional instruments, the rasp alone is preferably used to reduce moderate and small humps after the skin has been lifted off and the periosteum elevated. The osteotome is used rarely to first remove an upper layer of bone during reduction of a very large hump (▶ Video 8.1, ▶ Video 8.2). The instrument is then placed horizontally over the caudal edge of the bony hump (▶ Fig. 8.6). The desired height of the bone depends on that of the cartilaginous middle nasal third if this has already been lowered (see Chapter 9). The osteotome can otherwise be used to gently push intact cartilage over the nasal dorsum downward, immediately anterior to the bony interface (▶ Fig. 8.6).

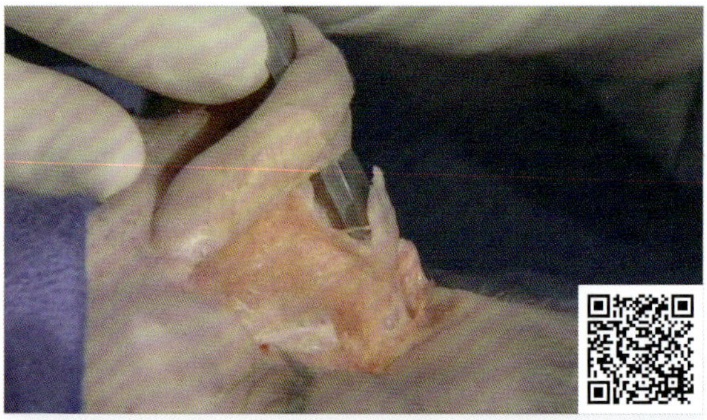

Video 8.1 Hump removal with conventional instruments (cadaver head).

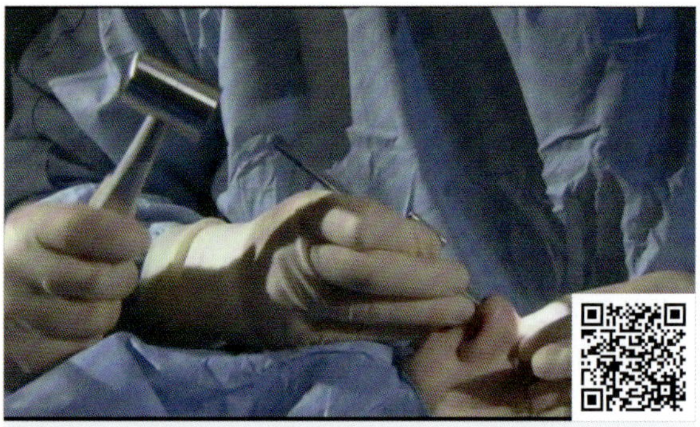

Video 8.2 Hump removal with conventional instruments (clinical case).

In this maneuver, the Rubin osteotome is advantageous (▶ Fig. 8.7). It is gripped between the thumb and forefinger. The working edge of this instrument has rounded shoulders that do not injure the hypodermis.

The objective of this osteotomy is not necessarily complete reduction of the hump in one step, but rather symmetrical removal of most of the bony hump; the final height is then achieved using the piezo technique or a rasp. As a precautionary measure, the osteotome is therefore initially directed at a point above the radix that is somewhat higher than the intended height of the bony nasal dorsum, but never lower.

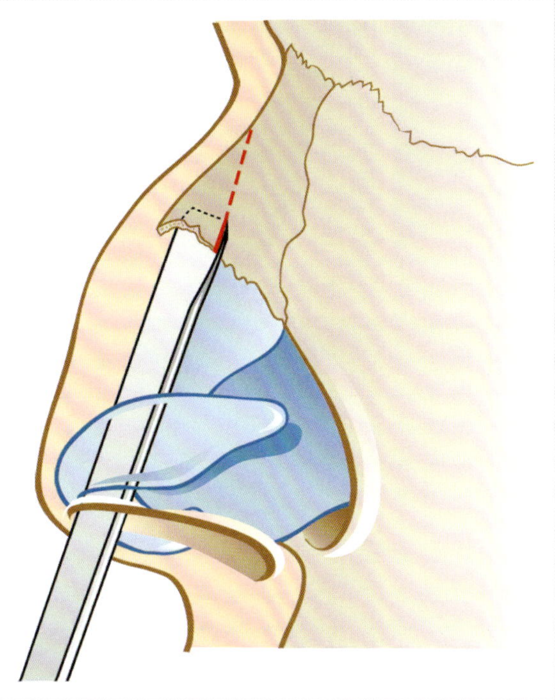

Fig. 8.6 Hump removal with an osteotome. The bony hump is resected at the desired level with the Rubin osteotome. The cartilaginous hump is first pushed down with the instrument, or has already been corrected beforehand.

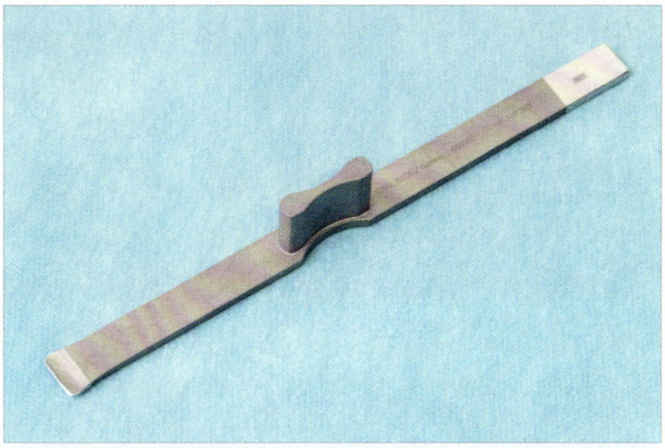

Fig. 8.7 The Rubin osteotome. The osteotome can be well guided by gripping its handle; the rounded "shoulders" at its tip protect the subcutaneous tissue during its passage through the bone (KARL STORZ SE & Co. KG, Tuttlingen, Germany).

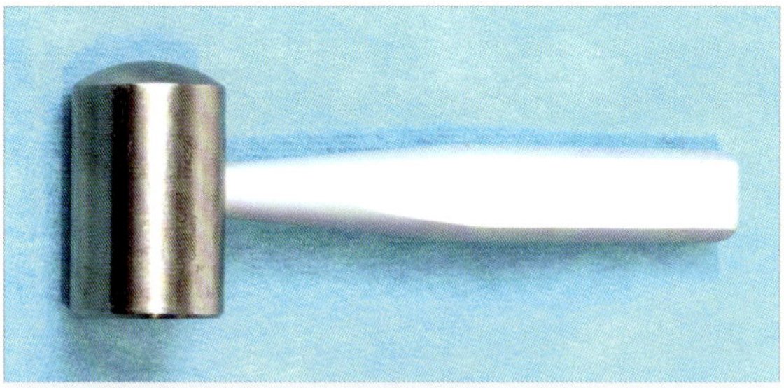

Fig. 8.8 Rhinoplasty osteotomy mallet. Only the side with the flat surface is used for working with the osteotome and chisel (KARL STORZ SE & Co. KG, Tuttlingen, Germany).

✔

Overreduction of the bony nasal dorsum and the cartilaginous framework is far more difficult to correct than undercorrection, either during the primary procedure or at revision surgery. Overcorrection of dorsal humps must therefore be avoided at all costs.

The direction and symmetric position of the instrument is controlled by the surgeon, while the assistant drives it forward – only when instructed to do so by the surgeon – **with two strokes of the flat surface** of a metal mallet (▶ Fig. 8.8; ▶ Fig. 8.9). The assistant is instructed to aim the mallet at the osteotome precisely at a **right angle** so as to advance the instrument in a straight line and in order not to lose the direction (▶ Fig. 8.9a, b).

The slightly widened, rounded shoulders on the head of the Rubin osteotome make it easier for the surgeon to palpate the position and direction of the instrument through the skin with the left thumb and index finger, without fear of injuring subcutaneous tissue (see ▶ Fig. 8.9a).

✔

Rhinoplasty instruments such as osteotomes and chisels cut through bone easily and smoothly only if they are very sharp. These instruments must therefore be sharpened before each use, and a whetstone (Arkansas stone) should ideally be available on the instrument table (▶ Fig. 8.10).

The resected hump can be removed with an instrument such as the Blakesley nasal forceps (see ▶ Fig. 5.4) once the osteotomy is complete.

Further procedures such as the correction of minor irregularities or controlled, continued lowering of the nasal dorsum are performed with a coarse or fine rasp, or a diamond rasp (▶ Fig. 8.11, ▶ Fig. 8.12a, b, ▶ Fig. 8.13). Small bony humps are only reduced with a rasp, rather than an osteotome. This allows far more controlled and stepwise removal.

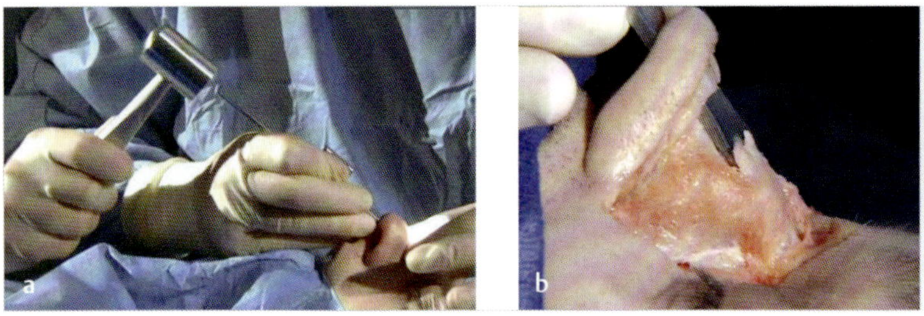

Fig. 8.9 Hump removal. (a) Hump removal with osteotome and mallet. The mallet hits the chisel at right angles; the assistant only strikes twice, at every request of the surgeon. **(b)** Hump removal demonstrated in a cadaver specimen after removal of the skin.

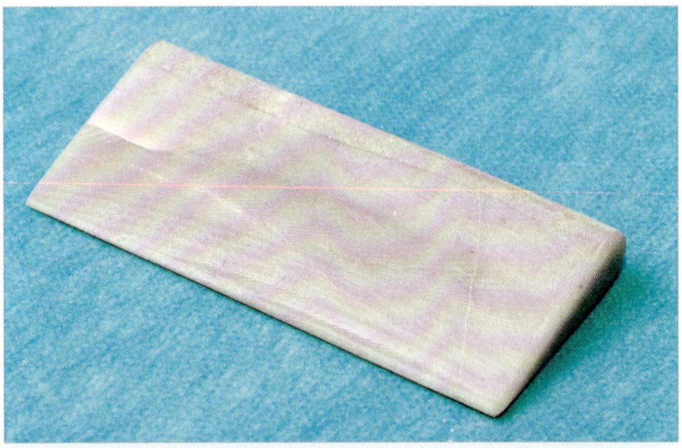

Fig. 8.10 Whetstone for the chisel. The sterilizable stone is used to resharpen chisels immediately before use (KARL STORZ SE & Co. KG, Tuttlingen, Germany).

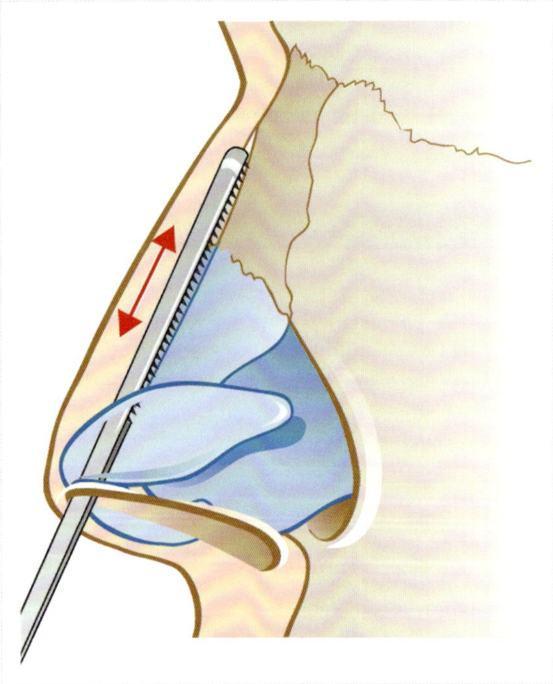

Fig. 8.11 Working on the bony nasal dorsum with the rasp. The rasp, which should be as sharp as possible, should be used with straight, pulling movements, and the outcome should be repeatedly rechecked visually and by palpation with a moistened glove. Overcorrection must be avoided.

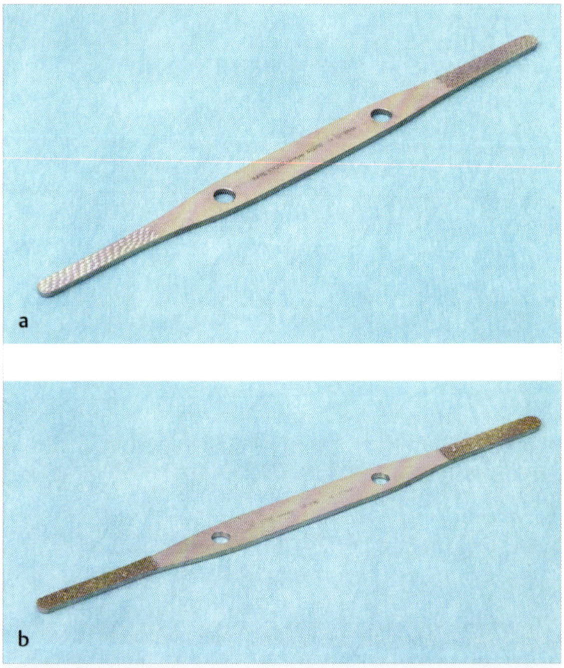

Fig. 8.12 Rasps. (a) Fine and coarse rasps (KARL STORZ SE & Co. KG, Tuttlingen, Germany). **(b)** Diamond rasp (KARL STORZ SE & Co. KG, Tuttlingen, Germany).

8.2.2 Paramedian, Lateral, and Intermediate Osteotomies Using the Chisel

The purpose of osteotomies of the nasal bones is to mobilize the lateral nasal walls toward the midline – i.e., to bring them closer together, thus narrowing the nasal framework. This is usually necessary if a nose is too wide to start with, or if it appears too wide after hump removal. Symmetrical osteotomies are usually performed, and an asymmetrical procedure may be appropriate only in patients with crooked noses (regardless of the technique used; see section 19.1).

A chisel was classically used for osteotomy in rhinoplasty for decades. It is primarily guided by palpation under the skin during the closed and open techniques, rather than under direct vision as is the case with

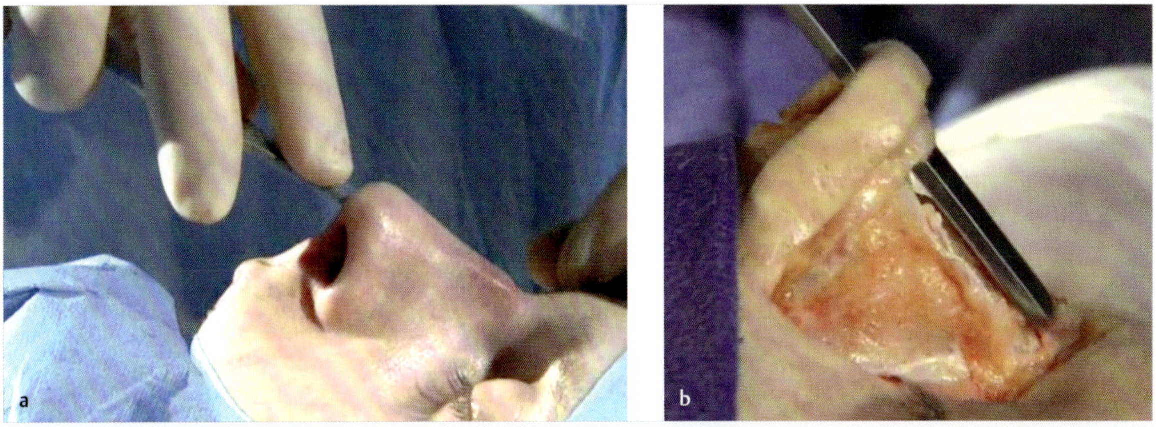

Fig. 8.13 **Working with the rasp. (a)** Handling a rasp (in the closed approach). Manipulated bone cannot be directly visualized, in contrast to the piezo technique with the open approach. **(b)** Working with the rasp on a cadaver specimen after removal of the skin.

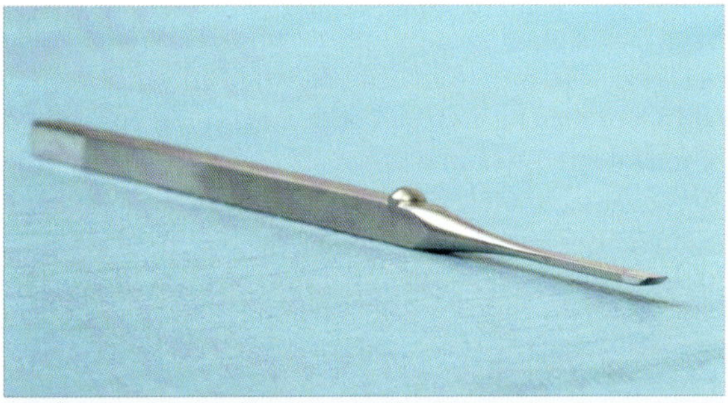

Fig. 8.14 This **3-mm chisel** is preferable for osteotomies (KARL STORZ SE & Co. KG, Tuttlingen, Germany).

piezoelectric osteotomy (see section 8.3.2). A chisel with symmetrically sharpened edges is commonly referred to as an "osteotome" in rhinosurgery. A chisel with a beveled edge will easily follow an oblique path through bone when advanced with the mallet. Such chisels are particularly suitable for oblique or arcuately curved incisions.

I do not recommend chisels that have a "nose" at the tip. Although transcutaneous palpation is facilitated while guiding the instrument through bone, such devices may give rise to subcutaneous tissue trauma, excessive bleeding, and more postoperative swelling of the facial soft tissues.

Chisels 3 mm wide without a guiding nose are preferable (▶ Fig. 8.14). A 4-mm wide instrument may be rarely required for very dense bones. These chisels have a small knob on the handle, which facilitates targeted advancement of the instrument through bone.

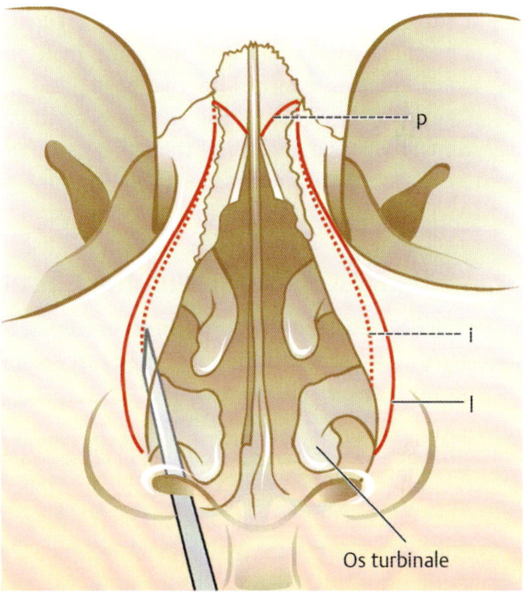

Fig. 8.15 Paramedian, lateral, and intermediate osteotomies using the chisel. The paramedian (p) and lateral (l) osteotomies meet at the level of the medial canthus or just below it. If necessary, an intermediate osteotomy (i) needs to be made before the lateral one.

Using a chisel, two osteotomy lines are combined for complete fracture of the nasal bones: the paramedian and the lateral osteotomy (▶ Fig. 8.15). It should be noted that complete osteotomy of the nasal wall results in a completely mobile bone fragment, which in principle is at risk of "falling" into the nasal cavity in the absence of any support.

Although this is an infrequent occurrence, the associated risk of unwanted overcorrection during hump reduction should not be underestimated. It is therefore crucial during chisel osteotomies to ensure that the fragment to be osteotomized is adequately adherent to the overlying soft tissues of the lateral nose, to prevent uncontrolled descent into the nasal lumen. This contrasts with piezoelectric surface osteoplasty, which usually requires complete exposure of bone.

The soft tissues are therefore only pushed off the nasal dorsum, rather than the bony lateral walls, during hump removal with a chisel, and only to the extent necessary for manipulation of the bone forming the nasal dorsum. The soft tissues and periosteum remain intact over the bone at the lateral aspect, allowing the lateral osteotomies to be blindly performed with the chisel under the skin, which remains attached to the bone like in a "closed" approach (see Chapter 16). The chisel osteotomy is very similar for open and closed rhinoplasty, but with regard to clear viewing differs considerably from the extended open approach using the piezo technique.

8

Paramedian Osteotomy Using the Chisel

The paramedian osteotomy using the beveled edge of the chisel starts in the paraseptal space of the nasal dorsum, in the angle between the septum and the (separated) upper lateral cartilage (paraseptal cleft), with the cutting edge on the outside and the beveled side in close contact with the septum. The paramedian osteotomy then follows the septum, initially in a straight line parallel to the midline in the direction of the nasal radix (▶ Video 8.3; ▶ Fig. 8.15, ▶ Fig. 8.16, ▶ Fig. 8.17a, b).

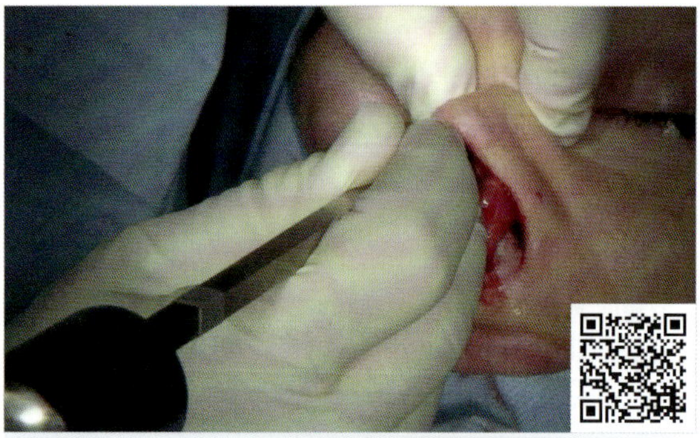

Video 8.3 Conventional paramedian and lateral osteotomies with the open technique (clinical case).

In order to obtain a straight incision, the surgeon has to grip the chisel handle at a slightly outwardly inclined angle. The assistant hits the end of the chisel twice with the flat surface of the mallet at a right angle, only when instructed by the surgeon – as is the case with hump removal (▶ Fig. 8.17a, b; see also ▶ Fig. 8.9a). The chisel is then turned slightly laterally in an arc before reaching the level of the medial canthus. The left index finger palpates the position and direction of the chisel through the skin. The surgeon then lifts the handle, which is still directed outward, progressively toward the midline in order to move the tip of the chisel further laterally.

The highest point of the osteotomy is just above the medial canthus, which in principle completes the classic paramedian osteotomy. However, the paramedian osteotomy may be continued as an upper lateral osteotomy from this point by turning the cutting edge of the instrument (without removing or reinserting it) from the inside out. The chisel is then guided under palpation from top to bottom in a lateral direction until roughly the upper third of the lateral osteotomy line is also severed (▶ Fig. 8.18). The advantage of this approach is that only a short lateral osteotomy is required for completion of the osteotomy lines.

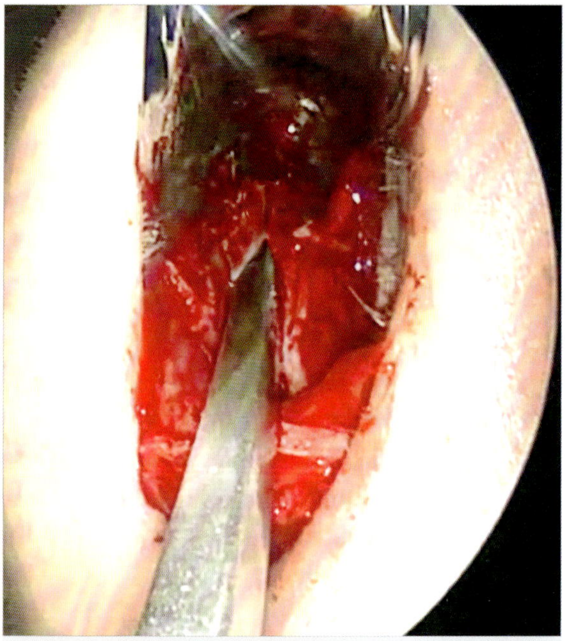

Fig. 8.16 Left paramedian osteotomy, intraoperative view. The paramedian osteotomy is carried out in a line right next to the septum. The chisel is placed exactly at the site of separation of the upper lateral cartilage from the septum.

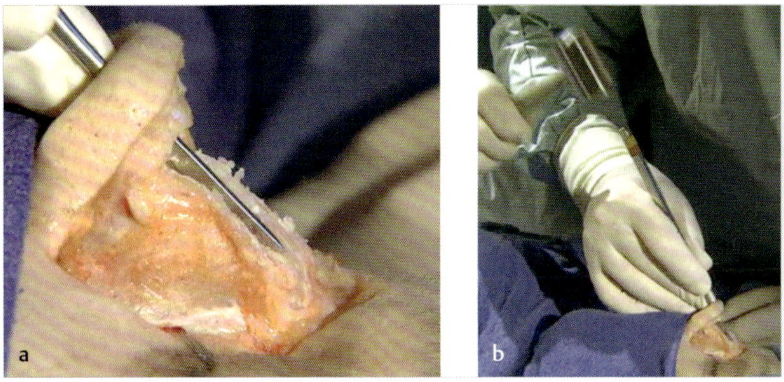

Fig. 8.17 Guiding the chisel during paramedian osteotomy. (a) The chisel severs the bone in a straight line right next to the septum before turning laterally at the level of the medial canthus. **(b)** The assistant hammers with moderate blows as instructed by the surgeon. Demonstrated in a cadaver specimen after removal of the skin.

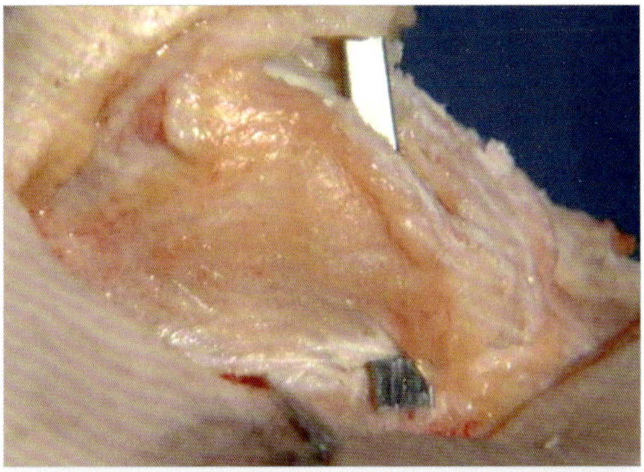

Fig. 8.18 Paramedian and superolateral osteotomy. The chisel is advanced to complete the upper segment of the lateral osteotomy after completion of the paramedian osteotomy. Demonstrated in a cadaver specimen after removal of the skin.

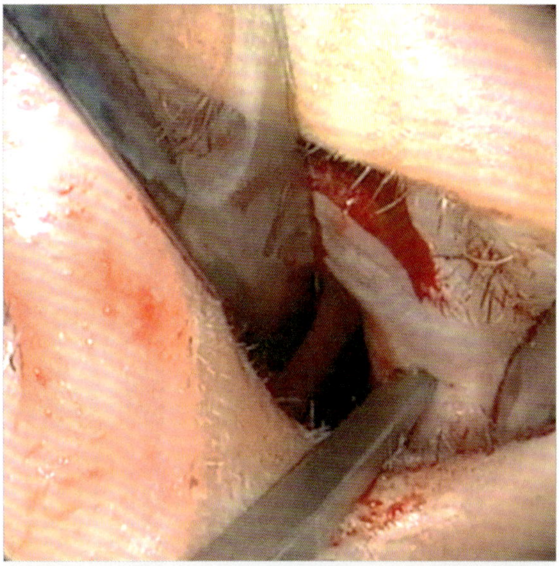

Fig. 8.19 Lateral osteotomy. In both the open and closed access routes, the lateral osteotomy starts at the edge of the piriform aperture at the level of the head of the inferior turbinate.

Lateral Osteotomy Using the Chisel

A lateral osteotomy is a controlled fracture of the lateral nasal bone (or bony lateral nasal wall), which meets the paramedian osteotomy at its cranial aspect, in order to completely mobilize and then medialize the lateral nasal bones (see ▶ Fig. 8.15). A lateral osteotomy with a sharp 3-mm chisel starts at the edge of the piriform aperture at the level of the head of the inferior turbinate (▶ Video 8.3; ▶ Fig. 8.19).

The cutting edge of the chisel is placed medially, the bevel laterally. The instrument must be very sharp – this facilitates severing of the vestibular skin overlying the piriform aperture, and an initial separate scalpel incision can be dispensed with. Prior tunneling to elevate soft tissue and the underlying periosteum along the osteotomy line should be omitted; it is more traumatic than cutting through the bone with a thin-bladed, sharp chisel. The chisel again has a small button-like elevation on the shaft, which marks the sharp end of the instrument, while providing a guide for the right thumb (see ▶ Fig. 8.14).

The starting point for the osteotomy is not at the most lateral point of the lateral circumference of the piriform aperture, but slightly above it. A small, intact bony triangle at the base of the piriform aperture (highlighted in blue in ▶ Fig. 8.20) is named after R. Webster. Keeping it untouched helps avoid excessive narrowing of the nasal entrance as a result of the osteotomy and the subsequent medially directed shift of the bone.

The incision then continues within the lateral nasal wall, initially a little laterally toward the frontal process and facial surface of the maxilla, and then about halfway over the total distance turns again craniomedially ("high–low–high osteotomy"; see ▶ Fig. 8.15).

The bone usually fractures completely before the lateral osteotomy reaches the level of the medial canthus, since with my preferred approach the upper third of the lateral osteotomy has already been completed with the paramedian osteotomy (see ▶ Fig. 8.18). The chisel is otherwise advanced up to the radix of the nose in the manner already described – with blows from the assistant's mallet – until it meets the upper extension of the paramedian osteotomy running obliquely and laterally. It is not uncommon for a complete osteotomy to be identified by a change in the sound of mallet blows.

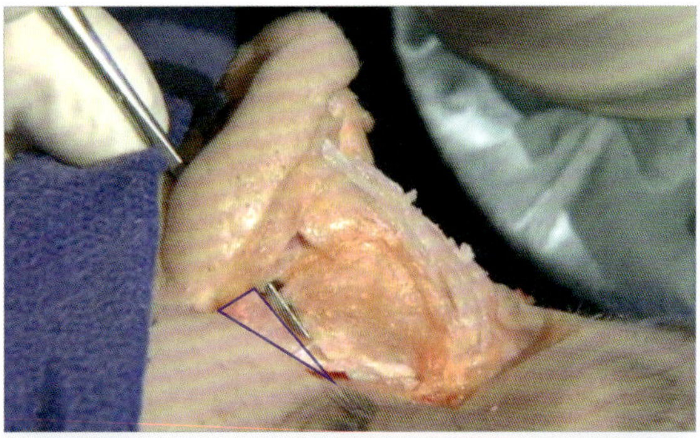

Fig. 8.20 Lateral osteotomy, Webster triangle. Lateral osteotomy with the chisel (demonstrated in a cadaver specimen after removal of the skin). The small bony triangle at the base of the piriform aperture (highlighted in blue) is named after R. Webster.

The completeness of osteotomies is checked by the surgeon by withdrawing the instrument and verifying the mobility of the bony nasal walls using both hands. This may result in a desirable fracture of residual bone between the osteotomy lines, which completes this step. On the other hand, if the fragments can neither be mobilized nor fractured, the osteotomy is still considered incomplete and the chisel has to be reinserted.

Fracturing bones along undesirable, unintended lines represents a real risk in chisel osteotomies, with unintentionally dislodged bone fragments requiring corrective procedures of the nasal dorsum. This risk is significantly lower using the piezo technique. However, this does not imply that excellent results cannot be achieved with a chisel and rasp (▶ Fig. 8.21a, b, ▶ Fig. 8.23a–d). What matters most is

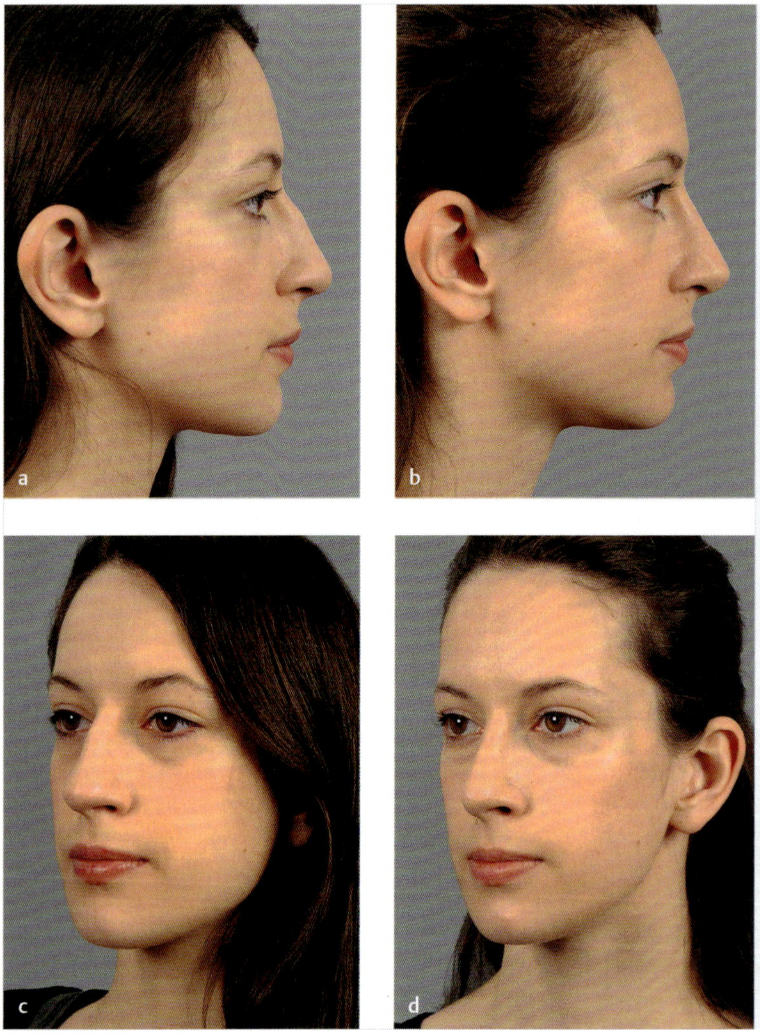

Fig. 8.21 Hump nose. (a, c) Nasal hump before surgery. **(b, d)** Postoperative status following endonasal correction with conventional instruments. (For correction of the tip in this patient, see also section 12.2.1, ▶ Fig. 12.19a, b).

8

that the surgeon should select the instruments that he or she is most comfortable with in a given case.

Palpable or visible edges along the lateral nasal slope following osteotomies can be carefully reworked with the chisel, but again not as efficiently and elegantly as with the piezo technique.

Intermediate Osteotomy

If the surgeon thinks a lateral osteotomy has been positioned far too medially, a second, slightly more lateral osteotomy may then be performed. The first is then the "intermediate" osteotomy, while the second is the actual "lateral" osteotomy (see ▶ Fig. 8.15, ▶ Fig. 8.22).

> ✓
>
> An intermediate osteotomy can be planned from the outset in patients with marked bulging of the lateral nasal wall or unusually large noses, so that the two lateral osteotomies give rise to a harmonious nasal slope (▶ Fig. 8.23a–d).

It goes without saying that the intermediate osteotomy is performed before the lateral osteotomy, since the latter gives rise to a mobile piece of bone that cannot be reworked using a chisel.

Postprocessing and fine work on the bone, if needed, continues until the final height of the nasal dorsum is achieved under visual guidance and palpation, using an instrument such as a fine diamond rasp (see ▶ Fig. 8.12b).

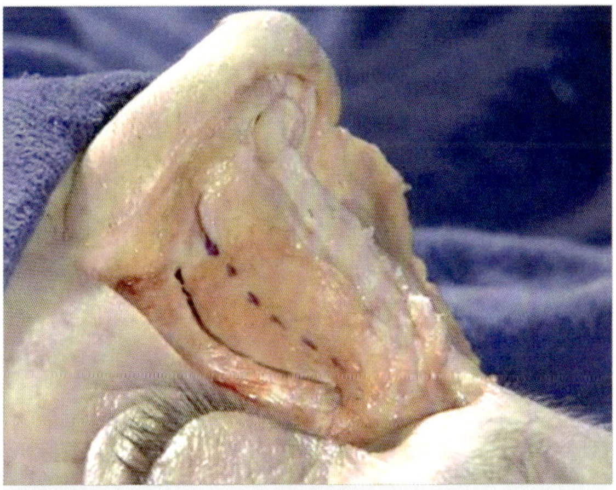

Fig. 8.22 Intermediate osteotomy. The dotted line between the medial (not marked) and the lateral osteotomy (solid line) indicates the course of an intermediate osteotomy.

This may be difficult if the osteotomies have resulted in excessively mobile lateral bony walls. The bones of the nasal dorsum may then be firmly gripped from the outside with one hand, while a rasp is simultaneously inserted under the skin. Again, the rhinoplasty mirror is very useful for determining the final nasal dorsal profile line (see ▶ Fig. 4.5a–c, ▶ Fig. 8.32).

8.3 The Piezo Technique

Surgical piezoelectric devices work on the principle of ultrasonic oscillation, with a frequency of over 20 kHz transmitted to a handpiece, which can be equipped with different inserts as required. I use the Piezosurgery Flex device (mectron s.p.a., Carasco, Italy), to which the following explanations and descriptions refer (▶ Fig. 8.24, ▶ Fig. 8.25).

> ✓
>
> Both disposable and reusable inserts are available. Disposable ones are recommended, as they are consistently effective. The surgeon's choice of insert may also depend on whether their work is governed by regulations that prescribe disposable instruments.

The high-frequency oscillating inserts cut or ablate hard tissue only (bone, hard cartilage) (▶ Video 8.4, ▶ Video 8.5). Soft tissue is not affected by the piezo technique, meaning that there is less risk of damage to vessels, nerves, and subcutaneous layers.

An integrated water irrigation system is required for cooling the handpiece, and it also cools tissue while flushing the surgical field. The sterile saline solution used for irrigation must be continuously suctioned. This is facilitated by a suction device integrated into the Aufricht retractor (▶ Fig. 8.26a) (suction retractor, Marina Medical Instruments Inc.). Alternatively, the irrigation fluid can be constantly suctioned off by an assistant, or by the operating room nurse using a separate suction device. Suction tubes should be equipped with a perforated plate to allow prompt interruption of the process if necessary (if tissue adheres to the tube, for instance) (▶ Fig. 8.26b).

The entire nasal framework – i.e., both nasal bones and the adjacent frontal process of the maxilla on either side – must be exposed laterally beyond the planned lateral osteotomies to allow hump removal, thinning of bone, and piezoelectric osteotomies. This **extended open approach**

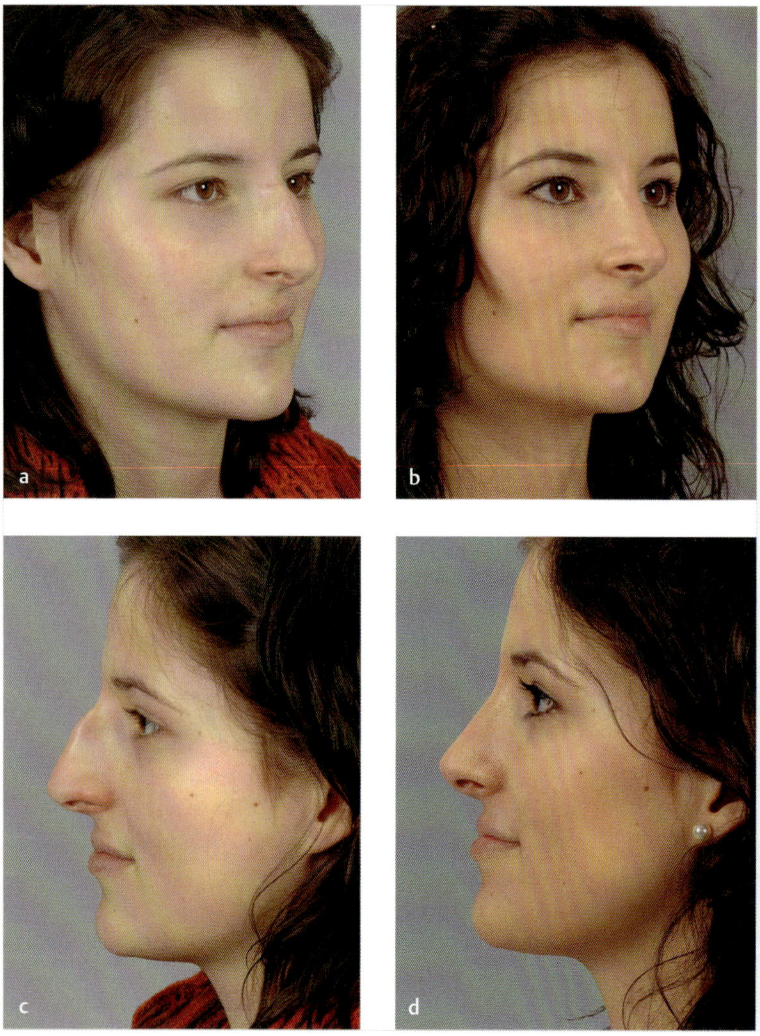

Fig. 8.23 Large, asymmetrical hump nose. **(a, c)** A large, asymmetrical hump nose. **(b, d)** Postoperative status following endonasal correction with conventional instruments, intermediate and lateral osteotomies.

8

using the piezo technique may be new to surgeons who are accustomed to classic instruments and less extensive elevation of the skin, but they are soon convinced of its advantages (▶ Fig. 8.27).

8.3.1 Hump Removal Using Piezo Technology (Osteoplasty)

The bone, and thus the hump, is removed using the MP1 (disposable) insert of the piezosurgery device. My surgical teams have termed this insert a "planer," as it achieves layered ablation of the surface (▶ Fig. 8.28, ▶ Fig. 8.29). The advantage of this instrument is its extraordinary precision. It also has a straight edge for even bone removal on the nasal dorsum and lateral aspects, in contrast to the round surface of a drill or a milling cutter. The medical industry is constantly developing new, more advanced attachments; interested users should keep themselves informed.

✓

Work is always carried out with good direct vision in the extended open approach using the piezoelectric device, provided that the irrigation fluid is continuously suctioned off directly at the tip of the instrument. This is a great advantage in comparison with the rasp, which inevitably obscures the bone on which work is being done.

The dorsal hump is reduced up to the desired level with the piezoelectric device, using very light pressure with pushing or pulling movements (▶ Video 8.4, ▶ Video 8.5; see ▶ Fig. 8.28). The orienting anatomical landmarks are the nasal radix cranially and the cartilaginous nasal framework caudally.

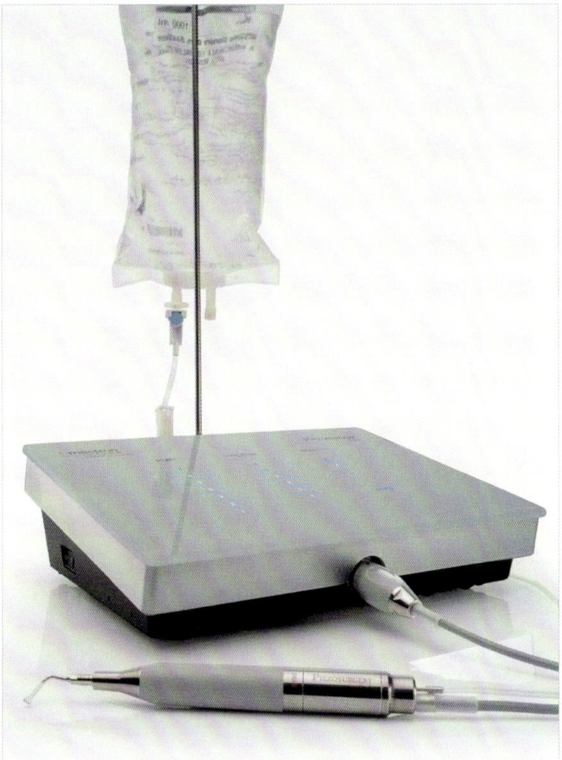

Fig. 8.24 Piezo surgery control unit and handpiece (irrigation system not shown). (Copyright mectron s.p.a., Carasco/Genoa, Italy. Reprinted with permission.)

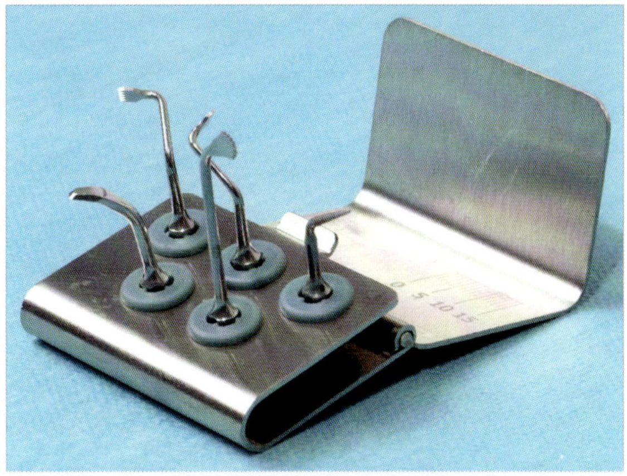

Fig. 8.25 Piezo inserts. The set with inserts most commonly used for the piezo technique (mectron s.p.a., Carasco/Genoa, Italy).

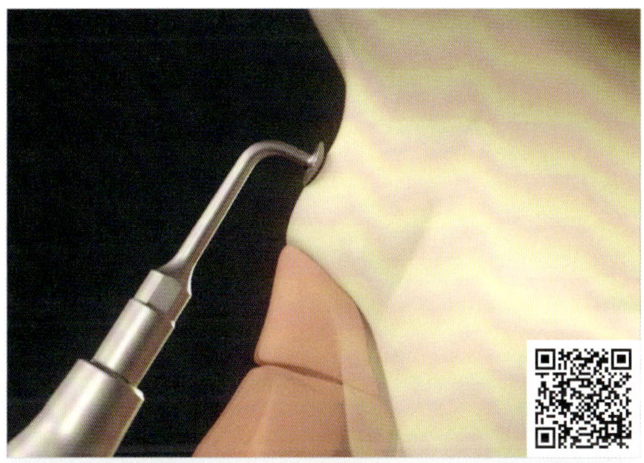

Video 8.4 Piezo technique in rhinoplasty (animated movie). (Copyright mectron s.p.a., Carasco/Genoa, Italy. Reprinted with permission.)

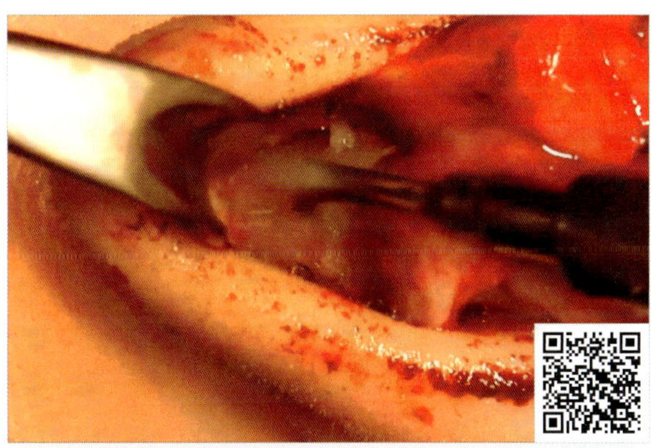

Video 8.5 Use of piezo instruments to correct the bony dorsum (clinical case).

Typical in this type of dorsal reduction is the exposure of progressively larger areas of the cartilaginous framework in the K-area of the nasal dorsum with progressive bone removal. The cartilage framework with the septum and attached upper lateral cartilages slides cranially to varying degrees under the bone (▶ Fig. 8.30). The piezo technique can also be used to elegantly thin wide nasal bones; lateral osteotomies can thus be dispensed with in suitable cases (▶ Fig. 8.31).

In addition to the direct visualization of the nasal dorsum, its desired height is repeatedly checked by palpation with a moistened glove over the index finger after temporary withdrawal of the Aufricht retractor and replacement of the skin. I also keep an eye on changes in the nasal profile in the rhinoplasty mirror across from me (▶ Fig. 8.32). Once the desired level has been reached, it is time for the lateral osteotomies. These can be dispensed with if the bony nasal framework is narrow (or has been thinned out using the piezo technique; see ▶ Fig. 8.31).

Correction of the height of the **cartilaginous** nasal framework follows in a later procedural step (see Chapter 9).

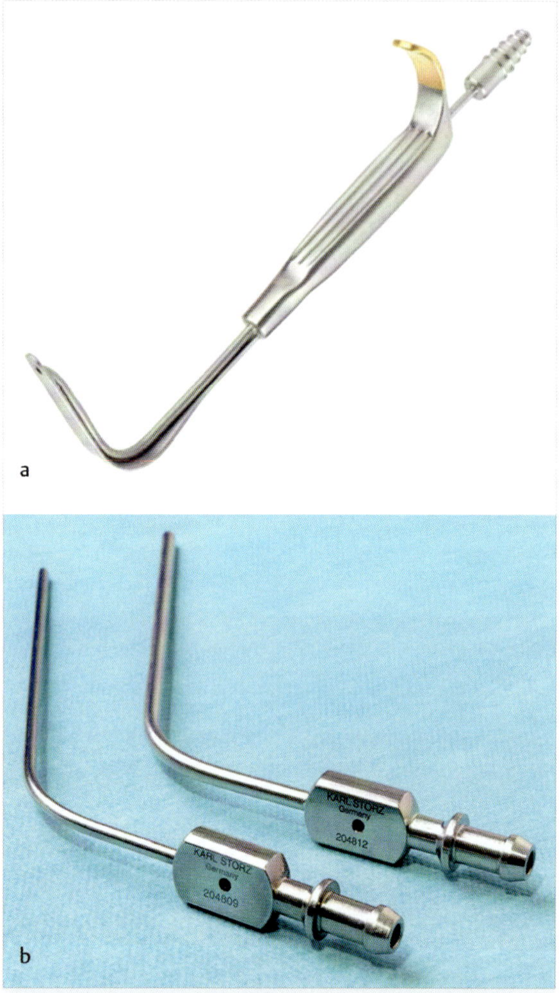

Fig. 8.26 Suction tubing. (a) Aufricht retractor with an integrated suction tube. ("Gerbault Suction Retractor," copyright Marina Medical Inc., Davie, Florida, USA. Reprinted with permission.) **(b)** Angled suction tubes in two sizes, with interrupter plate (KARL STORZ SE & Co. KG, Tuttlingen, Germany).

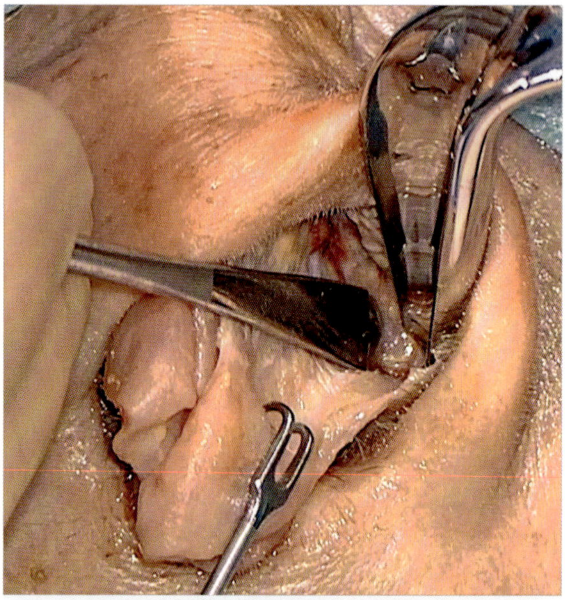

Fig. 8.27 Extended open approach. Periosteal elevation at the lateral aspect using the Freer elevator (sharp end; cadaver specimen) (see also ▶ Fig. 7.7). The vertical piriform attachments are severed (compare with ▶ Fig. 1.17).

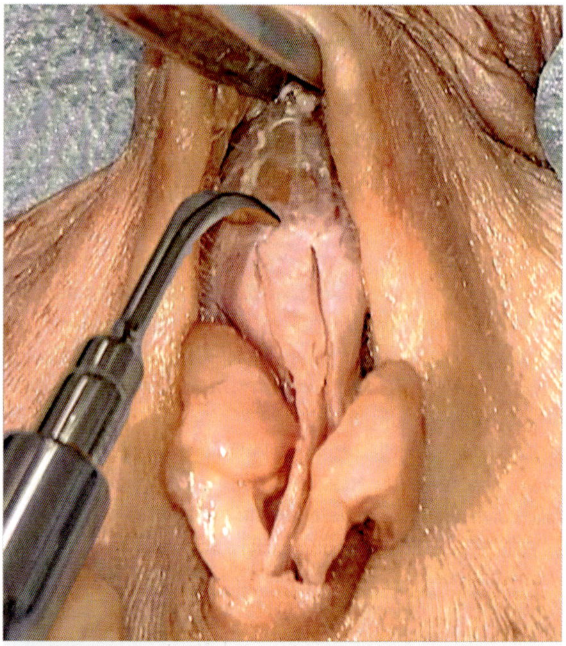

Fig. 8.28 Piezo technique. Hump removal using a "planer." Demonstrated in a cadaver specimen.

8.3.2 Piezoelectric Osteotomy with Surface Osteoplasty

✔

The aim of the procedure described here is to turn the bony side wall of the nose into a cranially pedunculated bone element that can be bent towards the middle in order to narrow the nose. In contrast to the procedure with the chisel, the bony side wall should not be completely cut around.

Safe use of the piezo technique in lateral osteotomies requires good exposure of the bones forming the nasal wall, extending from the nasal dorsum via the frontal process of the maxilla to the piriform aperture (*extended* open approach). If a closed access route is used for this procedure, which I do not recommend, adequate flushing must be reliably ensured in the narrow tissue tunnel in which one is working to avoid a thermal lesion of the subcutaneous tissue.

The osteotomy starts at the piriform aperture at the level of the insertion of the inferior turbinate. It follows the border between the nasal slope and the frontal process of the maxilla in a slight, laterally convex arc, but does not extend laterally into the maxilla (▶ Fig. 8.33, ▶ Fig. 8.34). It does not quite reach the level of the medial canthus cranially; the osteotomy then arches progressively toward the midline at this point, running at an angle of approximately 90° toward the edge of the nasal dorsum, which it usually stops short of.

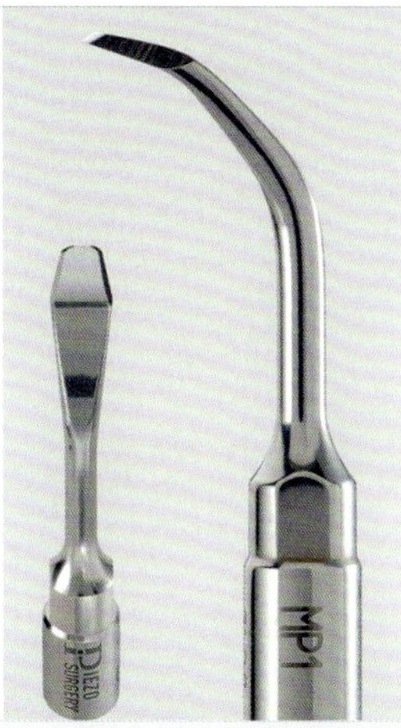

Fig. 8.29 The MP1 piezo insert – a disposable piezo "planer." (Copyright mectron s.p.a., Carasco/Genoa, Italy. Reprinted with permission.)

Specially designed, double-angled piezo inserts are recommended for lateral osteotomies, without which precision osteotomy to the lateral nasal wall is more difficult (▶ Video 8.4, ▶ Video 8.5; ▶ Fig. 8.34, ▶ Fig. 8.35). However, a straight vertical saw can also be used (see ▶ Fig. 8.39).

The classic combination of complete paramedian and lateral osteotomies that is commonly performed when hammer and chisel are used is not routinely carried out when a piezoelectric device is used. In contrast to the usual approach with hammer and chisel, the goal when using the piezo technique in some patients with a relatively narrow nasal bone and low hump is to achieve an isolated, somewhat shortened lateral osteotomy. Here the bony lateral wall remains attached at its mediocranial aspect to the nasal bone (see ▶ Fig. 8.33).

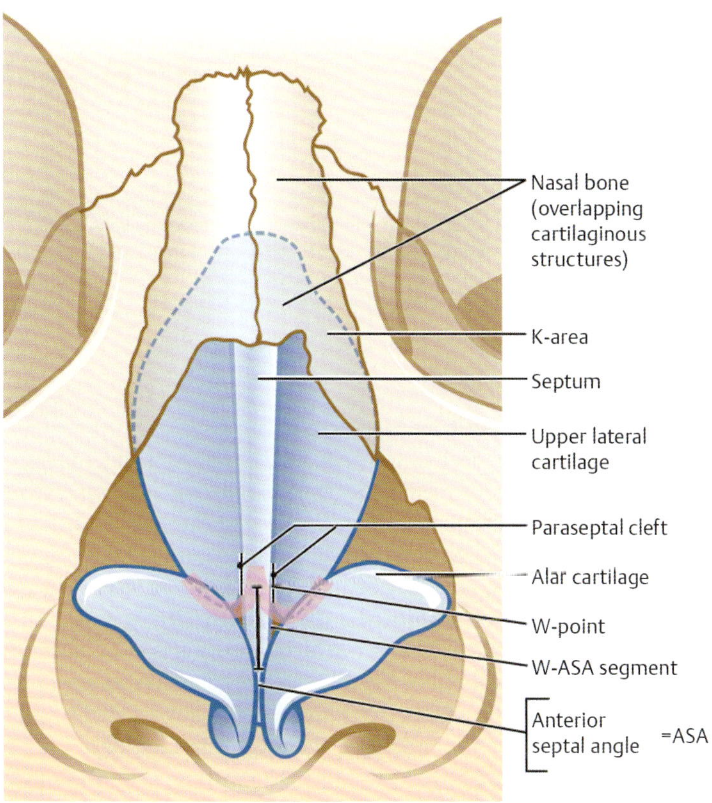

Fig. 8.30 Anatomy of the "K-area." A dorsal keystone area can be distinguished from the lateral keystone areas. Cartilage is increasingly exposed as the bone is removed at the site of overlap of bone and cartilage.

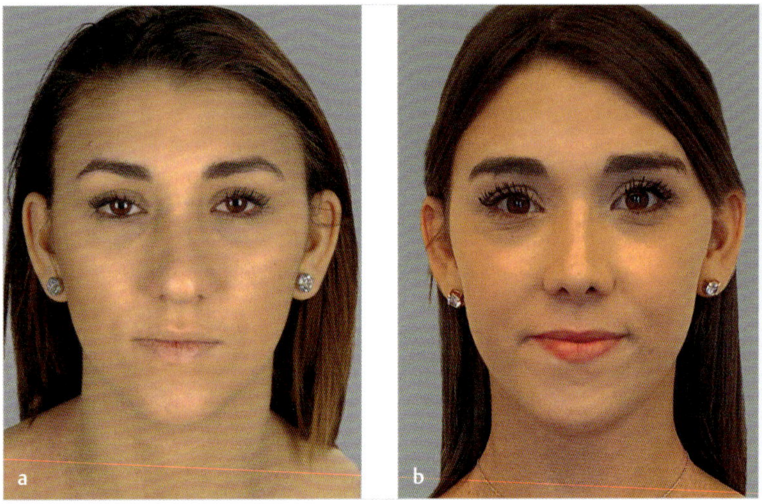

Fig. 8.31 Nasal dorsum correction without an osteotomy; case study. (a) Preoperative status. **(b)** Three years after rhinoplasty including hump removal with lateral thinning of the skeletal framework, without osteotomies.

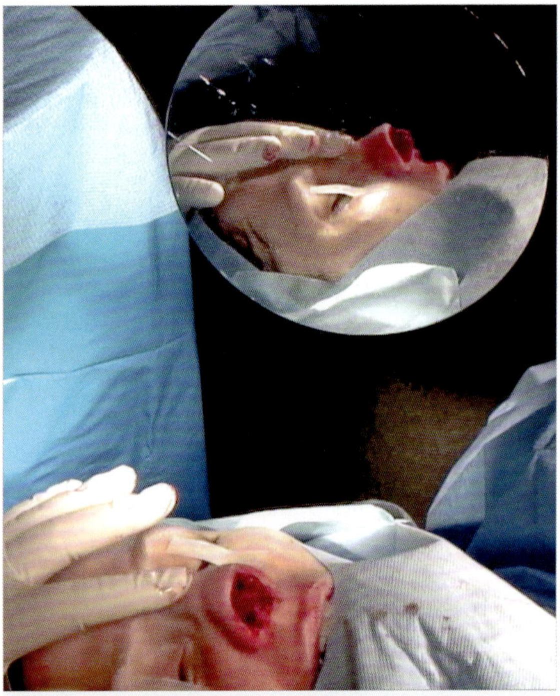

Fig. 8.32 Rhinoplasty mirror with holder. Palpatory examination of the nasal dorsal profile; visualization in the rhinoplasty mirror (see also ▶ Fig. 4.5a–c).

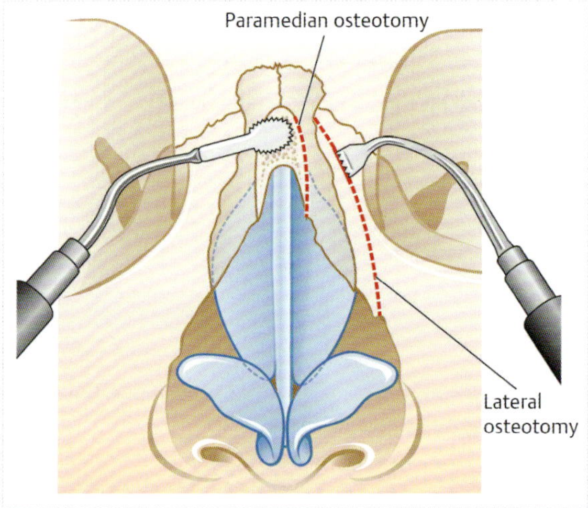

Fig. 8.33 Lateral and paramedian osteotomy with piezo technique (diagram). The lateral osteotomy extends from the piriform aperture to the lateral edge of the nasal dorsum. A short paramedian osteotomy may be added.

The lateral osteotomy is thus extended medially only far enough to facilitate deflection of the lateral nasal wall toward the midline while it remains attached to the nasal bone at its cranial aspect. This gives rise to a "bone flap" that is pedicled craniomedially on the nasal dorsum, which is rotated toward the midline to narrow the nose (▶ Fig. 8.36).

If the bone is severed with the piezo instrument, there is no need to worry about damaging the inner lining and mucous membrane. On the contrary, it is imperative to ensure that incisions made with the saw inserts of the piezoelectric device completely sever the thickness of the bone. Bony fragments remain immobile if these incisions are too superficial and incomplete. The bone is palpated with the Freer elevator to ensure it can be adequately medialized (▶ Fig. 8.37). In rare cases, a (shortened) paramedian piezoelectric osteotomy may be added (using the UNIVR insert) to facilitate medialization of dense nasal bones (▶ Fig. 8.38, ▶ Fig. 8.39). Strong bone at the lateral edge of the nasal dorsum can also be carefully thinned to

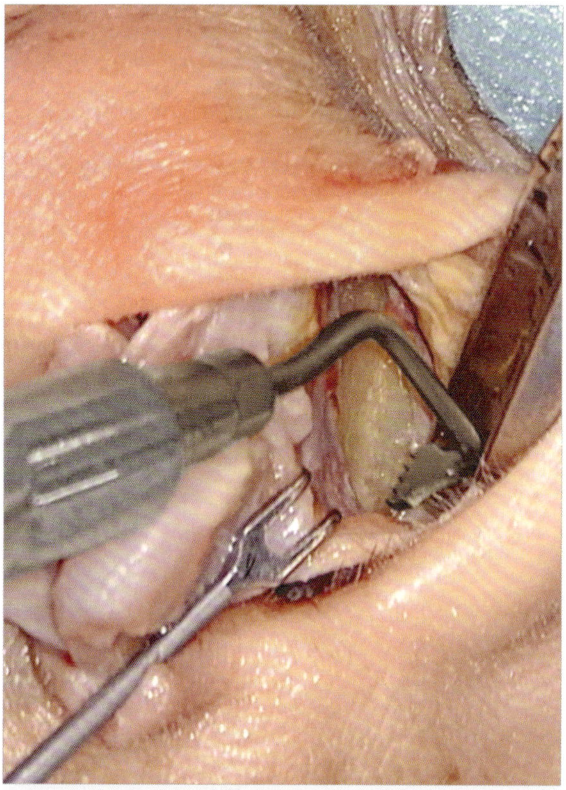

Fig. 8.34 Left lateral osteotomy with the piezo technique, angled insert MT2L-4.

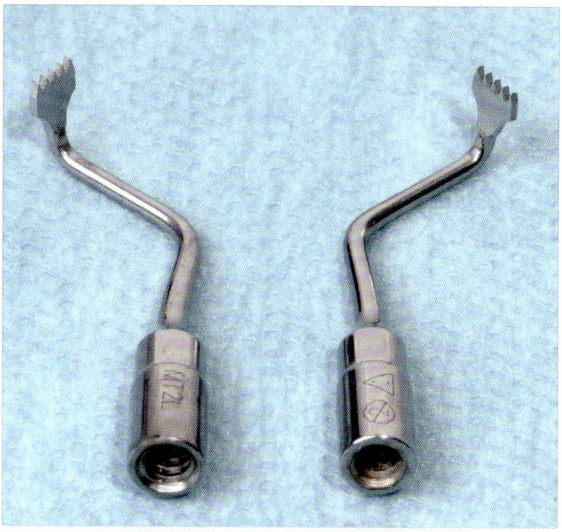

Fig. 8.35 Piezo inserts for right and left lateral osteotomy (mectron s.p.a., Carasco/Genoa, Italy).

facilitate bending, or to achieve the desired narrowing of the nasal dorsum.

> ✔
>
> The one great advantage of piezoelectric devices over conventional techniques is that they cut precisely through bone and do not give rise to bony splinters or undesired fracture lines. The risk of asymmetry and irregularities of the nasal dorsum is significantly reduced by not completely cutting around and mobilizing bony side walls, while ensuring better stability of the skeletal framework.

Visible edges along the osteotomy line and any other irregularities in the bony nasal framework are smoothed using the planer insert of the piezo device (MP1) (▶ Fig. 8.40).

Complete lateral and paramedian osteotomies, connected at their cranial ends and resulting in completely mobile lateral nasal walls, may be unavoidable in a very few cases when there is a particularly dense bony nasal framework. Since the bones forming the lateral nasal wall are no longer adherent to the overlying skin with the extended open approach, there is a theoretical risk that complete dissection around the nasal wall may cause the bone to “fall” into the nasal cavity, causing the nasal wall to collapse. However, the inner mucosal lining and parts of the inner periosteum of the nasal bones remain intact during a well-performed piezoelectric osteotomy, unlike a chisel osteotomy; the bony walls thus do not necessarily collapse into the nasal lumen, even with complete medial and lateral osteotomies. Nevertheless, complete lateral and paramedian osteotomies that are connected to each other are not the goal of the procedure described here.

The medialized, narrowed nasal walls are secured using a transverse mattress suture with 3–0 PDS thread, passed through boreholes. Two continuous boreholes through both lateral bony walls and the septum are usually sufficient. I use a drilling or finishing insert with the piezo handpiece for drilling (MF4; ▶ Fig. 8.41, ▶ Fig. 8.42).

A 3–0 suture is passed through the drill holes in the bone. For this purpose, a cannula (20 G, 0.9 × 40 mm) is first passed transcutaneously through two holes in the lateral walls from one side to the other; the 3–0 thread is then passed through the cannula lumen from side to side, after which the cannula is removed. The suture is knotted on one side once the same maneuver has been performed in the reverse direction, thereby securing the medialized bony nasal walls. The steps in this procedure are shown in ▶ Fig. 8.43a–j.

If the cartilaginous framework of the middle third of the nose with the upper lateral cartilages is wide, one of the two boreholes in the bone on either side may be dispensed with. The suture is then passed through the bone

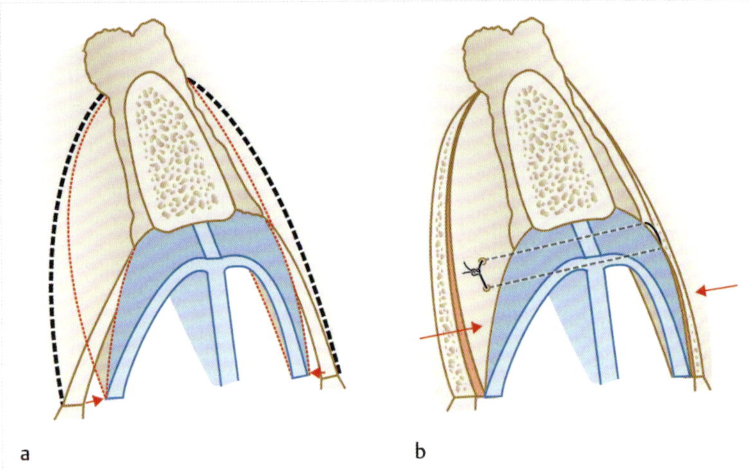

Fig. 8.36 Narrowing of the nasal framework using the piezo technique. (a) The cranially pedunculated bone can be bent medially. **(b)** A transverse mattress suture is passed through the boreholes. It secures the medialized bony and cartilaginous lateral walls of the nose.

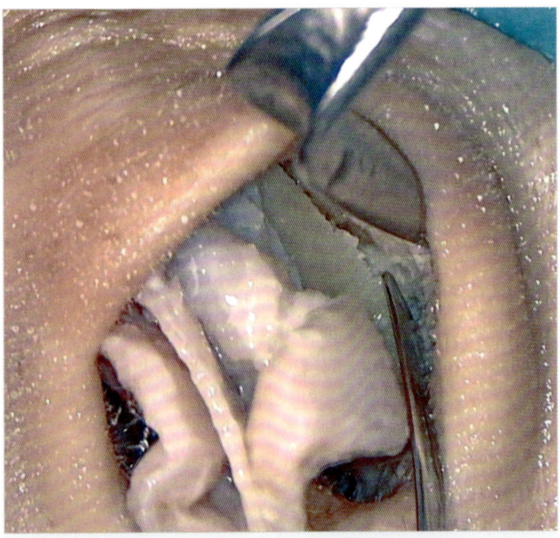

Fig. 8.37 Checking the mobility of the bony lateral wall. Medialization of the lateral wall after a lateral piezoelectric osteotomy is tested using a Freer elevator.

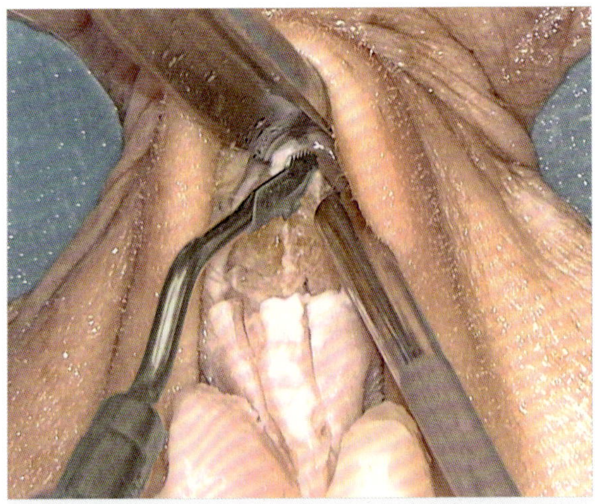

Fig. 8.38 Paramedian piezoelectric osteotomy with the MT9–13 vertical saw. The UNIVR saw may be used alternatively.

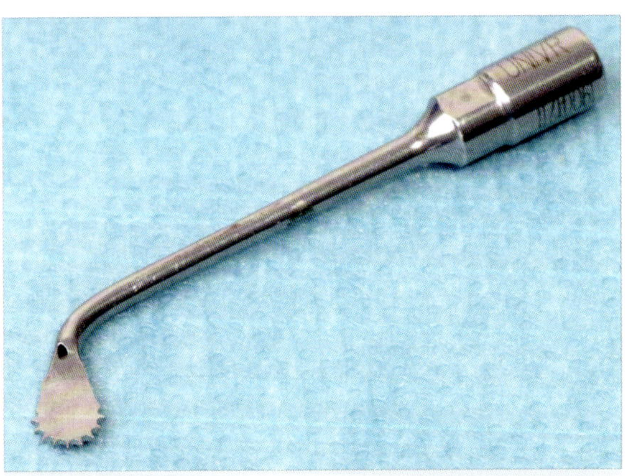

Fig. 8.39 The UNIVR vertical piezo saw insert. The channel opening for effluent irrigation fluid is clearly visible (mectron s.p.a., Carasco/Genoa, Italy).

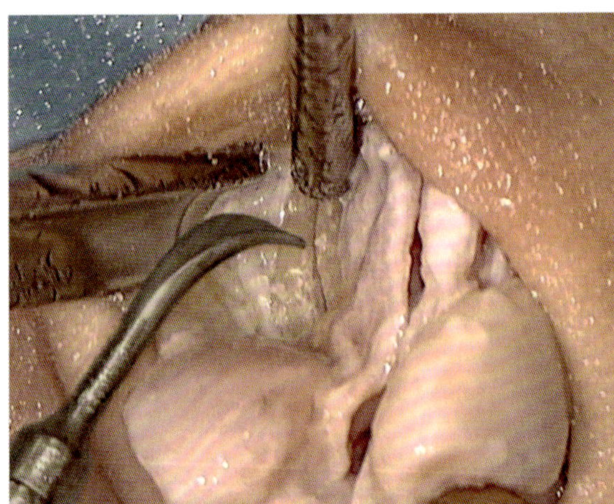

Fig. 8.40 Smoothing of bone edges. Bone edges are smoothed using the piezo MP1 planer.

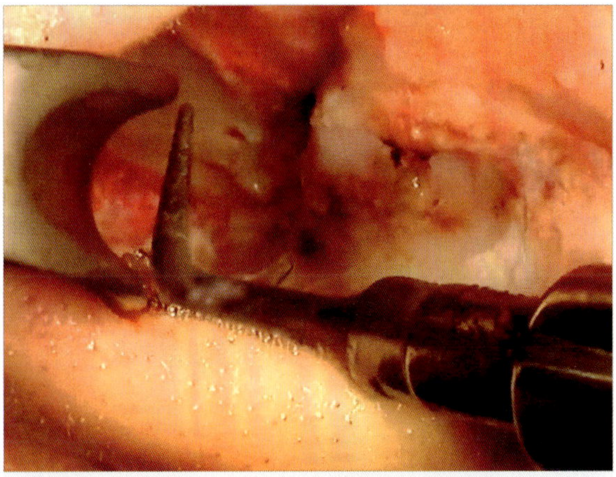

Fig. 8.41 Boreholes in the bony lateral wall. Two holes are usually made in the bony walls bilaterally with the MF4 piezo finishing insert.

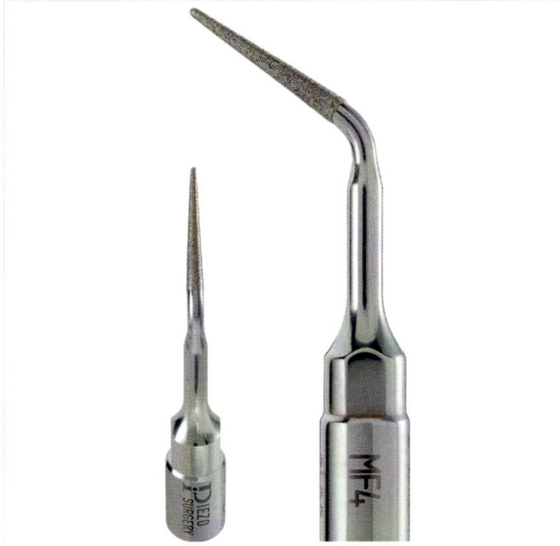

Fig. 8.42 The MF4 piezoelectric finishing insert. The angled MF4 piezoelectric finishing insert is better suited for making lateral boreholes than the manufacturer's straight drilling insert. (Copyright mectron s.p.a., Carasco/Genoa, Italy. Reprinted with permission.)

in one direction, but back through the cartilage. This suture then also supports the narrowed middle third of the cartilaginous vault (▶ Fig. 8.44).

Bone may be further reshaped using the piezoelectric device with the planer insert (MP1; see ▶ Fig. 8.29) even after placement of the bone suture, allowing procedures such as correction of irregularities, lowering of the nasal dorsum or the radix with deepening of the nasofrontal angle (▶ Fig. 8.45a, b), or further narrowing of the nose. This technique of surface reduction and lateral narrowing through osteotomies with piezo technology allows good control of the profile correction for moderate nasal humps (▶ Video 8.6).

Again, in suitable cases when there is a flat hump and narrow dorsum, pure surface treatment with piezo technology without lateral osteotomies may be sufficient (compare with ▶ Fig. 8.3a–d, ▶ Fig. 8.31a-d).

8.4 Dorsal Preservation Rhinoplasty: Push-Down and Let-Down Procedures

In comparison with the methods described so far, the "push-down" and "let-down" techniques follow a fundamentally different approach to lower the nasal dorsum and narrow the nasal framework. While the hammer and chisel are mostly used to do a "structure rhinoplasty" and the piezo technique is perfect for a "surface rhinoplasty" or "osteoplasty," preservation rhinoplasty with push-down and let-down can be classified as "foundation rhinoplasty." This describes the principle that resections are not primarily carried out on the dorsum of the nose, but on the base of the nasal framework, after which the entire nose can be lowered (▶ Video 8.4; see Video 6.1).

> ✔
>
> With the preservation technique, the cartilaginous bridge of the nose with the upper lateral cartilages often remains intact; the osseocartilaginous framework is then lowered as a unit.

These procedures have long been known, since the early twentieth century, but little significance was attached to them until they were recently highlighted by Yves Saban and others (see Bibliography below). The technique involves separating the entire nasal bone as a coherent element from the midfacial skeleton through a circumferential osteotomy at its base, composed of two lateral osteotomies and a radix osteotomy, followed by lowering of the dorsum below its original level, while the cartilaginous bridge of the nose remains connected to the bone. This procedure is made possible by resection of a well-defined osseocartilaginous strip of the septum under the nasal dorsum, the height of which determines the extent to which the nasal framework can be lowered (▶ Video 8.4; see ▶ Fig. 8.46, ▶ Fig. 8.47). At the same time, bone is removed at the lateral osteotomy line as needed to lower the framework. **Push-down**

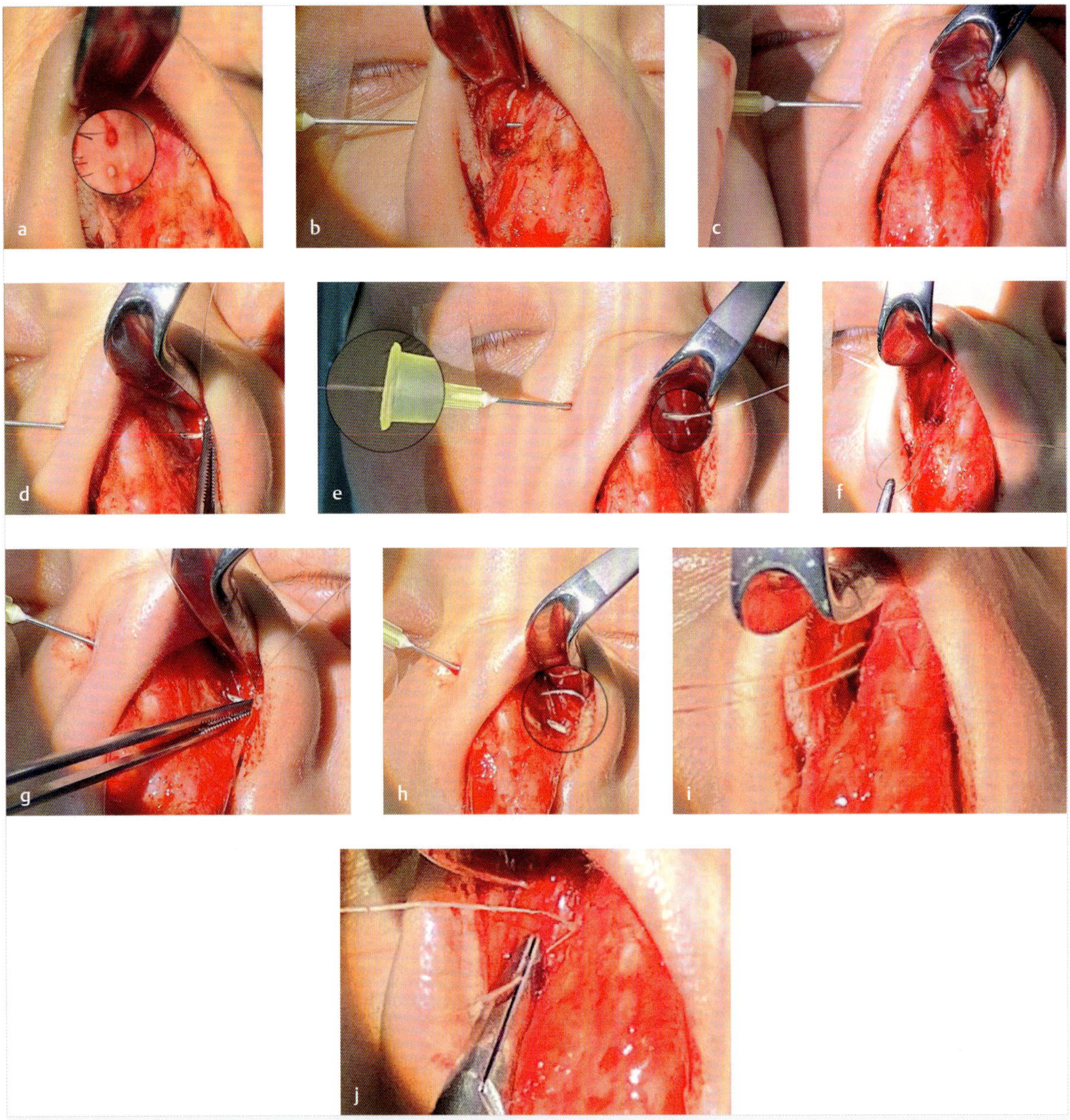

Fig. 8.43 Horizontal bone suturing of medialized lateral walls. **(a)** Two piezo boreholes in the right lateral nasal wall (under magnification). **(b)** A cannula has been inserted via the transcutaneous route into one of the drill holes. **(c)** Piercing the septum, the cannula emerges in the borehole on the opposite side. **(d)** A 3–0 PDS suture is inserted into the cannula lumen with bayonet forceps. **(e)** The thread is advanced until it emerges at the outer end of the cannula. **(f)** The cannula is extracted, and the right end of the suture is pulled out between the skin and the bone. **(g)** The cannula is reinserted transcutaneously through the same puncture site—this time through the second boreholes on either side. **(h)** The free end of the thread on the left is inserted into the cannula, as before. **(i)** The thread wraps around the two lateral bony walls after removal of the cannula and withdrawal of the second thread end between skin and bone. Both thread ends appear on the right between the skin and bone. **(j)** Knotting the suture secures the bony walls in a medialized position.

(▶ Fig. 8.46) thus involves septal height reduction in combination with lateral osteotomies on both sides and a transverse osteotomy at the nasal radix to connect the lateral bone cuts. In addition, a cartilage strip is removed from the septum and a bone segment of the perpendicular plate below the bony dorsum of the nose. This allows the nasal framework to be lowered in such a way that the bony walls are inserted into the stable bony frame formed by the piriform aperture.

The procedure is traditionally performed through the closed (endonasal) approach, but I prefer the open approach as described here, as it allows the use of piezo technology and extension to the hybrid procedure with additional surface processing (▶ Video 8.7).

Let-down (▶ Fig. 8.47) differs from push-down in that the bone is not only cut through by osteotomy but is also removed along the lateral osteotomy lines, creating a gap on either side. In simplified terms, one can imagine that the Webster triangle is resected (compare with ▶ Fig. 8.20). However, the bone usually has to be removed beyond this triangle and further cephalad at the osteotomy line in order to allow adequate lowering of the framework. Whereas during push-down the separated nasal framework is lowered below the level of the incised lateral bone edges, during let-down it drops down by the amount of resected bone to the level of the lower cut surface.

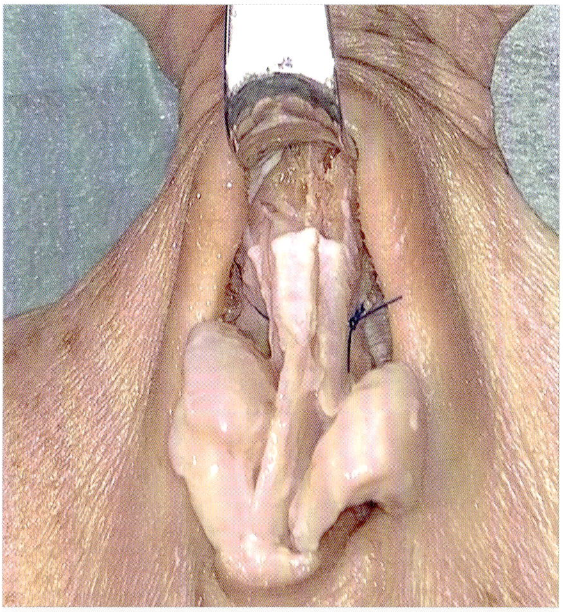

Fig. 8.44 Horizontal bone mattress suture through boreholes in the osseocartilaginous nasal framework. The suture is seen passing backward through the cartilage of the middle nasal vault, which may be indicated in cases when there is a wide cartilaginous framework (cadaver demonstration).

A characteristic feature of push-down and let-down techniques is that the nasal dorsum, and thus a nasal hump, are not necessarily directly manipulated, but are retained as a whole ("preserved") and only lowered to a defined extent (▶ Video 8.8; see also ▶ Fig. 10.40a–d).

In **preservation rhinoplasty**, particular attention is paid to the subdorsal septal segment, which needs to be cut out to allow for the let-down or push-down maneuver. The simplest variant is that of a subdorsal cartilage strip (high septal strip; ▶ Fig. 8.48a, b; see Video 6.1). The caudal incision into the septum's superior edge is made in the W-ASA segment near the W-point where the upper lateral cartilages insert on the septum (compare with ▶ Fig. 1.7).

The lowering of the hump only works if a strip of bone is also removed under the bony bridge of the nose. The resection of bone in this area needs to be very carefully dosed, and this step is done prior to the completion of the lateral and radix osteotomies in order to reduce the risk of fracture lines extending into the skull base from here. Depending on the extent of the hump and the intended lowering, a subdorsal osteotomy line is sufficient in some cases, while in other cases fragments have to be removed with the piezo technique or bone forceps. A preoperative sagittal computed tomography scan makes it easier to estimate in advance how much bone may have to be removed. In principle, a step-by-step approach is recommended in order to avoid overresection, which can lead to an excessive drop in the bridge of the nose, creating the appearance of an infantilized nose ("scooped-out dorsum").

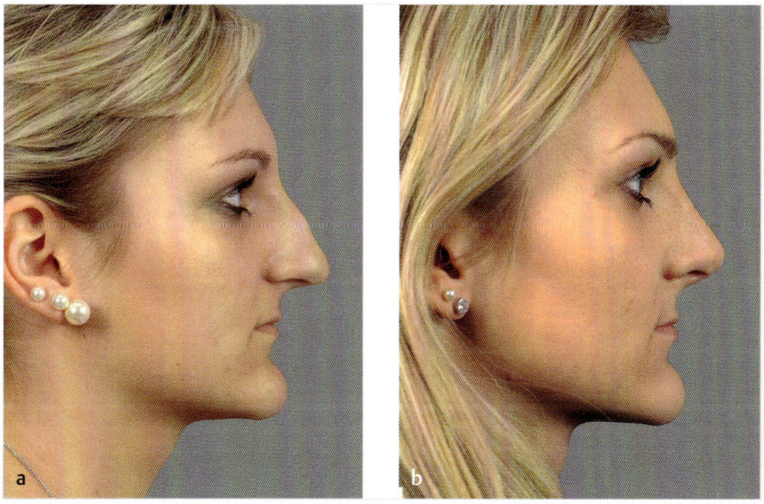

Fig. 8.45 Deepening of the nasofrontal angle. (a) A large hump nose with a flattened nasofrontal angle. **(b)** The piezo technique is particularly helpful in lowering the radix to reduce the nasofrontal angle.

The piezo technology is extremely helpful for the entire work on the bone during preservation rhinoplasty.

After work on the septum, the osteotomies on the nasal framework are completed, and the subdorsal osteotomy in the bone is connected to the radix osteotomy.

Another way to lower the cartilaginous dorsum is to cut a subdorsal square or triangular cartilage strip under the bridge of the nose, which is then moved caudally (▶ Fig. 8.49a, b). Vertical incisions in this cartilage flap just below the highest point of the hump during descent allow for extension of the cartilaginous bridge of the nose and loss of the cartilaginous arch that forms the hump. In this case, the lowered bridge of the nose can be fixed with sutures aside the rest of the septum, thanks to the preserved subdorsal cartilage strip (▶ Fig. 8.49b).

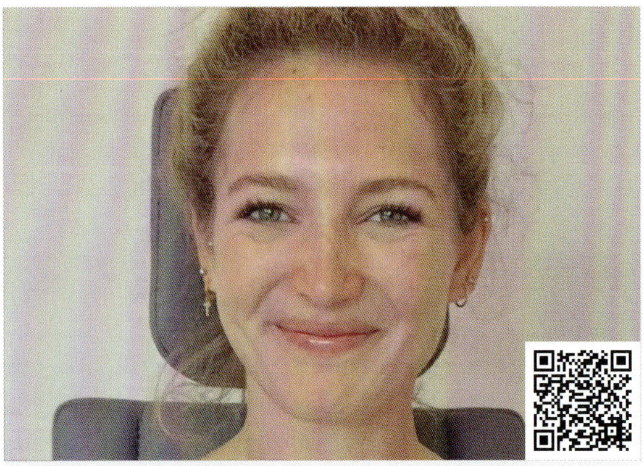

Video 8.6 Result after surface rhinoplasty plus lateral osteotomies using the piezo technique.

On the other hand, if one removes a strip of cartilage under the subdorsal septal cartilage, which has been excised in an almost rectangular shape, then the lowered dorsal cartilage element is set up with the bridge of the nose exactly on the lower cut edge of the septum and can be sutured in this position (known as a "Tetris" procedure after Neves; see the Bibliography below; ▶ Fig. 8.50a, b).

In contrast to the subdorsal strip, the **Cottle method** of lowering the bridge of the nose excises one vertical strip of cartilage and a horizontal one on the underside of the septum (▶ Fig. 8.51a, b). Surgeons can make the individual selection of the procedure dependent on whether and to what extent a septal deviation needs to be corrected in each case, or whether and how much cartilage graft material they plan to take from the septum.

With the maneuvers described here on the bone and cartilage, it is possible to correct not only a hump but also a crooked nose and to preserve the bridge of the nose by moving the entire nasal structure from the deviated position to the midline and fixing it with sutures (▶ Fig. 8.52 and case example ▶ Fig. 8.56 a-d).

In order to allow the cartilaginous and bony structures of the nose to spread open and straighten when the hump is lowered with the preservation procedure, the

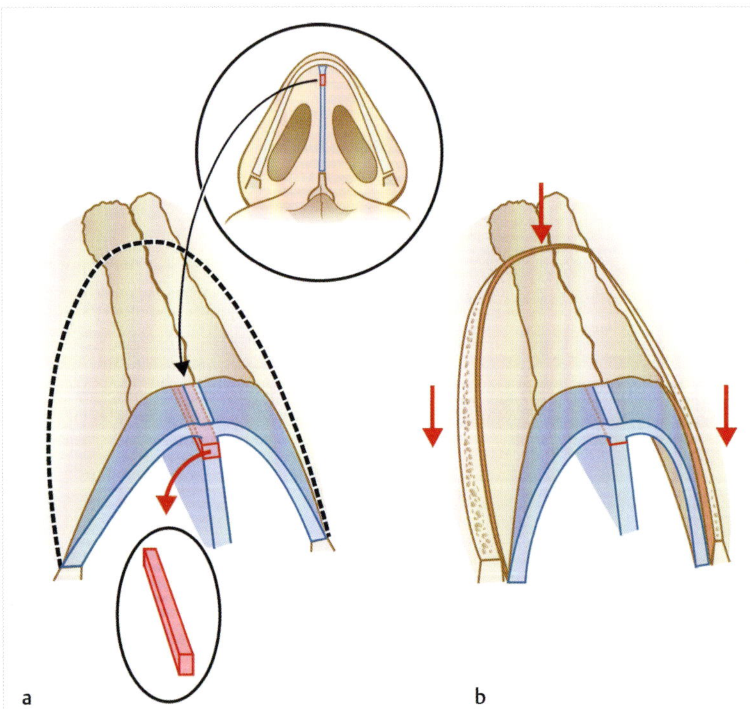

Fig. 8.46 Push-down. The entire bony nasal dorsum is mobilized by osteotomy **(a)** and moved down with the hump using the push-down technique, by pushing the nasal framework into the lower bony frame **(b)**. The prerequisite for success is the resection of a bone-cartilage strip from the septum below the nasal dorsum (highlighted in red in **(a)**).

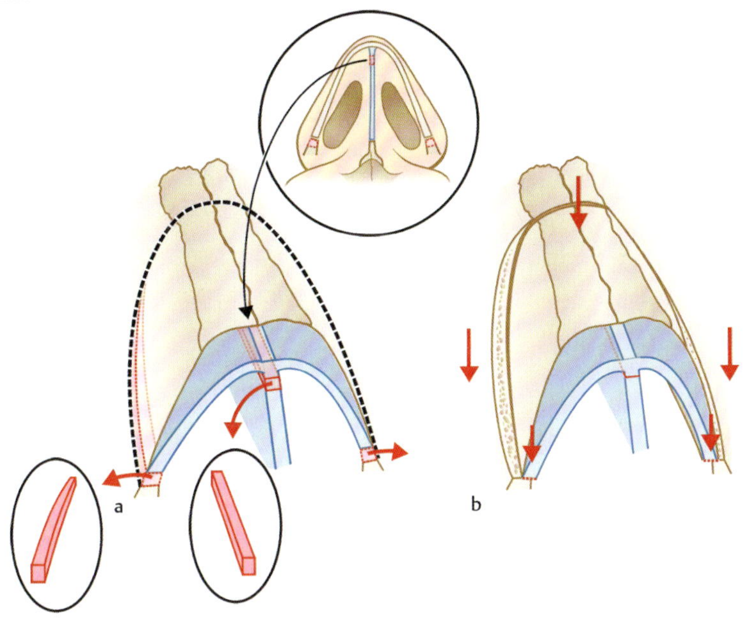

Fig. 8.47 Let-down. The bony framework with the hump after osteotomy and excision of bony strips **(a)** is "let down" to the lower edge of the bone **(b)**.

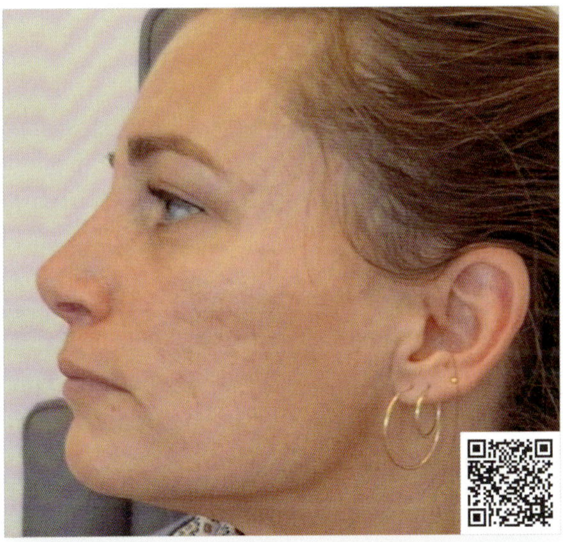

Video 8.7 Result after preservation rhinoplasty with the push-down technique.

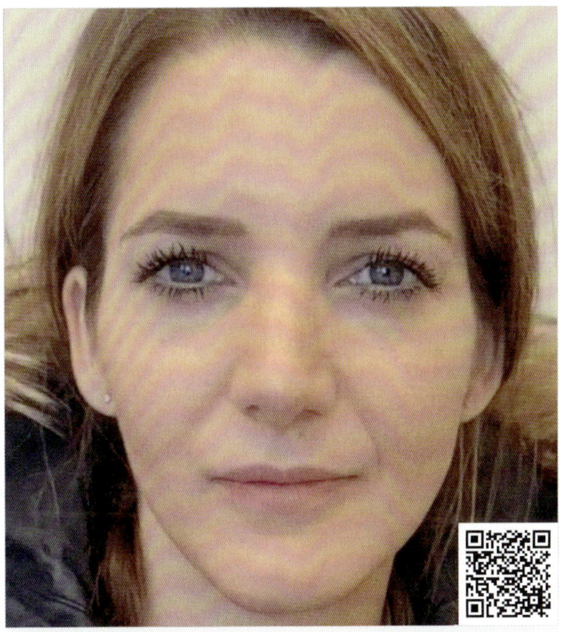

Video 8.8 Result after preservation rhinoplasty with the let-down technique.

upper lateral cartilage has to be separated from the bone laterally along the lateral keystone area. I call this lateral keystone release the "accordion maneuver" (also known as a "ballerina maneuver," after A. Göksel; ▸ Fig. 8.53a–c).

After push-down or let-down, the nasal dorsum can be fixed in the new position using the bone suture method as described above (see section 8.3.2; compare with ▸ Fig. 8.43a–j). In this case, however, it is sufficient to pass the thread of the mattress suture through the bone only once and through the cartilage framework for the second passage on the way back (compare with ▸ Fig. 8.44; see ▸ Video 6.1). The height of the caudal septum segment along the W-ASA line is adjusted after lowering of the hump.

In general, push-down and let-down lead to elevation of the tip of the nose in the sense of a rotation, as long as the connection between the upper and lower lateral

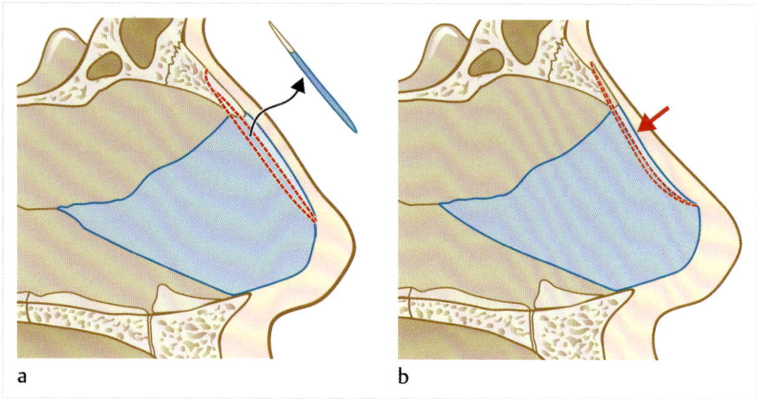

Fig. 8.48 High septal strip. (a) Outline of the subdorsal resection. **(b)** After lowering of the dorsum.

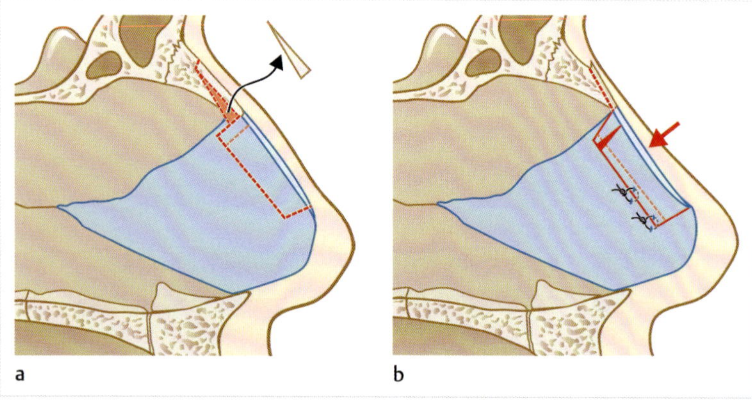

Fig. 8.49 Subdorsal square flap. (a) Outline of the incision. **(b)** After lowering of the dorsum. Note the vertical incision in the subdorsal cartilage flap, and subdorsal bone resection.

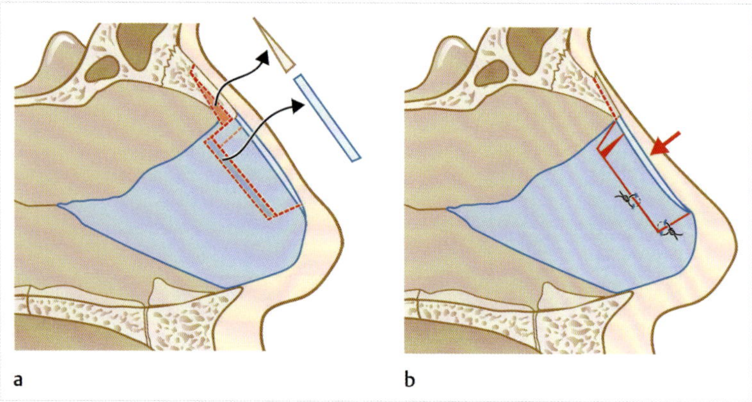

Fig. 8.50 The "Tetris" procedure (J.C. Neves). **(a)** Outline of the incision. **(b)** After lowering of the dorsum.

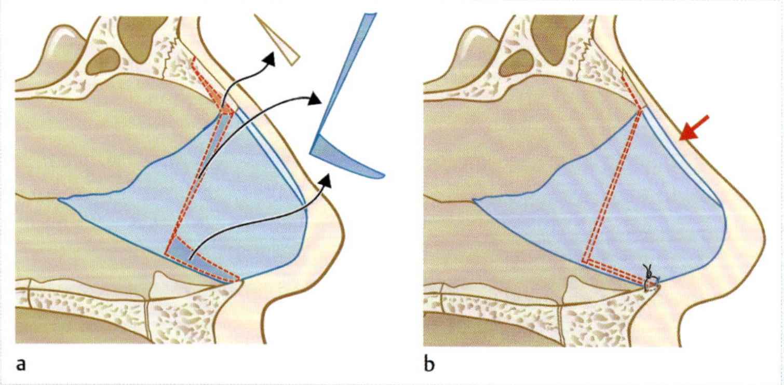

Fig. 8.51 The Cottle procedure. (a) Outline of incisions. **(b)** After lowering of the dorsum.

cartilages along the scroll area is maintained. The surgeon must then finally assess whether further corrections to the alar cartilages are necessary (see Chapter 10, Chapter 11, Chapter 12). It also needs to be assessed whether the hump has already been sufficiently corrected by the measures taken, or whether further surface corrections may be necessary to avoid "recurrence" of the hump (compare with ▶ Fig. 20.6a-f). Surface treatment with piezo technology can then give the hump correction the finishing touch (known as the "hybrid" technique).

With regard to the question of whether it is preferable to use a preservation technique with push-down or let-down, or whether a structural rhinoplasty or an osteoplasty with surface technique is more appropriate, the surgeon will be guided by what promises better results in his or her hands. Details in the profile of a humped nose offer further decision-making aids:

- If one looks at the profile of the bridge of the nose with a hump from the side, one can basically distinguish S-shaped and V-shaped contour lines (▶ Fig. 8.54a, b). A V-shaped contour offers better conditions for successful application of preservation rhinoplasty (▶ Fig. 8.55a–d), as well as a high radix in comparison with a low one.
- In the frontal view, a more narrow nose structure is better suited for this procedure than a very wide one.

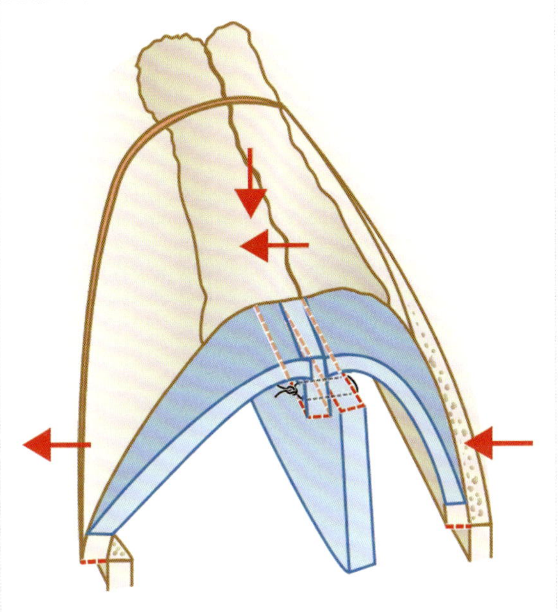

Fig. 8.52 Correction of a deviated nose with the preservation technique.

▶ Fig. 8.56a–d shows an example of a deviated nose with a V-shaped hump, corrected with a push-down procedure in combination with surface surgery using piezo technology. The septum was processed using the Cottle method (see also ▶ Video 8.7).

▶ Fig. 8.57a–d shows an example of a deviated nose with a slightly S-shaped hump, corrected with a let-down procedure in combination with surface surgery using piezo technology. The septum was processed with resection of a subdorsal strip (see also ▶ Video 8.8). ▶ Video 8.9 shows an example of a large nose that has been reduced using the let-down technique.

> ✔
>
> The most significant risks with push-down and let-down procedures are saddle nose or child-like flattening of the bridge of the nose with overcorrection, return or permanence of the hump as a dorsal convexity with undercorrection, and the formation of a step at the root of the nose with excessive reduction at the bony septum.

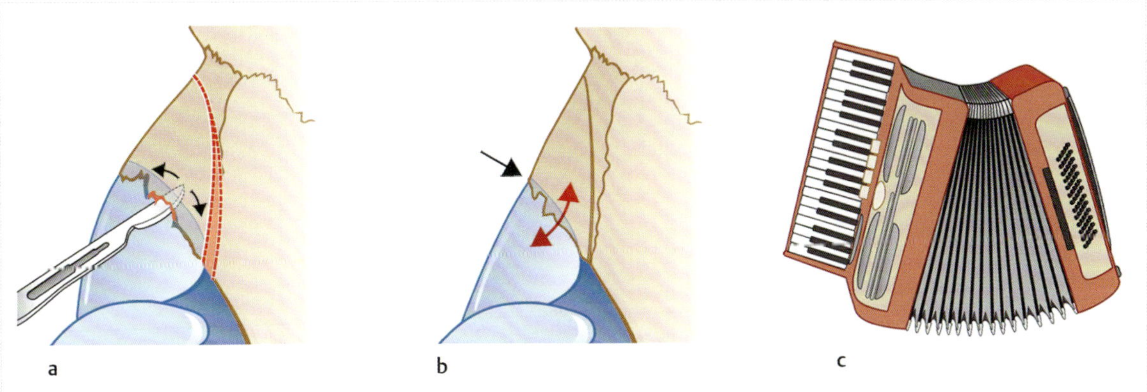

Fig. 8.53 Lateral keystone release for the "accordion maneuver." (a) The upper lateral cartilage is sharply separated from the bone of the piriform aperture. **(b)** The cartilage can now be moved against the bone, and the nasal dorsum can be lowered. **(c)** The movement is reminiscent of an accordion being pulled apart at the bottom.

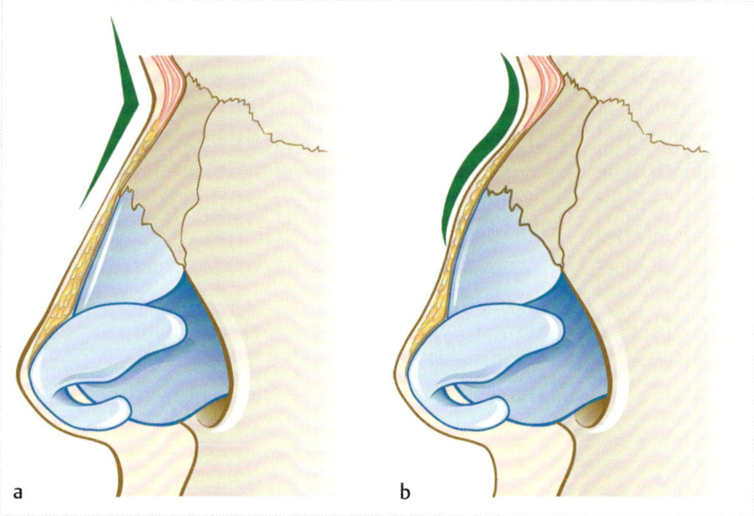

Fig. 8.54 V-shaped and S-shaped nasal dorsal contour lines. (a) A V-shaped nasal dorsal profile is considered favorable for a push-down or let-down procedure. **(b)** An S-shaped nasal dorsal profile will probably benefit more from a hybrid procedure with additional surface surgery.

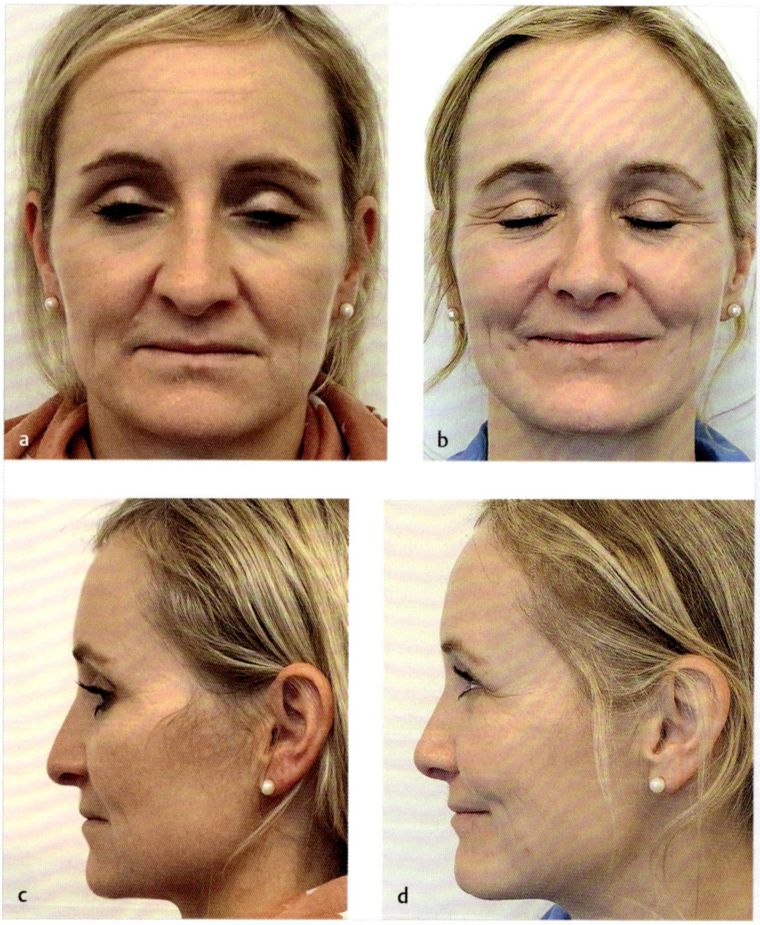

Fig. 8.55 V-shaped dorsum. (a, c) V-shaped elevation of the nasal dorsum, corrected with let-down technique **(b, d)**. Also note the improvement in nasal tip rotation.

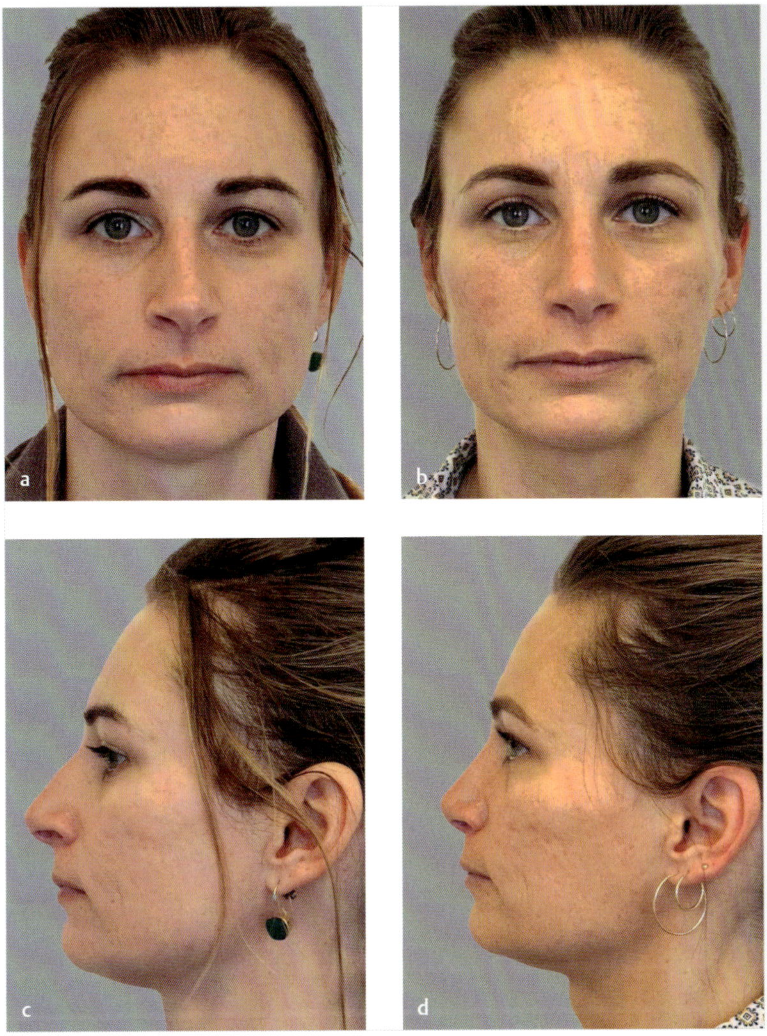

Fig. 8.56 Deviated nose with a V-shaped dorsum and hump. The patient underwent a rhinoplasty with a push-down procedure in combination with surface surgery using piezo technology. The septum was processed using the Cottle method. **(a, c)** Preoperative status. **(b, d)** Postoperative result (see also ▶ Video 8.7).

Less experienced surgeons in particular should bear in mind that the upper transverse osteotomy (radix osteotomy) is performed in proximity to the skull base, which carries a risk of injury to the cranial base, especially in patients with atypical anatomy.

Preservation rhinoplasty attempts to preserve not just the nasal dorsum but also the **ligaments** of the nasal framework, or to reconstruct them after surgery. This applies in particular to the vertical and longitudinal scroll ligaments, the interdomal and intercrural ligaments, the deep Pitanguy ligament (inserting into the depressor superficial nasalis muscle, DSN) and superficial Pitanguy ligament (inserting into the superficial orbicularis oris muscle, SOON; see ▶ Fig. 1.17; ▶ Fig. 8.58a, b, ▶ Fig. 8.59).

✓

Irrespective of the reconstruction of the Pitanguy ligament, it is worthwhile to close possible dead space at the end of the operation by an absorbable subcutaneous suture that connects the hypodermis to the cartilaginous dorsum at the level of the W-point, when the skin flap is moved back (see ▶ Video 6.1).

In appropriate cases, the preservation technique may also be used in reverse to augment the bridge of the nose. In this case, the bony and cartilaginous dorsum is mobilized with the same incisions, raised overall and underlaid with

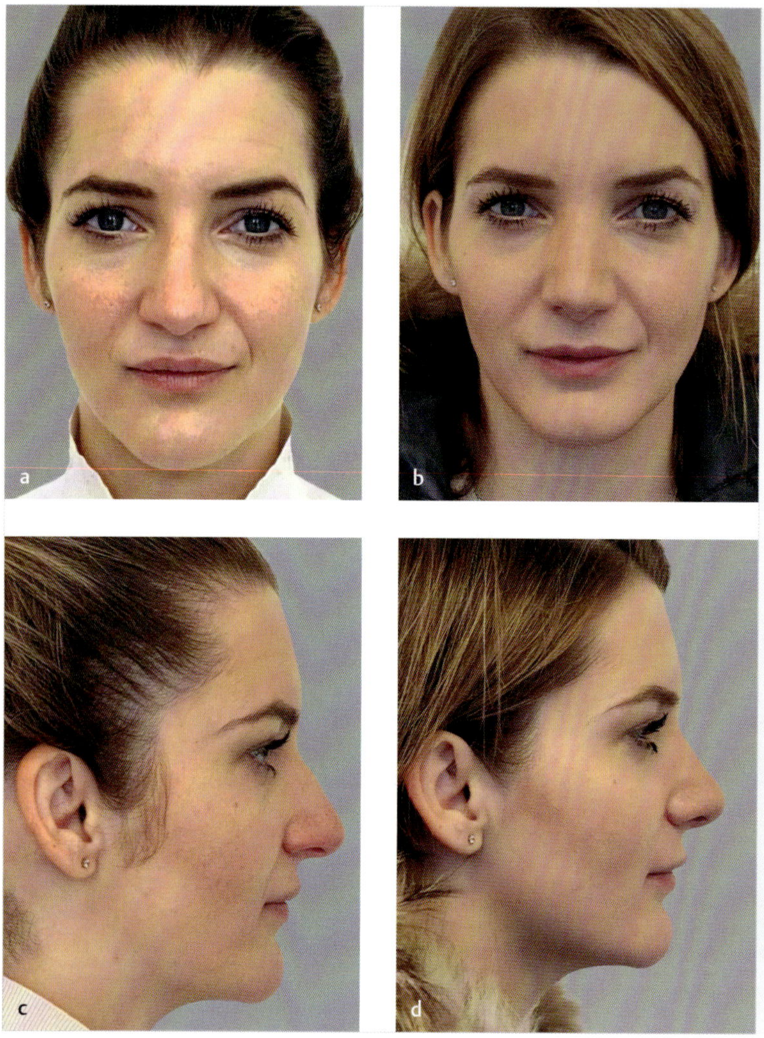

Fig. 8.57 Deviated nose with a slightly S-shaped dorsum and hump. The patient underwent a rhinoplasty with a let-down procedure in combination with surface surgery using piezo technology. The septum was processed with resection of a subdorsal strip. **(a, c)** Preoperative status. **(b, d)** Postoperative result (see also ▸ Video 8.8).

8

a graft, which brings the nasal framework to the new, desired height (Ferreira's "reverse spare roof technique"; see the Bibliography below).

8.5 Selection of Methods when Working on Bone

Given the variety of methods available for working on bone, the question arises as to when which method should be used.

If you do not have access to piezo technology, you will do the bone work with a chisel, osteotome and rasp; I know few colleagues who use an electric drill.

In addition, my experience on this topic leads me to the following assessments:

- For very minor work on the surface of the bony dorsum, the piezo technique is an ideal tool; an alternative is the rasp.
- If only a small hump is to be removed and only a slight narrowing of the nose is to be achieved, the piezo technique with only lateral osteotomies and bone suture is suitable (see section 8.3.2).
- A narrow nose with a small or medium-sized hump is suitable for preservation push-down or let-down, if necessary in combination with piezo surface treatment.
- The significant narrowing and reduction of a large, wide nose is achieved more reliably with classic instruments like hammer, chisel, and osteotome.
- For revisions that require re-osteotomies, I also prefer hammer and chisel because the existing scarring makes it difficult to use piezo instruments.
- This also applies to revisions for irregularities on the dorsum, which can often be smoothed out well with endonasal access and a rasp.

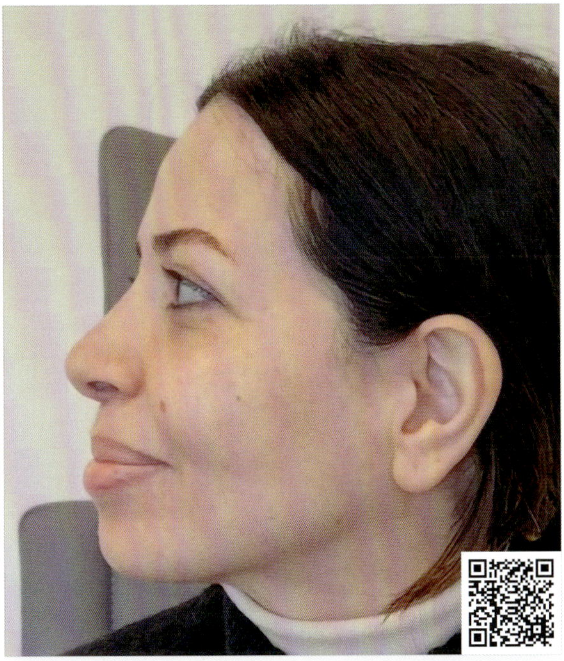

Video 8.9 A large nose corrected using the let-down technique.

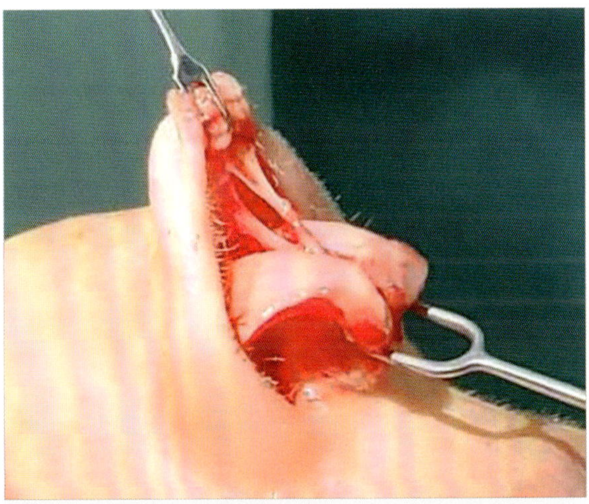

Fig. 8.59 Superficial and deep portions of the Pitanguy ligament. The two strands of the Pitanguy ligament cannot always be visualized so clearly intraoperatively.

Bibliography

Barelli PA. Long term evaluation of "push down" procedures. Rhinology. 1975; 13(1):25–32

Cakir B, Orereoğlu AR, Doğan T, Akan M. A complete subperichondrial dissection technique for rhinoplasty with management of the nasal ligaments. Aesthet Surg J. 2012; 32(5):564–574

Daniel RK, Palhazi P, Saban Y, Cakir B. Preservation rhinoplasty. 3rd ed. Istanbul: Septum; 2020

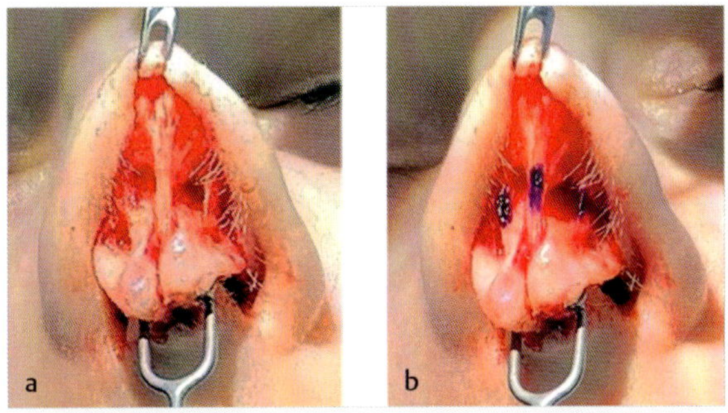

Fig. 8.58 Pitanguy and scroll ligaments. The Pitanguy and scroll ligaments **(a)** are color-coded intraoperatively **(b)**. The coloring facilitates correct reunion by suture after separation of these ligaments during the open procedure.

East C. Preservation rhinoplasty and the crooked nose. Facial Plast Surg Clin North Am. 2021; 29(1):123–130

Ferreira MG, Monteiro D, Reis C, Almeida e Sousa C. Spare roof technique: a middle third new technique. Facial Plast Surg. 2016; 32(1):111–116

Ferreira MG, Santos M. Preservation rhinoplasty in the saddle nose: the reverse spare roof technique. Facial Plast Surg Aesthet Med. 2022; 24(3): 168–170. DOI: 10.1089/fpsam.2022.0036

Gerbault O, Daniel RK, Kosins AM. The role of piezoelectric instrumentation in rhinoplasty surgery. Aesthet Surg J. 2016; 36(1):21–34

Göksel A, Patel PN, Most SP. Piezoelectric osteotomies in dorsal preservation rhinoplasty. Facial Plast Surg Clin North Am. 2021; 29(1):77–84

Göksel A, Saban Y, Tran KN. Biomechanical nasal anatomy applied to open preservation rhinoplasty. Facial Plast Surg. 2021; 37(1):12–21

Jin HR, Jeon YJ. Feasibility of Dorsal Preservation Rhinoplasty for Hump Nose Reduction in Asian Population. Facial Plast Surg Aesthet Med. 2024 Nov-Dec;26(6):748–755

Neves JC, Arancibia-Tagle D. Avoiding aesthetic drawbacks and stigmata in dorsal line preservation rhinoplasty. Facial Plast Surg. 2021; 37(1):65–75

Neves JC, Tagle DA, Dewes W, Ferraz M. A segmental approach in dorsal preservation rhinoplasty: the Tetris concept. Facial Plast Surg Clin North Am. 2021; 29(1):85–99

Özücer B, Çam OH. The effectiveness of asymmetric dorsal preservation for correction of I-shaped crooked nose deformity in comparison to conventional technique. Facial Plast Surg Aesthet Med. 2020; 22(4):286–293.-Epub 2020 May 13. PMID: 32392429

Patel PN, Most SP. Overview of dorsal preservation rhinoplasty. Facial Plast Surg Clin North Am. 2023; 31(1):1–11

Saban Y. Rhinoplasty: lessons from "errors": from anatomy and experience to the concept of sequential primary rhinoplasty. HNO. 2018; 66(1):15–25

Saban Y, Daniel RK, Polselli R, Trapasso M, Palhazi P. Dorsal preservation: the push down technique reassessed. Aesthet Surg J. 2018; 38(2):117–131

San Nicoló M, Berghaus A. [Advantages of piezoelectric technology in rhinoplasty]. HNO. 2019; 67(11):836–842- [Article in German]

Sullivan PK, Harshbarger RJ, Oneal RM. Osteotomies. In: Gunter JP, Rohrich RJ, Adams WP, eds. Dallas rhinoplasty. Vol. 1. St. Louis: Quality Medical Publishing; 2002:595–614

Toriumi DM. Subdorsal cantilever graft for elevating the dorsum in ethnic rhinoplasty. Facial Plast Surg Aesthet Med. 2022; 24(3):143–159

Toriumi DM, Kovacevic M. Dorsal preservation rhinoplasty: measures to prevent suboptimal outcomes. Facial Plast Surg Clin North Am. 2021; 29 (1):141–153

Zholtikov V, Ouerghi R, Kosins A. Dorsal Modification: Practical Applications in Rhinoplasty. Aesthet Surg J. 2024 Nov 15; 44(12):1258–1270. doi: 10.1093/asj/sjae148. PMID: 38992914

9 The Cartilaginous Middle Vault

The **cartilaginous middle third** of the nose extends from the “K-area” – the osseocartilaginous transition zone – to the caudal edge of the septum. The cartilaginous septum and the upper lateral cartilages therefore form the essential part of the middle third of the nose.

9.1 Considerations on the Sequence of Surgical Steps

After processing of the bony framework, this middle section of the nasal framework is addressed in the next surgical step, or after septoplasty.

> ✓
>
> If the surgeon has chosen a preservation technique, the cartilaginous bridge of the nose with the upper lateral cartilages often remains intact; the osseocartilaginous framework is then lowered as a unit (see section 8.4).

The alar cartilages in most cases are now entirely separated from one another in the midline. This is associated with the transection of the interdomal and intercrural ligaments. However, these ligaments can also be preserved in suitable cases, when the cartilage in that area can be left untouched (compare with ▶ Fig. 7.4a, b).

With the open technique, the Pitanguy ligament, with its superficial and deep portions, is usually already severed (compare with ▶ Fig. 1.17, ▶ Fig. 8.58, ▶ Fig. 8.59), but it can be restored at the end (▶ Fig. 9.1). The cartilaginous nasal dorsum, extending from the anterior septal angle to the bony dorsum, is then visualized following dissection of the medial crura of the alar cartilages and the caudal edge of the septum. A small “**membranous septum**” that lacks any supporting cartilage is present between the medial crura of the alar cartilages and the caudal edge of the septum. Vestibular skin defects must be avoided during dissection in this region (see Chapter 7; ▶ Fig. 7.3a, b).

The surgeon then proceeds with **septoplasty** or **harvesting of septal cartilage** if cartilaginous grafts are required during surgery. These procedures are described in Chapter 7. Rim and tip grafts harvested from septal cartilage are frequently required during rhinoplasty; preparation of the septum is therefore almost always part of the operation.

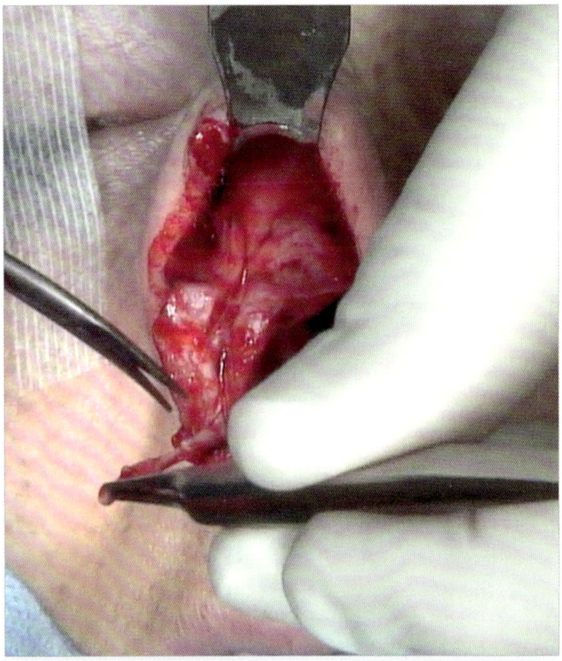

Fig. 9.1 Dissection of the Pitanguy ligament. The Pitanguy ligament can be regarded as part of the superficial musculoaponeurotic system (SMAS) in the midline.

If a preservation rhinoplasty is being carried out, then at this point subdorsal preparation with subdorsal strip resection or incisions is performed after adequate detachment of the septal mucosa (see section 8.4).

Separation of the mucoperichondrium and all further steps are performed as described in Chapter 7.

> ✓
>
> The open approach allows far better visualization of the septum than a hemitransfixion incision. I therefore prefer the open access route in patients with marked, complex septal deviations, especially in combination with deviated noses, and in those requiring correction of large septal perforations.

9.2 Reduction of the Cartilaginous Hump

Correction of the height and width of the cartilaginous nasal dorsum is very often part of a primary rhinoplasty.

9

Only very limited cartilaginous hump reduction should be undertaken by horizontal separation of the upper edge of the septum and the upper lateral cartilages "in one piece". The nasal dorsum may appear too wide if reduced in height by more than a millimeter or two. There is also a risk of exposing the nasal cavities between the upper lateral cartilages and the septum, with a resultant "open roof" deformity that requires further corrective surgery.

A more reliable approach for reducing more prominent humps involves separating the upper lateral cartilages from the septum (▶ Video 9.1), followed by gradual height reduction and reconstruction of the nasal dorsum.

The mucosa is first detached on both sides at the angle between the upper lateral cartilages and the septum. Beginning at the caudal septum and the anterior septal angle, the top edge of the septum in direct contact with the cartilage is traced, while a search is made for the attachments of the upper lateral cartilages at the W-point (compare with ▶ Fig. 1.7). A pair of fine, pointed scissors is inserted into the angle between the septum and the upper lateral cartilage (paraseptal cleft; ▶ Fig. 1.7), below the insertion of this cartilage and directly in contact with it. The mucosa – usually firmly adherent to the cartilage – is then separated from the angle between the upper lateral cartilage and the septum, using cutting and spreading movements, occasionally dissecting only with the tip of the scissors (▶ Fig. 9.2).

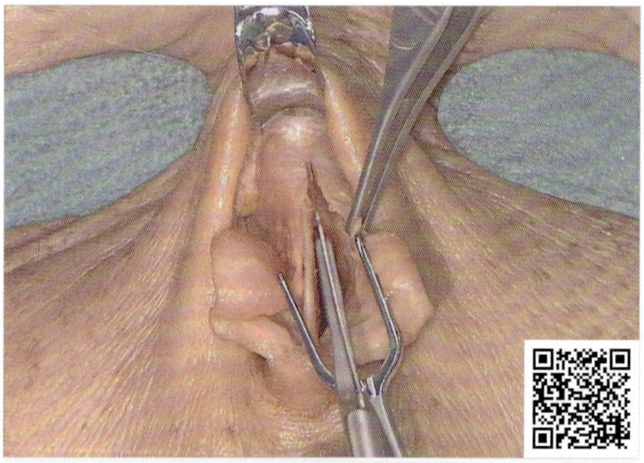

Video 9.1 Separation of the upper lateral cartilages (cadaver head).

Omitting mucosal separation and separating the upper lateral cartilages from the septum along with adherent mucosa exposes the nasal cavity and favors infections. This may also give rise to heavy bleeding from the mucosal edge, which may be difficult to control. The mucosa can be further loosened by removing it with a fine, sharp raspatory (▶ Fig. 9.3, ▶ Fig. 9.4).

Once dissection is complete, a no. 15 blade, placed flat against the septum and with the blade pointing upward, can be inserted into the tunnel-like space under the attachment of the upper lateral cartilage. This separates the upper lateral cartilage from the septum in one smooth movement, while the mucosa remains intact. The Aufricht retractor lifts the skin while protecting it from blade-induced injuries (▶ Fig. 9.5).

Separation of the upper lateral cartilage from the septum does not result in exposure of the nasal cavities if the mucosa has been previously mobilized; instead, a

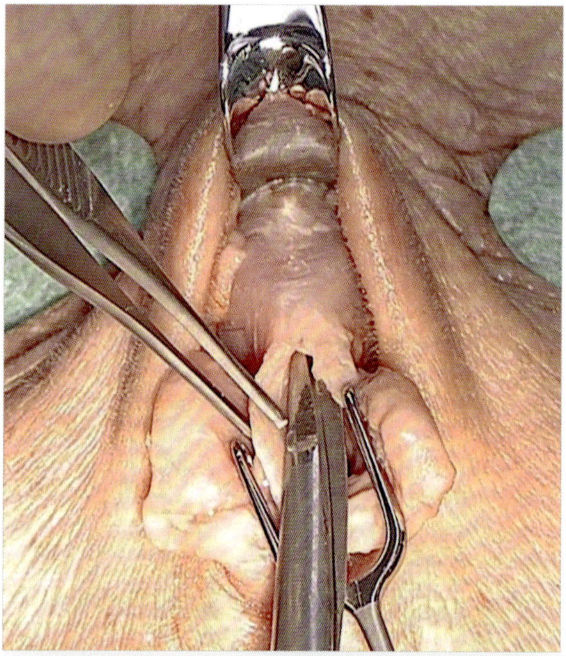

Fig. 9.2 Dissection of the attachment of the upper lateral cartilages to the septum with scissors. The mucous membrane in the angle between the septum and the left upper lateral cartilage is loosened with a pair of scissors, starting from the paraseptal cleft along the W-point–anterior septal angle (W-ASA) line.

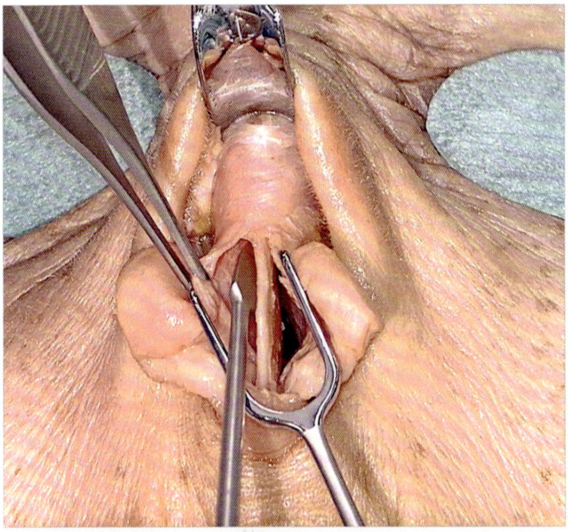

Fig. 9.3 Dissection of the attachment of the upper lateral cartilage with a fine raspatory. Adherent mucous membrane in the angle between the septum and upper lateral cartilage may occasionally be easier to loosen using a fine, sharp raspatory rather than a pair of scissors.

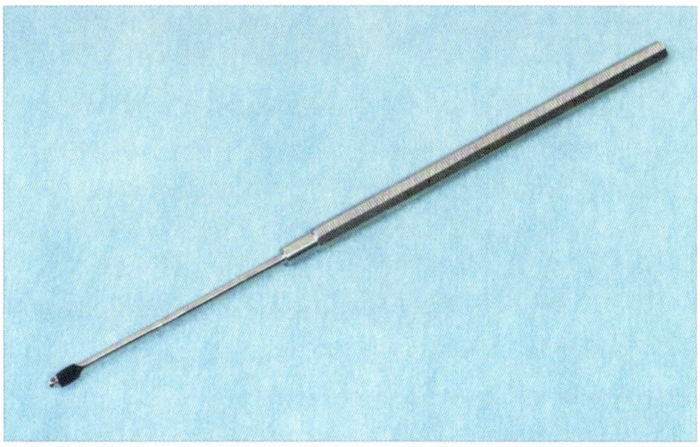

Fig. 9.4 Fine, sharp raspatory (KARL STORZ SE & Co. KG, Tuttlingen, Germany).

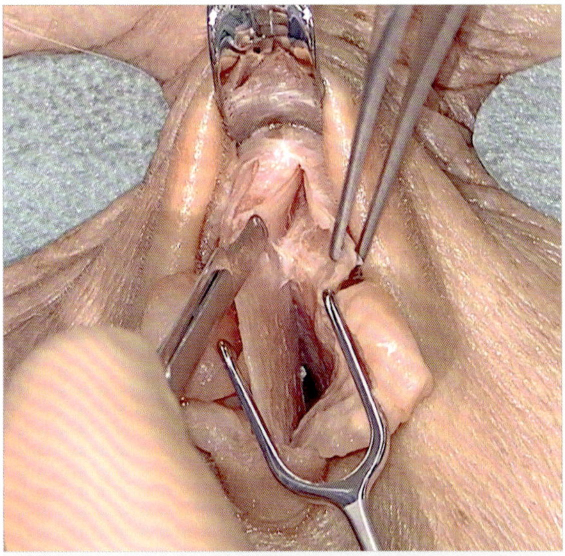

Fig. 9.5 Separation of the upper lateral cartilage from the septum. The left upper lateral cartilage is separated from the septum using a no.15 blade. The previously dissected mucous membrane remains intact.

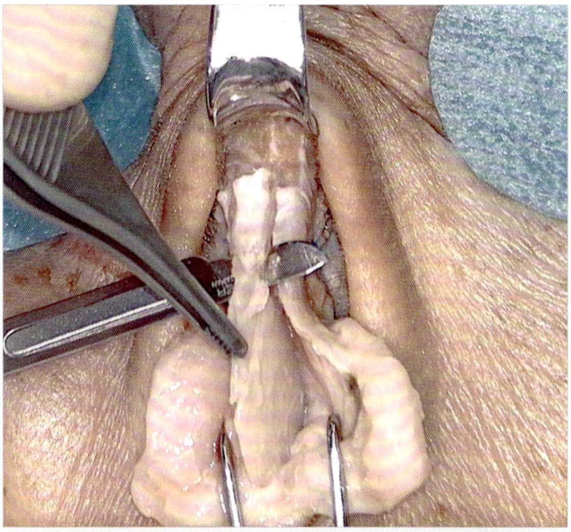

Fig. 9.6 Reduction of the cartilaginous hump. The cartilaginous hump is reduced by gradual ablation of the top edge of the septum with a size 15 blade until the appropriate height is achieved.

space is created between the septum and the upper lateral cartilage, bounded inferiorly by the separated mucoperichondrium (▶ Fig. 9.5). A cartilaginous strip can be inserted into this space later, if necessary, to prevent excessive narrowing of the nasal dorsum and to stabilize the middle nasal vault (autospreader flap or spreader graft; see section 9.3, 9.4).

Once the lateral cartilages have been separated from the septum, the hump is removed. The height of the septum, which has now been separated from the upper lateral cartilages, is reduced first. Even with large humps, care needs to be taken to proceed very carefully and to first remove only the somewhat widened top edge of the septum with the former attachments of the upper lateral cartilages (▶ Fig. 9.6). Even partial resection of this wide edge may be sufficient for low humps.

> It must be borne in mind that the position of the nasal tip is frequently corrected later, and excessive reduction of the nasal dorsum may only be evident when the tip is lifted or rotated. Caution is therefore required while reducing the hump; temporarily raising the tip with a pair of tweezers helps simulate the postoperative outcome.

It is advisable to occasionally put the skin flap back during hump resection, to provide an intraoperative overview and simulate the final position of the tip with a pair of tweezers. The surgeon can thus assess the overall appearance of the nasal dorsum relative to the nasal tip and can better decide on the extent of further hump reduction. The rhinoplasty mirror that is mounted or hand-held opposite the surgeon on the operating table is very helpful in this respect, as it allows adequate assessment of the nasal profile from the opposite side (see ▶ Fig. 4.5a–c).

The bony framework is also further reduced, if necessary, until the final height of the nasal dorsum is achieved. The piezo technique is particularly suitable for these finishing touches on the bone (▶ Fig. 9.7a, b).

> It is extremely important to bear in mind the harmonious appearance of the bony and cartilaginous profile of the nasal dorsum, as well as the objectives based on the simulated images discussed with the patient.

The cut edges of the separated upper lateral cartilages are adjusted once the bony nasal dorsum and the top edge of the cartilaginous septum have been reduced to the desired height; this affects both the height and also the width of these lateral cartilages, which also defines the width of the entire middle third.

In some cases, it is not necessary to refine the height of the cut edges of the upper lateral cartilages, and if their width also conforms to that of the bony framework, they do not require correction. The separated upper lateral cartilages only need to be reattached to the septum with double mattress sutures in these uncomplicated cases. More often, however, the edges of the upper lateral cartilages stand too high after correction at the upper edge of the septum and have to be shortened before, or rather after, being sutured to the septum.

> Again, with preservation rhinoplasty, the above steps are often not used, as this technique lowers the bridge of the nose overall without directly correcting anything on the cartilaginous bridge of the nose (see section 8.4).

Ablation of the cartilaginous hump reduces both the height and width of the cartilaginous nasal dorsum, and care must be taken to avoid excessive narrowing of the middle third. Autospreader flaps or spreader grafts may therefore be used if necessary.

9.3 Autospreader Flaps

Autospreader flaps are an excellent option for avoiding excessive narrowing of the nasal dorsum after ablation of

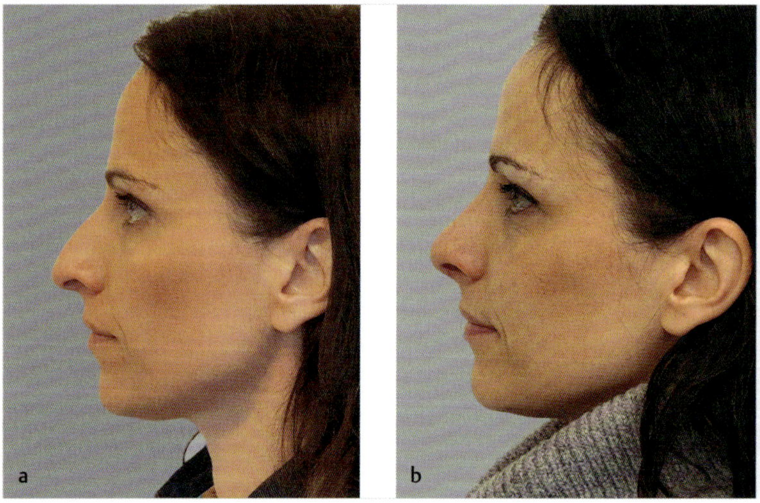

Fig. 9.7 Predominantly cartilaginous hump; case study. (a) Predominantly cartilaginous hump. **(b)** Post rhinoplasty with hump removal. Correction of the "Chinese hat" deformity at the nasal alar edge using rim grafts should also be noted.

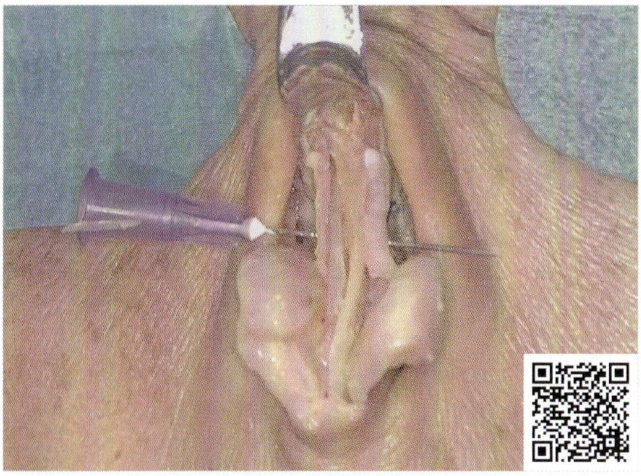

Video 9.2 Autospreader flap and spreader graft (cadaver head).

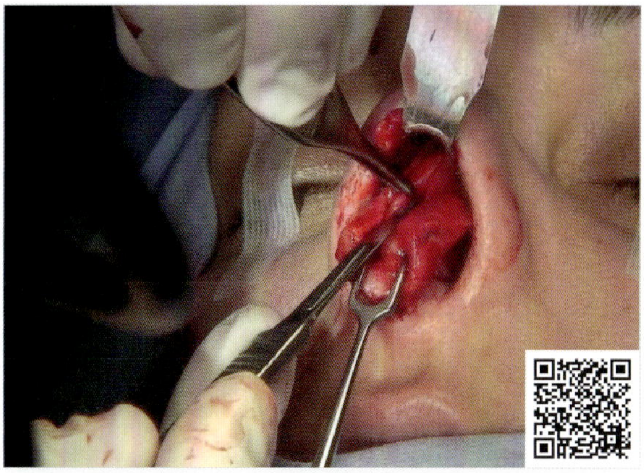

Video 9.3 Reduction of septal height and autospreader flaps (clinical case).

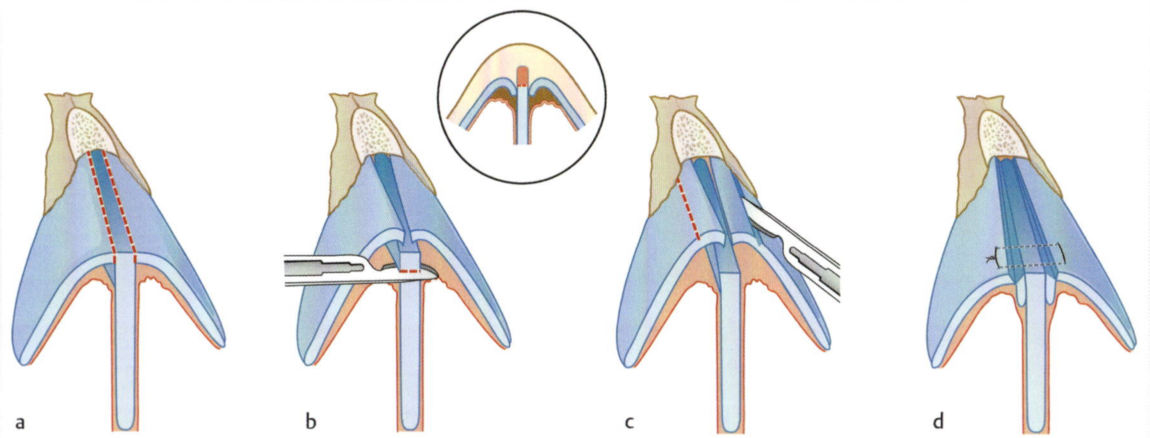

Fig. 9.8 Autospreader flaps. (a) The mucosa is detached as a whole at the attachment of the upper lateral cartilages to the septum. The upper lateral cartilages are separated from the septum using a clean cut. The bony nasal dorsum has already been lowered to the desired level. **(b)** Reduction in the height of the upper edge of the septum, adapted to the height of the corrected bony dorsum. The separated upper lateral cartilages remain intact. **(c)** The upper lateral cartilages are scored (not severed) along a line that marks the new edge of the nasal dorsum. This scoring can be omitted if the cartilage is delicate. **(d)** The upper lateral cartilages are folded medially next to the septum and fixed with one or two horizontal mattress sutures.

a cartilaginous hump; separate cartilage transplants (**spreader grafts**) may not then be required (▶ Video 9.2, ▶ Video 9.3; ▶ Fig. 9.8a–d). The separated upper lateral cartilages must not be shortened as a prerequisite, being initially positioned slightly higher than the upper edge of the septum. The edges of the cartilages are then folded lengthwise toward the septum on either side, while inserting the cut edge next to the septum, with subsequent fixation by one or two transverse 5–0 mattress sutures (with long-term absorbable suture material such as polyglyconate – e.g., Maxon – or polydioxanone – e.g., PDS) (▶ Fig. 9.8, ▶ Fig. 9.9). The upper lateral cartilages thus come to lie at the height of the septal edge.

Longitudinal scoring accentuates the crease line for the cartilaginous spreader flaps, which results in a sharply defined nasal dorsum, facilitates medialization of the folded cartilages, and prevents an excessively wide appearance of the nasal dorsum (see ▶ Fig. 9.8c, d).The procedure primarily prevents excessive narrowing of the middle third while aligning and stabilizing the nasal dorsum in the midline, which also helps straighten crooked noses (▶ Fig. 9.10a–d).

The course of action can be modified in rare cases in such a way that the edges of the upper lateral cartilages are not lowered next to the septum, but are placed over the septal edge (▶ Fig. 9.11). This method can be used to remodel a wide and flat nasal dorsum into one that is narrower and higher – contrary to the original purpose of spreader flaps. These flaps may therefore obviate the need for grafts for augmentation of the nasal dorsum in such cases (▶ Fig. 9.12). However, spreader flaps derived

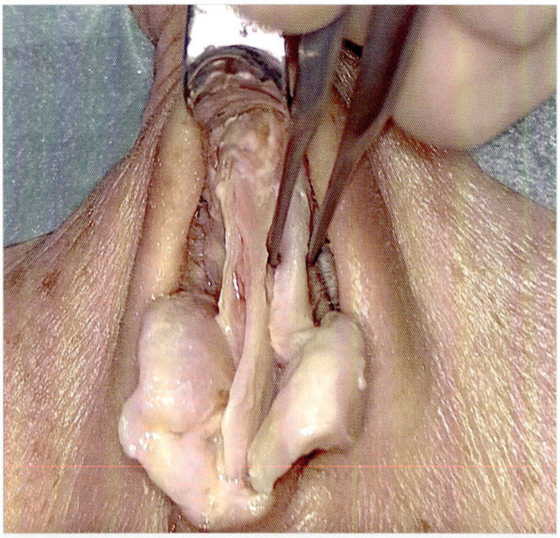

Fig. 9.9 Left autospreader flap. The edge of the upper lateral cartilage is folded toward the septum.

from the lateral cartilages cannot be used if the protrusions of upper lateral cartilages are too delicate and thin, and **spreader grafts** must be used if necessary.

9.4 Spreader Grafts

Spreader grafts can be placed to stabilize, straighten, or widen the nasal dorsum if autospreader flaps cannot be used because they are too delicate or small, or if they are unavailable – as in patients undergoing revision surgery (▶ Video 9.2, ▶ Video 9.4; ▶ Fig. 9.13).

As with spreader flaps, the aim is to reinforce the middle thirds of the nose with cartilaginous strips placed between and sutured to the top edge of the septum and the separated upper lateral cartilages. Spreader grafts of variable length and thickness can be placed on one or both sides, depending on the objective and individual needs. It is often advantageous to allow these cartilaginous grafts to extend into a paramedian osteotomy, if present (performed for hump removal or other reasons).

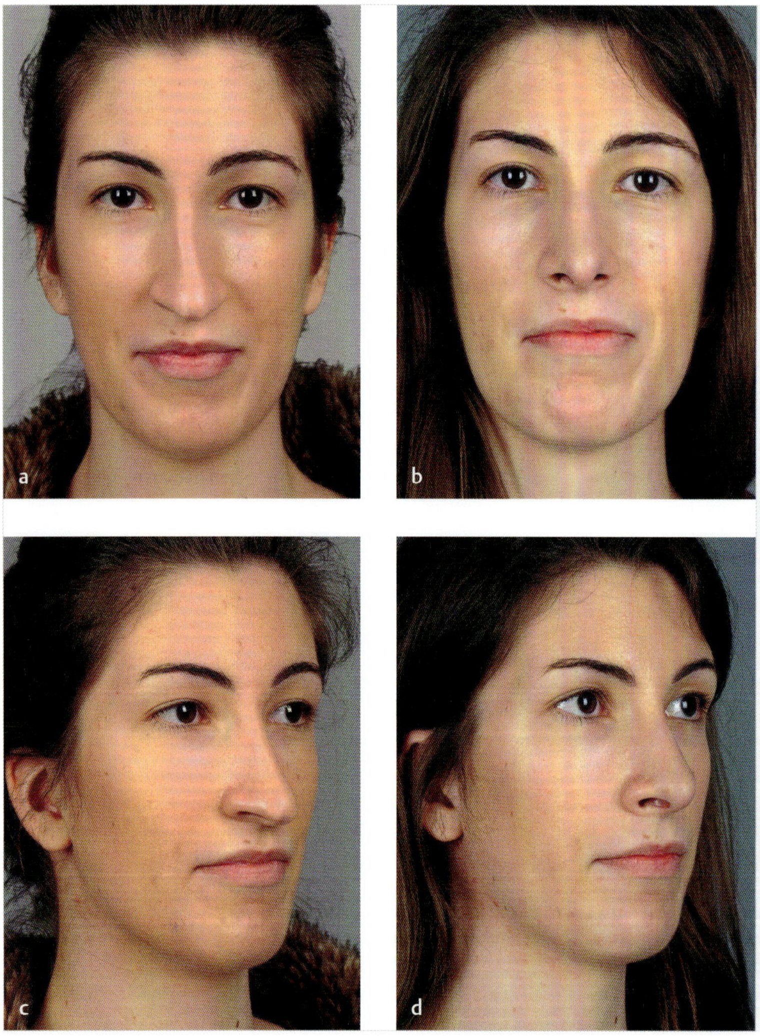

Fig. 9.10 Autospreader flaps for correction of a crooked nose. (a) Preoperative frontal view, **(c)** preoperative oblique view from the right. **(b, d)** Postoperative views. The autospreader flaps help straighten the nose while preventing it from becoming too narrow.

9

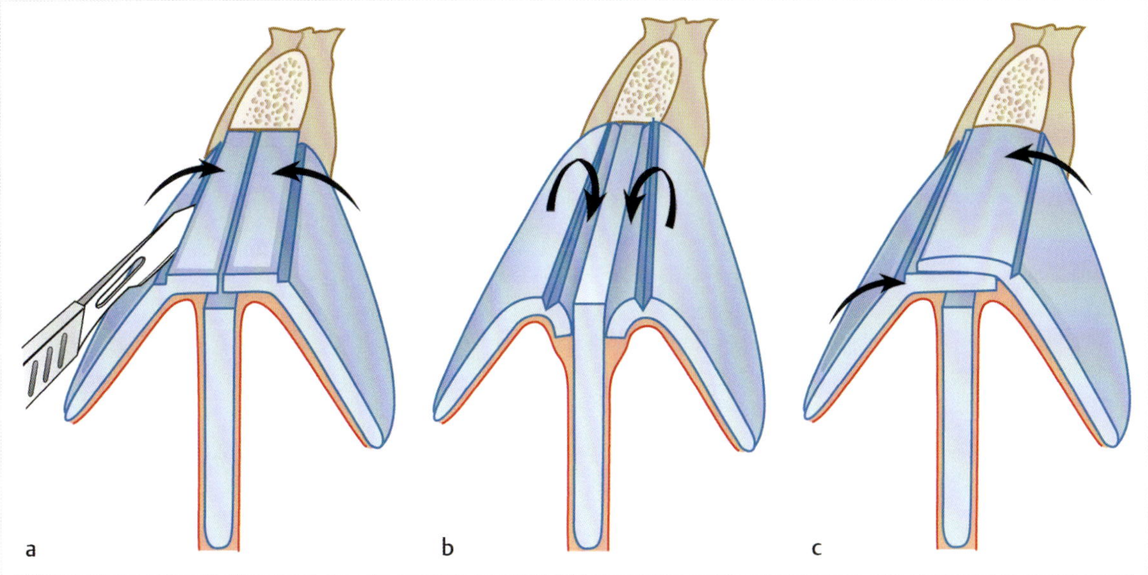

Fig. 9.11 Autospreader flaps for augmentation of the nasal dorsum. As an alternative to the classic autospreader flaps, which involve folding down of the cartilage in the midline next to the septum **(a, b)**, the surplus medial segments of the separated upper lateral cartilages can also be placed on top of each other to elevate the nasal dorsum **(c)**.

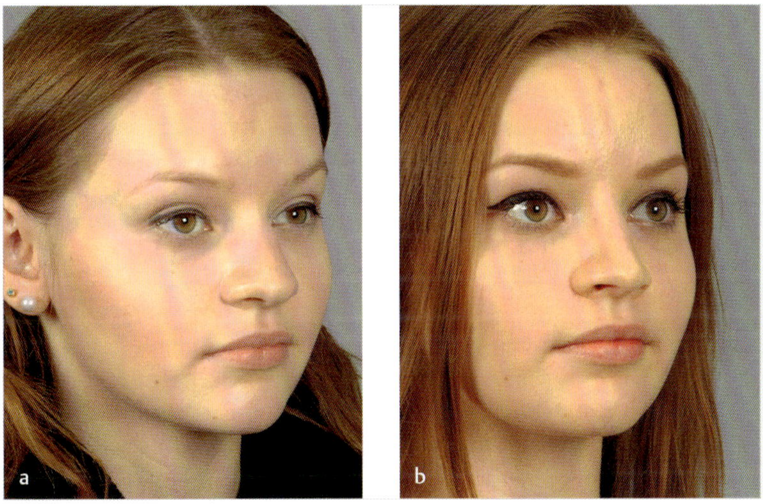

Fig. 9.12 Raising the nasal dorsum with autospreader flaps. Raising and narrowing the nasal dorsum with overlapping autospreader flaps (see also ▶ Fig. 9.11c). **(a)** Preoperative. **(b)** Postoperative.

9

> Spreader grafts extending into the bony nasal vault contribute effectively to straightening of a crooked nose, while ensuring better stability and evenness of the nasal dorsum, especially in the “K-area.”

These grafts are ideally fixed with two horizontal mattress sutures (e.g., 5–0 Maxon or PDS), which pass through all five layers in both directions: upper lateral cartilage and spreader graft on one side, and septum, spreader graft, and upper lateral cartilage on the other (▶ Fig. 9.14).

> While working on the septum, the surgeon should ensure that any excised cartilaginous material is preserved as compact, longitudinal pieces that can be used later — e.g., as a spreader graft. Small fragments are not suitable for this purpose.

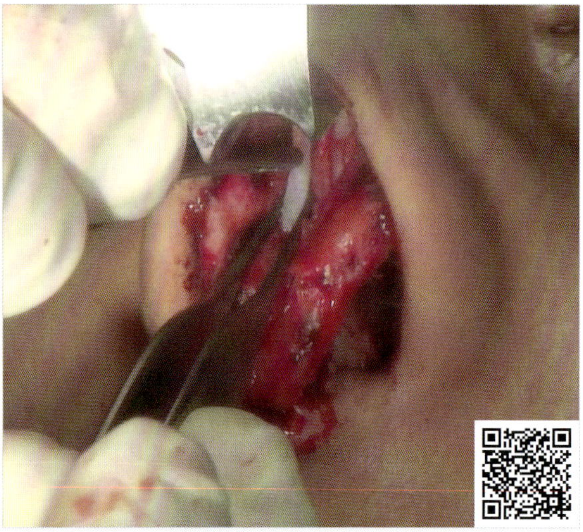

Video 9.4 Spreader grafts (clinical case).

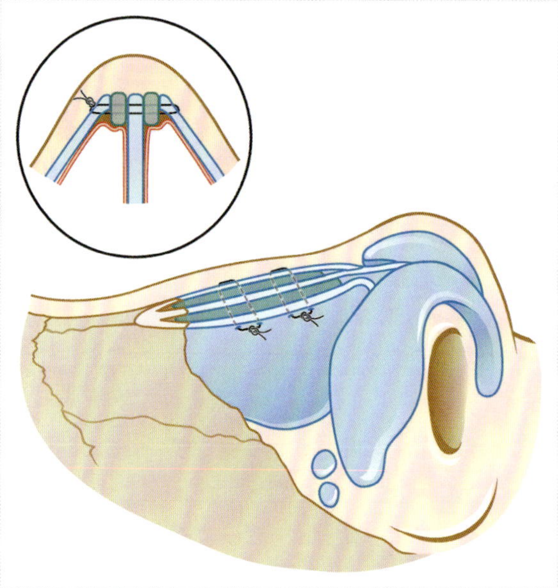

Fig. 9.13 Spreader grafts. An elongated cartilaginous strip is inserted on one or both sides between the upper lateral cartilage and the septum and fixed with horizontal mattress sutures.

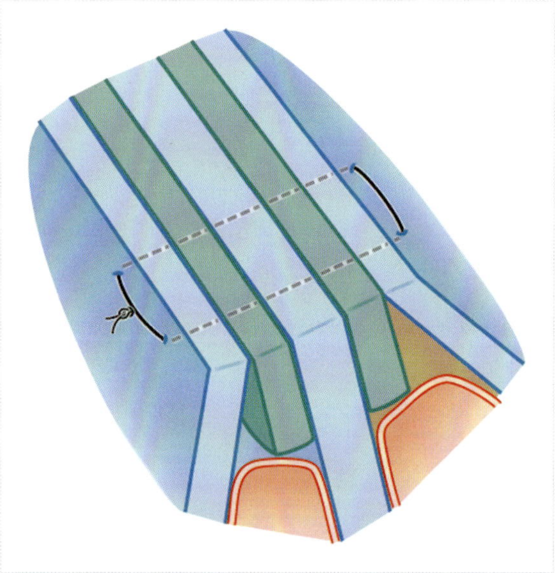

Fig. 9.14 Fixation of spreader grafts. Spreader grafts are secured in place with horizontal mattress sutures. Passing the suture over the surface of the cartilage hinders subsequent reworking of that surface with the scalpel.

The autospreader flaps and spreader grafts can be temporarily fixed with a transversely placed fine needle before suturing of the cartilage (▶ Fig. 9.15a–c).

9.5 Narrowing of the Cartilaginous Nasal Dorsum Without Height Reduction

It is not uncommon for a wide nasal dorsum to need narrowing in the middle cartilaginous third of it without concomitant height reduction (as in the case of hump removal). The nasal dorsum is elegantly and relatively easily narrowed in such instances by excising a narrow, roughly longitudinal to oval cartilaginous strip parallel to the septum on either side at the attachment of the upper lateral cartilages to the septum (▶ Fig. 9.16, ▶ Fig. 9.17a, b, ▶ Fig. 9.18a–f). The mucous membrane in the angle between the upper lateral cartilages and the septum is first mobilized and spared.

The upper lateral cartilages are finally reattached to the septum with one or two horizontal mattress sutures, which narrows the cartilaginous nasal dorsum without any height reduction.

9.6 Spanning Sutures

Spanning sutures between the upper lateral and/or alar cartilages on either side elevate the lateral cartilages to widen or stabilize the nasal valve region. These are therefore primarily functional sutures. The suture first passes through one lateral cartilage and is then brought over the nasal bridge to the other side, where it passes through the cartilage in the opposite direction (▶ Fig. 9.19). Knotting the thread ends typically results in elevation of the lateral cartilages, which then form a larger angle with the septum. This opens up the nasal valve and ideally improves nasal breathing.

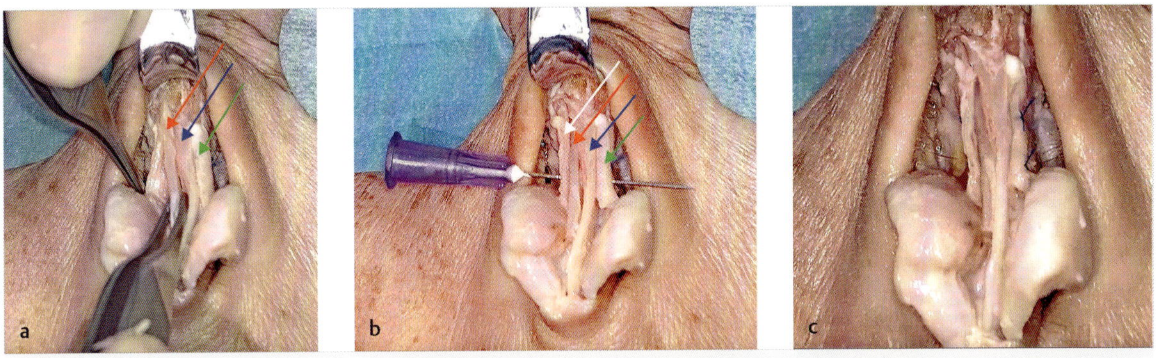

Fig. 9.15 Fixation of autospreader flaps and spreader grafts. (a) Insertion of a spreader graft (red arrow) on the right, between the septum (blue arrow) and the upper lateral cartilage (ULC); left autospreader flap (green arrow). (Demonstrated in a cadaver specimen.) **(b)** Temporary fixation of the spreader graft (right) and autospreader flap (left) with a fine cannula. White arrow: right ULC; red arrow: spreader graft; blue arrow: septum; green arrow: spreader flap. **(c)** Securing the spreader graft (right) and autospreader flap (left) with double horizontal mattress sutures.

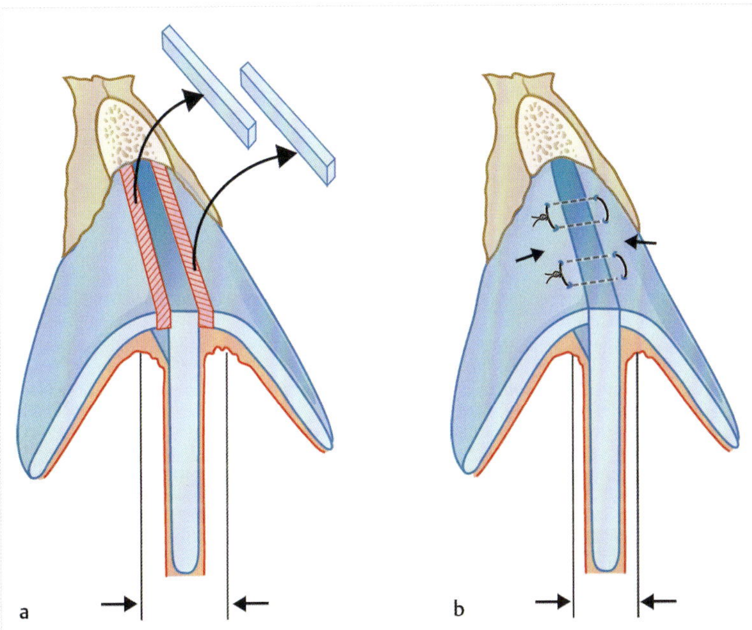

Fig. 9.16 Narrowing of the cartilaginous nasal dorsum. (a) Narrowing of the cartilaginous nasal dorsum without height reduction by resecting paramedian cartilaginous strips on either side, followed by reattachment to the septum **(b)**.

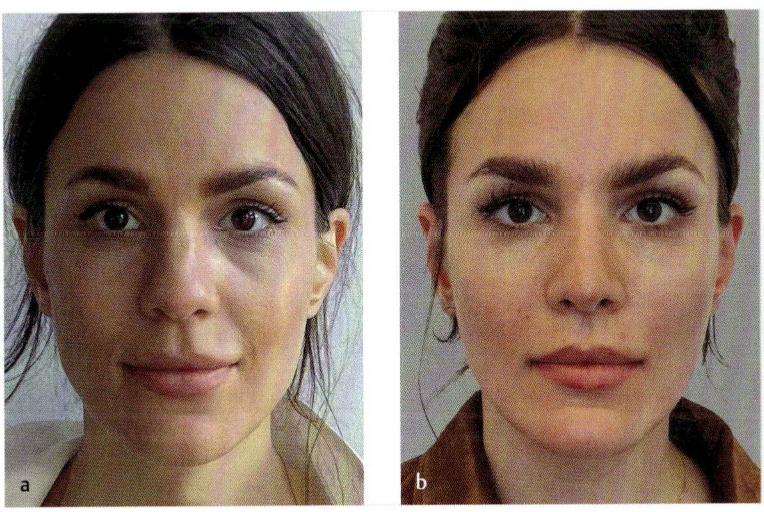

Fig. 9.17 Narrowing of the cartilaginous dorsum; case study 1. (a) Preoperative frontal view. **(b)** Postoperative frontal view.

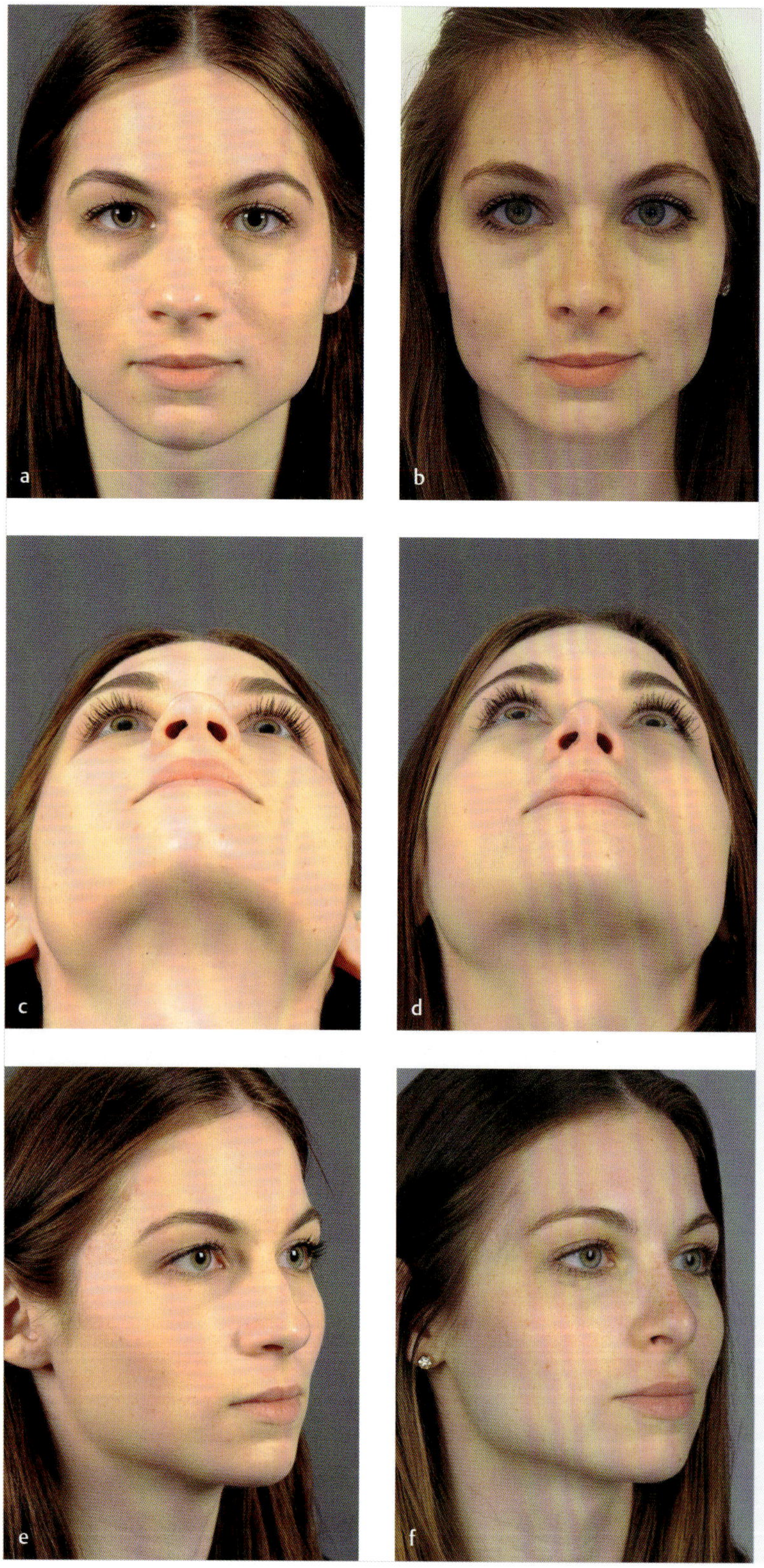

Fig. 9.18 Narrowing of the dorsum; case study 2. (a, c, e) Preoperative appearance. **(b, d, f)** The result after rhinoplasty. The tip was also refined, in this case with a delicate tip graft.

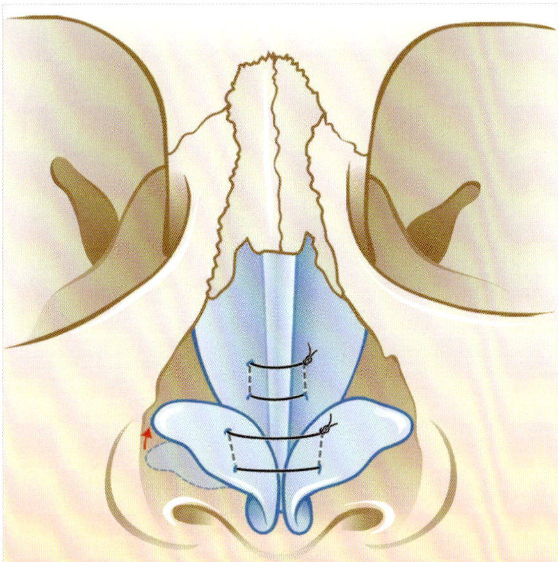

Fig. 9.19 Spanning sutures. Spanning sutures between the upper lateral or alar cartilages elevate the lateral cartilages and may contribute to opening of the nasal valve.

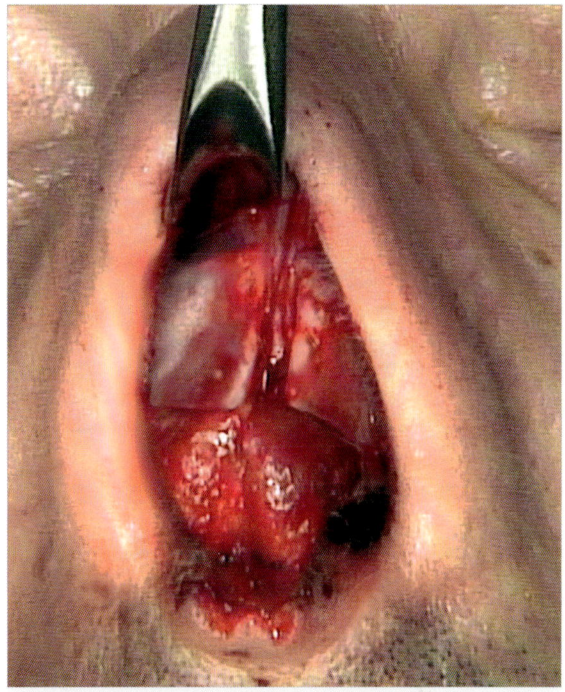

Fig. 9.20 Lateral batten graft. An upper lateral batten graft on both sides, harvested from conchal cartilage in this case.

9.7 Upper Lateral Batten and Strut Grafts

Lateral batten or strut grafts are indicated from a cosmetic or functional point of view for reinforcement of the lateral wall of the nose at the level of the upper lateral cartilage or the lateral crus of the alar cartilage. **Batten grafts** are fixed as "onlay grafts" to reinforce or replace attenuated or absent lateral cartilages on the outer aspect of the lateral nasal wall (▶ Fig. 9.20). Strut grafts, on the other hand, are placed as supports under the cartilage (compare with section 10.3).

The surgeon needs to find the right balance between stability and graft volume. These grafts must not be too delicate if they are meant to ensure stability. They should also not be too voluminous and cosmetically unappealing, or narrow the lumen of the nasal cavity and thus impair nasal breathing.

Lateral batten or strut grafts are valuable tools in reconstructive surgery of the upper and lower lateral cartilages when correctly indicated and of the appropriate size.

9.8 Butterfly Grafts

Butterfly grafts are approximately diamond-shaped grafts and are usually harvested from auricular cartilage. They are placed in the center of the upper edge of the septum in the region of the inner nasal valve. The "butterfly wings" between the upper lateral and lower lateral cartilages on either side then serve to stabilize and expand the inner valve region (▶ Fig. 9.21).

9.9 Composite Graft for the Lateral Wall

Composite grafts harvested from the auricle may replace the upper lateral cartilage if both the cartilage and the inner lining of the lateral nasal wall are deficient. However, these grafts heal less reliably than purely cartilaginous transplants (▶ Fig. 9.22).

Both layers heal better when this type of transplant is firmly connected to the covering nasal skin with mattress sutures for about a week. The sutures can be knotted on the outside over a silicone film to avoid pressure marks on the skin.

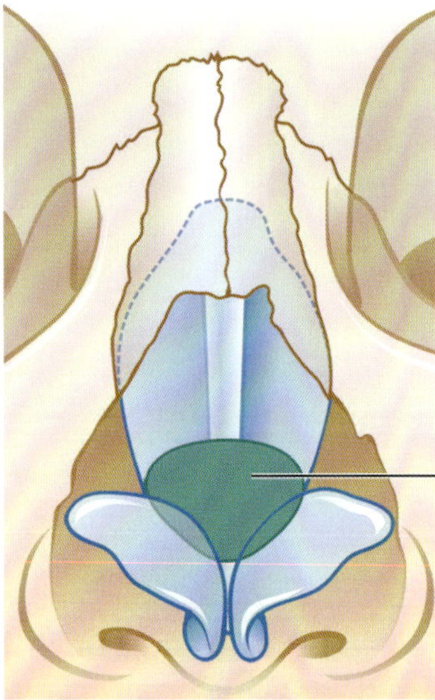

Fig. 9.21 Butterfly graft. The butterfly graft for stabilization of the nasal valve may vary in size depending on individual requirements.

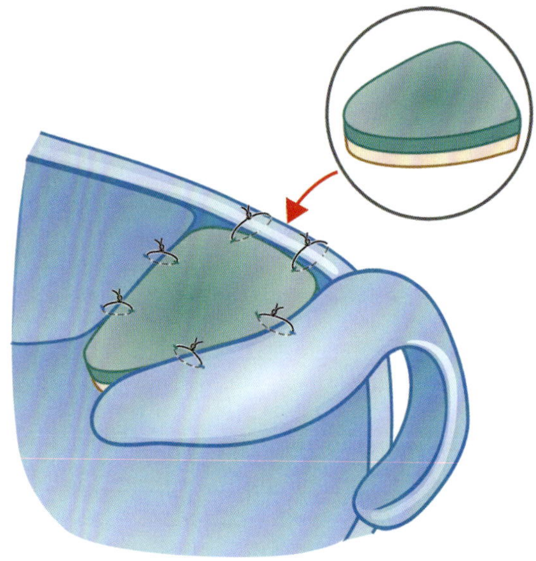

Fig. 9.22 Composite graft for the lateral nasal wall. A composite graft, including cartilage and skin harvested from the ear, for reconstruction of the lateral nasal wall and inner lining.

9

Bibliography

Abdelwahab M, Patel PN. Conventional resection versus preservation of the nasal dorsum and ligaments: an anatomic perspective and review of the literature. Facial Plast Surg Clin North Am. 2021; 29(1):15–28

Abdelwahab M, Patel PN, Kandathil CK, Most SP. Effect of midvault reconstruction versus preservation on lateral nasal wall stability. Facial Plast Surg Aesthet Med. 2021; 23(6):482–484

Boccieri A, Macro C, Pascali M. The use of spreader grafts in primary rhinoplasty. Ann Plast Surg. 2005; 55(2):127–131

Gruber RP, Park E, Newman J, Berkowitz L, Oneal R. The spreader flap in primary rhinoplasty. Plast Reconstr Surg. 2007; 119(6):1903–1910

Gruber RP, Perkins SW. Humpectomy and spreader flaps. Clin Plast Surg. 2010; 37(2):285–291

Harris MO, Baker SR. Management of the wide nasal dorsum. Arch Facial Plast Surg. 2004; 6(1):41–48

Kim L, Papel ID. Spreader grafts in functional rhinoplasty. Facial Plast Surg. 2016; 32(1):29–35

Kovacevic M, Riedel F, Göksel A, Wurm J. Options for middle vault and dorsum restoration after hump removal in primary rhinoplasty. Facial Plast Surg. 2016; 32(4):374–383

Sheen JH. Spreader graft: a method of reconstructing the roof of the middle nasal vault following rhinoplasty. Plast Reconstr Surg. 1984; 73(2):230–239

Sykes JM. Management of the middle nasal third in revision rhinoplasty. Facial Plast Surg. 2008; 24(3):339–347

Sykes JM, Tapias V, Kim JE. Management of the nasal dorsum. Facial Plast Surg. 2011; 27(2):192–202

10 Corrective Surgery of the Lower Lateral Cartilages (LLC)

10.1 Variant Forms of the LLC

The configuration of the lower lateral cartilage plays an important role in the overall appearance of the nose. Common and typical deformities of the lateral crura are shown in ▶ Fig. 10.1a–f. ▶ Fig. 10.2 shows an example of unilateral concavity of the lateral crus, and ▶ Fig. 10.3 shows asymmetry of the alar cartilages. The LLC may be fragile, and it is rare for it to be unilaterally absent or show aplasia (▶ Fig. 10.4). Interestingly, findings of this type may be clinically inconspicuous and only become apparent during the operation.

Traumatic lesions of the alar cartilages are predominantly iatrogenic and due to rhinoplasty. Accidents play a minor role, and primarily include bites or lacerations. Tumor-related defects – e.g., after resection of basal cell carcinoma – occur more frequently. The most common corrective procedures on the LLC in primary rhinoplasty are described below (see also Chapter 12, ▶ Table 12.2).

10.2 Narrowing of the Lower Lateral Cartilage

Narrowing of the nose and reduction of wide alar cartilages is very commonly performed during primary rhinoplasty. Precision surgery of the cranial (i.e., cephalic) aspect of the lateral crus requires separation of the outer skin far laterally to the lateral edge of the cartilage, as well as severing of the cephalic rim along the S-shaped junction of the upper and lower lateral cartilages (the scroll complex; see Chapter 1, ▶ Fig. 1.8) (▶ Video 10.1).

With the advent of preservation rhinoplasty, efforts were intensified to preserve the horizontal and vertical scroll ligaments when dissecting the cephalic border of the alar cartilage. This can be done by dissecting the perichondrium from caudal to cranial directly on the exposed cartilage and dividing the LLC below the insertion of the scroll ligaments. However, a possible disadvantage of this approach is that the alar cartilage,

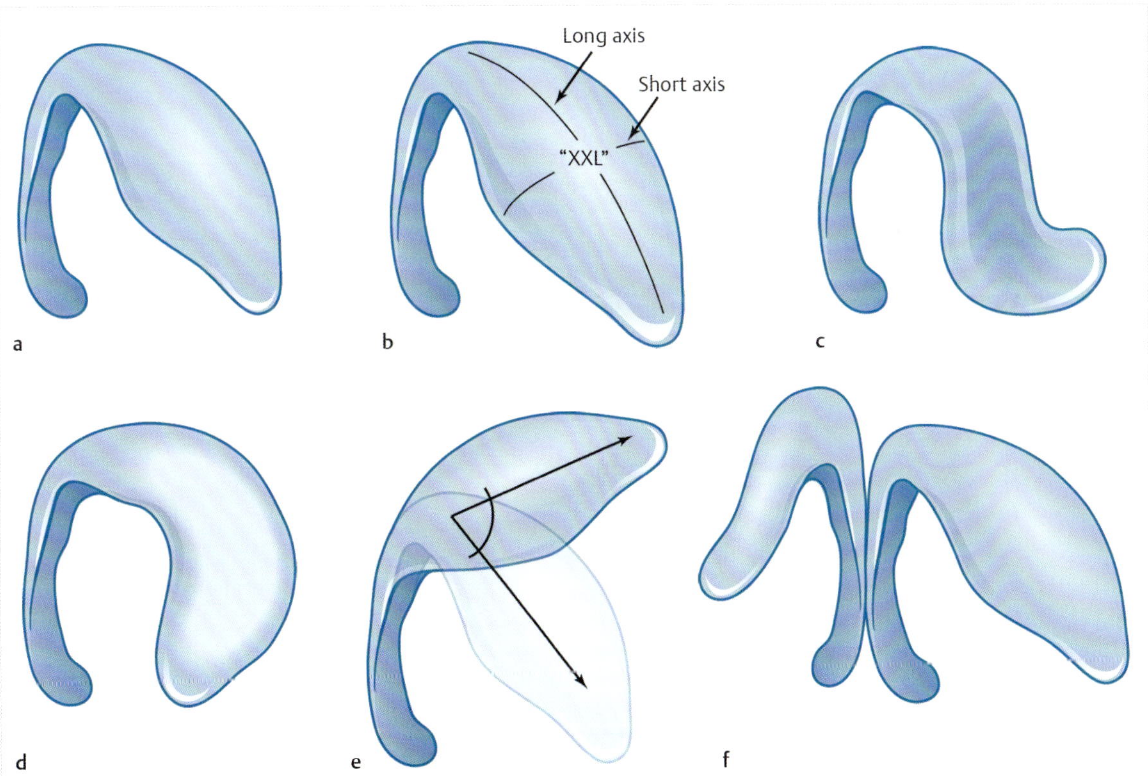

Fig. 10.1 Shape disorders of the lower lateral cartilages. (a) Normal appearance. **(b)** Oversized on both the long and short axes. **(c)** Marked concavity (see ▶ Fig. 10.2). **(d)** Marked convexity (spherical/"bulbous," or box-like/"boxy"). **(e)** Malpositioned; too medially aligned. **(f)** Asymmetrical (see ▶ Fig. 10.3).

10

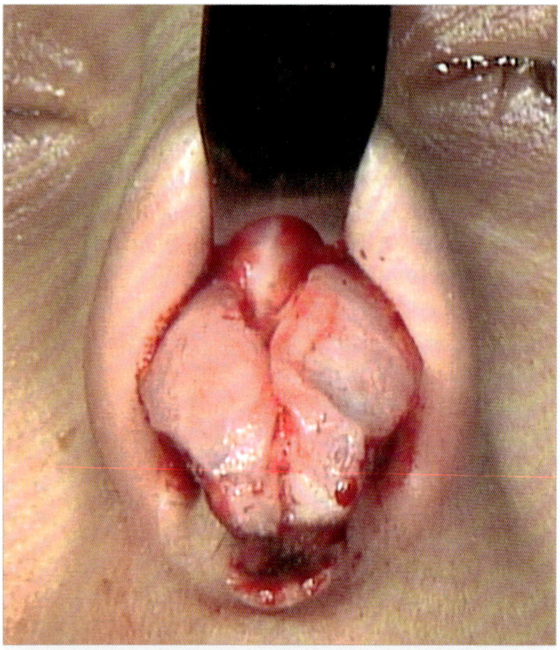

Fig. 10.2 Concavity of the lower lateral cartilage. Only the left lower lateral cartilage is involved in this case, resulting in an asymmetrical appearance.

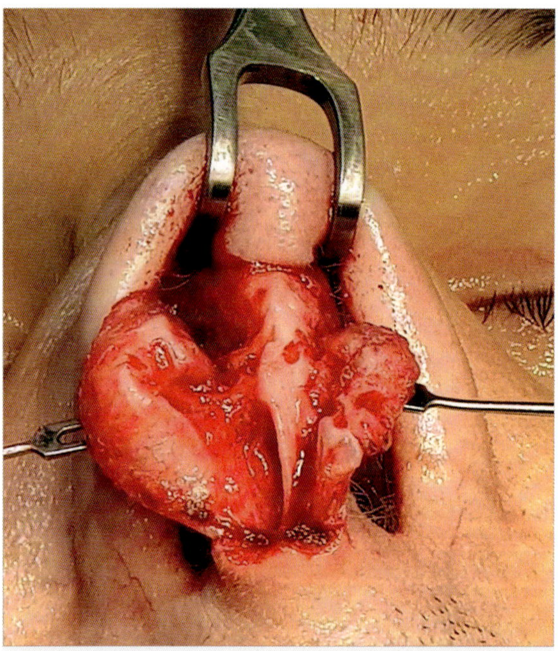

Fig. 10.4 Aplasia of the left alar cartilage. A rudimentary left alar cartilage is present. An anomaly of this extent was not visible on the nose.

which has been completely freed from perichondrium, loses stability.

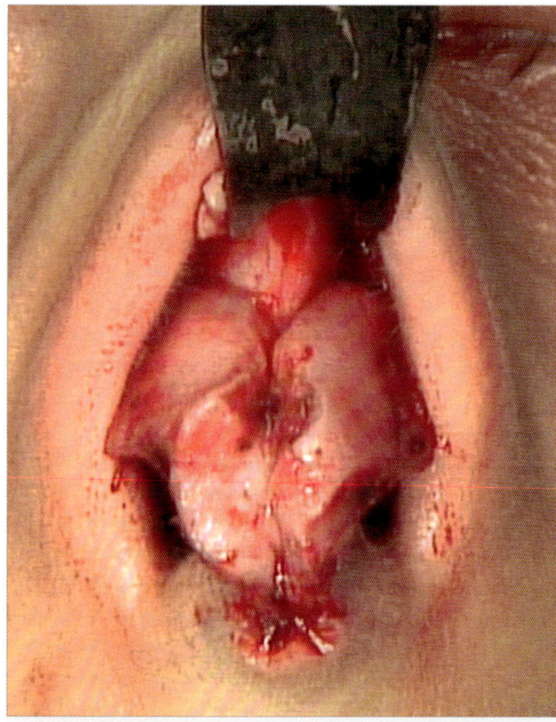

Fig. 10.3 Asymmetry of the alar cartilages. The cartilaginous framework frequently shows asymmetries of this type, but this does not necessarily lead to visible asymmetry of the nose.

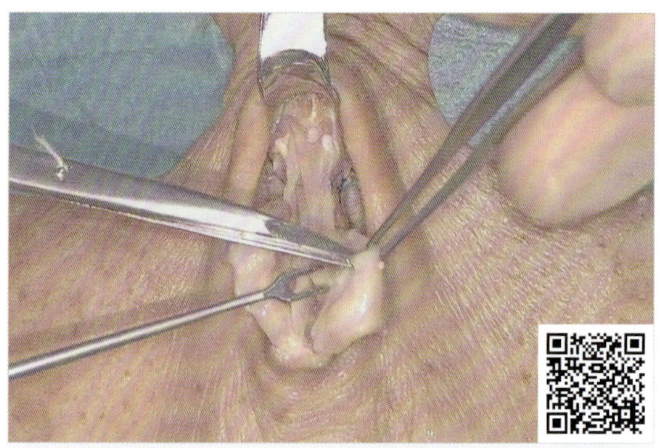

Video 10.1 Dissection of the lateral crura, cephalic resection, with marking of the domes (cadaver head).

Another way to preserve these scroll ligaments is to first expose and mark them, then cut them at the elevation of the skin flap, in order to later reconnect them by suture at the marks (see ▶ Fig. 1.17, ▶ Fig. 8.58b).

After separation of the lower from the upper lateral cartilage along the scroll line, the vestibular skin is then carefully separated from the LLC with a pair of pointed scissors, using the open technique (▶ Fig. 10.5).

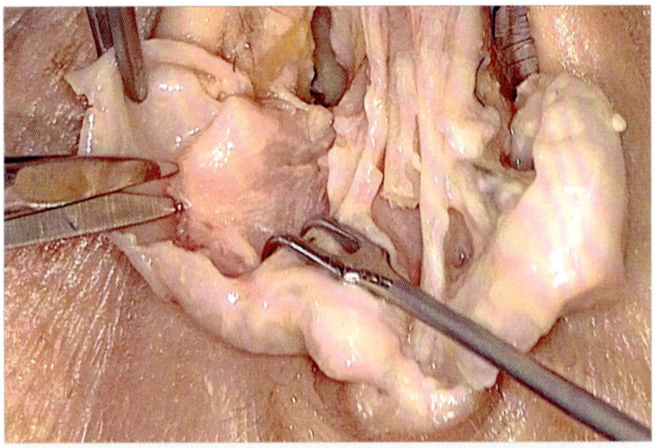

Fig. 10.5 Dissection of the lower lateral cartilage. The sensitive vestibular skin on the inner aspect of the lower lateral cartilage is carefully dissected after separation of the lower from the upper lateral cartilage along the intercartilaginous fold (alar scroll). Note the delicate two-pronged hook that stretches the vestibule skin medially (cadaver specimen).

> This dissection is greatly facilitated if an assistant stretches the vestibular skin of the lower lateral cartilage further medially using a fine two-pronged hook, while the surgeon gently grasps the cartilage with forceps and pulls it laterally (▸ Fig. 10.5).

This maneuver is not always easy, as the vestibular skin is thin and frequently tightly adherent to the cartilage. This delicate skin may tear in the process, and in the event of a major tear should be immediately repaired with rapidly absorbable 6–0 sutures to prevent ascending infection.

The inner lining can be wholly or partly separated, depending on further planned interventions on the alar cartilage.

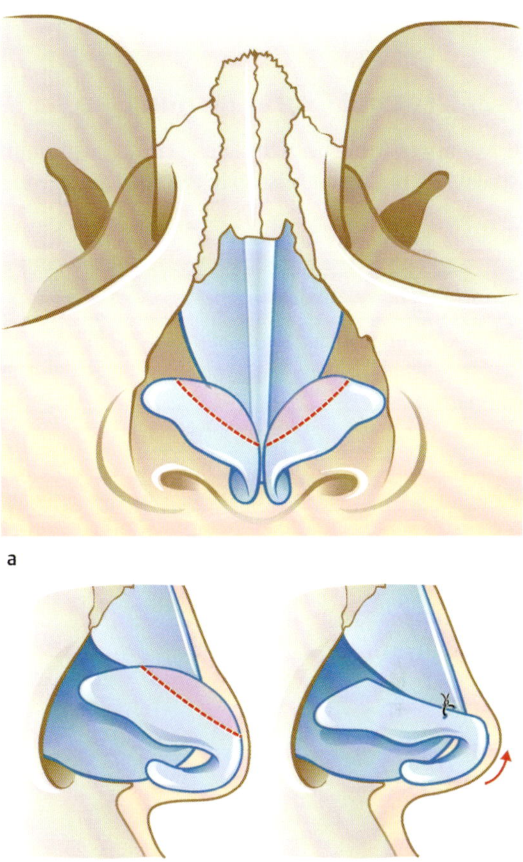

a

b c

Fig. 10.6 Cephalic resection. Shortening of the cranial (cephalic) alar rim **(a, b)** results in narrowing of the supratip region and cranial rotation of the nasal tip, especially with an additional suspension suture of the lateral crura to the middle thirds of the cartilaginous vault **(c)**.

10.2.1 Cephalic Resection

Very large and wide nasal alae are usually due to the presence of excessive cartilaginous tissue at the cephalic (cranial) aspect of the lateral crura; this condition has been corrected for decades by resecting and discarding the "excess" cartilage (▸ Video 10.1, ▸ Fig. 10.6a–c).

This "cephalic resection" or "cephalic trim" effectively corrects an excessively wide supratip region in most cases and continues to form part of the surgical routine for many rhinoplasty surgeons. However, when it is overdone, it can give rise to an undesirable postoperative outcome, such as depression of the alar wings or constriction in the region of the nasal valve and obstructed nasal breathing – especially secondary to an intercartilaginous incision using the "closed" technique.

The prevailing opinion is that **excessive resection** of the nasal vault in general, and particularly of the lower lateral cartilages, can lead to undesirable permanent functional and cosmetic damage. **Reshaping** and forming of the cartilage are therefore preferable to resection. However, a narrow marginal strip of floppy, usually unstable and functionless cartilage only is often resected from the cephalic rim of the lower lateral cartilage (▸ Fig. 10.7; see Video 6.1, Video 10.1), but significant narrowing is not the objective of this procedure.

Again: reshaping rather than resection of the lower lateral cartilages is desirable. The lateral crural turn-in flap serves this purpose, and can be regarded as similar to the autospreader flap on the upper lateral cartilage in the middle third of the nasal vault (see section 9.3, ▶ Fig. 9.8, ▶ Fig. 9.9).

10.2.2 Lateral Crural Turn-in Flap

The extent of narrowing of the lateral crura is determined by the width of the caudal strip of the alar cartilage to be preserved.

> ✓
> The intact residual caudal strip of the lower lateral cartilages must be equal in size on either side.

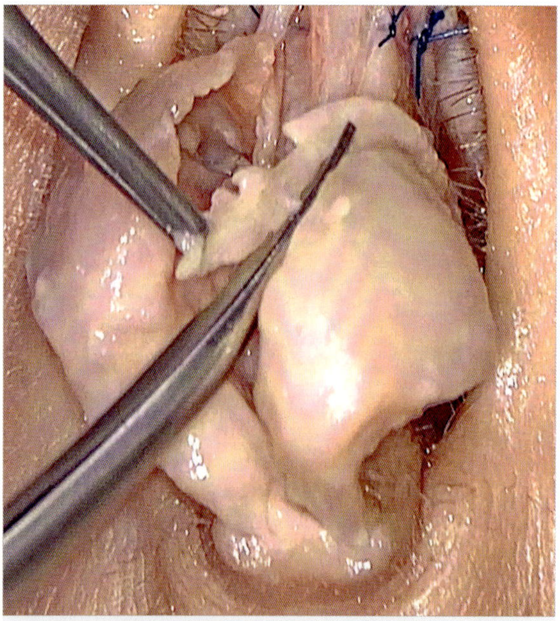

Fig. 10.7 Minimal cephalic resection. Resection of a narrow strip of floppy, functionless cartilage from the cephalic edge of the left lower lateral cartilage. cartilage (cadaver specimen).

As frequently mentioned in the literature, this cartilaginous strip should not be narrower than 6 mm in women and 8 mm in men, but may vary considerably from case to case depending on the individual's anatomy (▶ Fig. 10.8a, b).

> ✓
> To simplify matters, the width of the shaft of the no. 15 blade can be used as a rough measurement for the width of the intact strip of alar cartilage. This speeds up the measuring process, since the scalpel is in the surgeon's hand anyway and provides symmetry.
> A special measuring device is therefore not required (▶ Fig. 10.9).

A newly available Adson–Brown forceps with a millimeter scale is another elegant and precise means of measuring the lower lateral cartilage (▶ Fig. 10.10).

The cartilage is superficially scored along the line thus determined for the remaining width of the alar cartilage, until its cephalic segment can be folded inward while still adherent to the caudal segment (▶ Fig. 10.11), thereby creating the turn-in flap of the LLC (▶ Fig. 10.12a, b; ▶ Video 10.2, ▶ Video 10.3; see Video 6.1). This cartilaginous flap is completely rotated to obtain the **classic 180° variant**, after which it is flatly applied to the inner aspect of the preserved lower lateral cartilage. Both cartilaginous layers are finally secured in this position with one or two long-term absorbable mattress sutures with 5–0 or 6–0 polyglyconate or polydioxanone (e.g., Maxon or PDS). The rest of the lower lateral cartilage thus becomes narrower and is more stable, due to the double layer of cartilage.

In comparison with simple cephalic resection, the turn-in flap technique in patients with voluminous alar cartilages and excessive lateral crura reduces the postoperative risk of

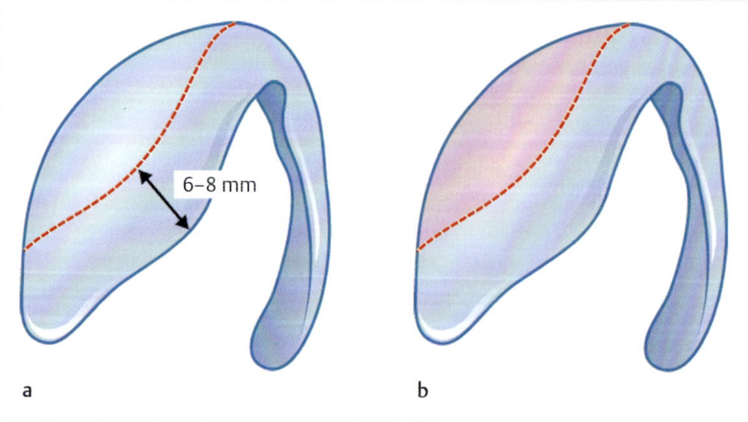

Fig. 10.8 Reduction of the lateral crus. **(a)** A caudal strip of cartilage, which may be slightly narrower in females than in males, remains untouched. **(b)** The area marked in red is usually remodeled and not resected.

10

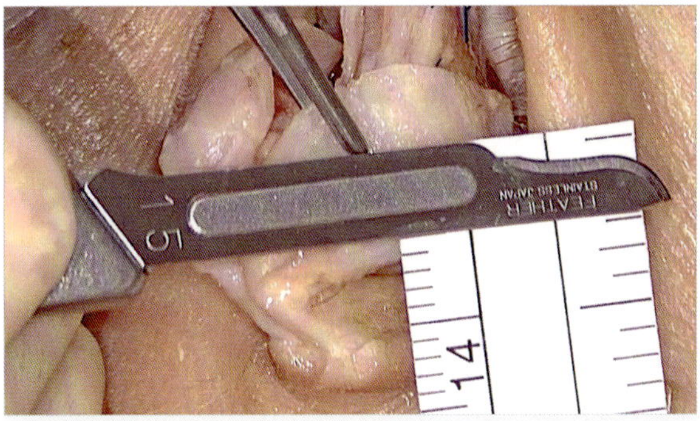

Fig. 10.9 Width of the intact alar cartilaginous strip. The width of the scalpel blade shaft can be used as a measure of size at the lower lateral cartilage.

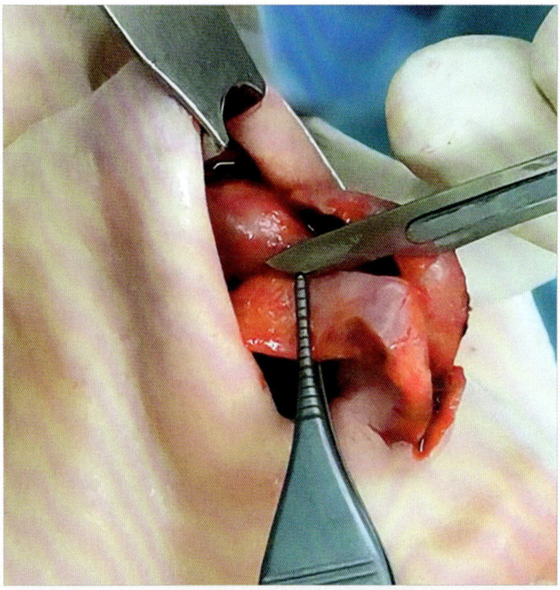

Fig. 10.10 Adson–Brown forceps with a millimeter scale. The scale on the forceps allows millimeter-precise measurement of the width at the alar cartilage (KARL STORZ SE & Co. KG, Tuttlingen, Germany).

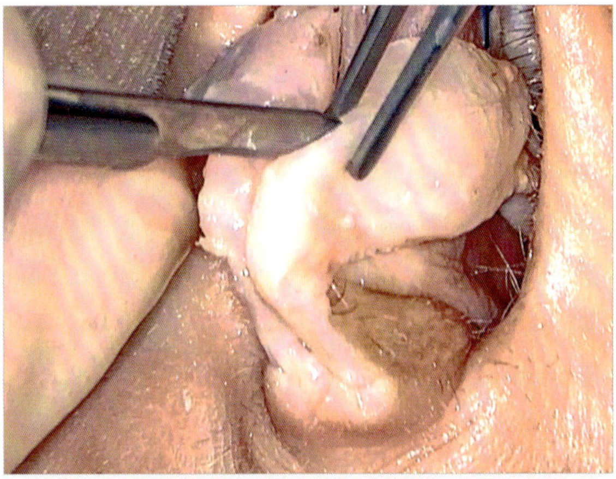

Fig. 10.11 Scoring the lower lateral cartilage. The crease line is scored into the lower lateral cartilage, which demarcates the lateral crural turn-in flap.

fragile, collapsible alar cartilage with associated valve incompetence (▶ Fig. 10.13a–d, ▶ Fig. 10.14a, b, c1).

Another great advantage of the lateral crural turn-in flap is its ability to correct concavity of the lateral crus. Although conversion to obvious convexity may not always be possible, concavity of the cartilage is usually largely eliminated by this method and alternative, more costly techniques for correcting it are often unnecessary.

10.2.3 The 90° Lateral Crural Turn-in Flap

Diverging from the classic form described above, a simplified turn-in flap with even greater benefits can be used. In fact, this cartilaginous flap can be further modified if complete rotation to the inner aspect of the remaining caudal cartilaginous strip is dispensed with and the flap is rotated by a mere 90° instead (▶ Fig. 10.14c2, d). It is then not necessary to detach the inner skin lining over a large area. The lateral crura are narrowed to the same extent if the flap at the cephalic rim of the alar cartilage is rotated by 90° instead of 180° (▶ Fig. 10.14c2). The cartilaginous flap is fixed at an approximately right angle, which provides better valve stability while preventing excessive flattening of the nasal alae ("hinged flap" after Sazgar; ▶ Fig. 10.14c2, d).

The folded cartilaginous strip in this variant of the turn-in flap should also be sutured to secure its position. The valve region can be further reinforced by inserting a cartilaginous strip as a lateral crural strut graft into the angle between the turn-in flap and the caudal strip of the alar cartilage and securing it with sutures (▶ Video 10.4; ▶ Fig. 10.14c3, ▶ Fig. 10.15a, b). This modification is also very advantageous for correcting lateral alar concavity and weakness (▶ Fig. 10.16a–d).

10.2.4 Lateral Crural Turn-out Flap

The counterpart of the lateral crural turn-in flap, the lateral crural turn-**out** flap, is less well known. In this, the cranial part of the lower lateral cartilage is turned outward instead of inward (▶ Fig. 10.17a–c). In principle, a turn-out flap is useful in the presence of a particularly wide lower lateral cartilage. However, if the surgeon is intending to reinforce the caudal edge of the lateral crus by outward rotation of the cartilaginous flap, this has not been very successful in my experience. An additional rim graft needs to be applied,

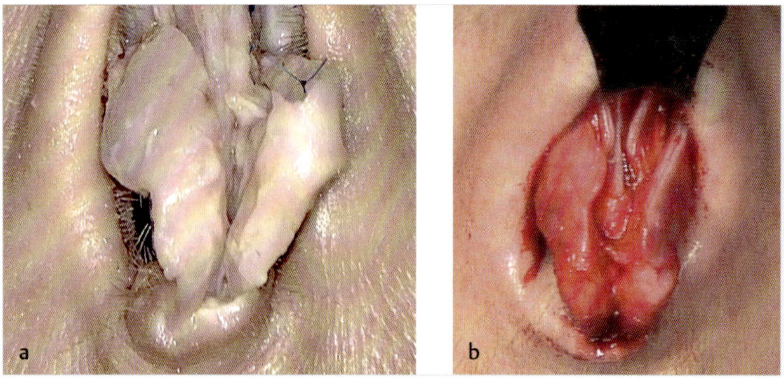

Fig. 10.12 180° lateral crural turn-in flap. **(a)** The turn-in flap has been folded in on the left and affixed with a suture in a cadaver specimen. **(b)** The intraoperative situation, showing the delicate, superficially incised line on the patient's right LLC, where the turn-in flap is not yet folded, and the already folded turn-in flap on the left side.

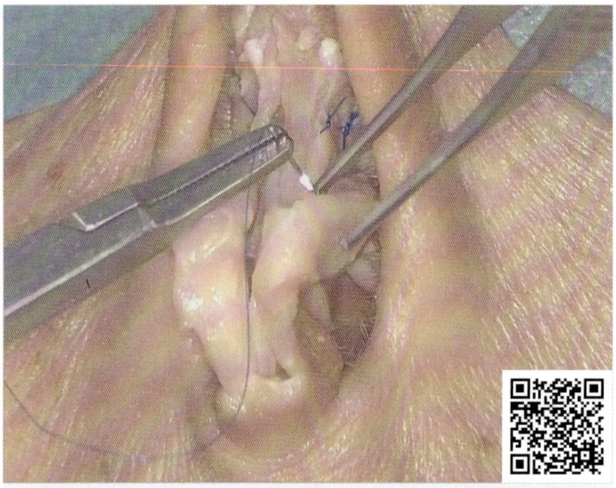

Video 10.2 Lateral crural turn-in flap (cadaver head).

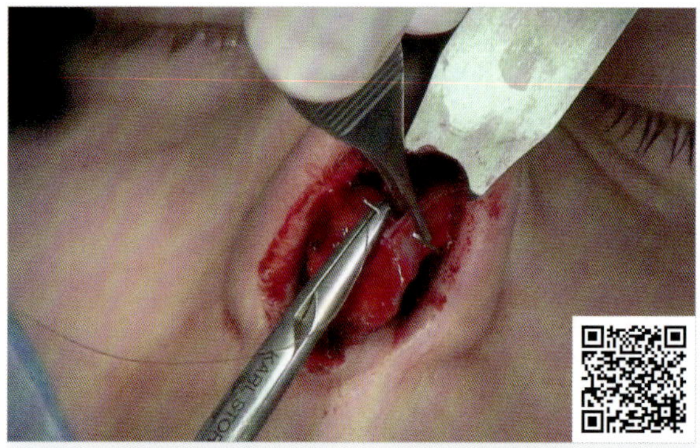

Video 10.3 180° lateral crural turn-in flaps (clinical case).

if necessary, even if the scored crease for the cartilaginous flap lies relatively far caudally.

10.3 Stabilization of the Lower Lateral Cartilage: Lateral Crural Batten, Strut, and Rim Grafts

Grafts are used to provide greater stability and contouring of the lower lateral cartilage. The lateral **strut** graft is applied to the inner aspect of the lower lateral cartilage (▶ Fig. 10.18a), whereas the lateral crural **batten** graft is affixed to the outer aspect of the lateral crus (▶ Fig. 10.18b). The **rim** graft is applied to its caudal rim (▶ Fig. 10.18c). All of these grafts serve to stabilize the lower lateral cartilage, and they are therefore beneficial in patients with weak nasal valves and nostrils.

> ✔
>
> Strut or batten grafts applied to the cephalic edge of the lower lateral cartilage are more suitable for stabilization of the inner nasal valve; rim grafts reinforce the outer nasal valve.

Careful preoperative evaluation should identify the region of the lateral wall that requires reinforcement (see section 3.2.2). This determines the type and position of the grafts, which can also be used in combination (e.g., a lateral strut graft with a rim graft).

In addition to providing stability, **rim** grafts also determine the profile of the alar rim. They are therefore frequently used to lower or accentuate an alar rim (retracted nasal ala; compare with ▶ Fig. 9.7a, b, ▶ Fig. 10.22a–d). These grafts are placed in small subcutaneous pockets usually created with fine, pointed scissors on the raised nasal skin flap along the nasal alar rim, extending from the marginal incision at the level of the dome (▶ Fig. 10.19a–f; see Video 6.1). Before the scissors are inserted, "tunneling" using a cannula with stylet is very useful – e.g., venous catheter Vasofix, 16 G (▶ Fig. 10.19a–c), which is advanced subcutaneously along the alar rim before the graft bed is expanded with scissors.

Fine, pin-shaped rim grafts are inserted into these pockets. These can be fixed with 6–0 polyglactin 910 (e.g., Vicryl Rapide) sutures to the subcutaneous soft tissue of the alar rim; and/or with 6–0 polydioxanone (e.g., PDS) to the caudal rim of the lower lateral cartilage.

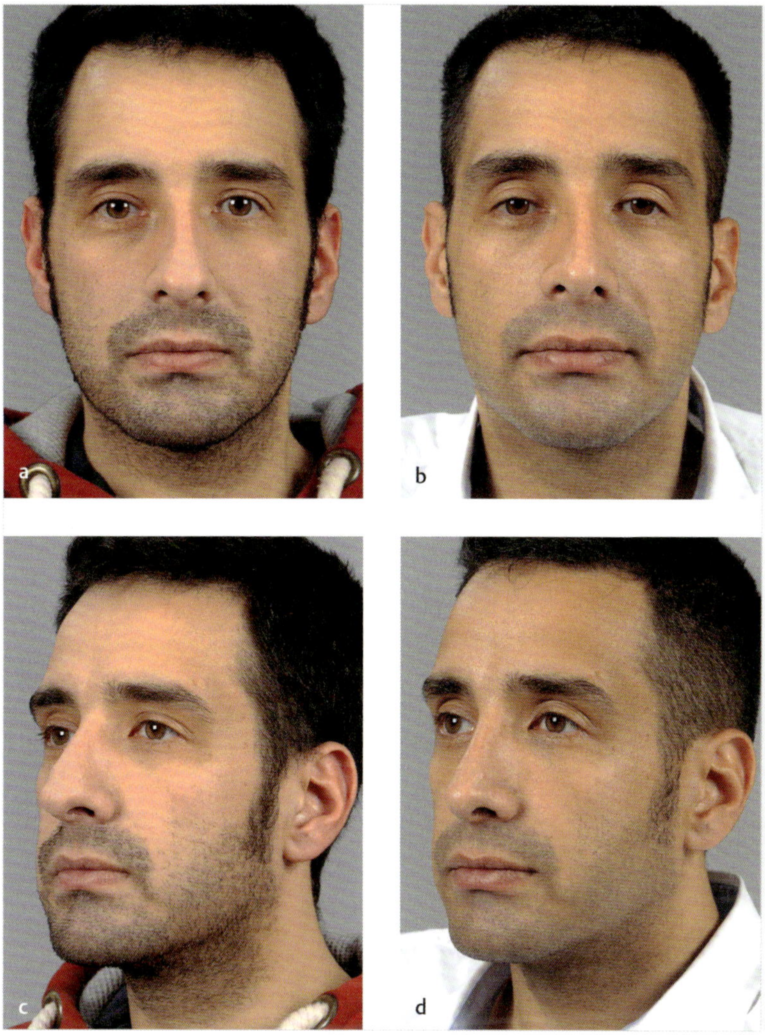

Fig. 10.13 Lateral crural turn-in flap; case study. (a, c) A large, overprojected hump nose with a boxy nasal tip and high anterior septal angle ("tension nose"); frontal and oblique left views. **(b, d)** Post rhinoplasty. Reshaping of the tip with wedge resection of the domes and lateral crural turn-in flaps.

10

> ✓
>
> Sutures applied to the subcutaneous tissue of the nostril must not be placed too superficially below the skin, as this may result in mild but troublesome skin retraction or dimple formation on the nasal tip.

Initially, during insertion these grafts remain a little longer than necessary at the medial aspect so that they can be trimmed to the required size after suture fixation (▶ Fig. 10.19f).

The graft bed for rim grafts can also be prepared using the closed technique and proceeding from lateral to medial. Medial suture fixation of the inserted cartilaginous strip is not required in these cases, with only the lateral access to the tunnel-like graft bed being closed with a rapidly absorbable suture (▶ Fig. 10.20a, b).

A cartilaginous strip sutured to the medial segment of the lower lateral cartilage has been termed an "articulated rim graft" (after Rick Davis). After being affixed to the medial segment of the LLC, the grafts are inserted into a subcutaneous pocket at the alar rim. Grafts of this type not only lower and strengthen the nasal alar rim (▶ Fig. 10.21a, b, ▶ Fig. 10.22a–d), but also prevent or correct retraction of it in the transition zone between the medial and lateral crus. This resembles the effect of facet grafts (see section 12.2.2, ▶ Fig. 12.36 a,b).

> ✓
>
> All procedures on the nasal dorsum should be complete before suture fixation of rim grafts; repeated elevation of the skin flap (for working on the nasal dorsum) leads to dislocation of these grafts from their soft-tissue pockets. The somewhat tricky insertion would then have to be repeated, with a risk of injuring the fragile cartilage.

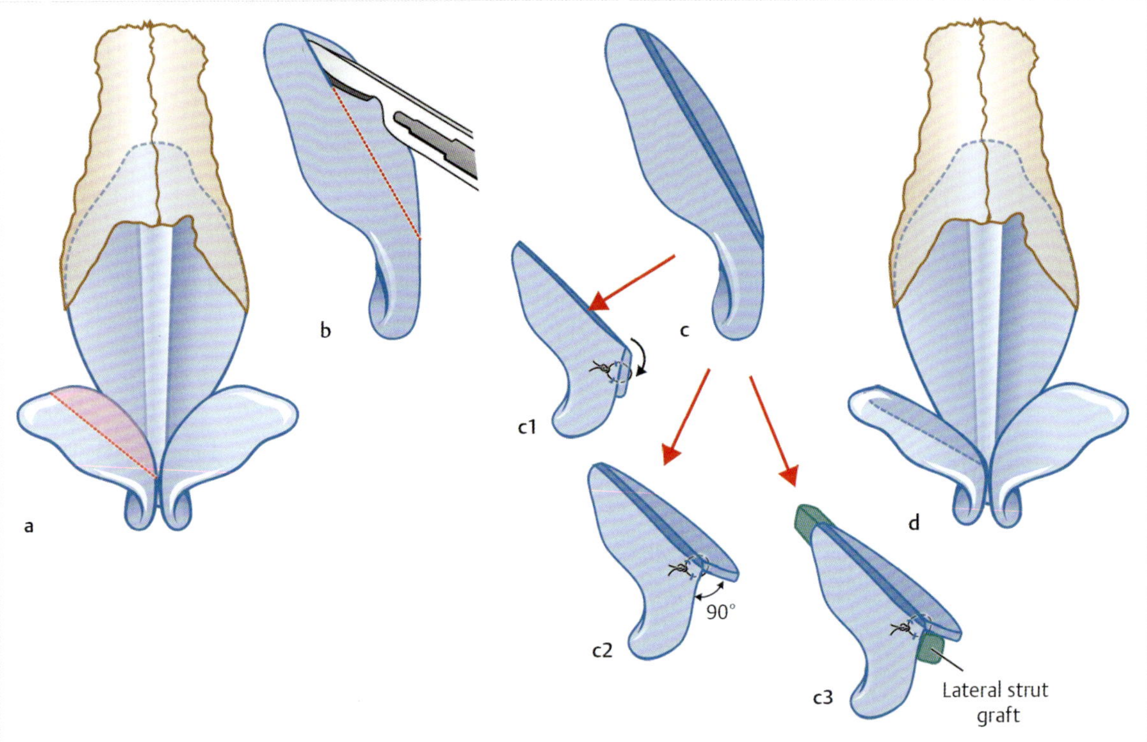

Fig. 10.14 Lateral crural turn-in flap: variations. The lateral crural turn-in flap helps correct the shape and position of a voluminous lower lateral cartilage, while maintaining or improving stability. **(a, b)** The lateral crus is superficially scored along its longitudinal axis. **(c)** The cephalic segment is folded. **(c1)** The flap is rotated by 180° in the classic variant. **(c2)** The 90° rotation simplifies the process. **(c3)** A lateral strut graft can be inserted into the angle between the cartilaginous surfaces for additional stabilization. **(d)** This results in a narrower but more stable lower lateral cartilage.

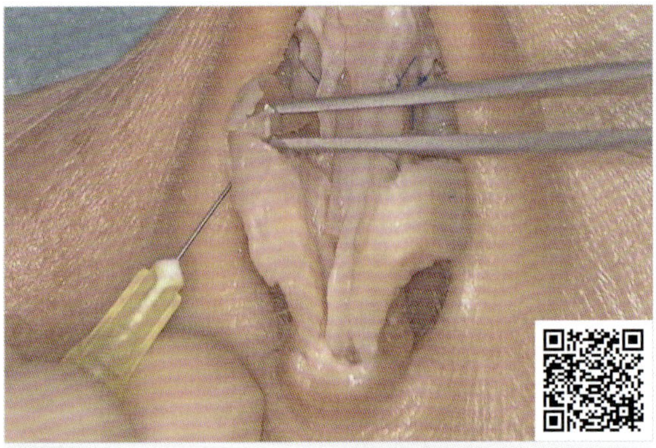

Video 10.4 Lateral crural turn-in flap and lateral strut graft (cadaver head).

Larger rim grafts can also be applied for better stabilization of the caudal alar rim, which may be viewed as a combination of batten or strut grafts and rim grafts (rim batten graft/rim strut graft; ▶ Video 10.5; ▶ Fig. 10.23, ▶ Fig. 10.24a, b). These grafts should sit laterally at the edge of the piriform aperture if they are to support the nasal alae.

If a need to place these grafts is foreseeable, a rim incision can be used as an alternative to a marginal incision. The rim incision provides better surgical access to the lateral aspect of the caudal alar rim than the more commonly used marginal incision (see section 6.5, ▶ Fig. 6.10).

10.4 Elongation of the Lower Lateral Cartilage: Lateral Crural Extension Graft

A cartilaginous graft that serves to laterally extend a short lateral crus is termed a lateral crural extension graft (see ▶ Fig. 10.18d). While the grafts described above, intended for **reinforcement** of the alar cartilage, have to be adequately long for placement along the lateral crus, a graft for lateral **elongation** only has to be applied to roughly the lateral third – although it must extend significantly beyond the lateral extent of the alar crus by the required distance to achieve true lengthening. However, grafts used for reinforcement can also be associated with lateral lengthening.

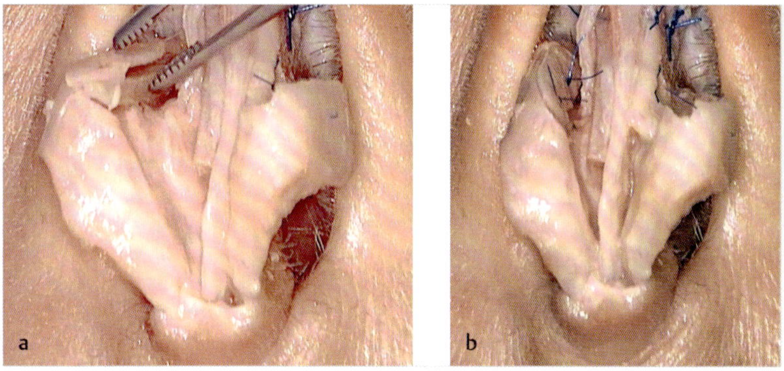

Fig. 10.15 Lateral crural turn-in flap with a lateral crural strut graft. Insertion of a lateral crural strut graft under the turn-in flap on the right for additional stabilization. **(a)** The graft has been placed. **(b)** After double suture fixation of the graft.

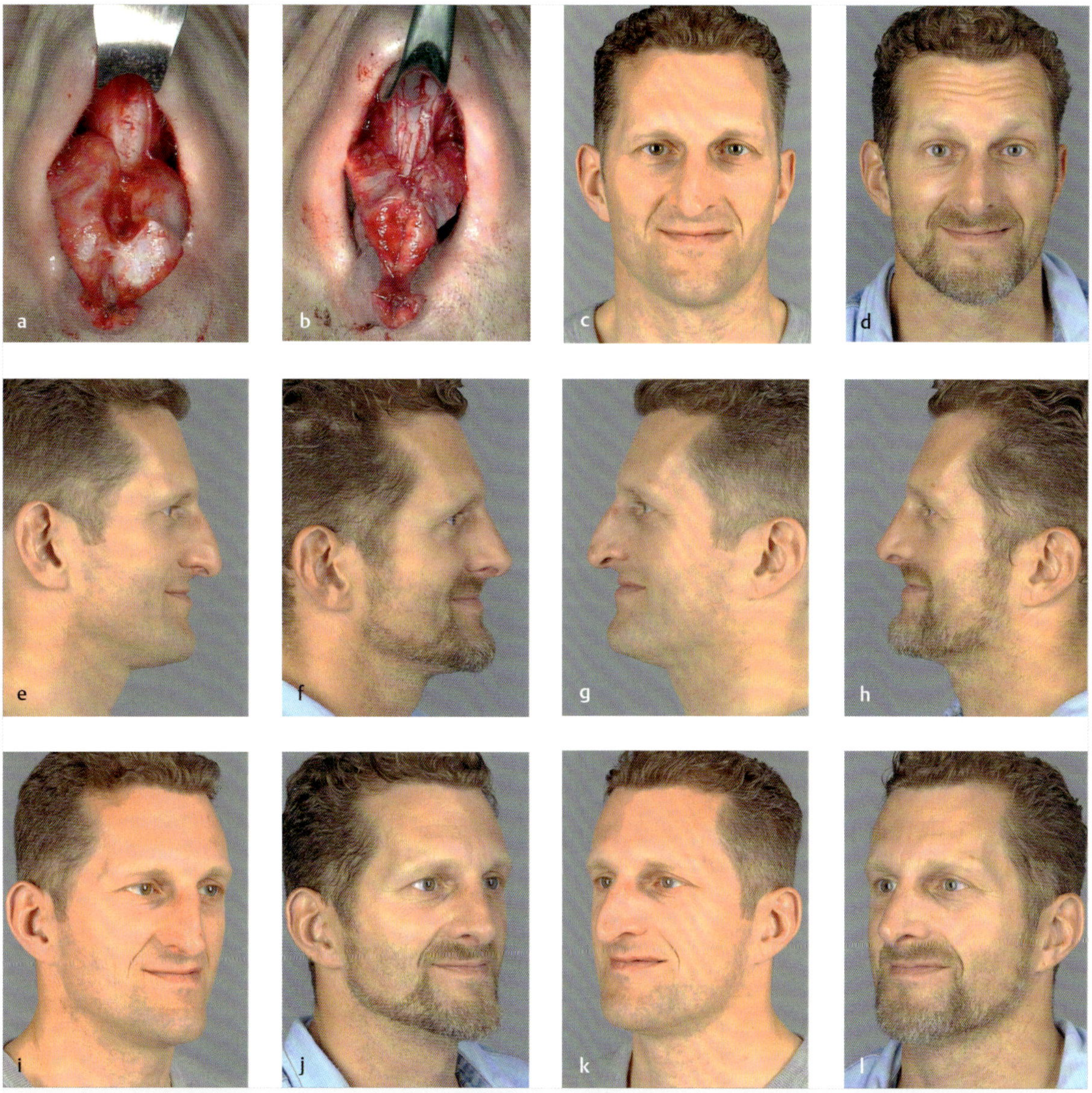

Fig. 10.16 Turn-in flap with strut and batten grafts. Concavity of the left lower lateral cartilage intraoperatively. **(a)** Before correction. **(b)** After correction with a turn-in flap with an integrated lateral crural strut graft and application of a flat outer batten graft. Same patient, **(c, e, g, i, k)** preoperatively and **(d, f, h, j, l)** postoperatively.

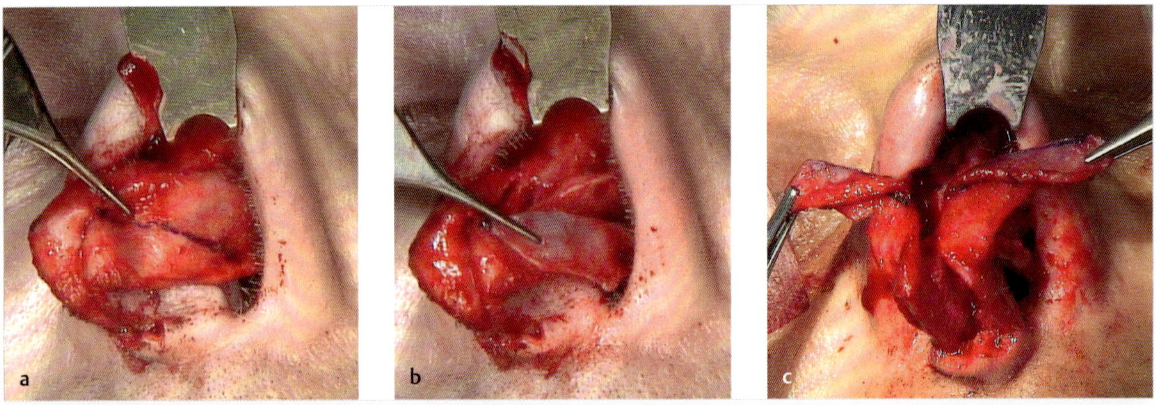

Fig. 10.17 Lateral crural turn-out flap. (a) The crease line has been delineated. **(b)** Outwardly rotated cartilaginous flap from the cranial rim of the lateral crus. **(c)** Bilateral turn-out flaps.

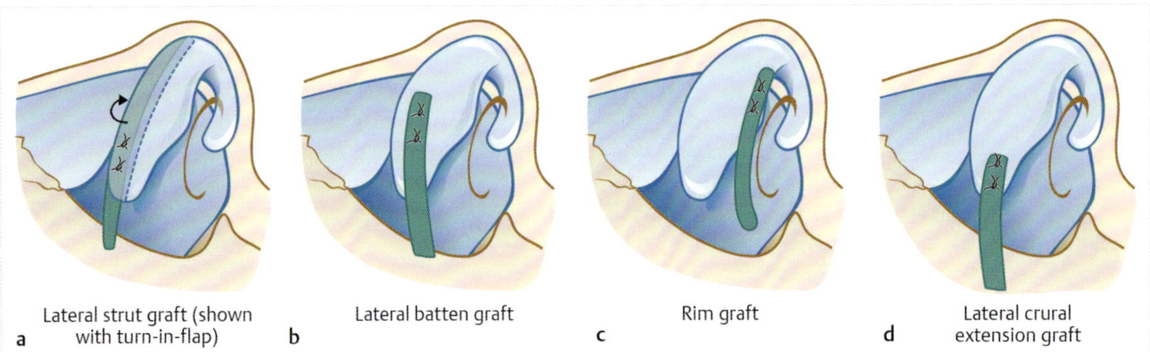

Fig. 10.18 Grafts for the lower lateral cartilage. Cartilage grafts for reinforcement of the lower lateral cartilage. All of the variants can be optionally combined with a turn-in flap. **(a) Lateral strut graft.** The cartilaginous strip is affixed to the inner aspect of the alar cartilage, with or without a turn-in flap. **(b) Lateral batten graft,** affixed to the outer aspect. **(c) Rim graft.** Reinforcement of the caudal rim of the alar cartilage. **(d) Lateral crural extension graft.** Lateral extension of the alar cartilage.

10

10.5 Shortening of the Lower Lateral Cartilage

Overprojection of the nasal tip is often associated with excessively long lateral and probably medial crura of the alar cartilages. Shortening the alar cartilage may be appropriate in these cases.

10.5.1 Lateral Crural Overlay

The lateral half of the cartilage first has to be detached from its inner skin covering before one proceeds with this technique. The lower lateral cartilage is then divided transversely with a smooth cut at the transition from its medial third to the lateral third. The medial edge of this incision can then be displaced to overlap the lateral edge, which inevitably leads to a reduced nasal tip projection. The overlapping cartilaginous edges are then secured in the new position with a mattress suture (▶ Fig. 10.25a, b, ▶ Fig. 10.26a–c, ▶ Fig. 10.27a, b). If a turn-in flap has been created beforehand, a 1–2-mm wide portion of the cartilage flap may have to be resected on the lateral segment in the area of the overlap in order to allow the displacement of the overlay (▶ Fig. 10.28a, b, ▶ Fig. 10.29a–d). A lateral crural overlay can then be combined with both the 90° and the 180° variants of the turn-in flap.

✔

Instability of the lateral crus cannot be ruled out after the overlay procedure, especially if the cartilage is fragile. This can be avoided by correcting the projection using alternative methods of nasal tip reduction (see also Chapter 12).

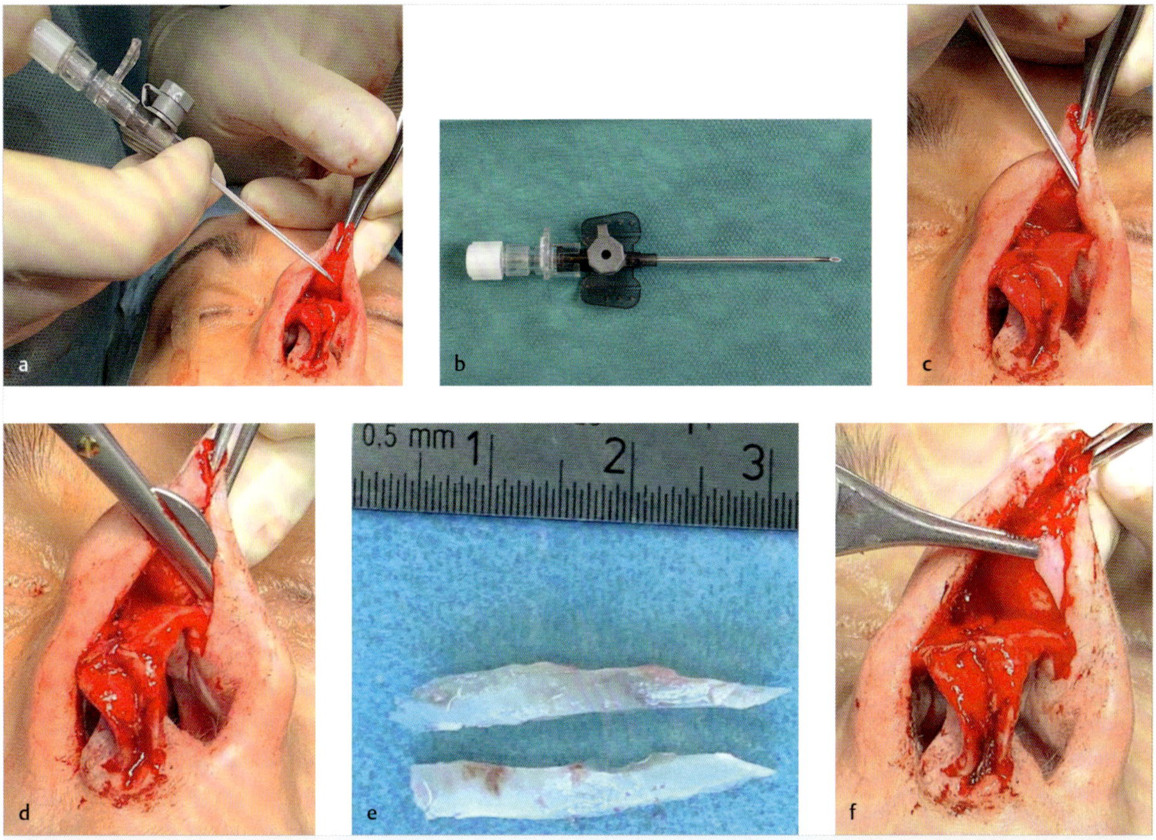

Fig. 10.19 Placement of rim grafts. (a–c) Creation of a tunnel-shaped pocket along the alar rim for insertion of a rim graft. **(b, c)** The graft bed is opened with a Vasofix 16 G venous catheter with a cannula. **(d)** Expansion of the tissue pocket with a pair of fine, pointed scissors. **(e)** Symmetrically trimmed rim grafts for both sides (septal cartilage). **(f)** Insertion of the rim graft into the prepared graft bed at the alar rim. Any excess length of the transplant is shortened at the end.

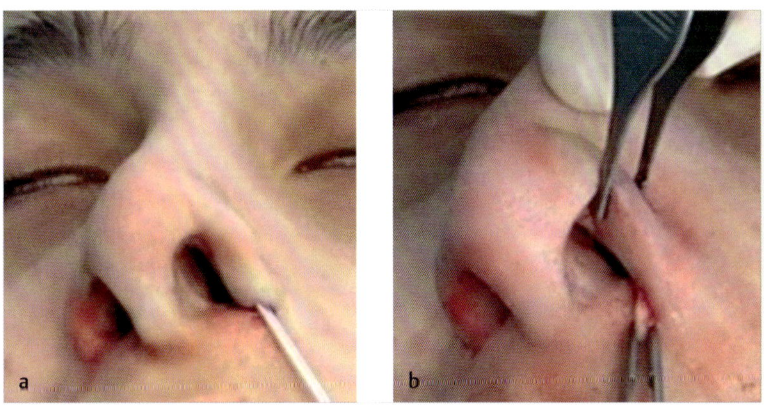

Fig. 10.20 Endonasal placement of a rim graft. (a) Lateral incision and preparation of the graft site. **(b)** Inserting the graft.

10.5.2 Lateral Crural Strip Resection

An alternative to the lateral crural overlay for shortening the lower lateral cartilage is a simple transverse strip resection from the cartilage, with subsequent coaptation of its edges using an end-to-end suture. This technically simpler variant does not have the mild stabilizing effect provided by the overlapping overlay suture, and thus increases the risk of instability in the lower lateral cartilage.

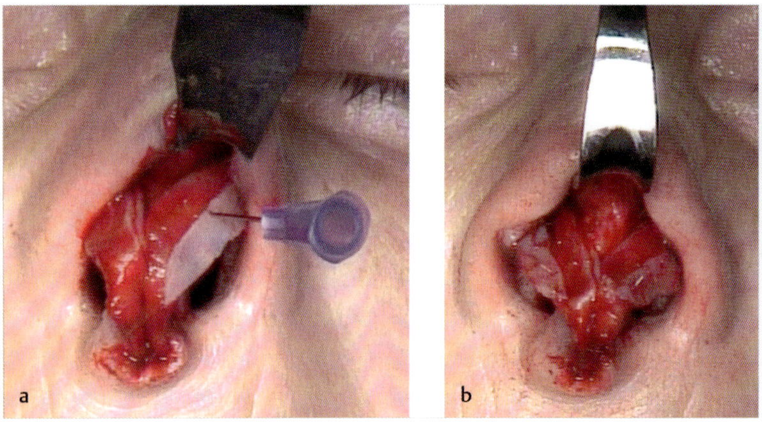

Fig. 10.21 Fixation of rim grafts. **(a)** Temporary fixation of a rim graft with a fine cannula to facilitate suture fixation. **(b)** After bilateral suture fixation and final trimming to the appropriate size.

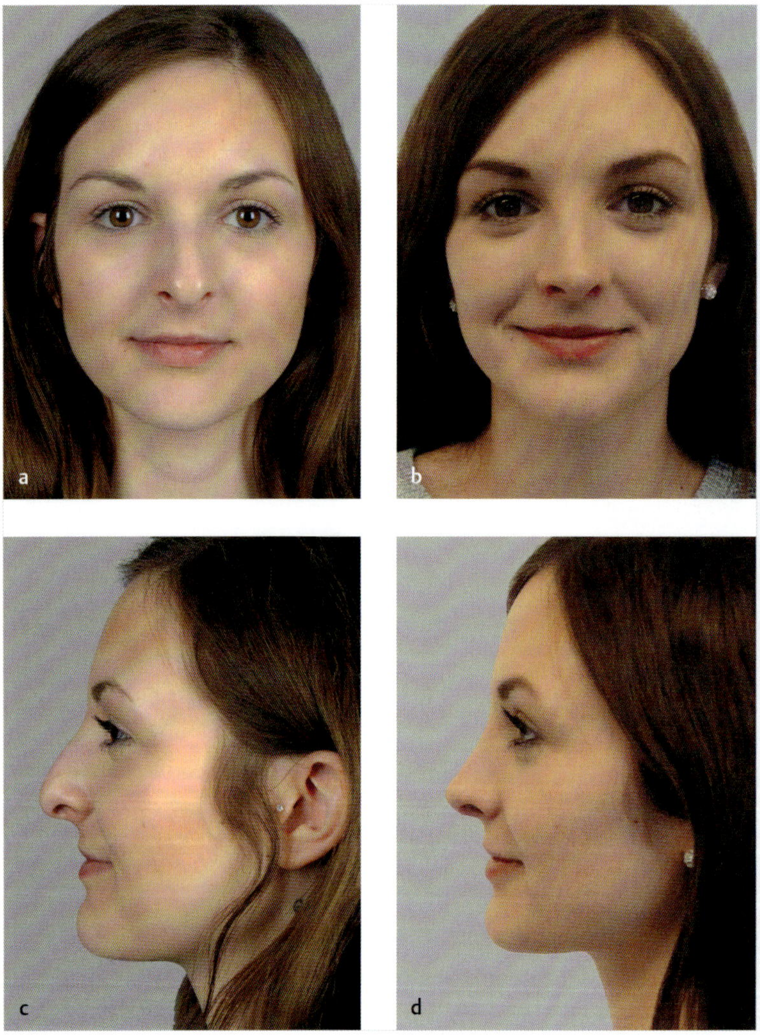

Fig. 10.22 Correction of retracted alar rim with rim grafts; case study. (a, c) Hump nose; wide, drooping tip with retracted alar rims ("Chinese hat" deformity). **(b, d)** After rhinoplasty with a tongue-in-groove procedure and rim grafts.

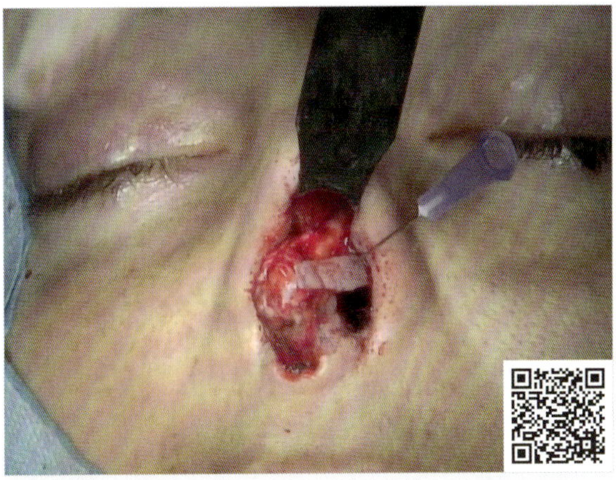

Video 10.5 Lateral crural batten–rim graft (clinical case).

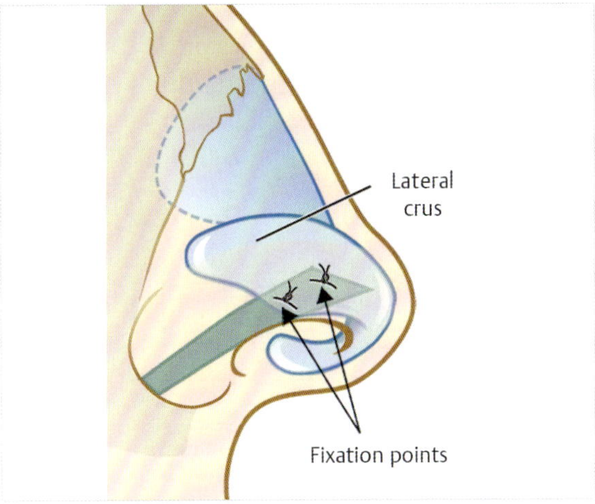

Fig. 10.23 Rim batten graft/rim strut graft. This variant, which is larger than the usual rim graft, is fixed to the lower lateral cartilage with one or two sutures. A rim strut graft has been depicted in the figure (inserted below the alar cartilage).

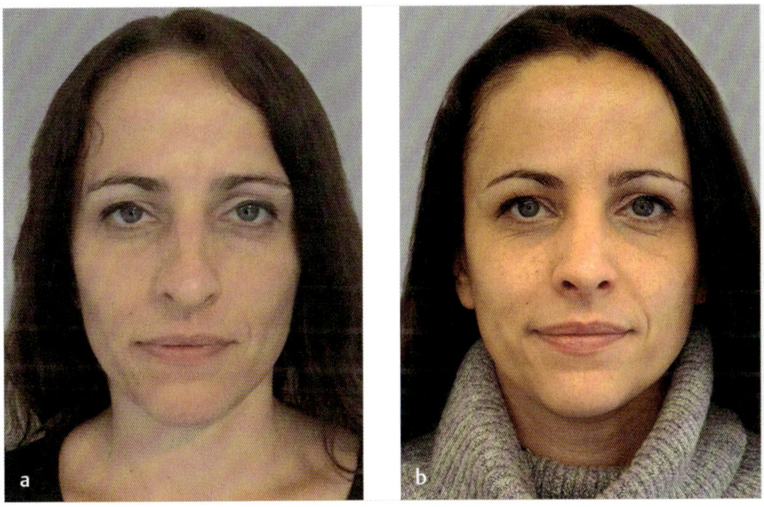

Fig. 10.24 Correction of the alar rim with a rim strut graft. (a) Retracted alar rims often give the face a stern, serious expression. **(b)** After correction with rim strut grafts (see also ▶ Fig. 9.7a, b).

10.6 Correction of Concavity of the Lower Lateral Cartilage

10.6.1 Lateral Crural Convexity Control Suture

It may be worthwhile to try to correct a subtle concavity of the lateral crus with a suture passing under the cartilage curved in the wrong direction (namely inward), which arches it outward by tying the suture – comparable to the Mustardé suture in the antihelical fold correction of the ear (▶ Video 10.6; ▶ Fig. 10.30a, b). Unfortunately, this suture is not always as effective in practice as the theory would suggest.

10.6.2 180° Lateral Crural Turn-in Flap

The concavity can be corrected with a greater chance of success using a lateral crural turn-in flap (see section 10.2.2), but the flap has to be rotated by 180° in order to correct the concavity. This is generally not as easy to do with a 90° variant.

10.6.3 Lateral Batten Graft

A lateral batten graft conforming to the desired shape can be placed if a lateral crural turn-in flap proves inadequate. This is applied as a septal or conchal cartilage graft to the lower lateral cartilage, as an onlay graft (▶ Fig. 10.31a, b, ▶ Fig. 10.32a, b, ▶ Fig. 10.33a–d).

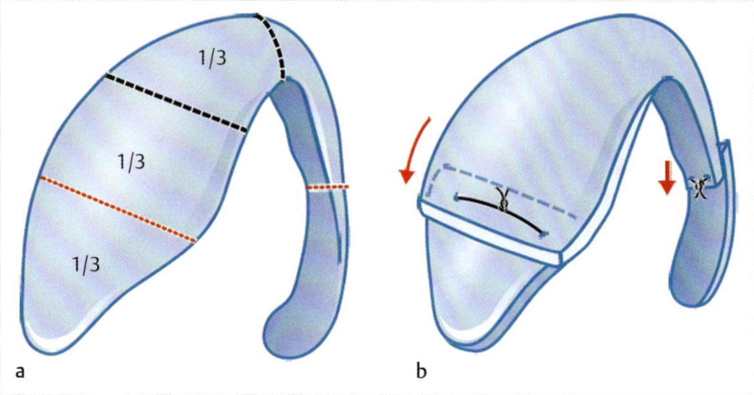

Fig. 10.25 Lateral and medial crural overlay. (a) The lateral crus is divided at the transition from the middle to the lateral thirds for the lateral overlap. **(b)** The medial segment is displaced over the lateral stump after mobilization of the inner skin covering, and fixed with sutures. The figure shows an analogous procedure on the medial crus (medial crural overlay).

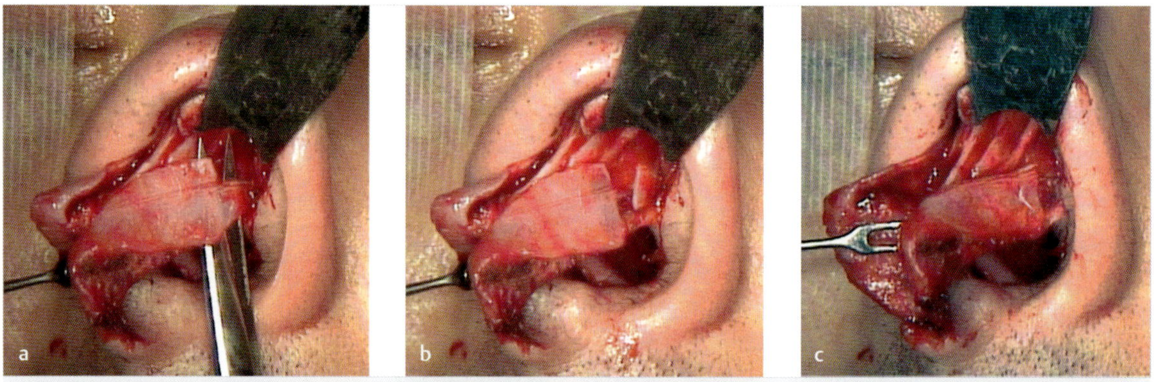

Fig. 10.26 Lateral crural overlay; intraoperative. (a) Dissection of the lateral third of the lower lateral cartilage. A turn-in flap has also been prepared. **(b)** Division of the lateral crus. **(c)** Overlapping of the middle over the lateral third of the lateral crus during suturing. Simultaneous placement of the turn-in flap. Note the shortening of the lateral crus, which results in decreased projection of the left alar cartilage.

10

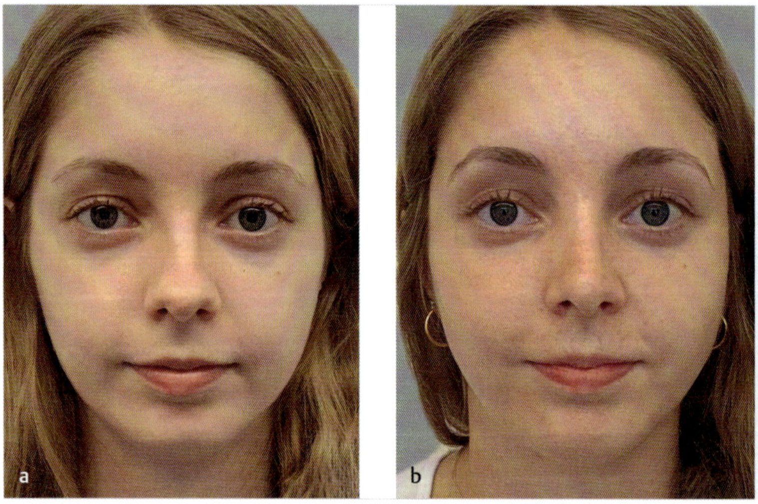

Fig. 10.27 Lateral crural overlay; case study. (a) Boxy, overprojected nasal tip. **(b)** After rhinoplasty with wedge resection of the domes and lateral crural overlay.

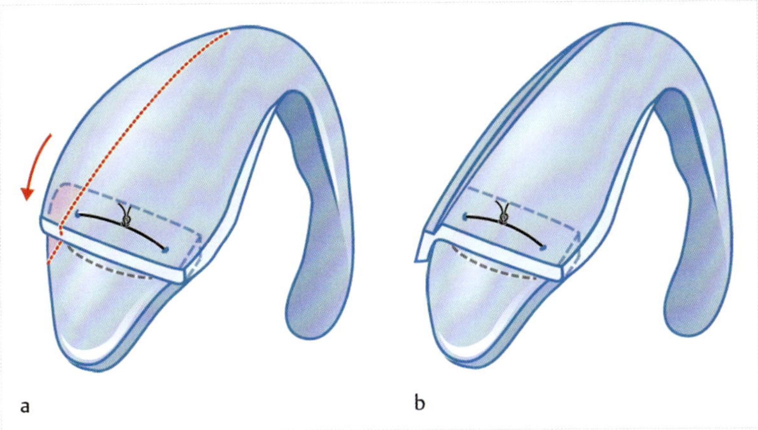

Fig. 10.28 Lateral crural overlay with lateral crural turn-in flap. **(a)** A small, troublesome cartilaginous triangle on the lateral stump has to be resected. **(b)** After that, the two procedures can be combined.

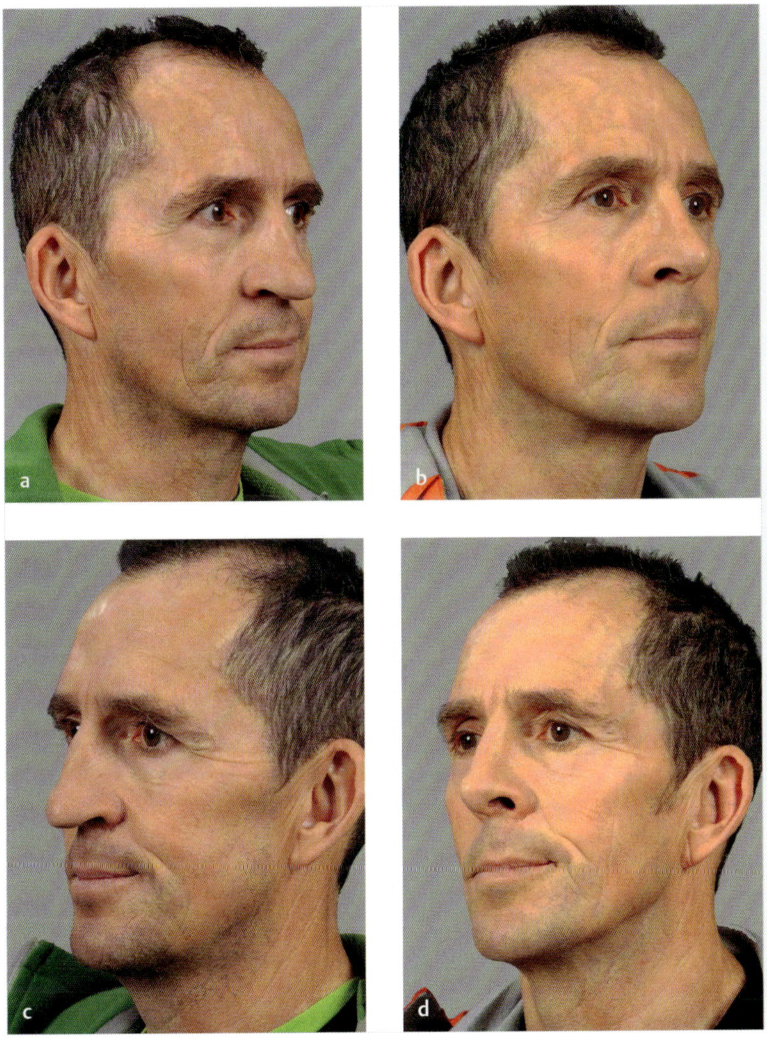

Fig. 10.29 Lateral crural overlay with lateral turn-in flaps; case study. (a, c) A markedly overprojected tip with "tip drop" and a narrow nasolabial angle. Right and left oblique views. **(b, d)** In this case, the lateral crural overlay was combined with lateral turn-in flaps and strip resections of the domes as corrective measures.

10.6.4 Interchange of the Lower Lateral Cartilages

A lateral crural concavity can also be corrected by bilateral resection with reciprocal exchange and refixation in a rotated position, in such a way that the crura are curved bilaterally outward.

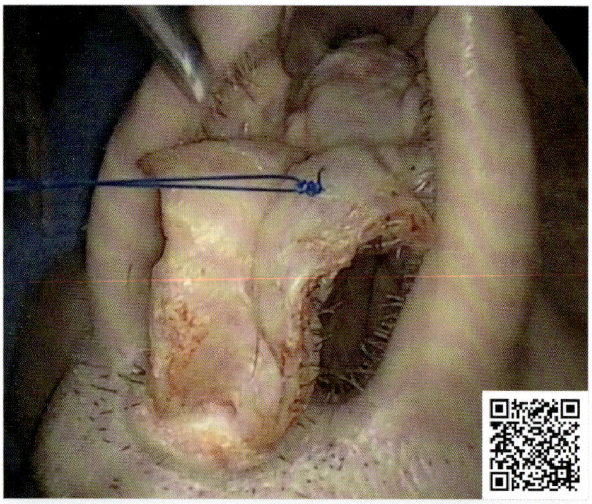

Video 10.6 Convexity control suture (cadaver head).

> ✓
>
> The turn-in flap, suture technique, and onlay graft are preferable, since the exchange procedure may give rise to undesirable instability in the alar cartilages.

10.7 Affixing the Lower Lateral Cartilage: Lateral Suspension Sutures

The definitive relationship between the nasal dorsum and the lateral crus must be defined once the surgeon is satisfied with the dimensions of the nasal tip. The point of intersection between the cephalic alar edge and the cartilaginous nasal dorsum is decisively important. Cranial migration of this point of intersection rapidly leads to increasing rotation of the nasal tip; conversely, caudal migration reduces the degree of rotation and lowers the tip (▶ Fig. 10.34a, b).

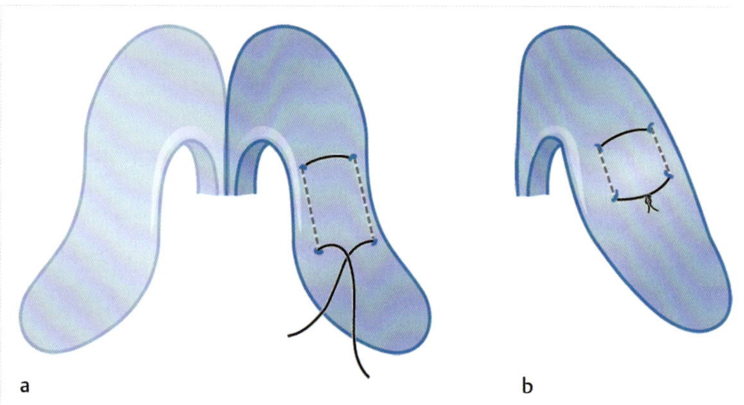

Fig. 10.30 Lateral crural convexity control suture. The suture **(a)** corrects the concavity of the lateral crus, with conversion to convexity at best **(b)**.

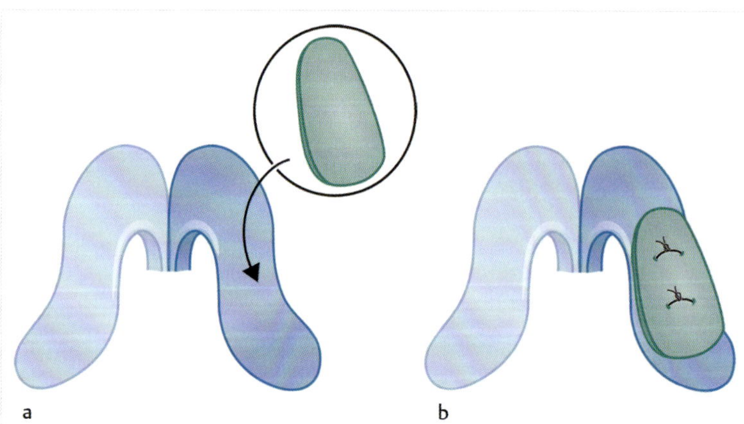

Fig. 10.31 Lateral batten graft to correct convexity of the lower lateral cartilage. The externally placed graft **(a)** transforms the concavity of the lateral crus into a convexity **(b)**.

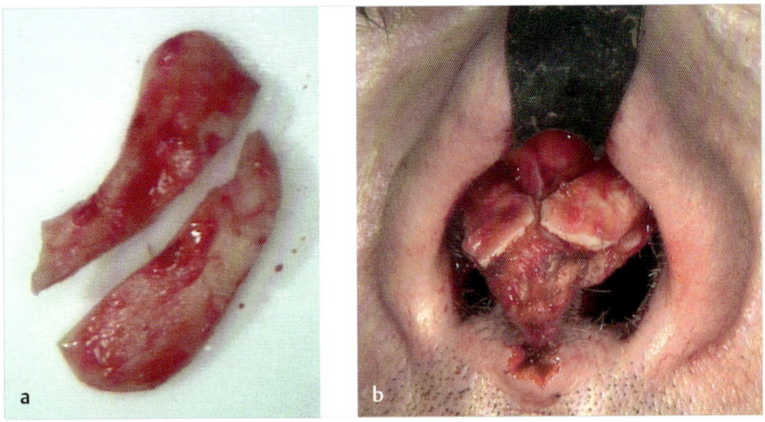

Fig. 10.32 Lateral batten grafts harvested from conchal cartilage; intraoperative. (a) The two grafts are obtained by longitudinal division from the cartilage of the cavum conchae of one side. **(b)** After bilateral suture fixation. Batten grafts of this size not only correct a concavity, but also help stabilize the lateral crus.

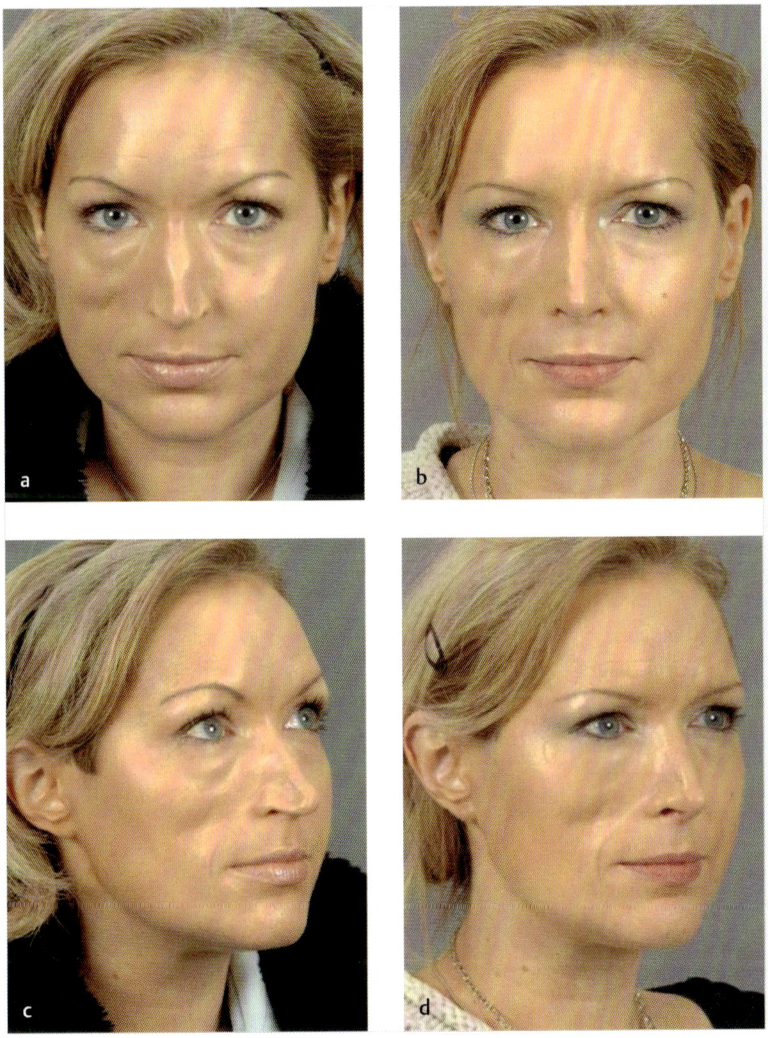

Fig. 10.33 Concavity of the nasal alae; case study. (a, c) Marked concavity of both nasal alae. **(b, d)** Corrected with lateral batten grafts. The case was aggravated by cutaneous lupus erythematosus, treated with cortisone.

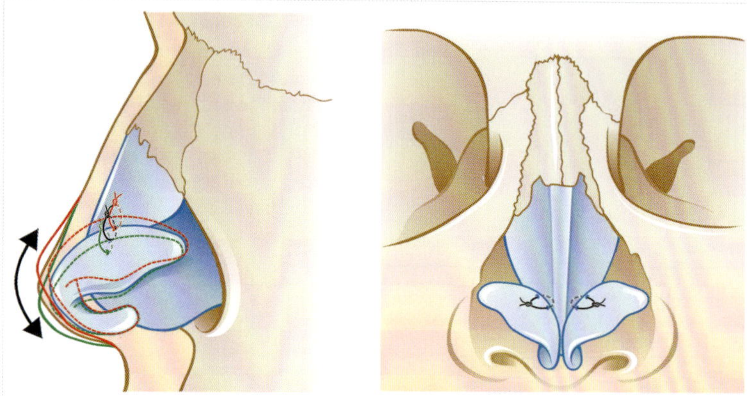

a b

Fig. 10.34 Lateral suspension suture. **(a)** The lateral suspension suture of the cephalic alar edge on the middle thirds of the cartilaginous vault controls tip rotation. A more caudally positioned suture results in lesser rotation (green); conversely, a more cranial suture results in greater rotation (red). **(b)** Frontal view.

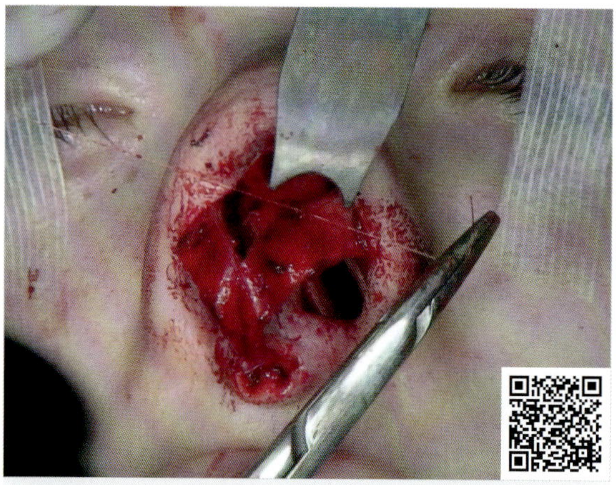

Video 10.7 Lateral crural suspension suture.

> ✓
>
> It is best not to use the Aufricht retractor, but rather to place the skin loosely over the nasal dorsum while determining the position of the nasal tip and suturing the alar cartilages to the middle third of the dorsum. The Aufricht retractor cranially retracts the nasal skin as well as the alar cartilages with the nasal tip, which may lead to incorrect assessment of the intraoperative findings. The nasal tip cartilage is then unintentionally sutured in an excessively rotated position, and this may only be recognized once the retractor has been removed and the skin replaced.

Lateral suspension sutures, using 5–0 polydioxanone (PDS) as suture material, fix the ideal point of intersection between the cephalic alar edge and the cartilaginous dorsum of the nose (▶ Video 10.7; ▶ Fig. 10.34a, b). One or two such sutures can be applied symmetrically between the alar cartilage and the septum–upper lateral cartilage complex, depending on the individual situation (▶ Fig. 10.35, ▶ Fig. 10.36a–d).

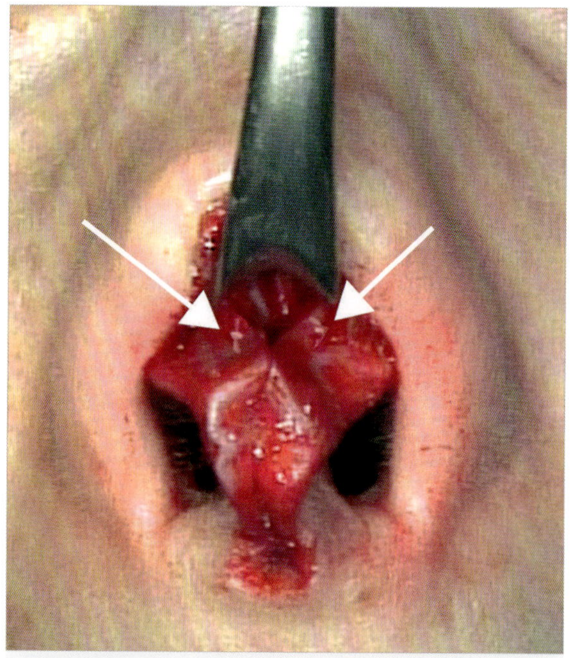

Fig. 10.35 Lateral suspension sutures; intraoperative. Bilateral lateral suspension sutures (white arrows). The suture fixes the intersection of the lower lateral cephalic edge and the cartilaginous dorsum of the nose.

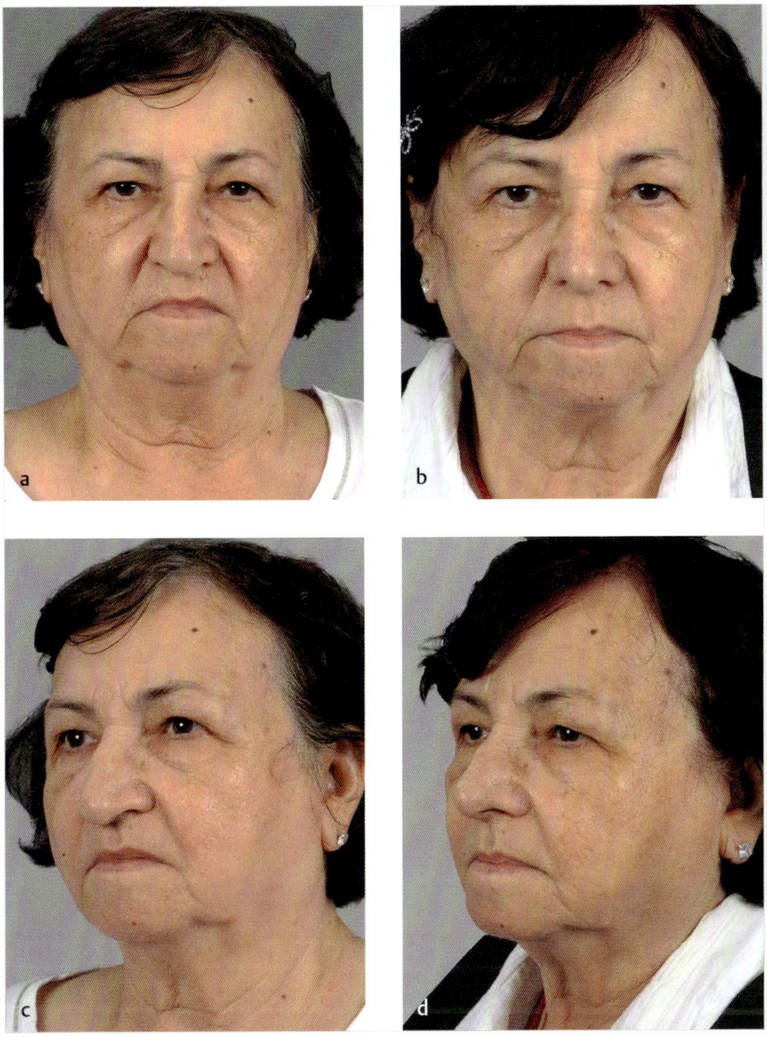

Fig. 10.36 Lateral suspension sutures; case study. (a, c) A drooping nasal tip with nasal valve incompetence; frontal and oblique left views. **(b, d)** Elevating and stabilizing the anterior nose with a septal extension graft and lateral suspension sutures has both functional and cosmetic effects.

> ✓
>
> It should be borne in mind that suspension sutures may elevate the caudal alar rim in such a way that the alar rims are positioned higher and appear retracted after the suture. This outcome is sometimes desirable (▶ Fig. 10.36a–d), but if the result is too pronounced one should not hesitate to undo the suture and replace it with another with a less marked effect, or do without it altogether. Alternatively, the tongue-in-groove method can be used to rotate the tip.

If already applied in the same case, the tongue-in-groove technique (see section 12.2.2) generally contributes significantly to tip rotation. Special care and restraint are advisable when applying additional lateral crural suspension sutures, which may further elevate the tip.

The single lateral suspension sutures on either side can be merged together in a joint bilateral suture to “suspend” the lateral crura on the middle thirds of the cartilaginous framework. The needle first passes through the cephalic rim of the lateral crus on one side, then through the septum–upper lateral cartilage complex, passing through the cephalic rim of the opposite side, and returns through the middle thirds of the cartilaginous vault back to the starting point, where it reenters the cranial alar rim (▶ Video 10.8, ▶ Video 10.9; ▶ Fig. 10.37). Knotting this suture generally results in narrowing of the supratip, while stabilizing the valve region. The tip may be rotated upward to a greater or lesser extent, depending on the position of the suture, which is

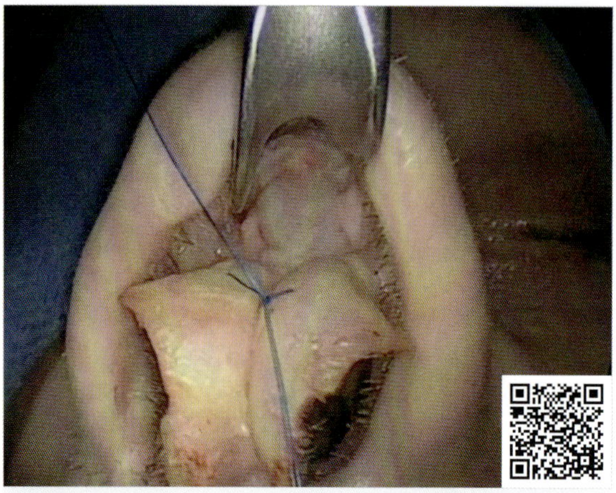

Video 10.8 Lateral crural binding and suspension suture (cadaver head).

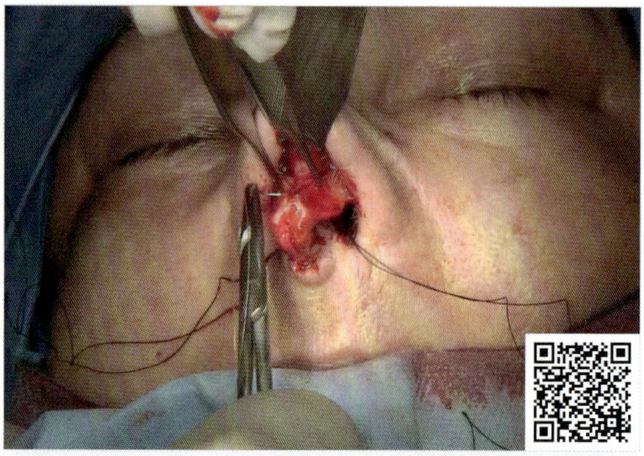

Video 10.9 Double suspension suture (clinical case).

usually a desirable effect. Again, retraction and elevation of the caudal alar rims due to this suture are not always desirable, and in case this happens the surgeon has to decide whether suture revision is necessary.

10.8 Elevation of the Lower Lateral Cartilages: Lateral Crura Spanning Sutures

In contrast to suspension sutures, bilateral spanning sutures between the upper and/or lower lateral cartilages elevate these lateral cartilages, thereby widening the nasal valve region. These are therefore primarily functional sutures. The suture first passes through one lateral cartilage, then **over the nasal dorsum** (and not through the septum) to the other side, and then through the cartilage in the opposite direction (▶ Video 10.10; ▶ Fig. 10.38).

Knotting of the suture ends typically leads to elevation of the lateral cartilages, which then form a larger angle with the septum. This opens up the nasal valve and ideally improves nasal breathing. These sutures are not regularly part of cosmetic rhinoplasty, but may prove valuable in individual cases.

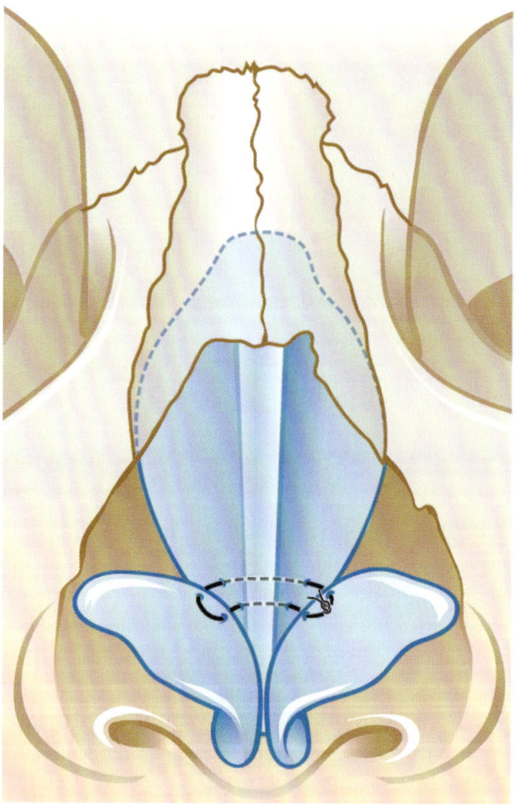

Fig. 10.37 Combined bilateral suspension sutures. Simultaneous bilateral suspension suturing of the lower lateral cartilages results in narrowing of the supratip.

10.9 Lowering of the Alar Rim

10.9.1 Repositioning of the LLC

With or without cranial malposition of the lateral crura, the nasal alar edges may be too elevated cranially. In these cases, the use of rim grafts may not be sufficient.

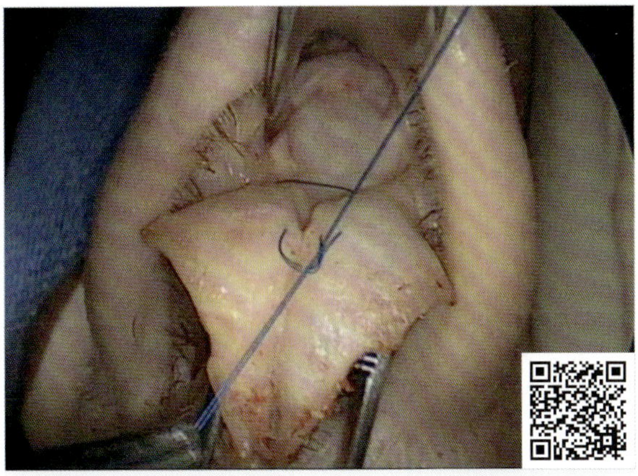

Video 10.10 Lateral crura spanning suture (cadaver head).

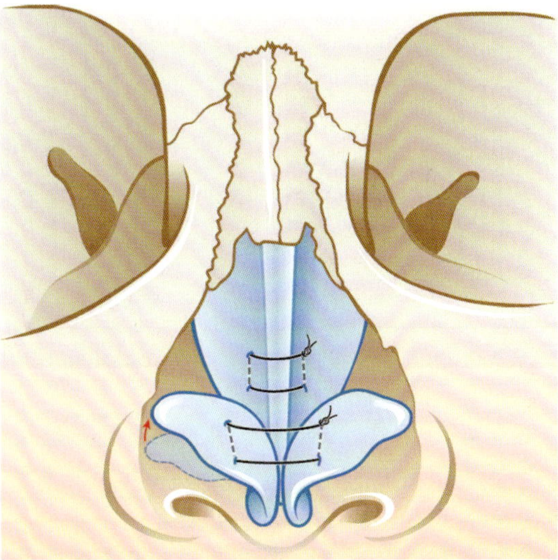

Fig. 10.38 Spanning sutures between the upper and lower lateral cartilages on both sides elevate the lateral cartilages.

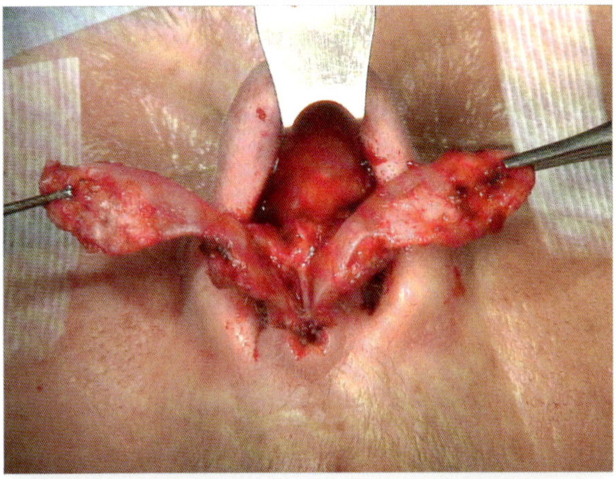

Fig. 10.39 Complete mobilization of the lateral crura for repositioning. The lateral crura are completely detached from the vestibular skin.

Complete lateral mobilization of the lateral crus, with subsequent rotation caudally, is then recommended in order to lower the edges of the nostrils (▶ Fig. 10.39; compare with ▶ Fig. 10.1e). Occasionally, the caudal edges of the lateral crura have to be trimmed symmetrically afterward (▶ Fig. 10.40 a-d).

10.9.2 Auricular Composite Graft

Composite grafts obtained from the cymba conchae are invaluable for correcting abnormalities of the nasal vestibule (see section 18.2.2). They can be used to widen a stenotic nasal vestibule, or – especially in patients with retraction due to scarring – to lower a retracted alar rim (▶ Fig. 10.41a–c). Composite grafts of this type are introduced via an incision on the inside of the nostril, parallel to the course of the nostril edge, after mobilization of the cut edges, and are fixed with absorbable sutures. Mattress sutures that press the graft firmly onto the outer skin covering for approximately 6–8 days promote healing. The suture may be passed over a protective silicone film in order to avoid pressure marks on the nasal ala. This procedure is particularly useful for reconstruction of the alar wing following trauma or tumor surgery (▶ Fig. 10.42a, b, ▶ Fig. 10.43a, b).

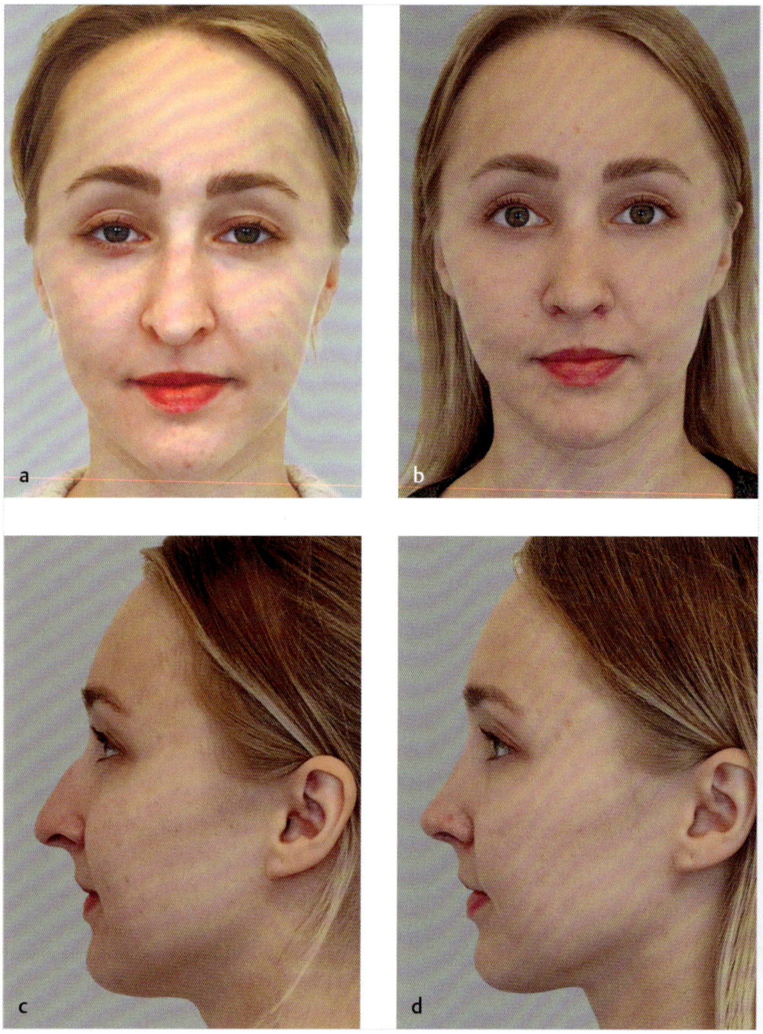

Fig. 10.40 Repositioning of the lateral crura; case example. (a, c) An elevated (retracted) alar rim preoperatively. **(b, d)** After lateral crura repositioning. The deviated nose with an S-shaped hump was corrected using the let-down technique with a subdorsal square flap.

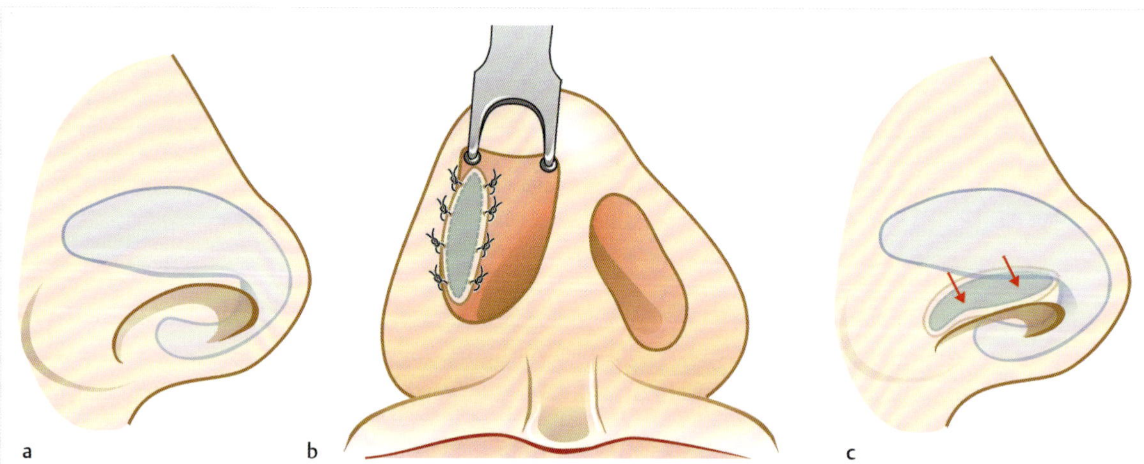

Fig. 10.41 Composite graft from the cymba conchae. (a) Lowering of a retracted alar rim using a composite graft harvested from the cymba conchae. The skin above the nasal opening on the inner aspect of the nostril is incised and dissected. **(b)** The skin–cartilage graft is inserted into the resultant defect, generally resulting in adequate lowering of the alar rim **(c)**.

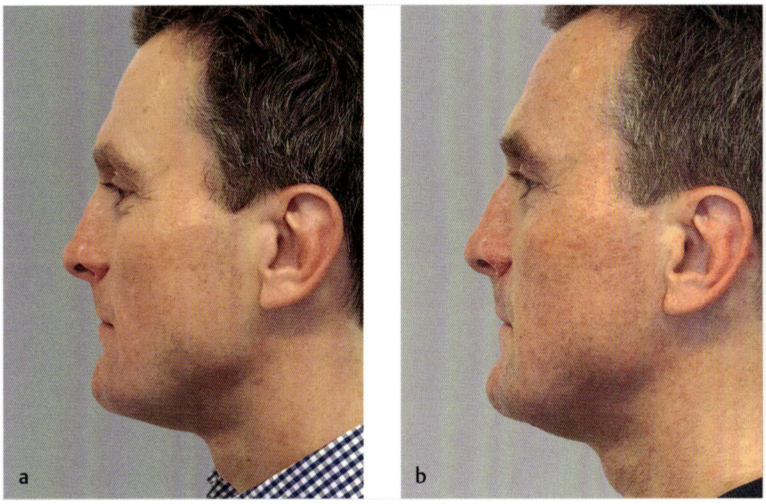

Fig. 10.42 Reconstruction of the retracted ala with a composite auricular graft; case study. (a) Notching of the alar rim in this case was due to tumor resection. **(b)** After reconstruction, with lowering of the alar rim using a composite auricular graft. A simple rim graft would not have solved the problem, since both the cartilage and skin required replacement.

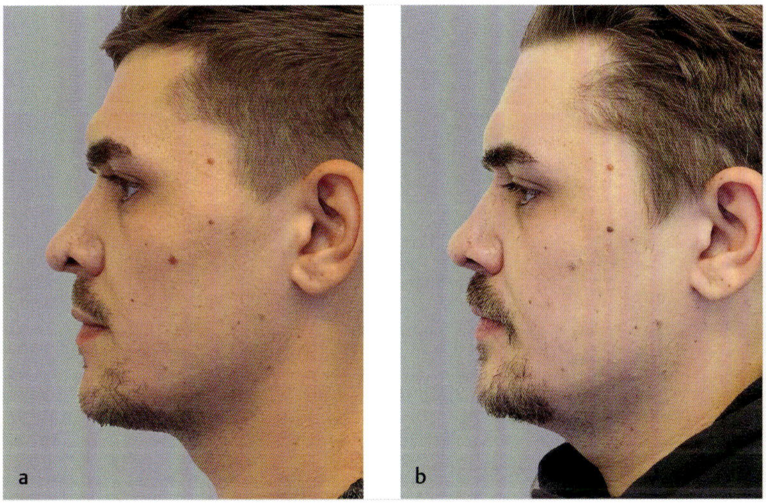

Fig. 10.43 Lowering of the alar edge with composite graft after trauma. (a) The patient was very disturbed by the triangular elevation of the alar edge after trauma ("Chinese hat" deformity). **(b)** Condition after rhinoplasty, including correction of the alar rim with composite graft from the ear.

Bibliography

Abdelhamid AS, Kimura KS, El Abany A, Kandathil CK, Most SP. Patient Outcomes in Lateral Crural Repositioning and Reconstruction in Revision Rhinoplasty. Facial Plast Surg Aesthet Med.. 2024; 26:9:14

Ballin AC, Kim H, Chance E, Davis RE. The articulated alar rim graft: reengineering the conventional alar rim graft for improved contour and support. Facial Plast Surg. 2016; 32(4):384–397

Barham HP, Knisely A, Christensen J, Sacks R, Marcells GN, Harvey RJ. Costal cartilage lateral crural strut graft vs cephalic crural turn-in for correction of external valve dysfunction. JAMA Facial Plast Surg. 2015; 17(5):340–345

Calloway HE, Heilbronn CM, Gu JT, Pham TT, Barnes CH, Wong BJ. Functional outcomes, quantitative morphometry, and aesthetic analysis of articulated alar rim grafts in septorhinoplasty. JAMA Facial Plast Surg. 2019; 21(6):558–565

Foda HMT, Kridel RWH. Lateral crural steal and lateral crural overlay: an objective evaluation. Arch Otolaryngol Head Neck Surg. 1999; 125(12): 1365–1370

Gruber RP, Peled A, Talley J. Mattress sutures to remove unwanted convexity and concavity of the nasal tip: 12-year follow-up. Aesthet Surg J. 2015; 35(1):20–27

Ilhan AE, Saribas B, Caypinar B. Aesthetic and functional results of lateral crural repositioning. JAMA Facial Plast Surg. 2015; 17(4):286–292

Kondo M, Orgain C, Alvarado R, Marcells GN, Harvey RJ. The effects of lateral crural tensioning with an articulated alar rim graft versus lateral crural strut graft on nasal function. Facial Plast Surg Aesthet Med. 2020; 22(4): 281–285

Langsdon P, Schroeder R, Rayess H, Clinkscales W. Lateral crural setback: a preservation technique to increase tip rotation. Facial Plast Surg Aesthet Med. 2022; 24(3):247–248

Sazgar AA. Horizontal reduction using a cephalic hinged flap of the lateral crura: a method to treat the bulbous nasal tip. Aesthetic Plast Surg. 2010; 34(5):612–615

Sazgar AA, Woodard C, Most SP. Preservation of the nasal valve area with a lateral crural hinged flap: a cadaveric study. Aesthetic Plast Surg. 2012; 36(2):244–247

Sazgar AA, Amali A, Peyvasty MN. Value of cephalic part of lateral crus in functional rhinoplasty. Eur Arch Otorhinolaryngol. 2016; 273(12): 4053–4059

Tripathi PB, Elghobashi S, Wong BJF. The myth of the internal nasal valve. JAMA Facial Plast Surg. 2017; 19(4):253–254

11 The Caudal Septum and Medial Crura of the Alar Cartilages: Corrective Surgery on the Columella

The structure of the caudal septum and medial crura has an effect on the contour of the columella and the position of the nasal tip, on its rotation and projection, as well as the appearance of the nostrils. The maneuvers described here are therefore extremely important for the outcome of rhinoplasty (see also Chapter 12, ▶ Table 12.3).

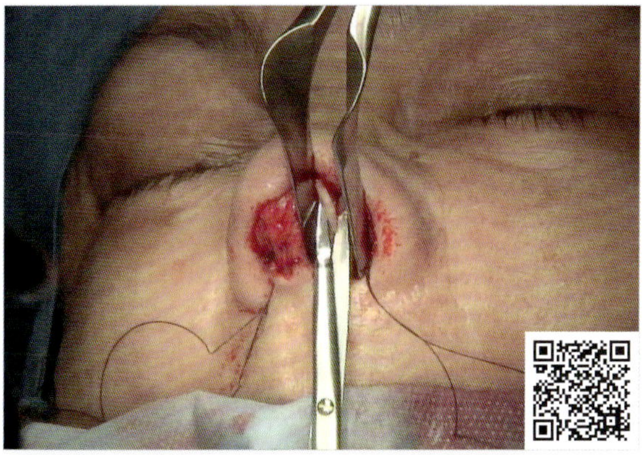

Video 11.1 Reduction of caudal septum through a hemitransfixion incision (clinical case).

11.1 Correction of the Caudal Septum

The caudal third of the septum forms part of the middle third of the nasal vault, but its configuration has a significant bearing on the position and to some extent the shape of the nasal tip. The caudal septum is therefore often corrected before work starts on the nasal tip and the alar cartilages. It is straightened and stabilized as required and maneuvered into the desired position and shape.

> ✓
>
> The caudal third of the septum constitutes an essential supporting element between the middle third and the nasal tip.

Typical septoplasty or harvesting of septal cartilage is performed first, if necessary (see Chapter 7), followed by correction of the caudal third of the septum. The surgeon therefore proceeds "from back to front."

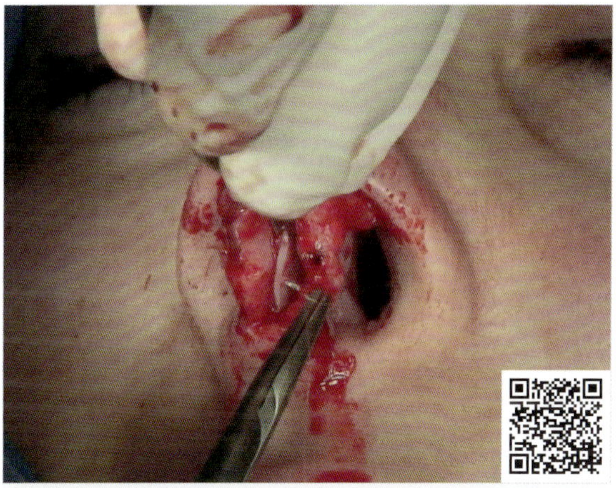

Video 11.2 Caudal septum reduction and tongue-in-groove procedure (clinical case).

11.1.1 Reduction of the Caudal Septum

The caudal edge of the septum may be shortened if the nose is too large, if tip retraction is desired, or if a drooping columella or a drooping nasal tip (tip drop) are present (▶ Video 11.1, ▶ Video 11.2).

The height of the anterior third is reduced by ablation of the **upper edge of the septum** along the W-point–anterior septal angle (W-ASA) line (see ▶ Fig. 1.7) using a no. 15 blade and leveling it with the nasal dorsum in its middle third. The surgeon must be aware that the height of the actual nasal tip is defined by the alar domes and not by the septum. The upper edge of the septum in the supratip region can be lowered slightly, particularly in women, to achieve a "supratip break" (see section 2.8). In contrast, the **caudal edge of the septum** helps define the columellar profile and can be divided into three parts (▶ Fig. 11.1):

- The contour of the upper third influences the position and rotation of the tip.
- The contour of the middle third determines the columellar profile.
- The contour of the lower third, together with the anterior nasal spine, determines the shape and angulation of the nasolabial angle (▶ Fig. 11.2).

Thus, cartilaginous strips may be resected from the upper, middle, or lower segments of the caudal edge of the septum, depending on the desired columellar profile. It should be noted that the full effect of resection of the septal edge often only becomes apparent late in the postoperative period, and retraction of the columella in the middle and upper thirds may increase over time. Such

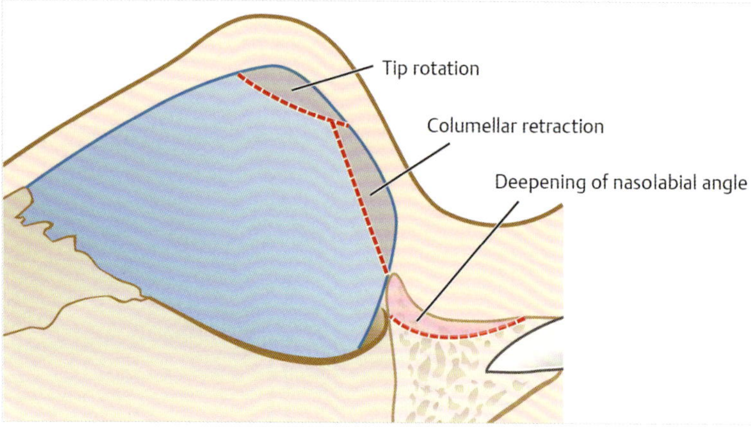

Fig. 11.1 Correcting the caudal edge of the septum. The extent and site of shortening of the caudal edge of the septum (and anterior nasal spine) vary depending on the needs in a given case.

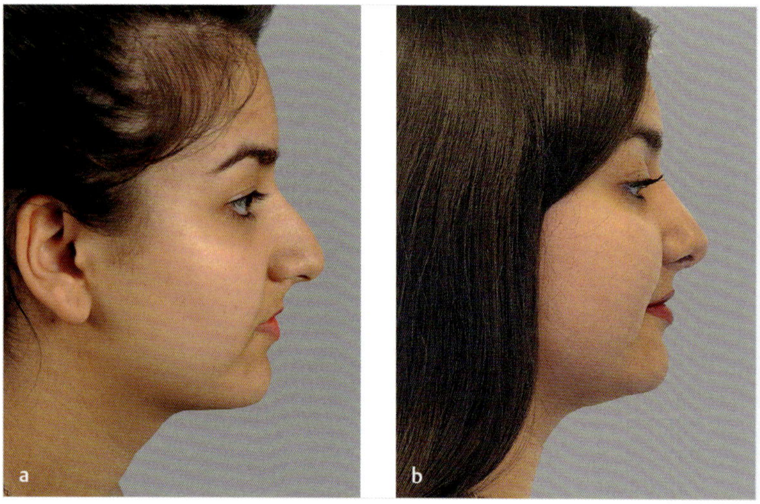

Fig. 11.2 Correction of the nasolabial angle; case study. (a) Poorly developed nasolabial angle. **(b)** Surgically corrected lower third of the caudal edge of the septum and anterior nasal spine.

resections should therefore be performed with due restraint. In order to achieve a long-term effect, removing one or two millimeters of cartilage at the caudal edge of the septum is often sufficient. Excessive reduction must be avoided, since the caudal septum constitutes an essential supporting pillar of the "tripod," which ensures stability of the anterior nose (see section 1.2.1, ▶ Fig. 1.11).

The caudal septum should provide permanent and stable support for attachment of the alar cartilages, which are worked on later.

11.1.2 Graft Augmentation of the Caudal Septum

The caudal septum may be weak or too short in patients with a history of trauma or prior nasal surgery, but also as a congenital variant. Reinforcement or even replacement of this cartilaginous plate is necessary in these cases to provide adequate support and stability to the alar cartilages and thus to the nasal tip. The caudal septum is reinforced or lengthened using cartilage grafts, often referred to as "columellar struts."

However, the various forms and alternatives of the columellar strut and their characteristics need to be examined in greater detail to allow better decision-making on how to use them. Grafts that enhance the profile of the caudal septum also determine the columellar shape. It is important to bear in mind that the further away a corrective procedure is performed from the visible profile – i.e., from the columellar skin – the less pronounced is its effect on the columellar shape. Grafts placed directly under the skin **anterior** to the medial crura of the alar cartilages have the most noticeable impact on the columellar shape. However, instability of the caudal edge of the septum carries a risk of posterosuperior retraction of the entire columella over time.

> The surgeon must therefore ensure stability of the edge of the caudal septum (or prevent loss of stability). Regardless of this, however, delicate grafts can also be placed directly under the columellar skin to modify the columellar shape (see section 11.2.6).

The septum primarily ensures the stability of the anterior nose; if necessary, a variety of grafts are available for this and are selected depending on the needs in each case (▶ Fig. 11.3a–d).

Free and Extended Columellar Strut Graft

A columellar strut graft is inserted between the medial crura of the alar cartilages in the columella, and not necessarily in direct relationship to the caudal edge of the septum (▶ Video 11.3). These transplants are available in two forms:

- **Free columellar strut graft** ("floating columellar strut," ▶ Fig. 11.3a): the graft sits between the medial crura of the alar cartilages and is not in contact with the anterior nasal spine.
- **Extended columellar strut graft** ("extended columellar strut," ▶ Fig. 11.3b): the graft sits on the anterior nasal spine.

Some surgeons use columellar strut grafts if the anterior nose does not appear stable enough to permanently support the tip in the desired position. However, the main reason for this instability is an inadequate caudal septum that requires reinforcement, which cannot be achieved with these free strut grafts. Septal lengthening or replacement grafts are therefore used far more frequently for an unstable anterior nose, as described below (septal extension graft, septal replacement graft, ▶ Fig. 11.3c, d).

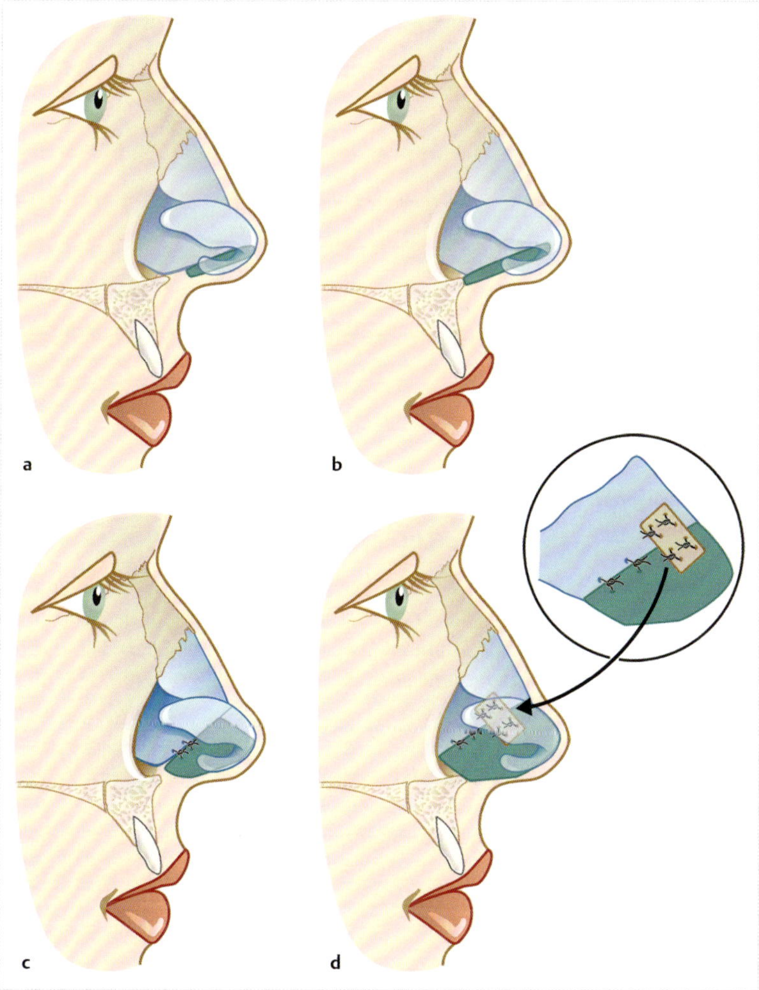

Fig. 11.3 Columella strut, septal extension, and septal replacement grafts. **(a)** Floating columellar strut. **(b)** Extended columellar strut. **(c)** Septal extension graft. **(d)** Septal replacement graft, showing splinting of the interface between an extension or replacement graft and the caudal septum.

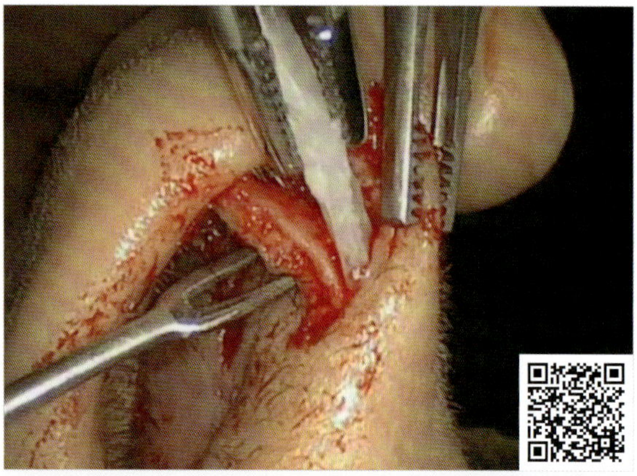

Video 11.3 Columellar strut through an endonasal columella rim incision (clinical case).

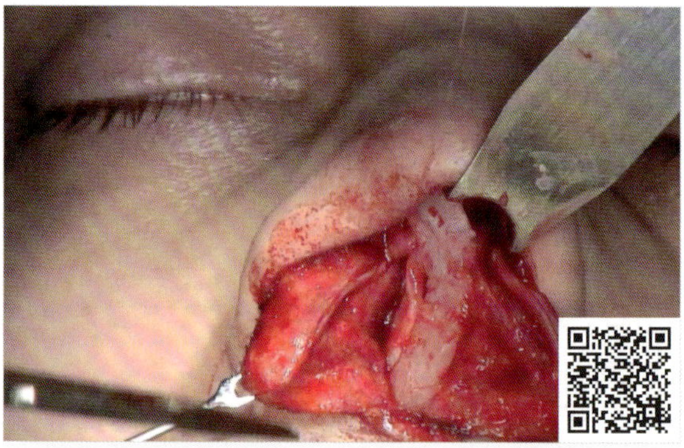

Video 11.4 Septal extension graft and tongue-in-groove procedure (clinical case).

A columellar strut graft only reinforces the medial crura of the alar cartilages. This type of strut has to be delicate to avoid excessive widening of the columella, which counters the stabilizing effect of a columellar transplant of this sort. In addition, the graft does not lie in contact with the caudal septum, and columellar retraction often cannot be prevented in the long term, despite this strut graft.

Patients in whom a columellar strut graft has been placed often describe a sensation of there being “a small, troublesome mobile foreign body” in the columella – the strut. Free columellar strut grafts of this type are therefore not so rarely removed during revision surgery – particularly since they do not contribute to stability.

11

Slim, elongated cartilaginous strips may nevertheless be indicated and inserted between the medial crura of the alar cartilages to correct an S-shaped or C-shaped deformity of the medial crura and thus of the columella (see ▶ Fig. 11.22).

A slim columellar strut graft that does not result in columellar widening is very useful for straightening of such deformities (see section 11.2.5 and ▶ Fig. 11.22a, b). However, to ensure stability of the anterior nose, grafts with a firm connection with the septum are preferable, such as the septal extension graft and septal replacement graft (▶ Fig. 11.3c, d).

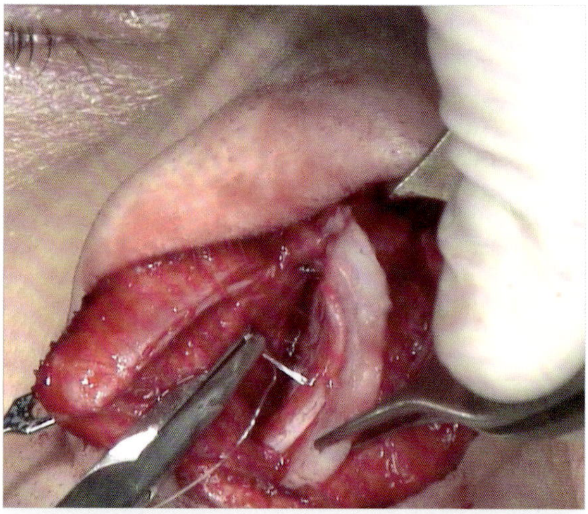

Fig. 11.4 Septal extension graft. Suture fixation of a septal extension graft, consisting of septal cartilage, to the caudal edge of the septum.

Septal Extension Graft

In contrast to the columellar strut, the **septal extension graft** lies in contact with the caudal edge of the septum, to which it is sutured (▶ Video 11.4; ▶ Fig. 11.3c, ▶ Fig. 11.4).

If the caudal edge of the septum is found too far posteriorly, a septal extension graft is placed precisely end-to-end and sutured to it, either with a few simple interrupted sutures, a continuous suture, or a so-called “figure-of-eight suture,” which describes a figure of eight between the transplant and the septal cartilage. The extension graft can also be sutured side-to-side to the caudal septum, depending on the situation.

If considered necessary, the interface between the septum and extension graft can be splinted using a thin, perforated, laterally applied bony plate (obtained from the perpendicular plate) or cartilage and affixed with sutures (see ▶ Fig. 11.3d). This graft thus securely augments the caudal edge of the septum, in contrast to the free columellar strut graft (▶ Fig. 11.5a, b).

First, a model made from the sterile cardboard of a suture package is fabricated and placed as a trial into the graft bed, to avoid any errors of judgment while harvesting an extension graft for the caudal septum. The cartilage graft is then cut to size based on this model. Septal cartilage is obtained from the posterior segment if possible, but auricular or costal cartilage can also be used.

These grafts usually lie in contact with the anterior nasal spine, to which they are sutured; this gives stability to the caudal septum and allows the medial crura of the alar cartilages to be securely sutured (tongue-in-groove technique; see section 11.2.2.

Septal Replacement Graft

A septal replacement graft differs from a septal extension graft essentially in that it is not attached to the caudal edge of the septum, which is not present. It may be attached to a rudimentary cartilaginous septum, for instance, or to the bony septum, or the transplant is only fixed in the dorsal K-area. This type of septal replacement graft has to be stable and of the correct size. However, it must not be too wide or too robust, to avoid functional or visible cosmetic disorders. Unless conserved cartilage is used, the graft can only be harvested from auricular or costal cartilage, since it replaces the deficient septum (▶ Fig. 11.6a, b, ▶ Fig. 11.7a, b).

Any physiological curvature on this cartilaginous transplant– if obtained from the conchal cartilage – must be corrected. Two strips of auricular cartilage with opposing curvatures can be sutured together for this purpose. This procedure increases the stability of the conchal cartilage and counters undesirable flexion. Costal cartilage is in principle often more suitable for this purpose, given its larger volume and better stability.

As already described for the septal extension graft, the use of a prefabricated pattern made of sterile cardboard is helpful for septum replacement. Septum replacement grafts are usually sutured to the anterior nasal spine; the suture can be passed through a small drill hole in the spine if it cannot be passed around the spur of the spine.

> ✔
>
> The surgeon must assess preoperatively whether harvesting of grafts from the auricular or costal cartilage is necessary, and the patient must be informed about this accordingly before the operation. Failure to do this can result in a problematic intraoperative situation, with inadequate material, and harvesting of cartilage without informed consent may have medicolegal implications.

The septum replacement graft may initially rise high between the medial crura, where it is sutured to securely support the alar domes; it will subsequently be shortened to the level of the domes. This graft stabilizes tip rotation and projection, but occasionally causes stiffness in the anterior nose, which is not well tolerated by all patients.

Opening the Nasolabial Angle: Premaxillary Grafts (Plunge Grafts)

The angle between the upper lip and the columella (nasolabial angle) influences the columellar contour. A persistently acute angle despite correction of the caudal septum and columella, or insufficient prominence

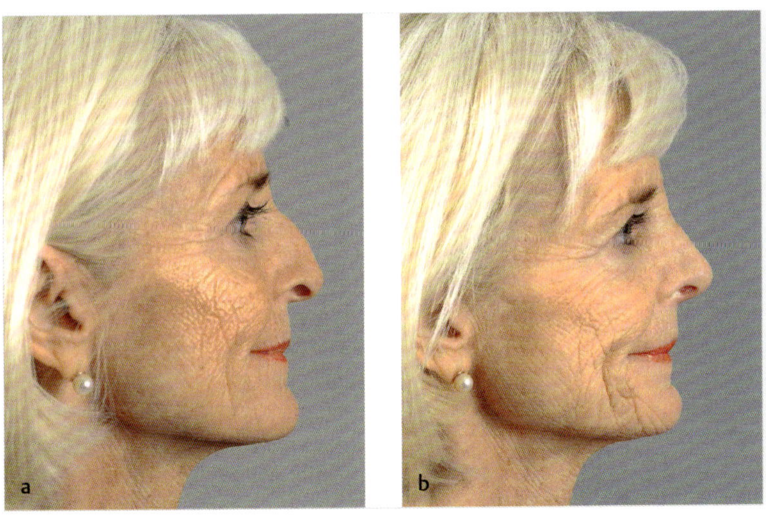

Fig. 11.5 Effect of the septal extension graft. (a) Retracted lower third of the columella, with a drooping tip and unstable and poorly developed caudal septum. **(b)** Effect of the septal extension graft on the nasolabial angle and stability of the anterior nose postoperatively.

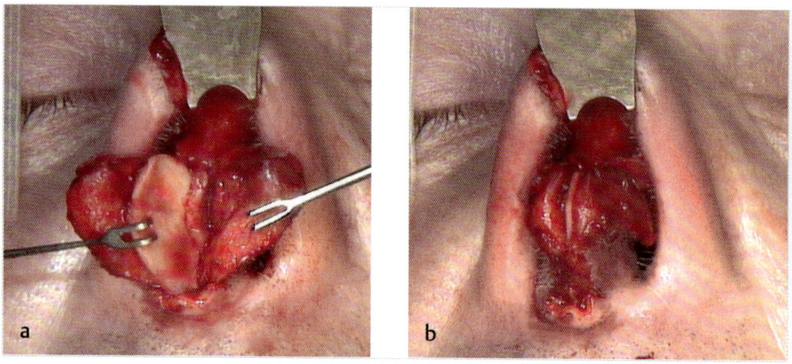

Fig. 11.6 Septal replacement graft. **(a)** Septal replacement graft harvested from conchal cartilage, sutured to a rudimentary cartilaginous septum. **(b)** Medial crura of the alar cartilages attached to the septal replacement graft.

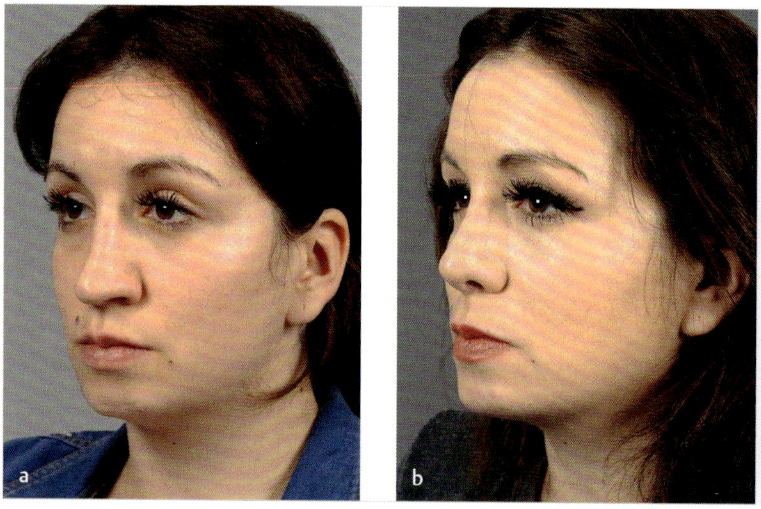

Fig. 11.7 Stabilization of the anterior nose with a septal replacement graft. **(a)** Unstable anterior nose, with drooping tip and narrow nasolabial angle and loss of the anterior septum following trauma. **(b)** Post rhinoplasty with a septal replacement graft harvested from conchal cartilage. Simultaneous correction of the chin scar using a multiple W-plasty.

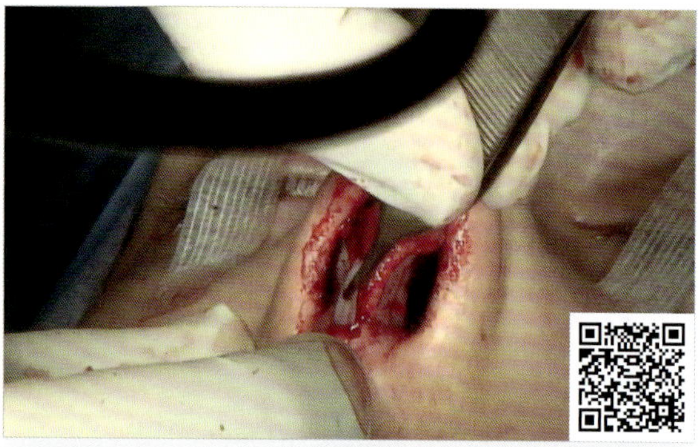

Video 11.5 Columella plunge graft (clinical case).

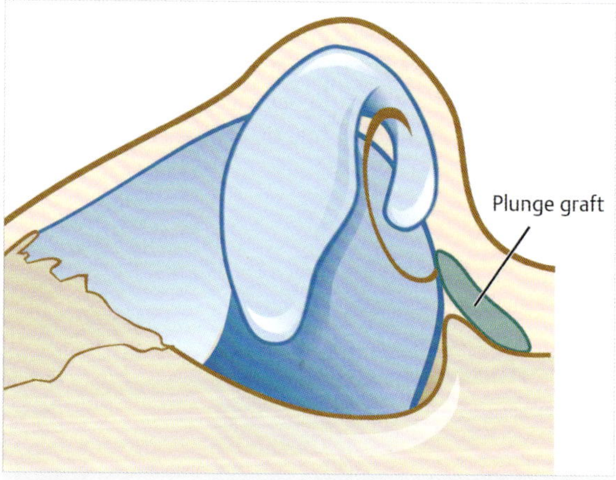

Fig. 11.8 Plunge graft. The plunge graft increases the nasolabial angle and is used for premaxillary augmentation.

of the lower third of the columella regardless of the above, may be remedied using graft material placed anterior to the maxilla and the anterior nasal spine (▶ Video 11.5). This can be done using either an open access route or a closed technique via a columellar rim incision. Either compact cartilaginous grafts, slightly softened by crushing if necessary, or fragmented, residual pieces of cartilage from other grafts can be used to augment the nasolabial angle. This graft material is then inserted with suitable forceps into a narrow premaxillary graft bed, prepared with a pair of delicate scissors, immediately anterior to the bone in the center of the nasolabial angle ("plunge graft," ▶ Fig. 11.8).

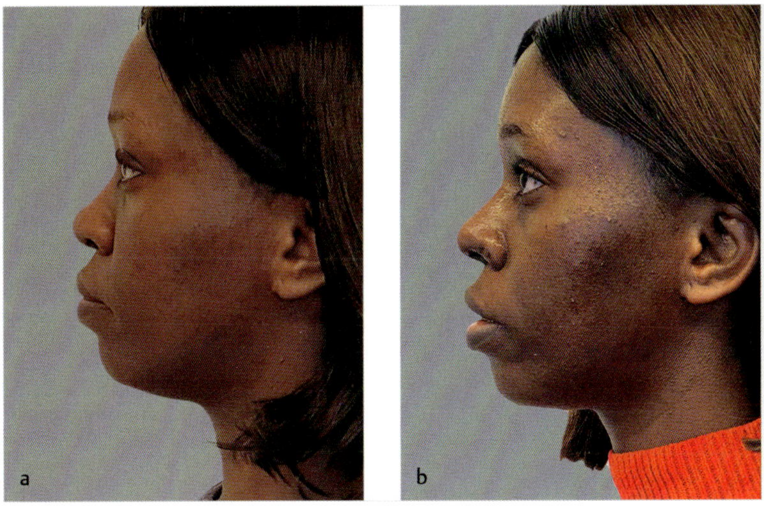

Fig. 11.9 Correction of the nasolabial angle with a plunge graft. (a) Narrow nasolabial angle. **(b)** Post rhinoplasty with septal and conchal cartilage grafts.

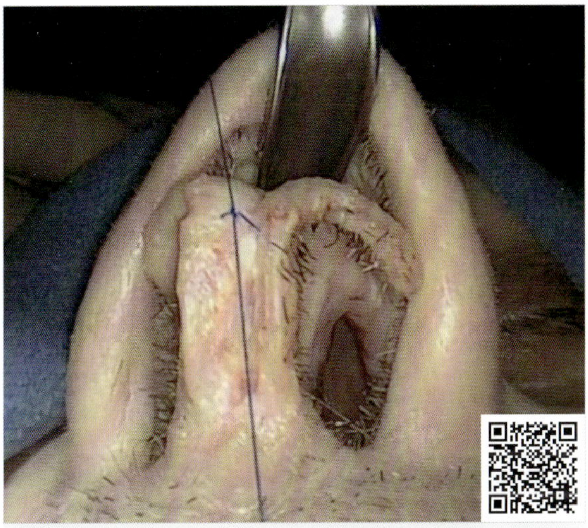

Video 11.6 High anterior suture of the medial crura (cadaver head).

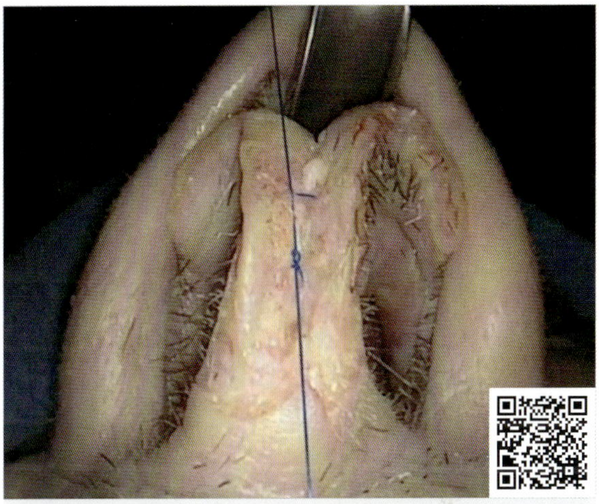

Video 11.7 Medial crural suture (cadaver head).

Additional fixation is usually unnecessary; however, tiny fragments can be fixed in a large graft bed using TachoSil (see also section 17.2), fibrin glue, or a few drops of blood (▶ Fig. 11.9).

11.2 Corrective Surgery of the Columella

The configuration of the medial crura of the alar cartilages and their relationship to the caudal edge of the septum affects the appearance of the columella and the nasal tip, and various suture techniques play a significant role in this.

11.2.1 Narrowing of the Columella: Approximating Suture of the Medial Crura

The columella is frequently wide, and should be narrowed. Widening is usually due to the presence of excessive soft tissue between the crura; removing this tissue and subsequent suturing and approximation of the crura results in a narrower columella (▶ Video 11.6, ▶ Video 11.7, ▶ Video 11.8; ▶ Fig. 11.10, ▶ Fig. 11.11a, b, ▶ Fig. 11.12a,b). The suture is placed at the level of the abnormality.

When this is an isolated finding in the medial crural **footplates**, it can be corrected using a **medial crura footplate suture** (▶ Video 11.9; ▶ Fig. 11.13a, b), or by partial resection of the footplates after dissection and exposure of these cartilages.

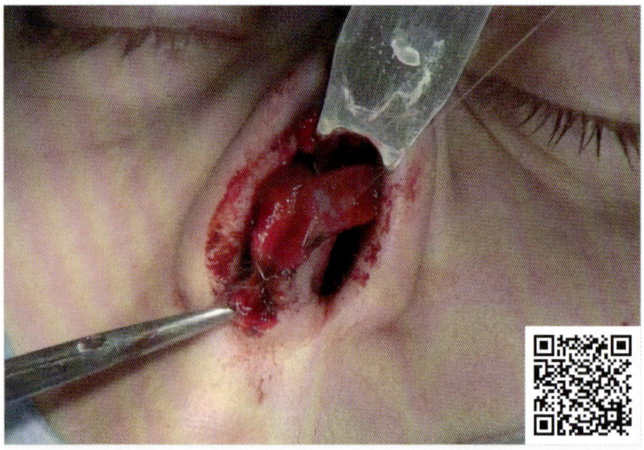

Video 11.8 Medial crural suture (clinical case).

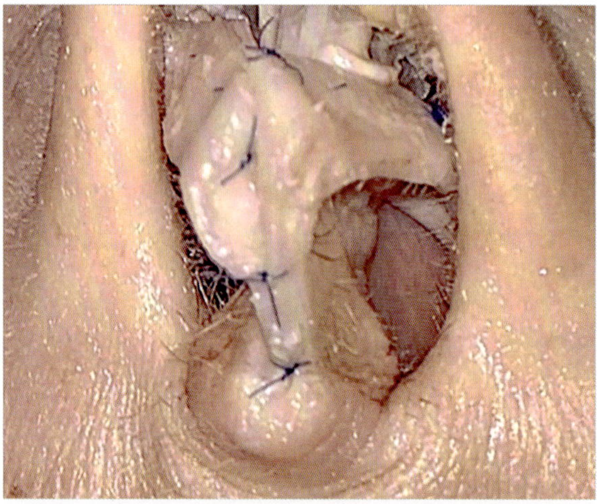

Fig. 11.10 Medial crural sutures to narrow the columella in its upper, middle, and lower thirds (medial crural footplates). (Demonstrated in a cadaver specimen.)

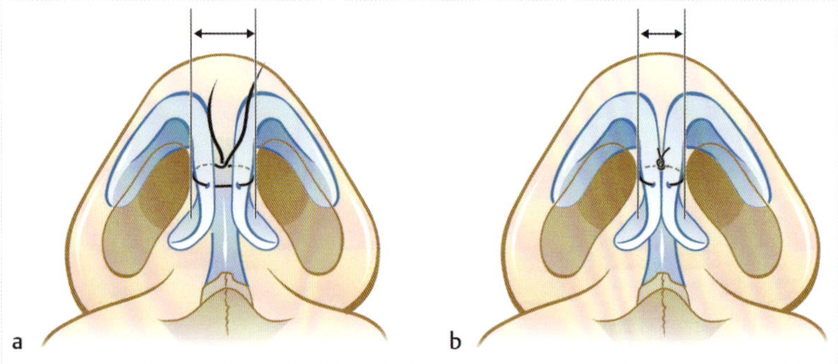

Fig. 11.11 Medial crural suture for columellar narrowing. (a) Before the suture. **(b)** After the suture.

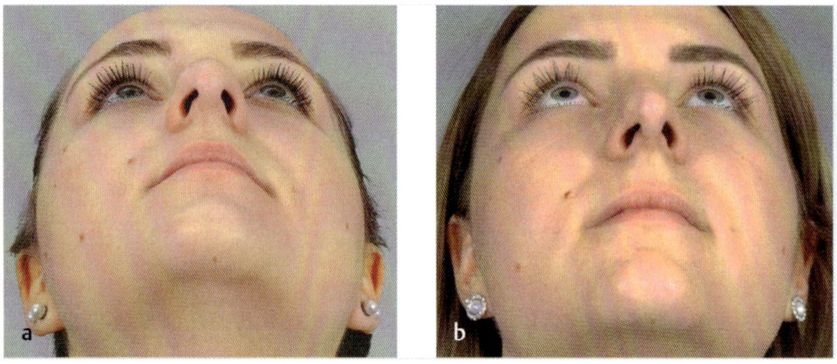

Fig. 11.12 Narrowing of the columella; case example. (a) Broad columella. **(b)** After narrowing with medial crural sutures.

> It should be noted that approximating the divergent caudal edges of the medial crura also rotates these edges anteriorly (▶ Fig. 11.14a, b). This may lead to an increase in the columellar projection, a "drooping columella," or undesirable enlargement of the nostrils in severe cases.

11.2.2 Correction of Columellar Projection and Rotation: Septum–Columella Suture and Tongue-in-Groove Technique

Sutures between the medial crura and the septum play an essential part in determining the columellar profile and position. The columella is raised by shortening the distance between these structures, which is particularly useful for correction of a drooping columella and "tip drop" with a ptotic nasal tip. An alteration of even one or two millimeters can cause a marked change (▶ Video 11.2, ▶ Video 11.10; ▶ Fig. 11.15a–d).

Anchoring the posterior edges of the medial crura to the caudal septum is very effective and is used quite often (**septum–columella suture**).

The **tongue-in-groove technique** (▶ Fig. 11.16a, b; see Video 6.1) is used to achieve even greater retraction of the upper third of the columella with rotation of the nasal tip. In this technique, the posterior edges of the medial crura slide lateral to the caudal edge of the septum and are thus more or less moved cranially and sutured in this position. This is how the term "tongue in groove" (or "tongue and groove") arose, originally used in woodworking – the tongue of one board slides into the groove of an adjacent board to stabilize the interface. In rhinoplasty, the tongue corresponds to the caudal edge of the septum, while the groove is formed by the medial crura of the alar cartilages.

11.2.3 Accentuating Tip Rotation: Combination of Lateral Suspension Sutures and Tongue-in-Groove Technique

Lateral suspension and a tongue-in-groove technique can be used in combination if indicated, since these procedures achieve different goals: lateral suspension lifts and fixes the lateral crura to the desired position (see section 10.7), while the tongue-in-groove technique elevates the medial crura. However, both of these procedures play a role in defining the position of the tip (▶ Fig. 11.17a–c, ▶ Fig. 11.18a, b, ▶ Fig. 11.19a–d).

> It should be noted that the addition of bilateral suspension sutures to enhance nasal tip rotation with a supplementary tongue-in-groove technique may have a positive additive effect at the tip, but overcorrection has to be avoided.

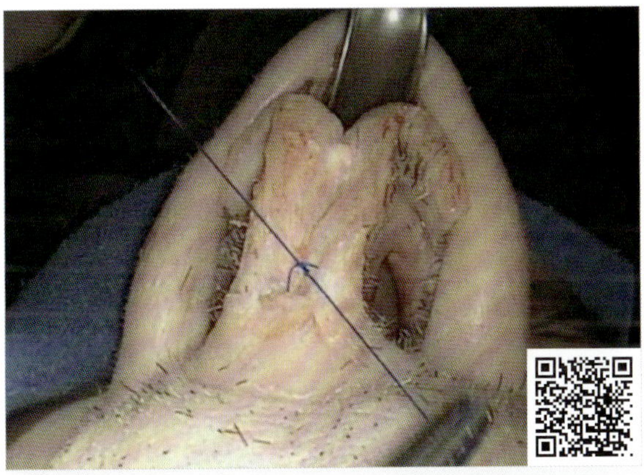

Video 11.9 Medial crural footplate suture (cadaver head).

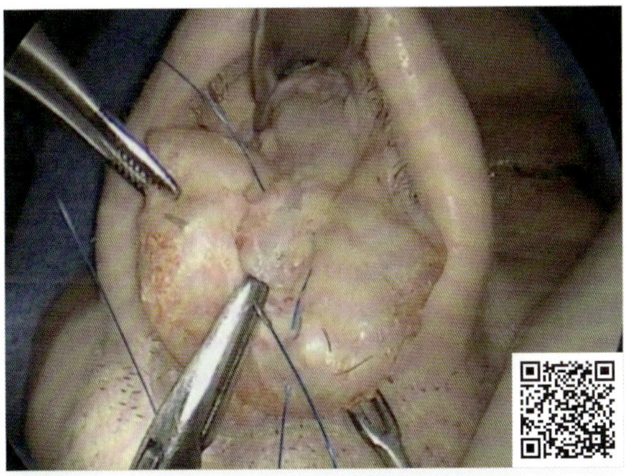

Video 11.10 Tongue-in-groove and tip rotation (cadaver head).

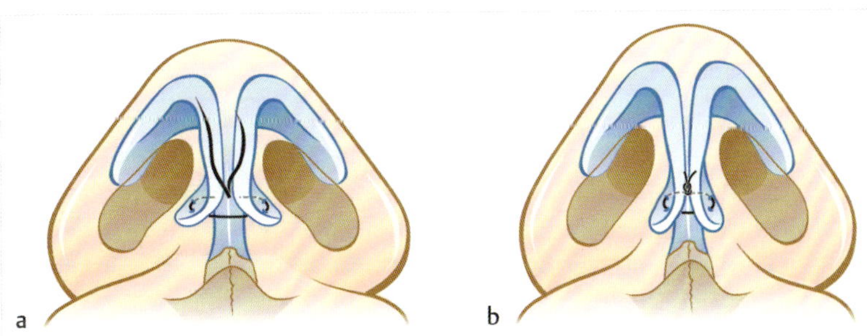

Fig. 11.13 Correction of protruding medial crura footplates. An approximation suture of the medial crura footplates **(a)** usually has a marked effect on the width of the columellar base **(b)**.

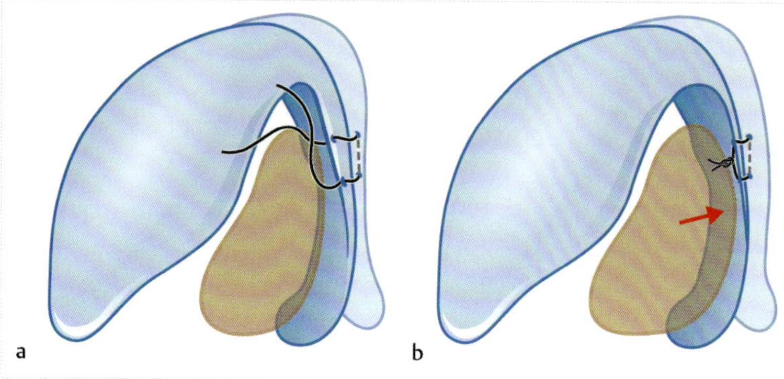

Fig. 11.14 (a, b) Narrowing of the columella. Approximation of the medial crura of the alar cartilages results in columellar narrowing, but may also enhance the projection of the columella, when the suture is placed on the caudal rim of the crura.

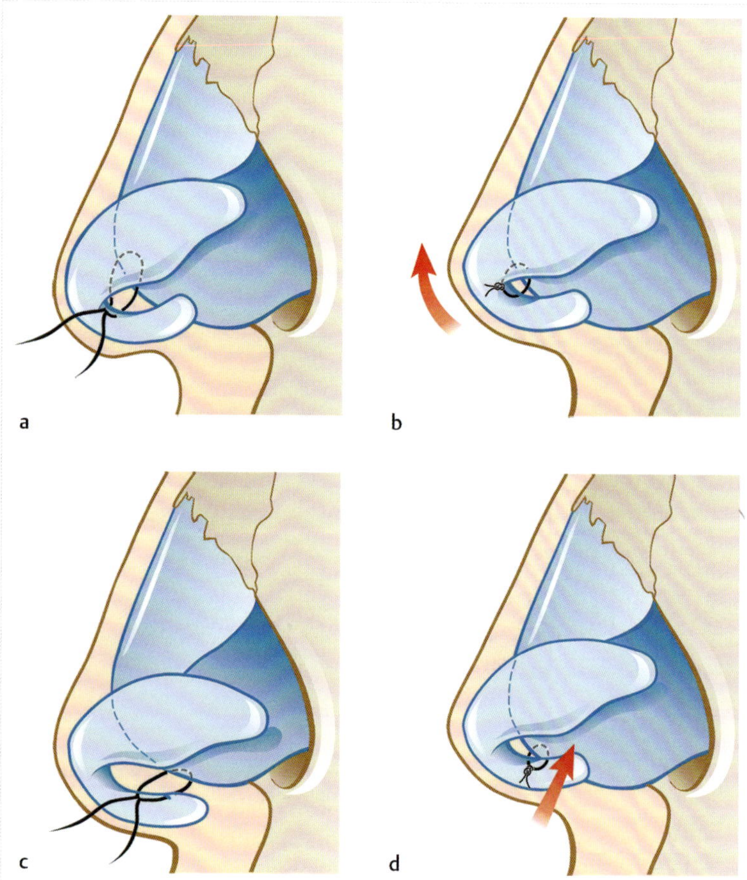

Fig. 11.15 Septum–columella suture, or tongue-in-groove procedure. Approximation of the medial crura of the alar cartilages to the caudal septum. **(a, b)** Tip rotation is more pronounced if the suture is positioned in the vicinity of the anterior septal angle. **(c, d)** A suture placed further posteriorly along the septal edge results in elevation of the columella and can be used to correct a drooping columella.

11

Extreme and persistent stiffness in the nasal tip due to the tongue-in-groove procedure is occasionally reported, but appears to be rare.

The extent of the tongue-in-groove procedure must always be adapted to meet the needs in the individual case. Suturing only through the outermost edge of the caudal septum may be sufficient, but is less effective than passing the needle through the septum 1 or 2 mm above the edge of the cartilage. It is advisable to briefly replace the nasal skin over the tip and test the best profile line of the columella using a pair of forceps before deciding on the extent of the procedure, while reviewing the resultant alteration of the nasal tip in the mirror.

The tongue-in-groove procedure may occasionally give rise to excessive skin folds laterally in the transition zone between the septum and columella, which may then be resected.

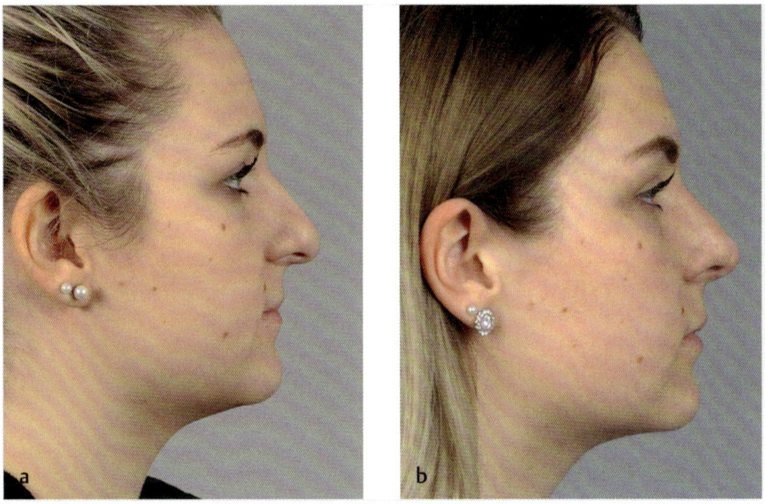

Fig. 11.16 Tongue-in-groove technique; case study. (a) Drooping nasal tip, with an unstable anterior nose. **(b)** Correction using an extension graft, tongue-in-groove technique, and a delicate tip graft.

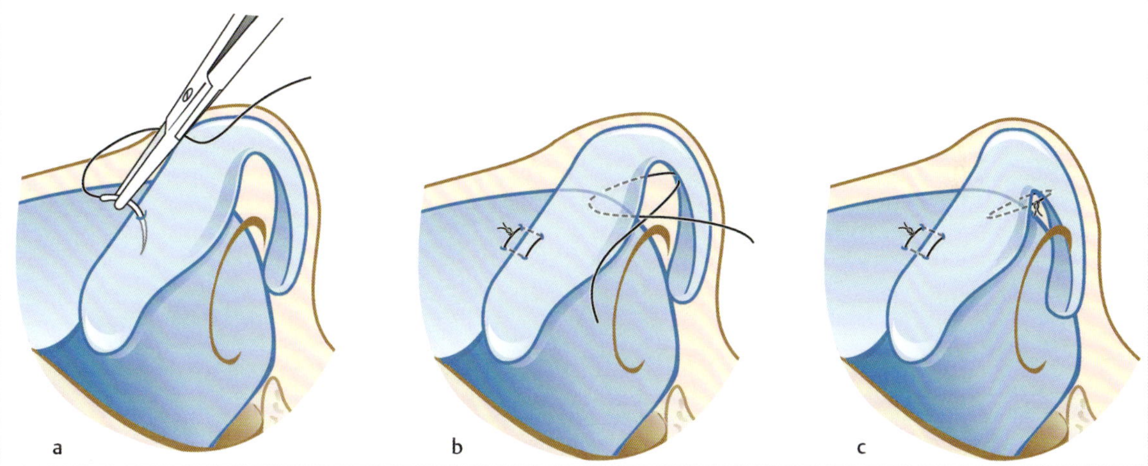

Fig. 11.17 Lateral suspension suture and tongue-in-groove technique. (a, b) The cephalic edges of the lateral crura of the alar cartilages are fixed to the middle third of the cartilaginous vault using a suspension suture. **(b, c)** The nasal tip is rotated, and columellar projection is reduced using the tongue-in-groove technique. This suture between the medial crura of the alar cartilages and the caudal septum allows the caudal septum to slide between the medial crura ("tongue-in-groove").

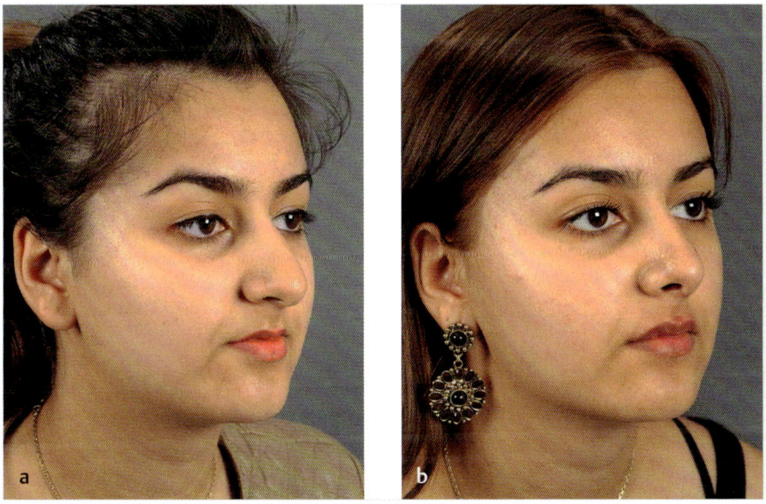

Fig. 11.18 Tongue-in-groove procedure and suspension sutures; case study. (a) Marked nasal tip overprojection and ptosis. **(b)** Corrected using the tongue-in-groove procedure in combination with suspension sutures.

11

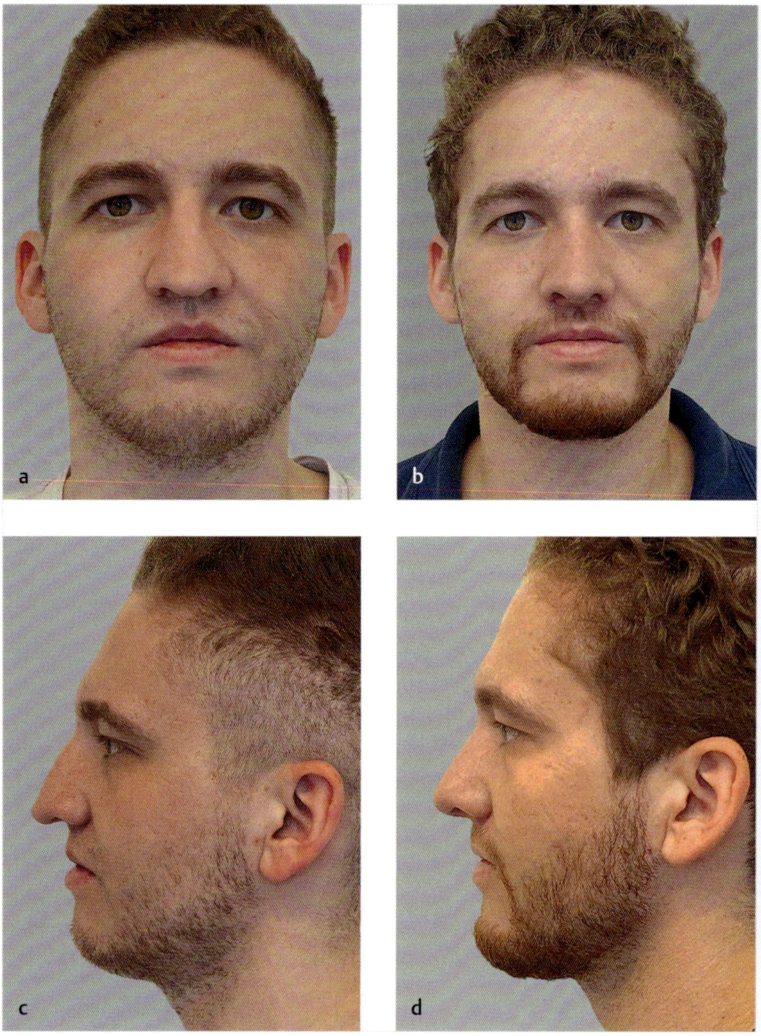

Fig. 11.19 Septal extension graft, lateral suspension sutures, and tongue-in-groove-procedure; case study. In this case, instability of the nasal tip complex was combined with overprojection and underrotation, requiring a septal extension graft, lateral crural suspension sutures, and a tongue-in-groove-procedure. Preoperative frontal **(a)** and side views **(c)**; result after rhinoplasty **(b, d)**.

Finally, asymmetry of the caudal edges of the medial crura can be corrected by minimal unilateral resection of the more prominent edge, while bilateral resection may be beneficial in isolated cases only.

Caution: These corrective procedures immediately alter the appearance of the columella, since they are performed directly under the mostly thin columellar skin.

11.2.4 Shortening of the Columella: Medial Crural Overlay

The height of the columella and thus nasal tip projection or rotation can be reduced by overlaying the excessively long medial crura of the alar cartilages. This procedure is equivalent to the lateral crural overlay of the lower lateral cartilages (see section 10.5.1; ▶ Fig. 11.20, ▶ Fig. 11.21). Medial crural overlay is used far less frequently in comparison with lateral crural overlay.

11.2.5 Straightening the Columella: Strut Grafts

A C-shaped or S-shaped curvature of the medial crura of the alar cartilages is frequently present, and the extent of it occasionally becomes evident only after separation of the skin flap. A flat, linear "floating columellar strut" is indicated in these cases and in those requiring widening of the columella (▶ Video 11.11; ▶ Fig. 11.22a, b; see also section 11.1.2 and ▶ Fig. 11.3a). The floating strut is then placed between the deformed crura and secured with a suture.

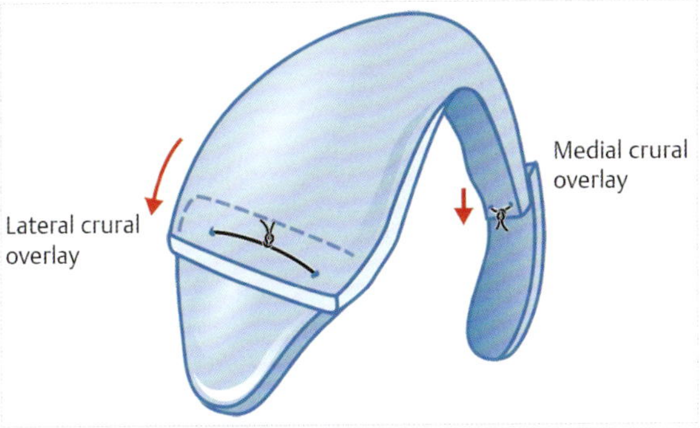

Fig. 11.20 Medial crural overlay (schematic diagram). The medial crus is divided, the apical stump is moved over the lower segment, and the segments are then sutured in the new, shortened position.

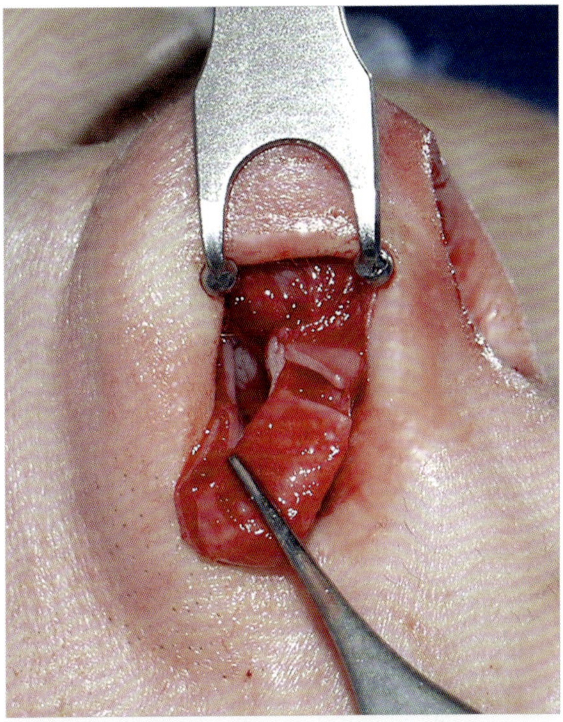

Fig. 11.21 Medial crural overlay, intraoperative view (using a closed technique); before suturing.

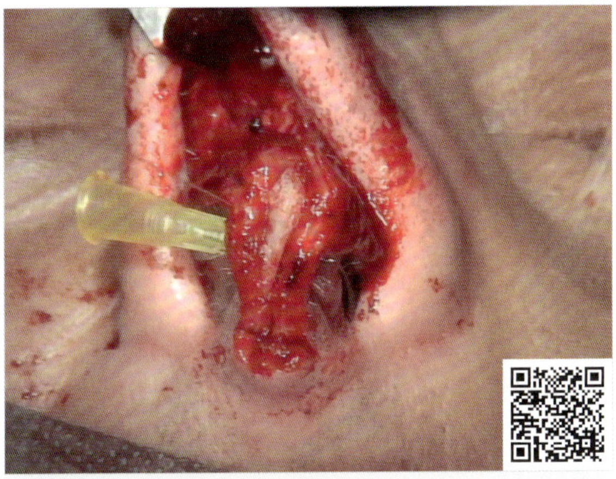

Video 11.11 Columella strut graft (clinical case).

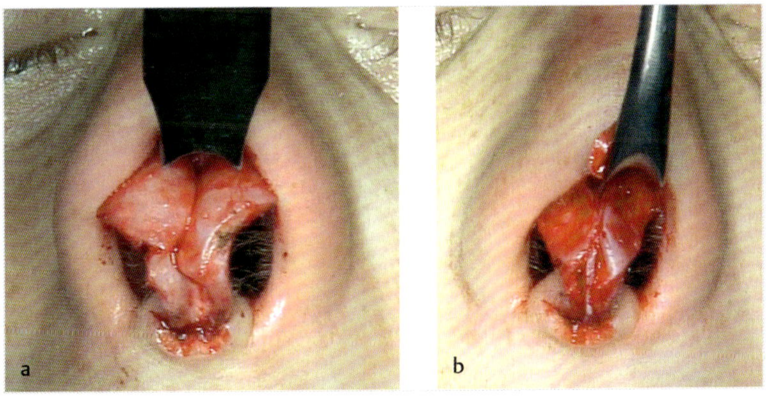

Fig. 11.22 Floating columella strut graft, intraoperative view. (a) S-shaped columellar deformity. **(b)** Straightening with floating columellar strut graft.

11.2.6 Correction of the Columellar Profile: Button Graft

A delicate strip of cartilage or "columellar button" may be placed anteriorly to the medial crura – akin to a tip graft – to enhance columellar projection or conceal an irregularity. Button grafts of this type may, for instance, help to shape the **angle of rotation** at the columella (▶ Fig. 11.23; see also section 1.2.1 and ▶ Fig. 1.12b).

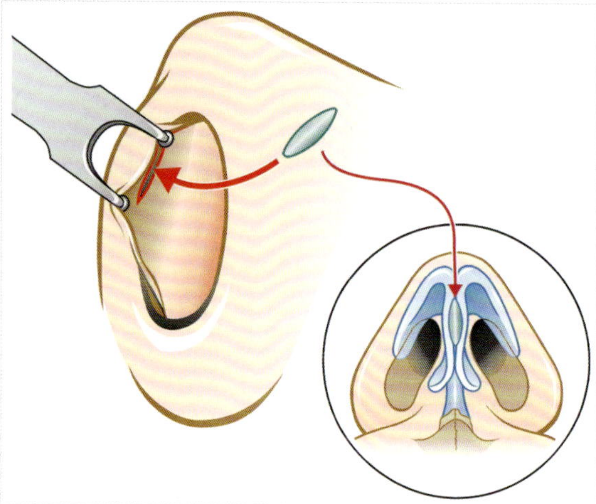

Fig. 11.23 Columellar button graft. A small cartilaginous graft is placed anterior to the edges of the medial crura. The procedure is shown using the closed technique.

If mild enhancement of the columellar profile is required as an isolated procedure, a button graft can be conveniently placed in a subcutaneous soft-tissue pocket via a columellar rim incision – i.e., using the closed technique.

Bibliography

Byrd HS, Andochick S, Copit S, Walton KG. Septal extension grafts: a method of controlling tip projection shape. Plast Reconstr Surg. 1997; 100(4): 999–1010

Cobo R, Caldas A. Caudal septum surgery techniques reviewed. Curr Opin Otolaryngol Head Neck Surg. 2017; 25(1):4–11

Datema FR, Lohuis PJ. The tongue-in-groove technique in primary and revision rhinoplasty. Facial Plast Surg. 2016; 32(4):416–423

Foda HMT. The caudal septum replacement graft. Arch Facial Plast Surg. 2008; 10(3):152–157

Kridel RW, Scott BA, Foda HM. The tongue-in-groove technique in septorhinoplasty. A 10-year experience. Arch Facial Plast Surg. 1999; 1 (4):246–256, discussion 257–258

Most SP. Anterior septal reconstruction: outcomes after a modified extracorporeal septoplasty technique. Arch Facial Plast Surg. 2006; 8(3): 202–207

Pastorek NJ, Bustillo A, Murphy MR, Becker DG. The extended columellar strut-tip graft. Arch Facial Plast Surg. 2005; 7(3):176–184

Patel KB, Mendonca DA, Skolnick G, Woo AS. Anatomical study of the medial crura and the effect on nasal tip projection in open rhinoplasty. Plast Reconstr Surg. 2013; 132(4):787–793

Rohrich RJ, Durand PD, Dayan E. Changing Role of Septal Extension versus Columellar Grafts in Modern Rhinoplasty. Plast Reconstr Surg. 2020; 145 (5):927e–931e

Sawh-Martinez R, Perkins K, Madari S, Steinbacher DM. Control of Nasal Tip Position: Quantitative Assessment of Columellar Strut versus Caudal Septal Extension Graft. Plast Reconstr Surg. 2019; 144(5):772e–780e

11

12 Correction of the Nasal Tip

Correction of the nasal tip is regarded as the most challenging procedure in rhinoplasty, not least because many details that are confined to a small space have to be optimally addressed in order to achieve an aesthetically appealing surgical outcome. The surgeon also has to have a well-developed aesthetic sense of appropriate proportionality and a thorough knowledge of regional anatomy. The saying, "if you've mastered the tip, you've mastered the nose!" is very appropriate here.

12.1 Introductory Remarks

Each of the three anatomical segments of the alar cartilages (medial, middle, and lateral crus) is addressed individually while working on the nasal tip, and the required correction and extent for each is determined (▶ Fig. 12.1). An overview of the range of available surgical options on the alar cartilages and the impact of these procedures on the corresponding structures is provided below (▶ Table 12.1, ▶ Table 12.2, ▶ Table 12.3). The procedures listed in the tables are explained in detail in the following sections.

The self-retaining Aufricht retractor is used when working on the alar cartilages, to facilitate bimanual dissection (see ▶ Fig. 6.23a–c), and the fine-toothed Adson forceps, serrated at the tip only (▶ Fig. 12.2), or the Adson–Brown tissue forceps with multiple teeth (▶ Fig. 12.3) can be used to gently grasp the cartilage.

The most frequently performed surgical maneuvers are described below. If the surgeon uses a preservation technique (see section 8.4), then in some cases – but not always – the push-down or let-down techniques already lead to an increase in the rotation of the tip. However, it still needs to be assessed in each individual case whether further measures on the alar cartilages are necessary for optimization.

12.2 Shaping of the Alar Domes

Nasal tip deformities must be classified as either abnormalities of shape or position. Abnormalities in the shape of the nasal domes (hypertrophy, bulbous shape, see ▶ Fig. 12.8a, ▶ Fig. 12.16a, ▶ Fig. 12.19a; boxy appearance, see ▶ Fig. 12.18a; asymmetry) are corrected directly at the domes, while an abnormal position of the nasal tip is rectified mainly by corrective measures on its periphery (e.g., on the lateral and medial crura of the alar cartilages or at the caudal edge of the septum).

Cartilage grafts are usually required for nasal tip augmentation, with the increase in volume enhancing tip rotation and/or projection. Patients who are undergoing primary rhinoplasty often have overly large, wide, or round nasal tips and cartilaginous domes. These should therefore be made smaller, narrower, and more pointed.

The alar cartilage domes should be first tentatively "pinched" using the Adson–Brown forceps into the de-

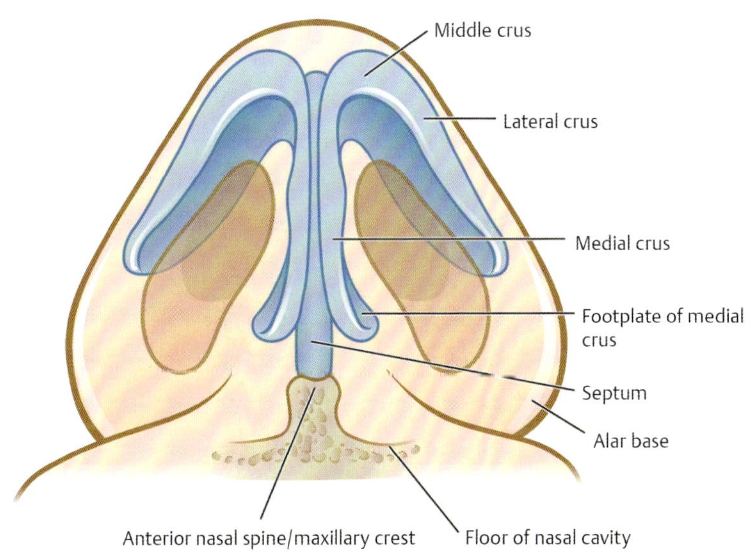

Fig. 12.1 Anatomy of the alar cartilages. From the surgical point of view, the alar cartilages are divided into three parts: medial, middle, and lateral crura.

12

Table 12.1 Procedures on the alar domes and their effects

	Procedures	Effects
Sutures	Domal (aka transdomal / intradomal / tip defining / dome creation) suture	Narrowing of the tip
	Dome-equalizing suture	Symmetrical positioning of the tip-defining points; stabilization
	Double dome suture	Combination of domal suture and dome equalizing suture in one: narrowing and symmetrical positioning; stabilization
Cutting / scoring procedures	Scoring in the dome • With domal suture	Marking the nasal tip-defining point; mild unrounding of the tip. • Marked accentuation of the tip
	Vertical dome division • With domal suture	Marked unrounding and accentuation of the tip. • Accentuation and narrowing of the tip; stabilization
	Wedge resection of the dome • With domal suture	Limited reduction of tip volume • Narrowing of the tip; stabilization
	Strip resection of the dome • With domal suture	Marked reduction of tip volume • Marked narrowing of the tip; stabilization
	All suture and cutting procedures with lateral crural steal	Cranial displacement of the nasal tip defining point; enhanced rotation
Grafts	Tip graft (shield graft); single or double layer	Augmentation of rotation and/or projection; contouring of the tip
	Blocking graft	Stabilization of a tip graft
	Cap graft	Enhanced rotation
	Domal strut graft	Domal support
	Facet graft	Reconstruction of facet, lowering of the anterior edge of the nostril; reduction of nostril size
	Tip spreader graft	Widening of the tip

sired new shape and position at the start of corrective surgery of the nasal tip (▶ Fig. 12.4), and the new nasal tip defining points of the alar domes should simultaneously be defined by very superficial marking or scoring. These marks provide guidance on the new shape and position of the domes during the subsequent surgical procedure. The new position of the nasal tip-defining points is reviewed using the forceps once the nasal dorsum and the upper and lower lateral cartilages have been corrected; the nasal skin flap can be tentatively replaced to simulate the surgical outcome as far as possible. As the new position of the domes initially is marked only by superficial scoring, it can later be modified if this proves more appropriate for a desirable outcome.

The nasal tip-defining points should finally lie above the level of the middle third of the nasal dorsum when the patient is supine.

With regard to the intensity of the effect, the surgeon has a graduated range of options for modifying the shape of the nasal tip to the desired extent (▶ Table 12.4). A choice can therefore be made from a wide range of available interventions for nasal tip correction. The following sections take a closer look at these options.

12.2.1 Suturing Techniques for the Nasal Tip

Dome Suture

A dome suture (synonyms: transdomal, intradomal suture; tip-defining suture; dome-binding suture; dome creation suture) is most commonly used for shaping of the domes, which accentuates or establishes the tip defining point (▶ Video 12.1, ▶ Video 12.2, ▶ Video 12.3; ▶ Fig. 12.5a–c). Superficial scoring of the cartilage at the tip-defining points helps define the new domes and facilitates symmetrical coaptation of the two sides. The suture material used for the nasal tip is 5–0, or more frequently 6–0 polydioxanone (e.g., PDS), or a comparable, long-term absorbable suture, depending on the firmness of the cartilage.

These tip-defining sutures are usually best applied in the cephalic segment of the dome (cephalic tip suture);

Table 12.2 Procedures on the lower lateral cartilages and their effects

	Procedures	Effects
Sutures	Lateral suspension sutures	Raising and fixation of lateral crura position; controlling tip rotation
	Lateral crural spanning suture	Elevation of lateral crura
	Lateral crural convexity control suture	Correction of lateral crural concavity
Cutting / scoring procedures	Cephalic resection	Narrowing the lateral crura and supratip area
	Lateral crural turn-in flap; 90° • 180° • With lateral crural strut graft	Narrowing and stabilization of the lateral crura • Helps with concavity • Support of lateral crura; helps with concavity
	Lateral crural overlay/lateral crural strip resection	Axial shortening of the lateral crura; reduction of tip projection
Grafts	Lateral strut graft	Lateral crural support
	Lateral batten graft	External splinting of lateral crus; correction of concavity
	Lateral crural extension graft	Axial elongation of lateral crura
	Rim graft	Augmentation, contouring, lowering, and stabilization of alar rim; nostril size reduction
	Rim batten graft	Splints caudal edge of lower lateral cartilage
	Rim strut graft	Supports caudal edge of lower lateral cartilage
	Composite graft	Filling of an internal alar skin–cartilage defect

Table 12.3 Procedures on the medial crura of the alar cartilages / on the columella, and their effects

	Procedures	Effects
Cutting procedures	Medial crural overlay / medial crural strip resection	Shortening of medial crura; reduction of tip projection/ rotation
	(Partial) resection of alar footplates	Narrowing of columella base
Sutures	Medial crura sutures	Narrowing of columella
	Medial crura footplate sutures	Narrowing of columella base
	Septum–columella sutures	Fixation of medial crura on caudal septum edge; columella retraction
	Tongue-in-groove procedure	Enhanced tip rotation, reduced projection; retraction of lobule
Grafts	Columella strut graft, floating; extended	Columella stabilization and straightening; support
	Septal extension graft / septal replacement graft	Reinforcement and lengthening of the nose; stabilization of columella
	Button graft	Correction and projection of columellar profile
	Plunge graft	Opening, rounding and projection of nasolabial angle

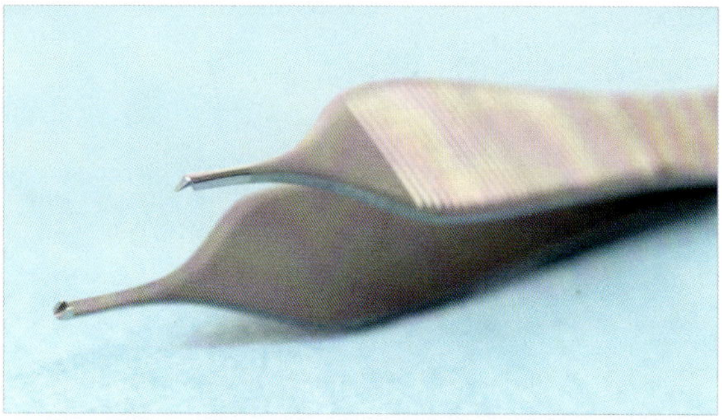

Fig. 12.2 Adson forceps. The Adson forceps securely grips fine cartilage in situ, and in the operating room it is better known as the "mouse-tooth forceps" (KARL STORZ SE & Co. KG, Tuttlingen, Germany).

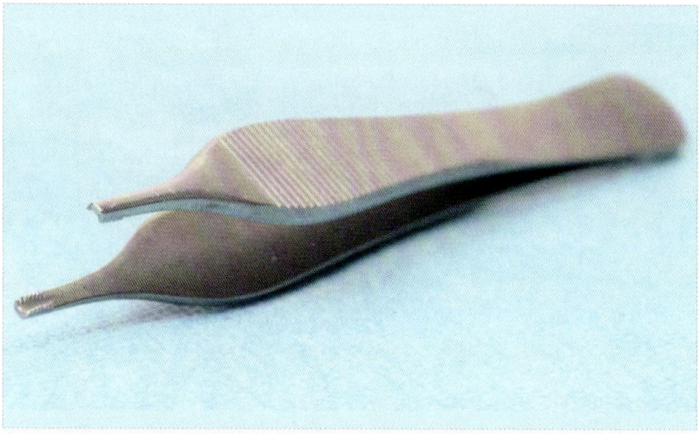

Fig. 12.3 Adson–Brown forceps. The Adson–Brown forceps have a larger row of "teeth" (KARL STORZ SE & Co. KG, Tuttlingen, Germany).

further caudally, they may induce (often undesirable) lowering of the caudal edge of the alar rim. ▶ Fig. 12.6a, b (diagram), ▶ Fig. 12.7a, b (in a cadaver specimen) and ▶ Fig. 12.8a, b (case study) show the typical effects of a transdomal suture.

> ✔
>
> The inner skin layer is not routinely dissected before the transdomal suture is applied, since detached skin often does not reattach itself well to the domal segment and it is then perceived by the patient as a troublesome, nodular foreign body in the roof of the nostril. The transdomal suture alone works just as well without separation of the skin, as long as it is not combined with any cartilage resection in the domal segment.

Several variants of the cephalic tip suture can be distinguished, particularly in relation to the elevation of the caudal edge of the alar cartilage (▶ Fig. 12.5a–c).

- In the standard variant, the thread describes a square (▶ Fig. 12.5a).
- A nearly triangular configuration as proposed by Kovacevic and Wurm (see Bibliography below) (▶ Fig. 12.5b).
- A particularly strong effect on the caudal edge of the alar cartilage is attributed to thread guidance on the inside of the cephalic tip (▶ Fig. 12.5c).

The suturing technique most suitable in the individual case can be identified by trying to shape the tip with tweezers (compare with ▶ Fig. 12.4). Of course, a thread that does not achieve an ideal result can be pulled out and replaced with another suture.

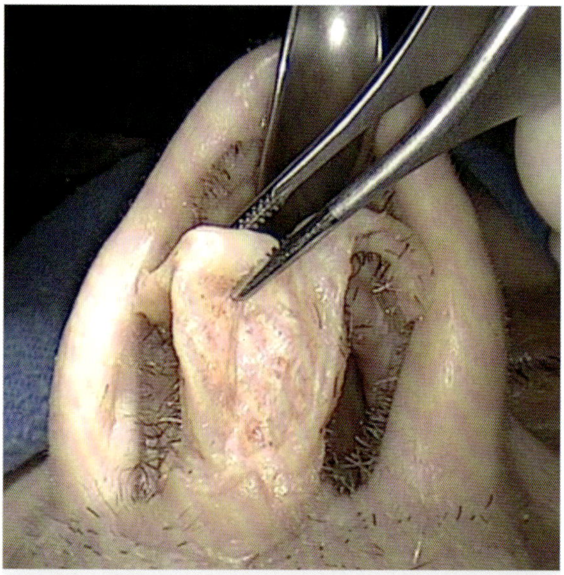

Fig. 12.4 Tentative shaping of the alar domes. Initially, the alar domes are tentatively shaped with forceps before the final corrective surgery is performed.

Dome Suture with Lateral Crural Steal

Lateral crural steal is relatively commonly used to accentuate upward rotation of the tip. The procedure involves shifting the alar dome buckle – which determines the nasal tip-defining point – laterally by a few millimeters onto the lateral crus of the alar cartilage (▶ Fig. 12.9). The medial crus thus lengthens cranially, at the expense of the lateral crus (▶ Fig. 12.10), leading to cranial rotation of the tip.

Table 12.4 Graduated scheme of operative procedures on the alar domes

Strength of the effect	Procedure
	• **No intervention** — the tip is perfectly shaped (very rare in rhinoplasty cases)
	• **Scoring** — accentuates the dome, barely helps narrow the tip
	• The **dome-equalizing suture** (interdomal suture) secures the surgically corrected alar domes in a symmetrical position.
	• A **domal suture** narrows a slightly wide, rounded, or boxy tip
	• **Lateral crural steal** shifts the nasal tip-defining point laterally on to the lateral crus. This leads to an increase in tip rotation
	• **Division of the dome** narrows the tip, accentuates the tip-defining points
	• **Wedge resection** of a triangular segment of cartilage in the dome reduces tip volume while narrowing the tip; always with domal sutures
	• **Strip resection** leads to even more narrowing and volume reduction of the tip; add domal sutures
	• **Tip grafts** augment the tip and can enhance rotation and/or projection, depending on their size and position.
	• **Blocking grafts** support tip grafts and augment their effect.
	• Other useful grafts for the nasal tip are listed in ▶ Table 12.1 and section 12.2.2.

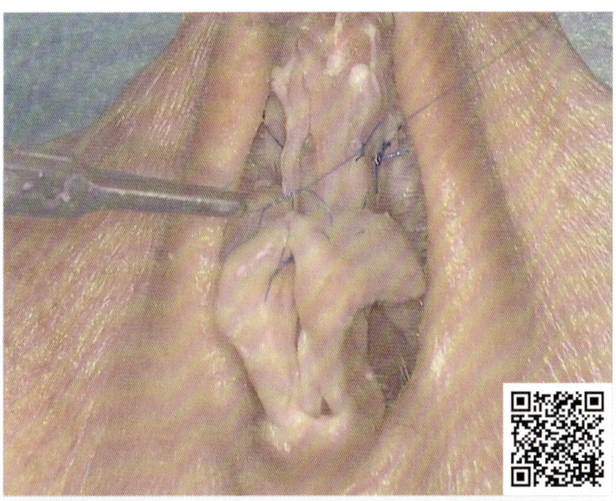

Video 12.1 Dome suture and supratip suture (cadaver head).

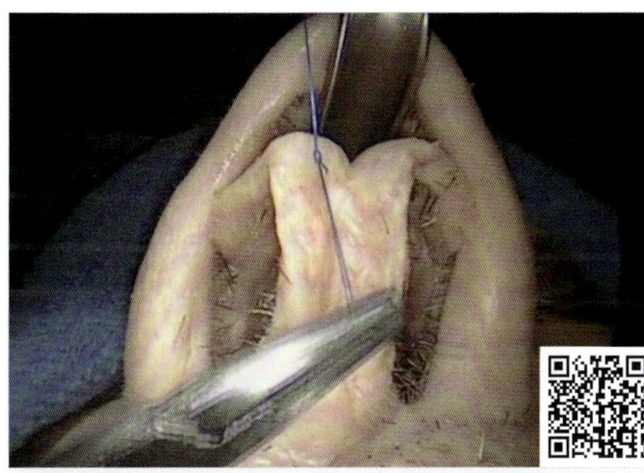

Video 12.2 Domal suture (cadaver head).

The corresponding **medial crural steal** is needed much less often; this derotates and lowers the tip.

Dome Suture with Dome Division

Complete division of the dome in the tip-defining point **narrows** the tip to a greater extent than scoring of its surface (▶ Fig. 12.11a, b, ▶ Fig. 12.12). However, complete division of the cartilage is associated with a risk of losing stability at the nasal tip. The stumps of the severed alar cartilage therefore always have to be restabilized by suturing.

Caution: With thin skin in particular, there is a risk that the contours of the cut edges of the domes following complete division may later become increasingly visible through the skin and in the worst case may give the tip a "pinched" appearance ("pinched nose").

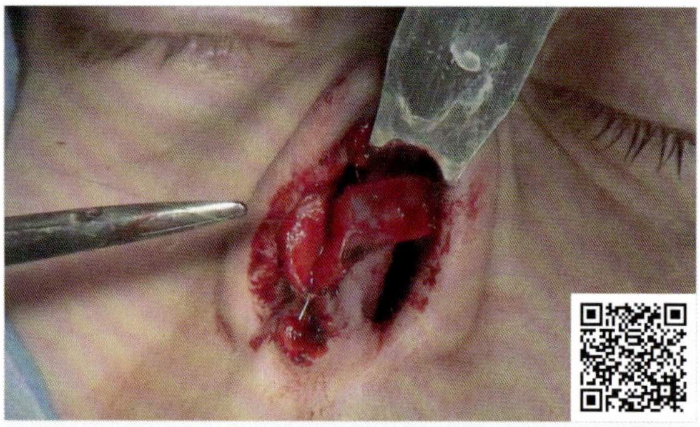

Video 12.3 Domal suture (clinical case).

This risk is mainly associated with end-to-side suturing of the lateral to the (higher) medial crus (▶ Fig. 12.11a, ▶ Fig. 12.12), known as the **Goldman technique**. This technique fell into disrepute due to the frequent development of aesthetically unappealing pinched nasal tips, but its use is occasionally justified, especially in patients with a thick-skinned nasal tip.

To avoid the undesirable consequence of visible edges, covering of the new tip with fascia or thin cartilage when using this technique in patients with thin skin is recommended.

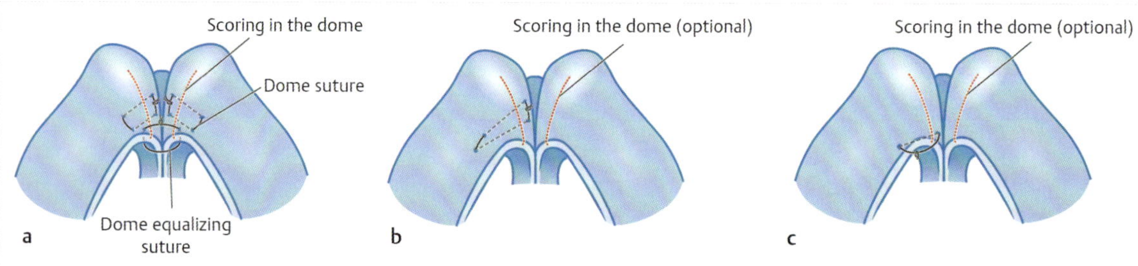

Fig. 12.5 Dome suture with variations and dome equalizing suture. (a) The most important sutures on the nasal tip are the dome suture to accentuate the alar domes, shown here as a square-shaped cephalic tip suture; and the dome-equalizing suture which secures the alar domes at the same height bilaterally. Top-down view. Superficial scoring, which facilitates shaping of the alar domes, may be omitted in patients with delicate cartilage. **(b, c)** Variants on the cephalic tip suture: **(b)** nearly triangular configuration, **(c)** inner cephalic tip suture.

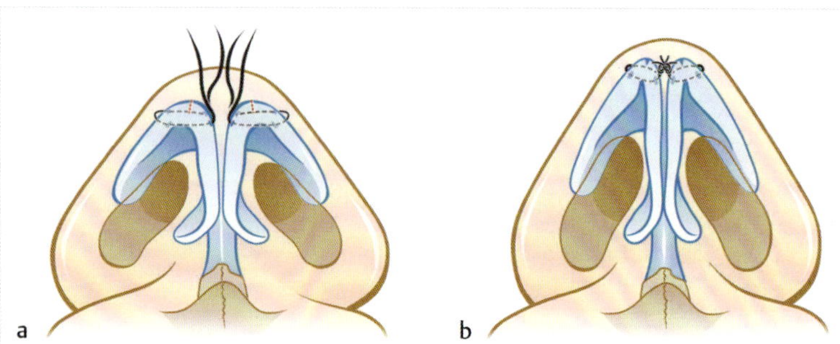

Fig. 12.6 Principle of the domal suture. The transdomal suture accentuates the nasal tip and is applied cranially above the tip-defining point in practice. **(a)** This suture leads to narrowing and a mild increase in nasal projection. **(b)** After knot fixation.

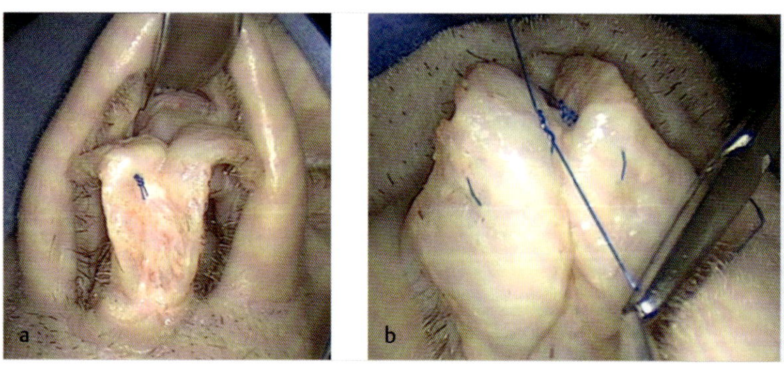

Fig. 12.7 Domal suture, in a cadaver specimen. **(a)** Transdomal suture on the right side. There is a distinctly accentuated tip-defining point in the alar dome. **(b)** Completed transdomal suture (right side), before knot fixation (left); top-down view. A blue, nonabsorbable suture was used in the specimen for demonstration purposes only.

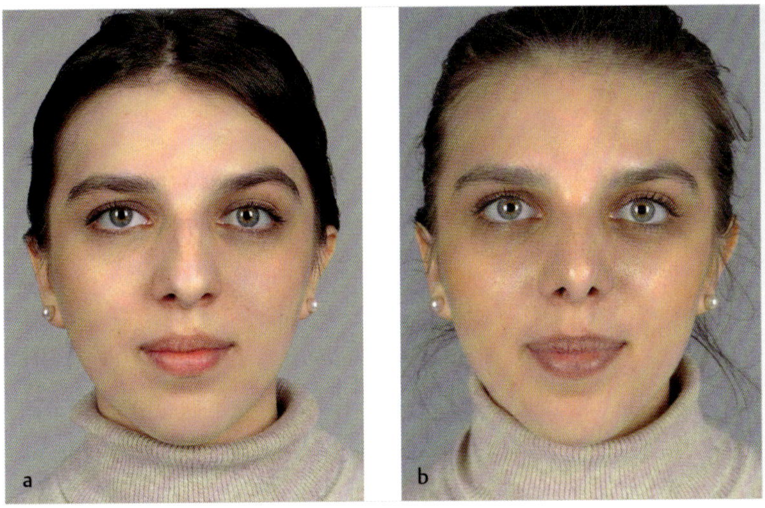

Fig. 12.8 Nasal tip correction with a domal suture, case study. (a) Flat, rounded nasal tip. **(b)** After rhinoplasty with tip correction using domal sutures.

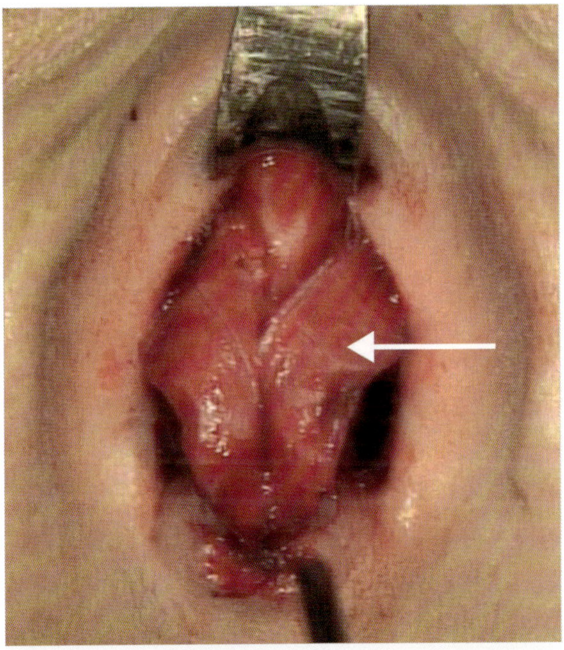

Fig. 12.9 Dome suture with lateral crural steal. Lateral crural steal on the left, with intact right alar cartilage: cranial displacement of the left nasal tip-defining point (arrow).

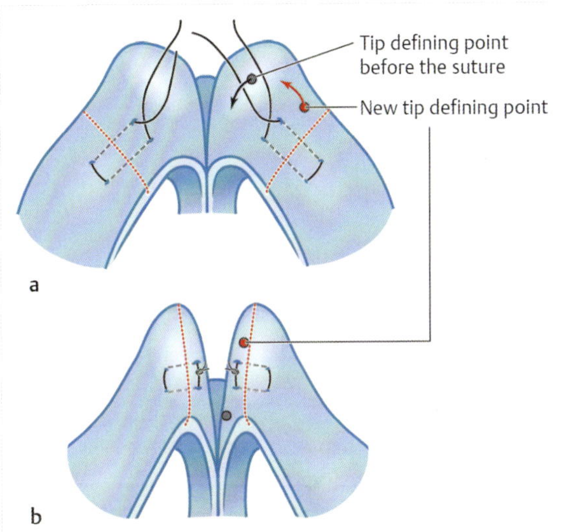

Fig. 12.10 Lateral crural steal (schematic diagram, top-down view). The nasal tip-defining point has been moved to the lateral crus of the alar cartilage. The dome is usually superficially scored in its new position, followed by a transdomal suture. **(a)** Before tightening the knot. **(b)** After tightening.

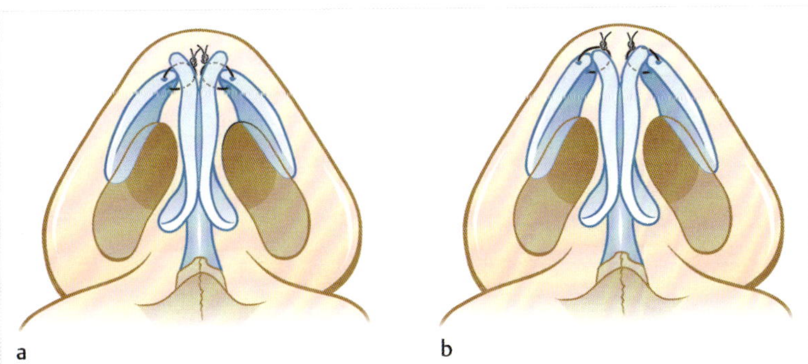

Fig. 12.11 Dome division (schematic diagram). Complete division of the alar domes, with subsequent transdomal suture. The lateral and medial crura can be sutured together end-to-side **(a)** or end-to-end **(b)** along their incised edges, resulting in narrowing of a wide tip.

12

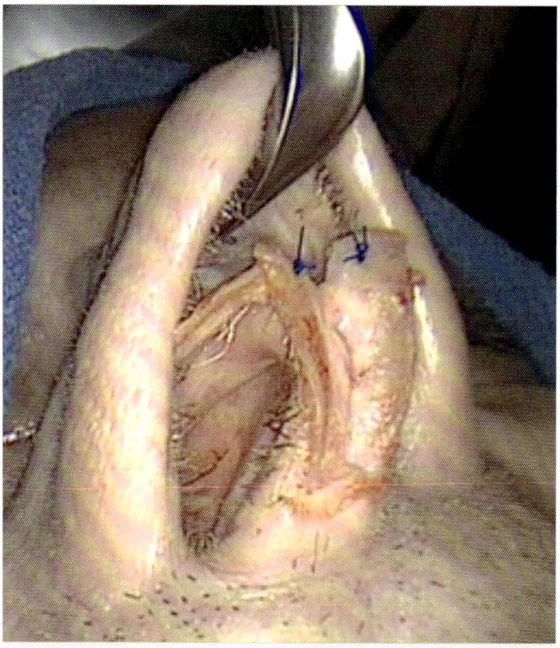

Fig. 12.12 Dome division and domal suture. Bilateral dome division and transdomal suture, demonstrated in a cadaver specimen.

Dome Suture with Dome Resection

Resection is required if volume reduction of the tip is desirable; wedge or strip resection can be performed, depending on the extent of the desired volume reduction (▶ Video 12.4; see Video 6.1; ▶ Fig. 12.13, ▶ Fig. 12.14). Wedge resection primarily affects the cephalic segment of the dome, while strip resection has a more pronounced effect on the width of the entire tip (▶ Fig. 12.15a, b).

> Dome division and wedge or strip resection effectively narrow and accentuate the contour of the nasal domes, but are not performed routinely. These procedures are indicated if the shape of the tip cannot be improved upon by other means — especially suturing techniques alone.

Continuity of the alar cartilage is preserved during wedge resection, and the risk of deformities such as a pinched nasal tip is therefore lower than with complete dome transection (▶ Fig. 12.16a–d). However, wedge resection also has a less pronounced effect on reducing the tip volume.

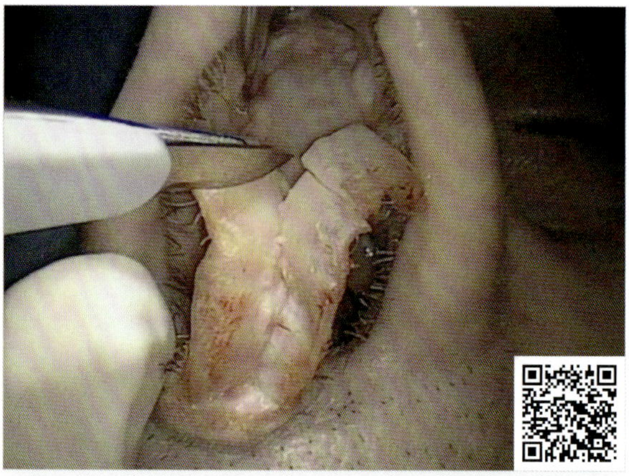

Video 12.4 Wedge and strip resection of the dome (cadaver head).

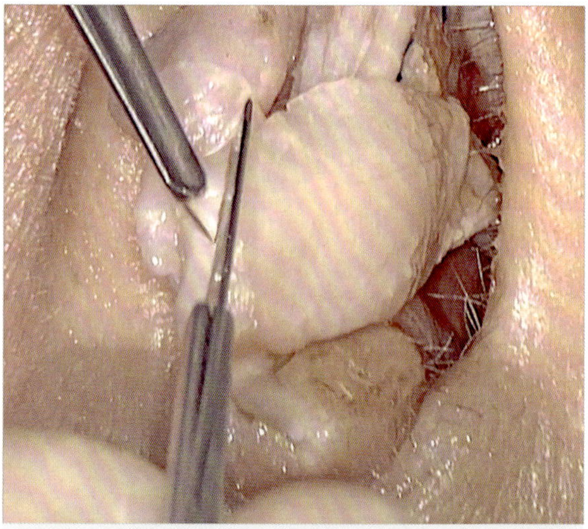

Fig. 12.13 Wedge resection. Triangular wedge resection of the dome in a cadaver specimen (left alar cartilage).

Whenever possible, scoring in combination with a dome suture is used for surgical corrections in the dome, and wedge resection is reserved for situations in which the suture is not sufficient. Complete division and strip resection are only carried out in patients with a marked nasal tip volume (▶ Fig. 12.17a–d, ▶ Fig. 12.18a,b, ▶ Fig. 12.19a,b). Alternatively, an over-projected but otherwise well-shaped nasal tip can be corrected by retrodisplacement using a lateral and/or medial crural overlay, while the domes remain intact (see sections 10.5.1, 11.2.4).

12

On the other hand, division of the dome may be both essential and effective in patients with thick skin to achieve visible narrowing and better tip definition.

Visible contours in patients with thin skin can be avoided by covering the dome with soft tissue – e.g., thin fascia or finely crushed cartilage. A delicate, flattened tip graft or cap graft may also effectively cover the edges of the alar domes and can simultaneously accentuate projection. These are only applied toward the end of the procedure (see section 12.2.2).

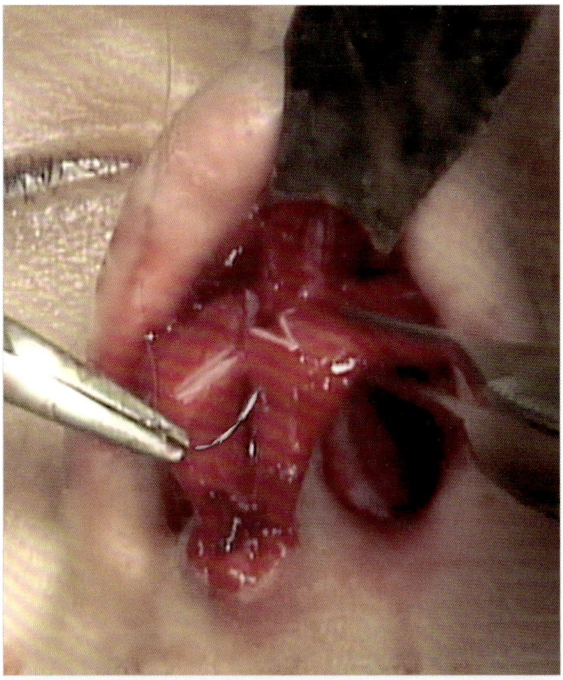

Fig. 12.14 Wedge resection of the dome. Left side, before the suture; right side, after transdomal suture.

Dome-Equalizing Suture

The alar domes are leveled to the same height following correction of the shape of the nasal tip. This is achieved with a suture just above the tip, connecting both supratip points at the same height – the "dome-equalizing suture" (synonyms: supratip suture, interdomal suture) (see ▶ Video 6.1Video 6.1, ▶ Video 12.1; compare with ▶ Video 16.11; ▶ Fig. 12.20; see ▶ Fig. 12.5a).

Double Dome Suture

The domal suture and the dome-equalizing suture (interdomal suture) can be combined as a double dome suture in suitable cases with structural symmetry (▶ Video 12.5, ▶ Video 12.6, ▶ Video 12.7, ▶ Video 12.8; ▶ Fig. 12.21a, b, ▶ Fig. 12.22).

The shaping of the tip is now far advanced, and the upper and middle thirds of the nasal vault and the nasal dorsum have also been surgically corrected. The surgeon should now occasionally move the skin flap back to check whether the overall picture corresponds to the plan.

> ✔
>
> The projection, rotation, and profile of the nasal tip are determined at this stage of the operation, and the relationship between the nasal dorsum and the nasal tip is examined by tentatively setting back the skin flap. Particularly valuable is a sterile metallic nasal mirror, which is either permanently mounted on the operating table opposite the surgeon or is available as a sterile instrument on the table, to be used when required (see ▶ Fig. 4.5a–c).

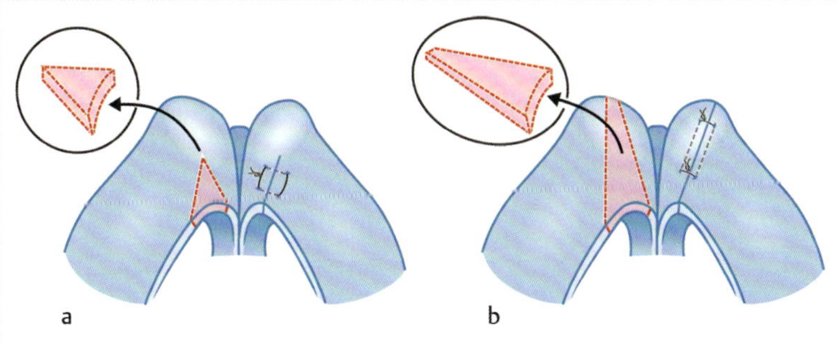

Fig. 12.15 Dome resection (top-down view). (a) Partial cephalic wedge resection of the dome (left side) followed by suturing (right side) adequately narrows and reduces the tip in most cases. **(b)** Narrowing of wide alar domes through complete division with strip resection (left), followed by domal suturing (right side): a very effective procedure for narrowing of the tip, but with a higher risk of visible sequelae ("pinching," asymmetry).

12

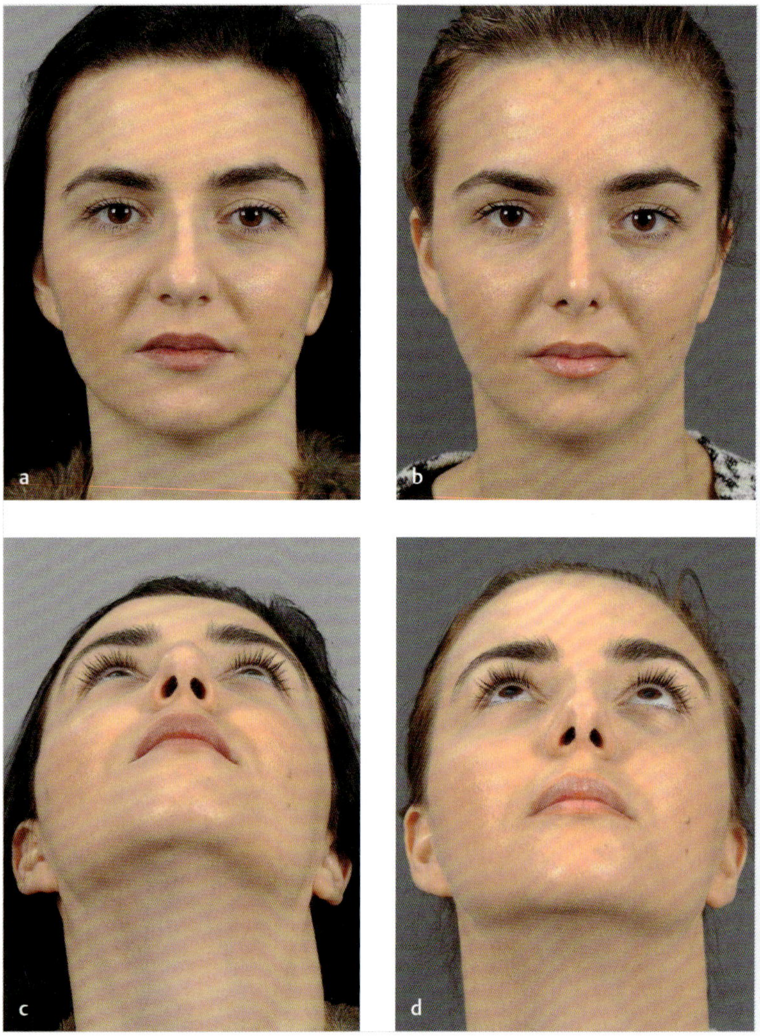

Fig. 12.16 Nasal tip correction using wedge resection; case study. (a, c) A relatively wide nasal tip with a subtle boxy appearance. **(b, d)** After correction with wedge resection of the alar domes.

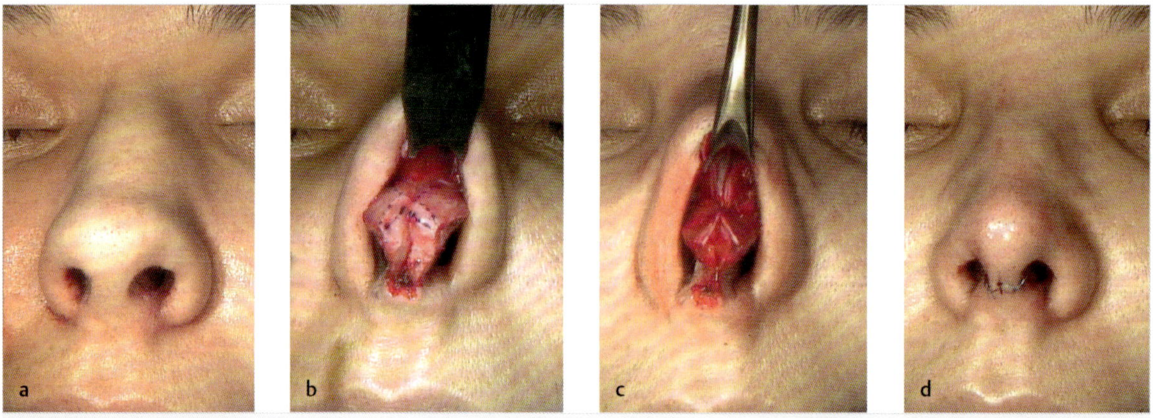

Fig. 12.17 Strip resection of the dome, intraoperative view. (a) Wide nasal tip, intraoperative view. **(b)** Strip resection delineated on the domes. **(c)** After dome resection and domal suturing bilaterally **(d)** Narrow nasal tip at the end of the operation.

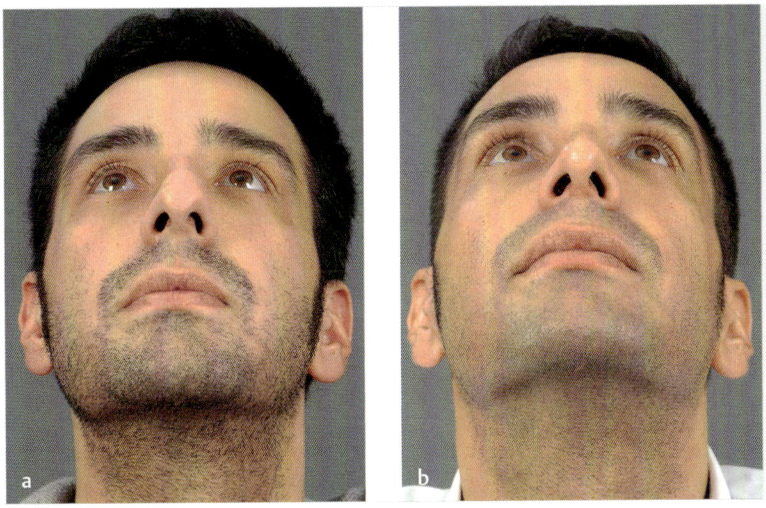

Fig. 12.18 Strip resection of the dome; case study 1. (a) A wide nasal tip, with a boxy appearance, in a male patient. **(b)** After rhinoplasty with strip resection of the domes.

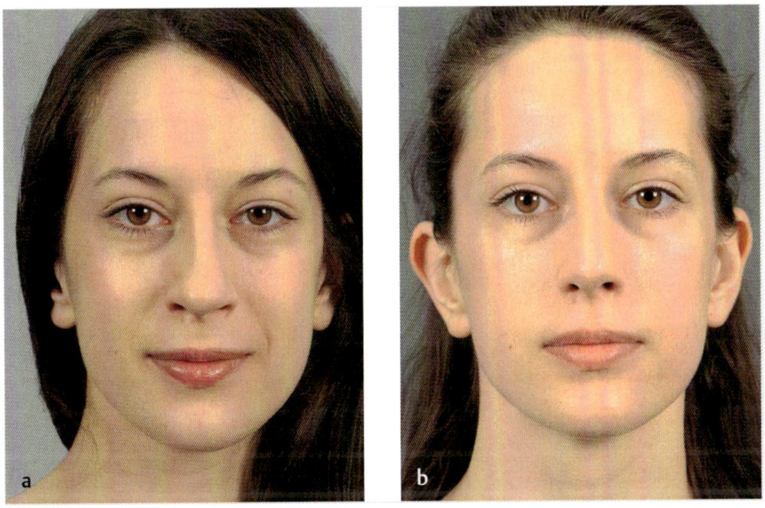

Fig. 12.19 Strip resection of the dome; case study 2. (a) A wide, bulbous nasal tip in a female patient. **(b)** After endonasal rhinoplasty using a delivery technique and strip resection of the domes.

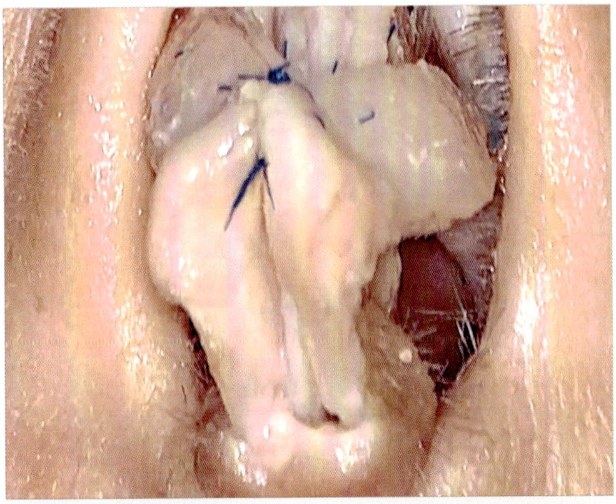

Fig. 12.20 Dome-equalizing suture. The supratip suture (dome-equalizing suture), here in addition to a bilateral domal suture, secures the symmetrical position of the nasal domes.

12.2.2 Grafts for the Nasal Tip

Nasal tip grafts are primarily required in order to enhance projection or rotation once the surgeon has exhausted all suturing techniques. In addition, even delicate tip grafts, rim grafts, and other grafts may significantly optimize the shape of the nasal tip. Tentative repositioning of the skin flap helps the surgeon decide in favor of or against such grafts.

Tip Graft

Tip grafts are invaluable for augmentation and optimal contouring of the nasal tip (▶ Video 12.9, ▶ Video 12.10, ▶ Video 12.11, ▶ Video 12.12; ▶ Fig. 12.23a–c, ▶ Fig. 12.24).

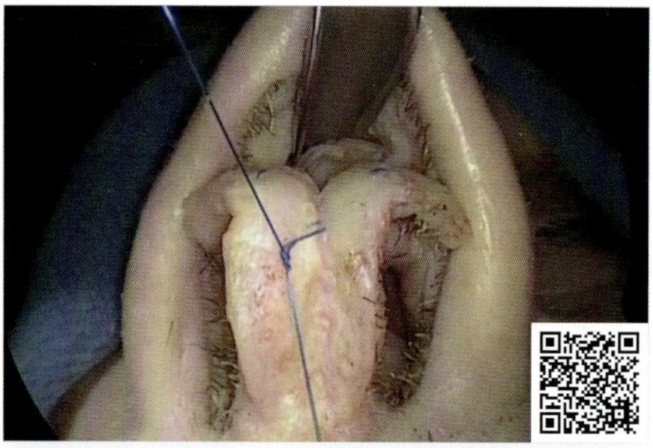

Video 12.5 Double dome suture (cadaver head).

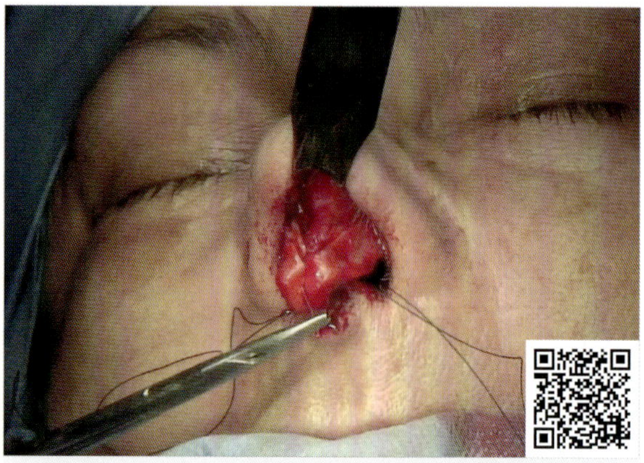

Video 12.6 Double dome suture (clinical case).

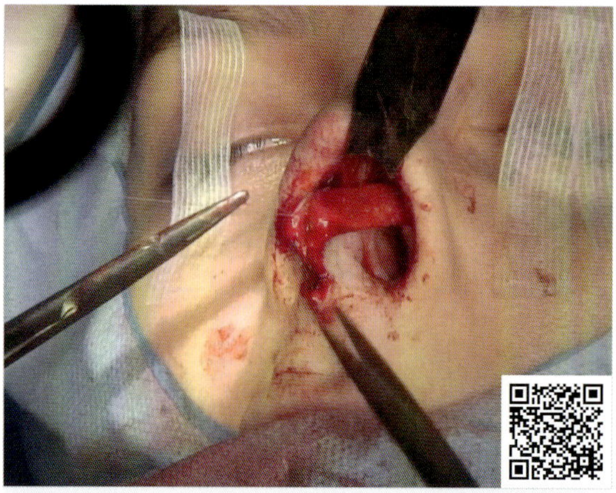

Video 12.7 Domal suture and double dome suture (clinical case).

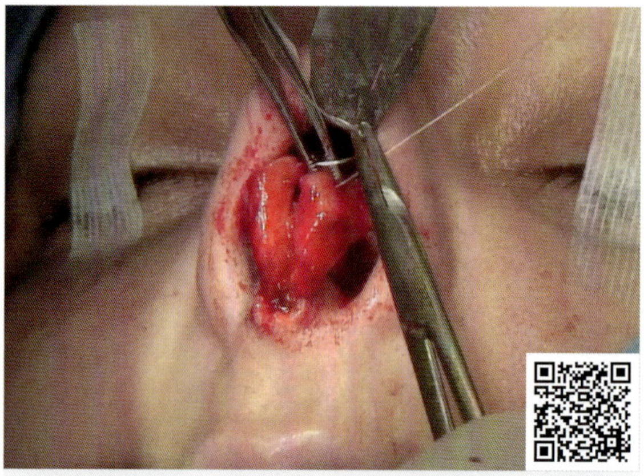

Video 12.8 Scoring of the dome, domal sutures, medial crural sutures, and double dome sutures (clinical case).

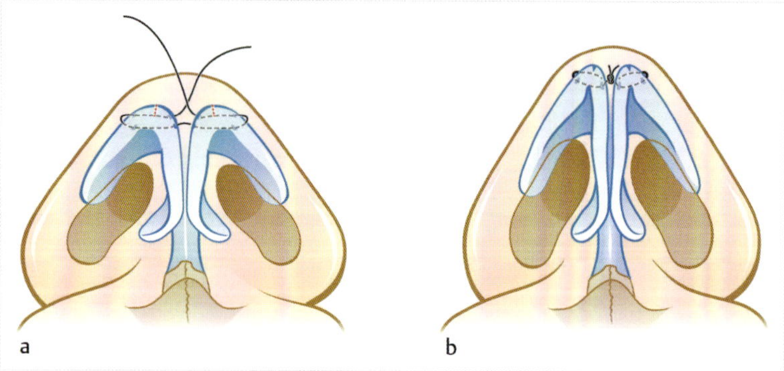

Fig. 12.21 Double dome suture (schematic diagram). **(a)** The combination of domal and dome-equalizing sutures (supratip suture; interdomal suture) in a single suture combines the effects of the two sutures: accentuation of the tip while securing the domes at the same height. **(b)** In practice, the suture is applied above the nasal tip defining point.

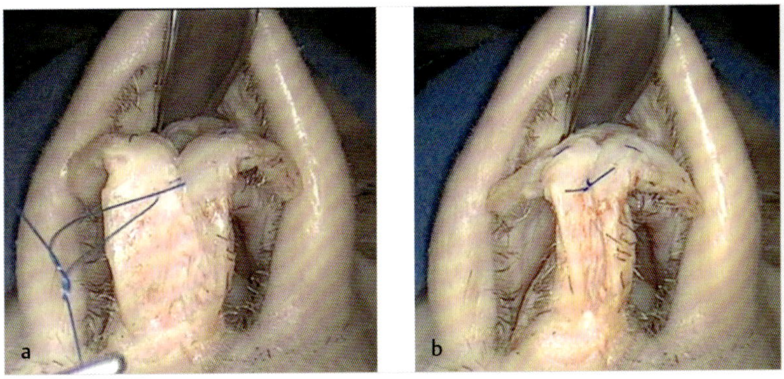

Fig. 12.22 Double dome suture, in a cadaver specimen. **(a)** Double dome suturing technique. **(b)** After knot fixation.

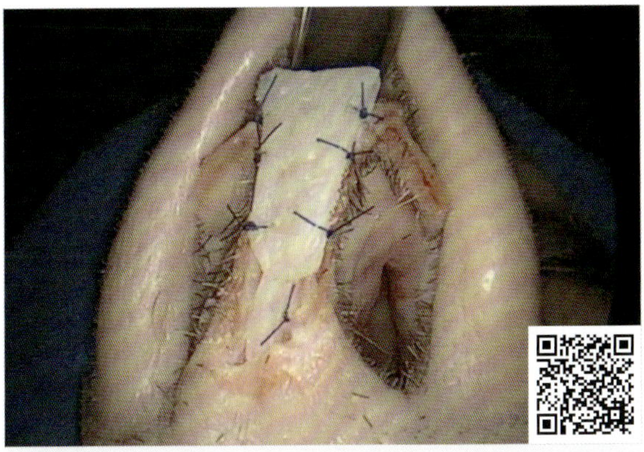

Video 12.9 Tip graft (cadaver head).

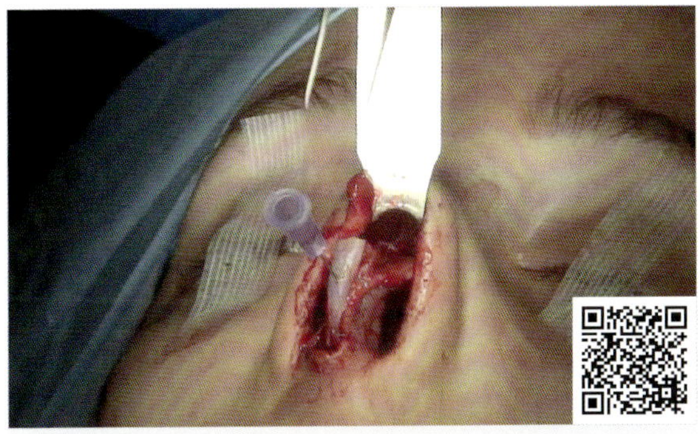

Video 12.10 Tip graft and trimming (clinical case).

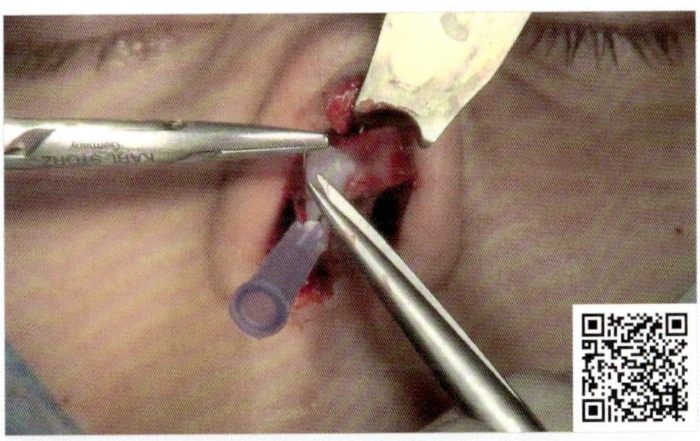

Video 12.11 Tip graft (clinical case).

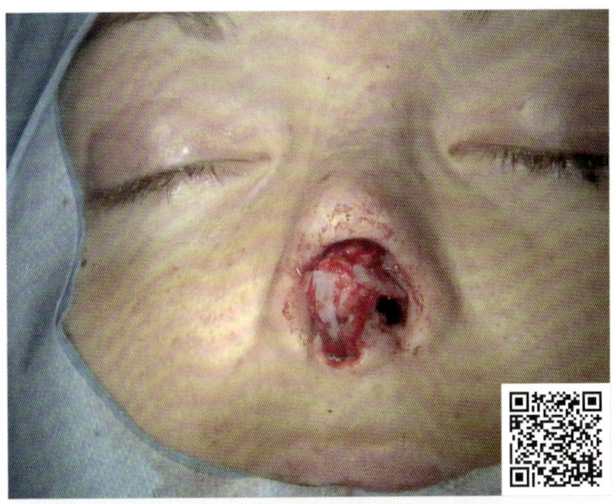

Video 12.12 Asymmetric tip graft (clinical case).

> A tip graft is by far the most reliable option for enhancing both nasal tip projection and rotation, apart from augmentation of the caudal septum.

The ideal material for such nasal tip grafts is septal cartilage, but these grafts can also be harvested from auricular and rib cartilage. However, rib cartilage is rigid and brittle, and is not ideal for reconstruction of the nasal tip.

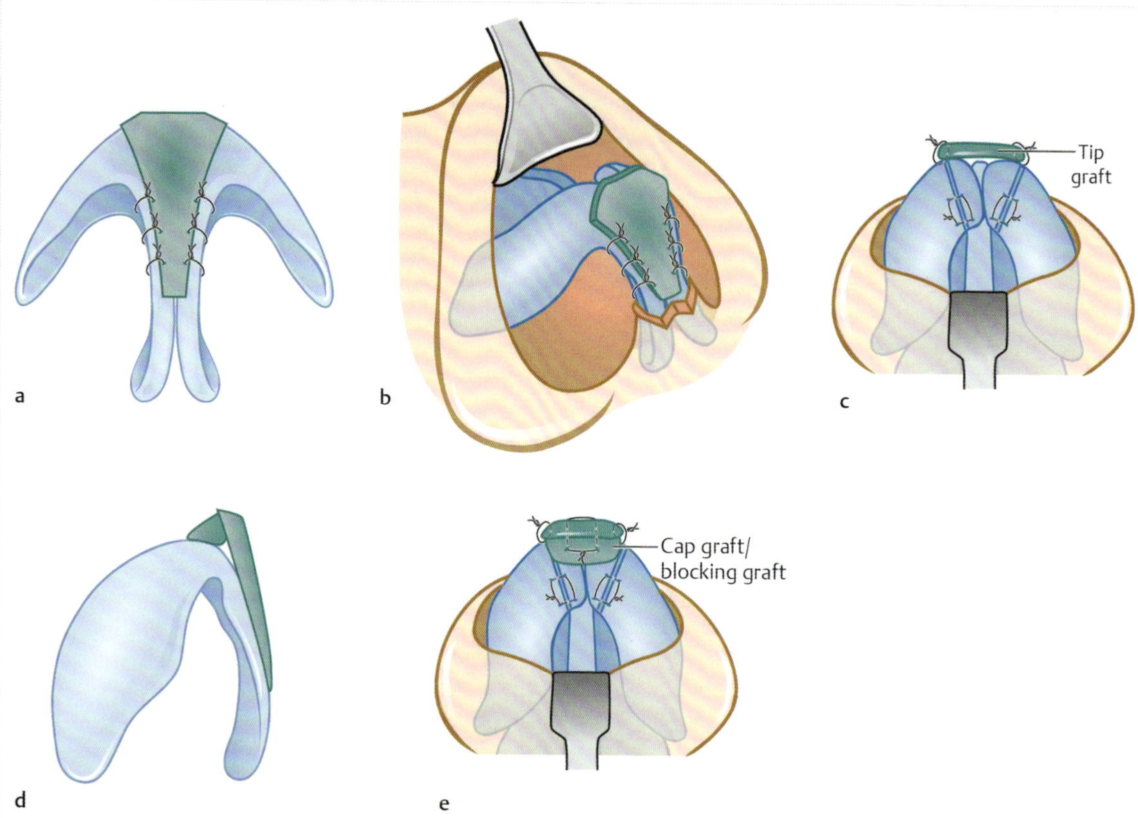

Fig. 12.23 Tip graft and blocking graft. The appropriately trimmed tip graft is affixed to the alar cartilage anterior to the domes with four to six delicate sutures. **(a)** Frontal view, **(b)** oblique view, **(c)** top-down view. A blocking graft can be applied if necessary. It stabilizes and reinforces the tip of the tip graft and prevents it from kinking posteriorly. **(d)** Side view, **(e)** top-down view. A blocking graft alone can also be regarded as a cap graft.

> ✔
>
> Auricular or septal cartilage is best chosen for the nasal tip during extensive reconstruction of the nose using a variety of cartilaginous material, while rib cartilage should be used for the rest of the nasal vault.

12

Tip grafts vary in shape depending on individual needs. They are always placed anterior to the nasal alar domes or the medial crura of the alar cartilages. ▶ Fig. 12.23 and ▶ Fig. 12.24 show a shape that is frequently used.

The shield-like nasal tip graft ("shield graft") for augmentation of the nasal tip should always initially be slightly higher than intended. The skin is tentatively put back over the nasal tip after suture fixation, so that the appearance of the tip can be reviewed after graft placement. An overly high tip graft, consequently leading to marked rotation, can easily be shortened as desired. However, correction is more difficult if the graft is too short. The graft then has to be separated and repositioned, or another tip graft has to be applied.

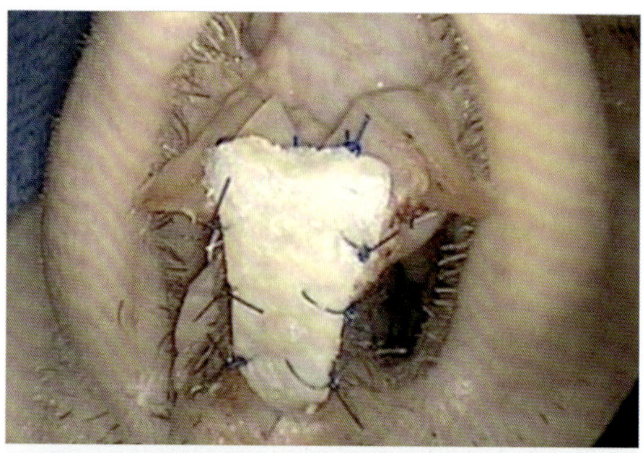

Fig. 12.24 Tip graft. Fixation of a tip graft on the alar cartilages; demonstrated in a cadaver specimen. In a real operation, finer suture material would be used.

Ideally, the tip graft must be handled on a stable surface on the instrument table. The cartilaginous graft may slip

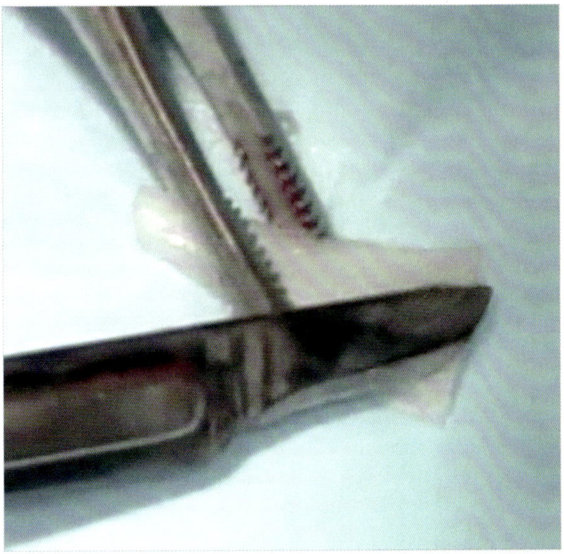

Fig. 12.25 Trimming a tip graft. The Adson–Brown forceps holds the cartilage securely without damaging it (KARL STORZ SE & Co. KG, Tuttlingen, Germany). The metal base plate has been covered with a paper towel.

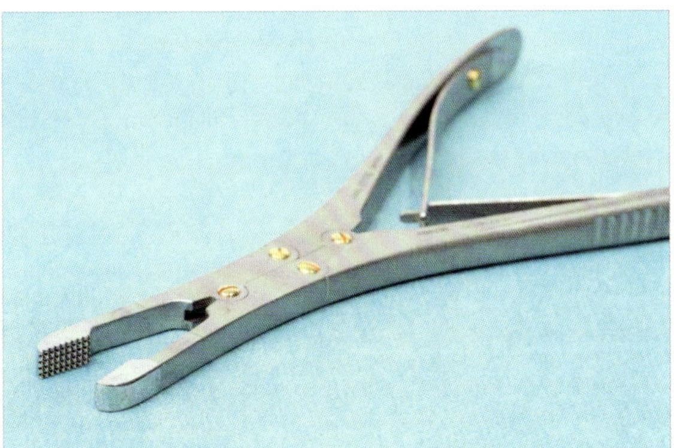

Fig. 12.27 A "crusher" for working on cartilage. The powerful, double-jointed instrument helps with gentle crushing and softening of cartilage transplants and their edges (KARL STORZ SE & Co. KG, Tuttlingen, Germany).

and then no longer be available for use, a risk associated with all such grafts. This situation may be problematic if only a small amount of material is available, and the surgeon needs to take the utmost care to prevent the loss of the piece of cartilage. It is best held securely with Adson–Brown tissue forceps with multiple teeth (see ▶ Fig. 12.3) while working with a sharp no. 15 blade (▶ Fig. 12.25). A slightly rough work surface is suitable, such as a matt metallic plate (▶ Fig. 12.26).

Fig. 12.26 Metal plate as a work surface. A metal plate with a matt surface for working on cartilage transplants (KARL STORZ SE & Co. KG, Tuttlingen, Germany).

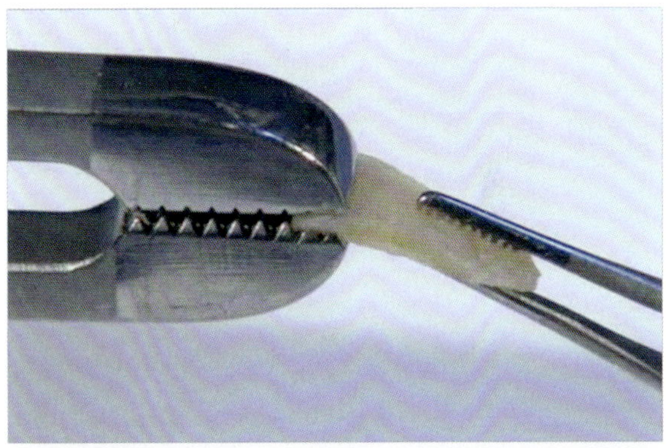

Fig. 12.28 Using the "crusher." The crusher is used to soften tip grafts and enhance their flexibility.

A large tip graft may give rise to undesirable prominence of the new nasal tip-defining points, particularly in patients with thin skin, and may even impair perfusion if the skin flap is under tension during wound closure on the columella. The rigidity of the upper edge of the graft must therefore be checked by palpation; thinning out this edge with a scalpel (see ▶ Fig. 12.25) or softening it very carefully by crushing with a suitable instrument without jeopardizing stability may be useful (▶ Fig. 12.27; ▶ Fig. 12.28).

Securing an appropriately trimmed tip graft with a very fine cannula (e.g., 27 G) in the desired position at the nasal tip has been shown to be very beneficial before it is fixed in situ with at least four, or possibly six delicate sutures (▶ Fig. 12.29). A 6–0 polydioxanone (PDS) suture is preferable for this procedure; permanent sutures should not be used.

> In principle, a robust, thick tip graft enhances projection (▶ Fig. 12.31a-d), while a long, high tip graft accentuates rotation (▶ Fig. 12.30a-c).

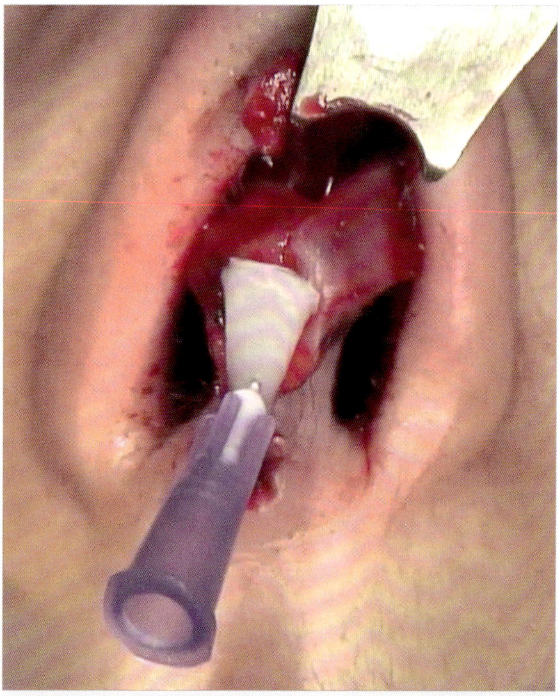

Fig. 12.29 **Needle fixation of a tip graft.** Temporary fixation of a tip graft prior to suturing.

If further augmentation of nasal projection is required after placement of a tip graft, a similar graft can be positioned anterior or posterior to the one previously applied and can be affixed with sutures (▶ Fig. 12.30c; see also ▶ Fig. 12.32, ▶ Fig. 12.33).

A tip graft may also be primarily used to accentuate the nasal tip defining points. A very thin tip graft can be selected in such cases to improve the profile of the nasal tip if concomitant enhancement of rotation or projection is not required.

Blocking Graft

Another transplant can be placed on the nasal dome behind an existing tip graft to prevent posterior bending of the graft tip (▶ Fig. 12.30c, ▶ Fig. 12.32, ▶ Fig. 12.33; see also ▶ Fig. 12.23d, e). This additional graft secures the rotation achieved by the tip graft. It supports the free upper end of the tip graft above the nasal tip and can also accentuate projection ("backing graft").

Cap Graft

In contrast to the typical tip graft, a cap graft is not placed anterior to the alar domes, but over them, akin to a cap. This can be compared to a blocking graft used without a tip graft (see ▶ Fig. 12.23e). Grafts of this type are cut into a roughly crescent shape and help raise the tip and enhance rotation. Occasionally, soft grafts of this type are used to cover sharp edges of nasal tips.

Tip Spreader Graft

The nasal tip may appear too narrow – particularly in patients who are undergoing revision surgery, less often in

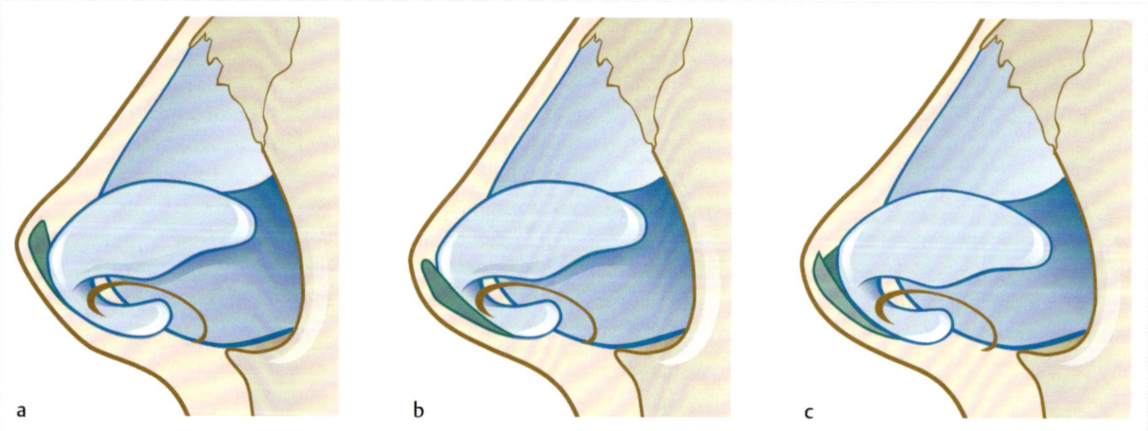

Fig. 12.30 **Tip graft variations. (a, b)** The length, thickness, and position of a tip graft determine the extent to which rotation or projection is enhanced by the graft. **(c)** If a single tip graft is inadequate, another can be added in front of or behind it. More than two grafts can be superimposed in exceptional cases.

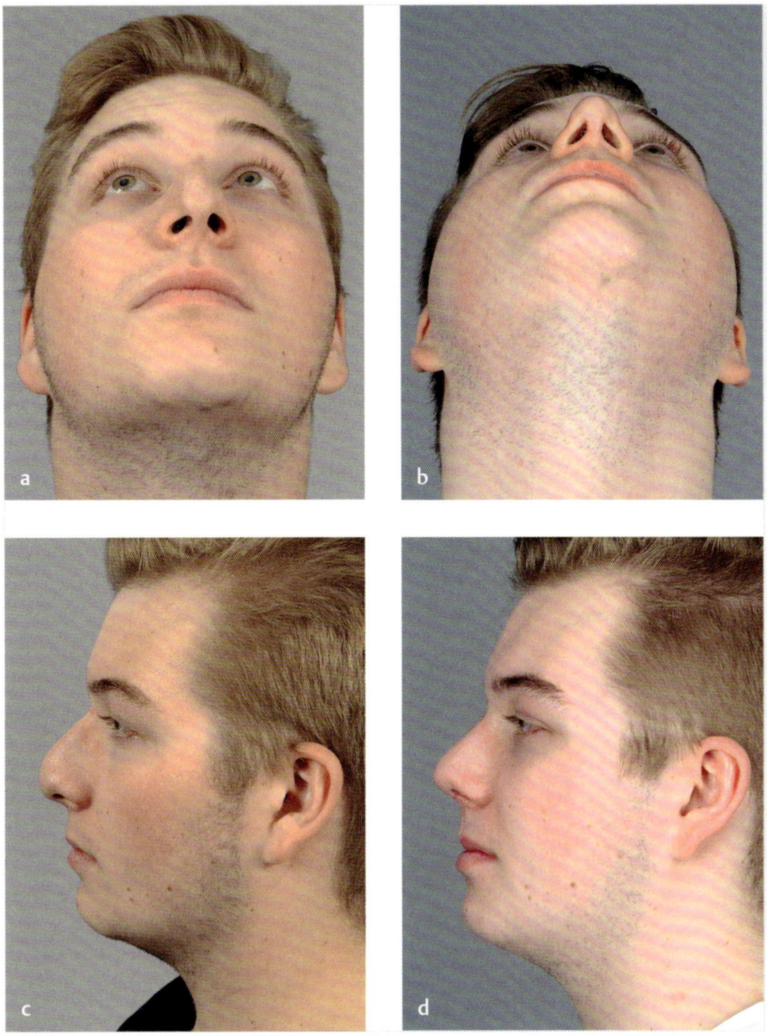

Fig. 12.31 Tip graft, case study. The tip graft enhances projection, rotation, and contouring of the nasal tip. **(a, c)** Nasal deformity, with underprojection of the tip and pollybeak-like convexity above the tip, after a traffic accident and before surgery. **(b, d)** After rhinoplasty.

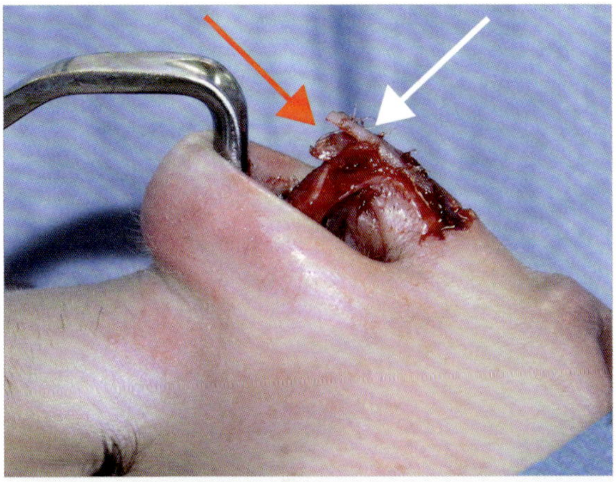

Fig. 12.32 Blocking graft, side view. The tip of the tip graft (white arrow) is stabilized using a blocking graft (red arrow).

those undergoing primary rhinoplasty – as a result of a narrow angle between the upper thirds of the medial crura (angle of divergence; see Chapter 1, ▶ Fig. 1.12 a). The alar domes thus lie too close together, with the nasal tip points being separated only by a short distance.

This appearance can be remedied using a small, triangular cartilaginous transplant, inserted and sutured between the domes or the upper third of the medial crura. In the process, the nasal tip points are pushed apart, depending on the dimensions of the graft, thus correcting the appearance of a pinched nasal tip (pinched nose; ▶ Video 12.13, ▶ Video 12.14; ▶ Fig. 12.34a, b, ▶ Fig. 12.35).

12

Facet Grafts

Facets are the small, roughly triangular, cartilage-free areas forming the anterior margins of the nostrils below

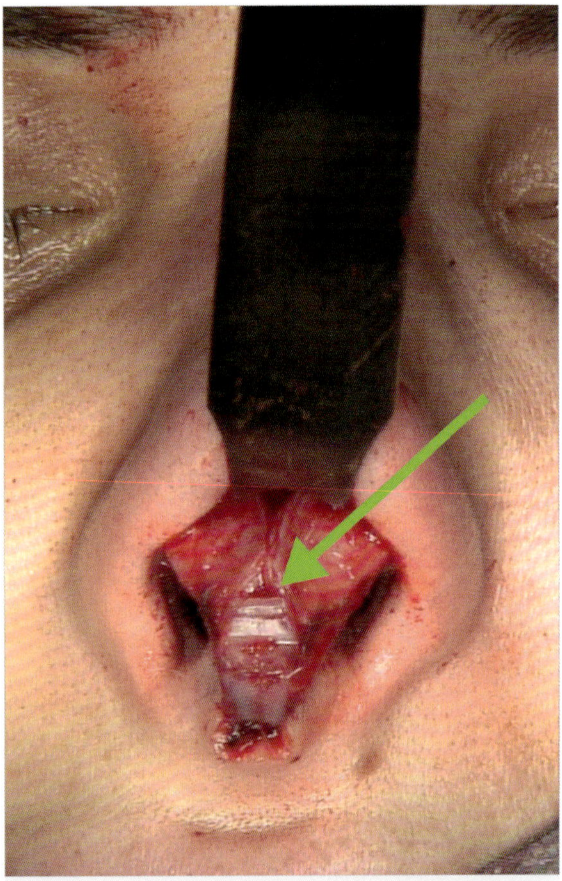

Fig. 12.33 Blocking graft, front view. The blocking graft (green arrow) is used to enhance the projection provided by the tip graft.

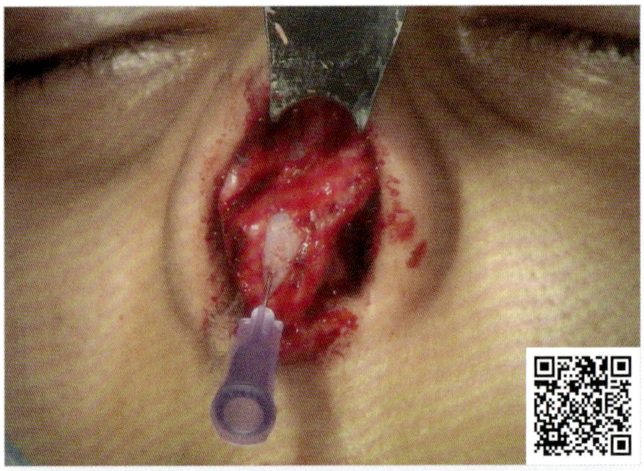

Video 12.13 Tip spreader graft (clinical case 1).

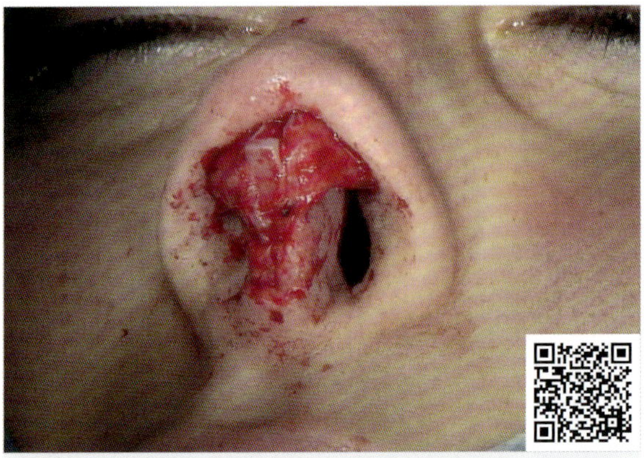

Video 12.14 Tip spreader graft (clinical case 2).

the domes, at the angle between the medial and lateral crura of the alar cartilages. Retracted facets, occasionally seen as an unwanted finding in patients after rhinoplasty, may lead to retraction of the cranial edge of the nostrils ("notching") or to large, vertically elongated nostrils. Triangular cartilage grafts are placed in the angle between the medial and lateral crura of the alar cartilage and affixed with fine 6–0 sutures to lower the upper edges of the nostrils in these cases – i.e., to fill in the facets (▸ Fig. 12.36, ▸ Fig. 12.37). This results in improved contouring of the facets, as well as lowering of the upper edges of the nostrils, and thus in a reduction in their size.

Domal Strut Grafts (Dome Bolsters)

The alar domes can be supported using small cartilage grafts, placed directly under the domes after detachment of the inner skin cover and affixed with dome sutures. These supporting grafts correct or prevent excessive narrowing of the dome due to intradomal sutures, especially in patients after wedge or strip resection (▸ Fig. 12.38, ▸ Fig. 12.39).

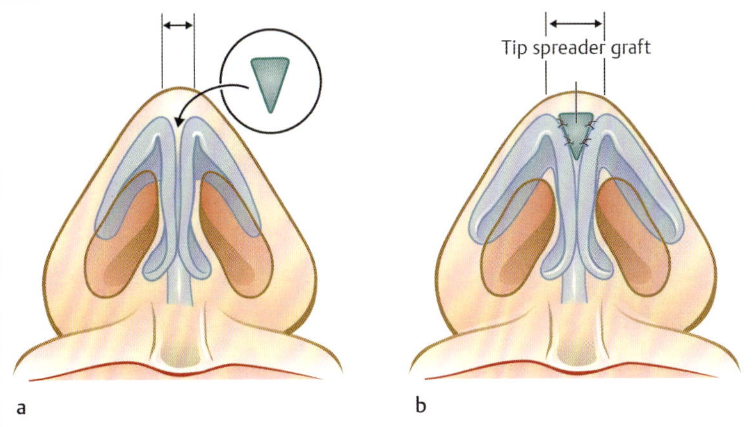

Fig. 12.34 Tip spreader graft. An approximately triangular wedge of cartilage is inserted between the mobilized domes of the alar cartilages **(a)** to increase the angle between the upper thirds of the medial crura **(b)**.

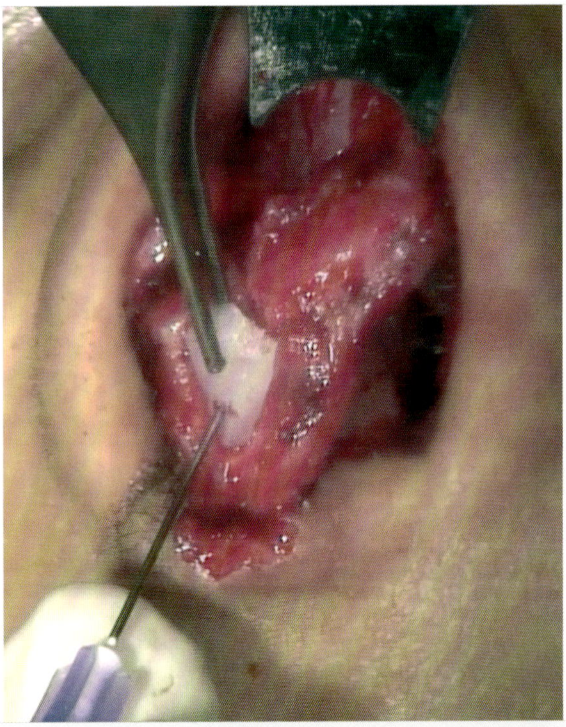

Fig. 12.35 Tip spreader graft, intraoperative view. Insertion of a tip spreader graft between the domes.

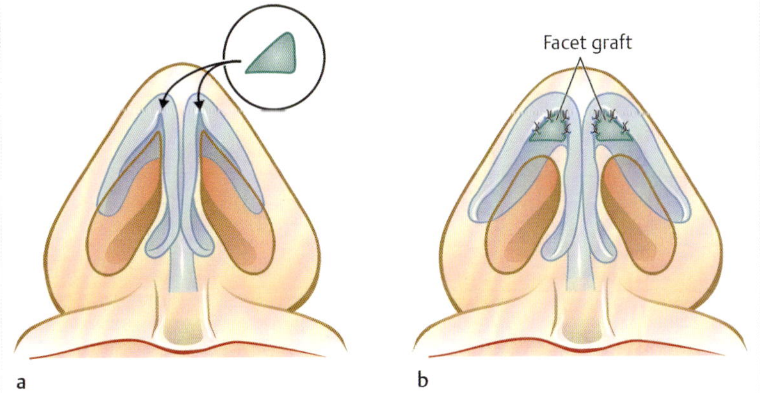

Fig. 12.36 a, b Facet grafts (schematic diagram). Facet grafts **(a)** help lower the upper circumference of the nostril **(b)**.

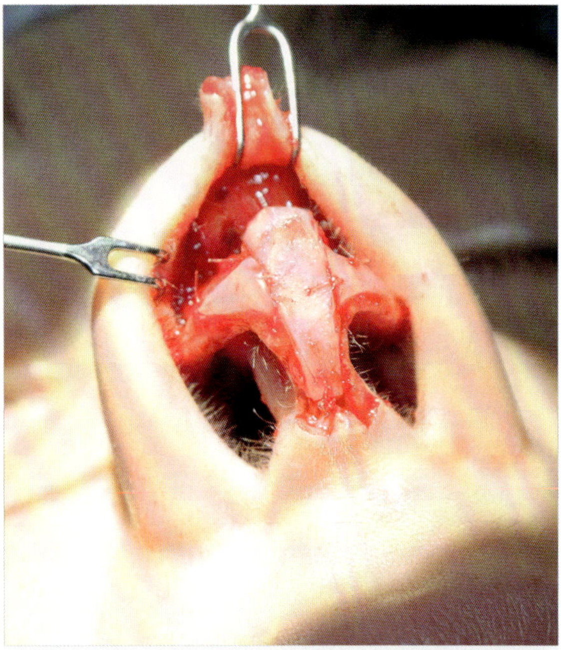

Fig. 12.37 **Facet grafts, intraoperative view.** Bilateral facet grafts, here in combination with a tip graft.

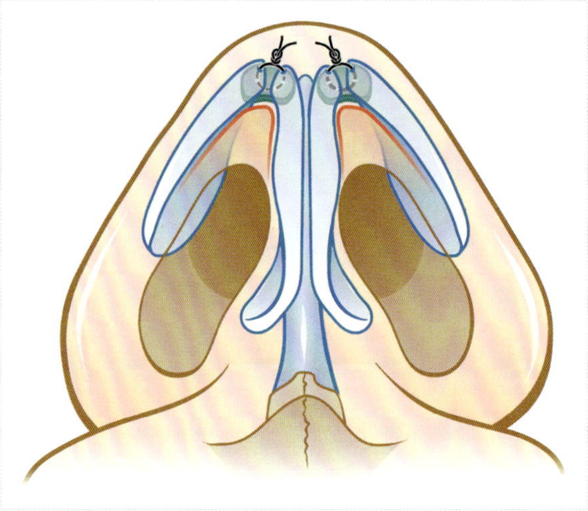

Fig. 12.38 **Domal strut grafts** (schematic diagram). Domal strut grafts support the domes and prevent excessive narrowing by domal sutures, with or without resection.

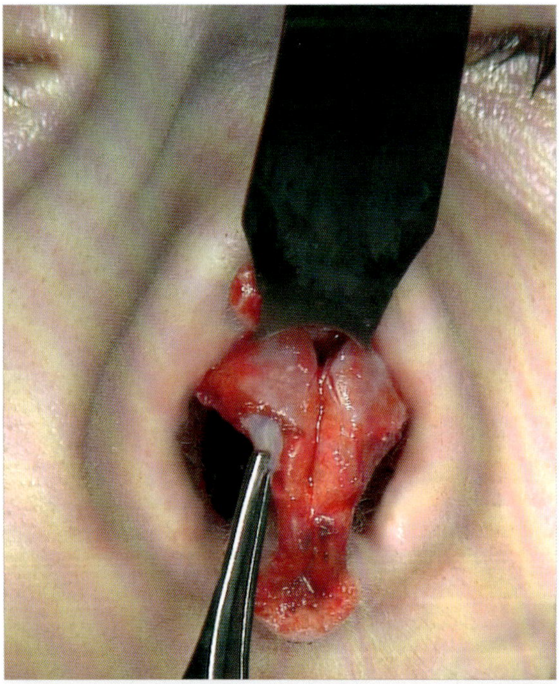

Fig. 12.39 **Domal strut grafts, intraoperative view.** Insertion of a domal strut graft into a graft bed between the vestibular skin and the alar domes.

Bibliography

Apaydin F. Projection and deprojection techniques in rhinoplasty. Clin Plast Surg. 2016; 43(1):151–168

Behmand RA, Ghavami A, Guyuron B. Nasal tip sutures part I: the evolution. Plast Reconstr Surg. 2003; 112(4):1125–1129, discussion 1146–1149

Cingi C, Bayar Muluk N, Winkler A, Thomas JR. Nasal tip grafts. J Craniofac Surg. 2018; 29(7):1914–1921

Constantian MB. The boxy nasal tip, the ball tip, and alar cartilage malposition: variation on a theme – a study in 200 consecutive primary and secondary rhinoplasty patients. Plast Reconstr Surg. 2005; 116(1): 268–281

Daniel RK. Rhinoplasty: open tip suture techniques: a 25-year experience. Facial Plast Surg. 2011; 27(2):213–224

Foda HMT. Nasal soft-tissue triangle deformities. Facial Plast Surg. 2016; 32 (4):339–344

Guyuron B, Behmand RA. Nasal tip sutures part II: the interplays. Plast Reconstr Surg. 2003; 112(4):1130–1145, discussion 1146–1149

Jang YJ, Hong HR. Augmentation shield grafts. JAMA Facial Plast Surg. 2015; 17(4):301–302

Kovacevic M, Wurm J. Cranial tip suture in nasal tip contouring. Facial Plast Surg. 2014; 30(6):681–687

Kridel RW, Soliemanzadeh P. Tip grafts in revision rhinoplasty. Facial Plast Surg Clin North Am. 2006; 14(4):331–341, vi

Rowe-Jones J. Refining the nasal tip – an anatomical approach. Facial Plast Surg. 2014; 30(2):113–122

Tardy ME, Jr. Graduated sculpture refinement of the nasal tip. Facial Plast Surg Clin North Am. 2004; 12(1):51–80

Toriumi DM. New concepts in nasal tip contouring. Arch Facial Plast Surg. 2006; 8(3):156–185

Toriumi DM. Nasal tip contouring: anatomic basis for management. Facial Plast Surg Aesthet Med. 2020; 22(1):10–24

12

13 Handling the Skin

13.1 General Considerations

The skin represents a kind of life insurance for the nose. A severely deformed or disfigured nose can still be reshaped by reconstructing the structures under the skin, as long as its skin covering is intact and stable. However, even complex corrections of the osseocartilaginous vault are of little use if the skin is irreversibly damaged or lost – the nose will continue to appear conspicuous as long as the skin cover is deficient or spoiled.

Classic methods of scar correction include special creams, laser or radiofrequency treatment, Z-plasty and W-plasty, local transposition and rotation flaps, or "bilobed flaps." Severe cases may require skin replacement using a forehead skin flap – meaning that, when there is pronounced nasal skin damage, the surgeon faces the demands of a (partial) nasal reconstruction procedure rather than a classic rhinoplasty. A comprehensive description of the methods used in such cases is beyond the scope of this book. It is therefore important to do justice to the exceptional importance of the skin in nasal surgery and to avoid injury at all costs.

On the other hand, some nasal shape abnormalities are occasionally due to peculiarities of the skin or subcutaneous tissue, and corrective surgery of the integument is unavoidable. This may be the case with "thick skin" – usually meaning highly voluminous subcutaneous tissue – or excessive, thin, and occasionally scarred skin. If the skin shows signs of superficial inflammation before rhinoplasty, prior treatment with a combination of cortisone and antibiotics in the form of a cream can be useful (e.g., fluocinolone acetonide and neomycin sulfate).

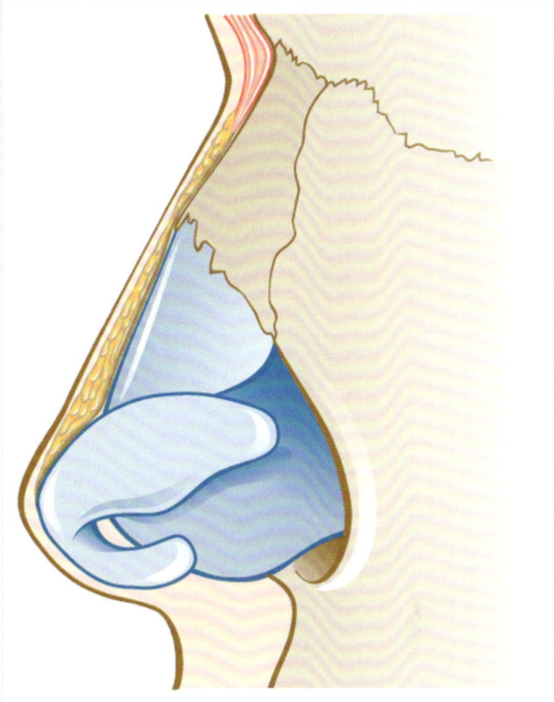

Fig. 13.1 Skin thickness over the nose. The subcutaneous tissue is thickest above the tip of the nose (supratip region), due to the presence of a fibroadipose tissue layer. Muscles add to the volume of subcutaneous tissue in the nasofrontal angle.

> ✓
>
> When rotated upward, a well-shaped cartilaginous nasal tip extends under the thicker skin of the former supratip region, which may obscure the delicate contours of the alar cartilages forming the tip. This can be prevented by thinning out the subcutaneous fibroadipose tissue, which determines skin thickness.

13.2 Thick Skin

The skin – or rather subcutaneous tissue – is thicker in the supratip region than at the nasal tip and over the bony nasal framework (▶ Fig. 13.1), The skin cover may be problematic:

- In patients with thick skin that completely obscures the shape of the cartilaginous vault or any surgical corrections in it.
- Following cranial rotation of a ptotic tip into the region with thicker skin.
- In patients with persistent postoperative soft-tissue swelling in the supratip area, with a risk of a "pollybeak deformity."

It should be noted that the fibroadipose subcutaneous tissue over the nose is typically responsible for "thickened skin," and usually not the dermis or epidermis itself (▶ Fig. 13.2). Although thinning of the dermis itself would be extremely risky, it can be done with careful handling of the subcutaneous fibroadipose tissue.

The degree of subcutaneous thickening can be assessed by reverting the skin flap over the left middle finger using the open technique. The fibroadipose tissue layer can then be gradually thinned out using a pair of fine, pointed

13

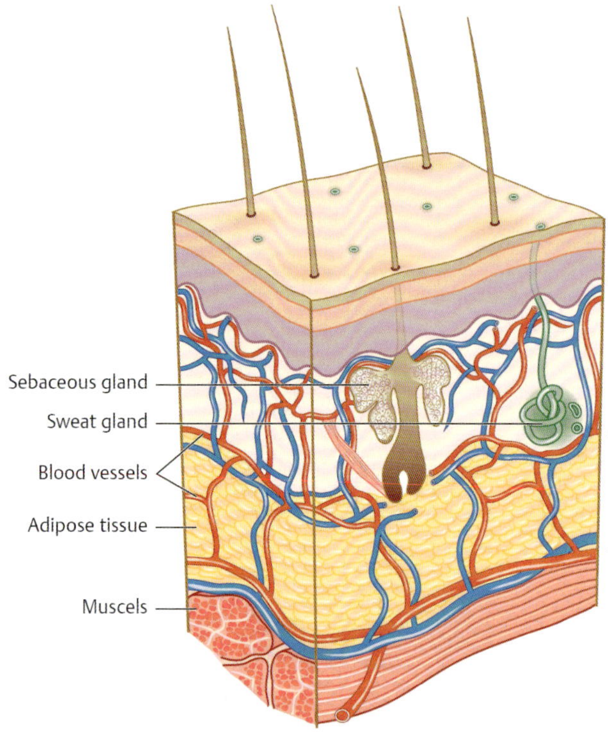

Fig. 13.2 Skin layers. The presence of subcutaneous adipose tissue should be noted.

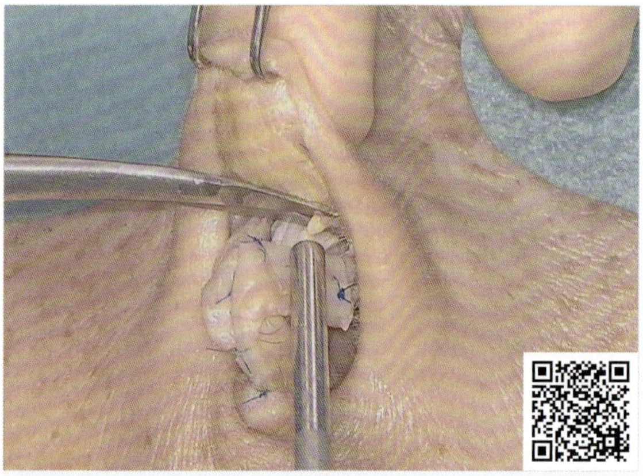

Video 13.1 Thinning of subcutaneous tissue (cadaver head).

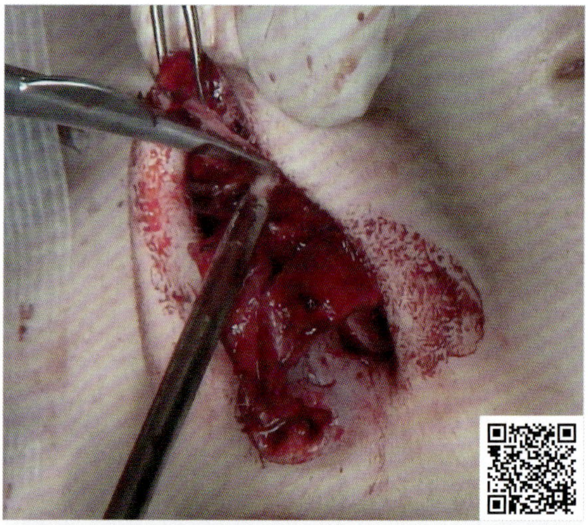

Video 13.2 Thinning of subcutaneous tissue (clinical case).

scissors (▶ Video 13.1, ▶ Video 13.2; see Video 6.1; ▶ Fig. 13.3). The procedure is constantly checked visually and by palpation to ensure that ablation does not extend into the dermis; extension into the subcutaneous vascular network may give rise to marked bleeding. Hemostasis is preferably achieved by applying moist compresses – failing which, fine bipolar forceps can be used at the lowest power setting possible to avoid thermal injury to the dermis (▶ Fig. 13.4).

✓

Entering the vascular network is avoided as far as possible during thinning of subcutaneous tissue, to avoid endangering the blood supply to the skin and to prevent cutaneous lesions and scars.

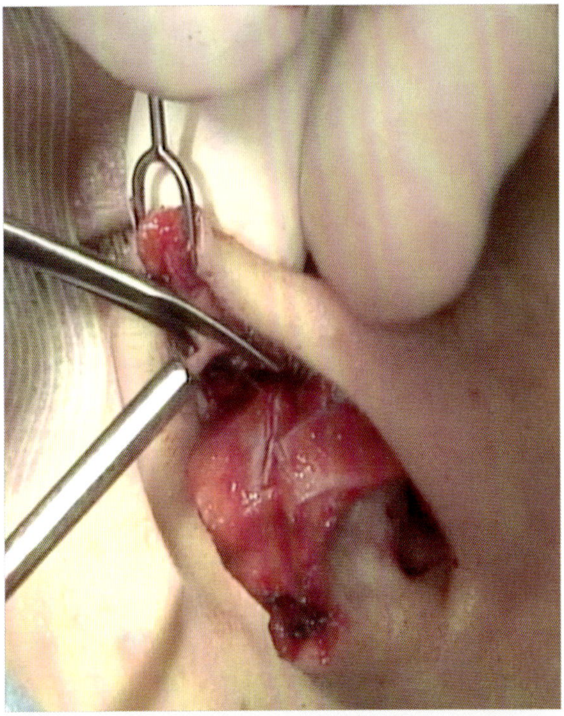

Fig. 13.3 Thinning of subcutaneous tissue. Thinning of the fibroadipose subcutaneous layer. Fine scissors are placed flat, and resected tissue is promptly suctioned off. The middle finger supports the skin.

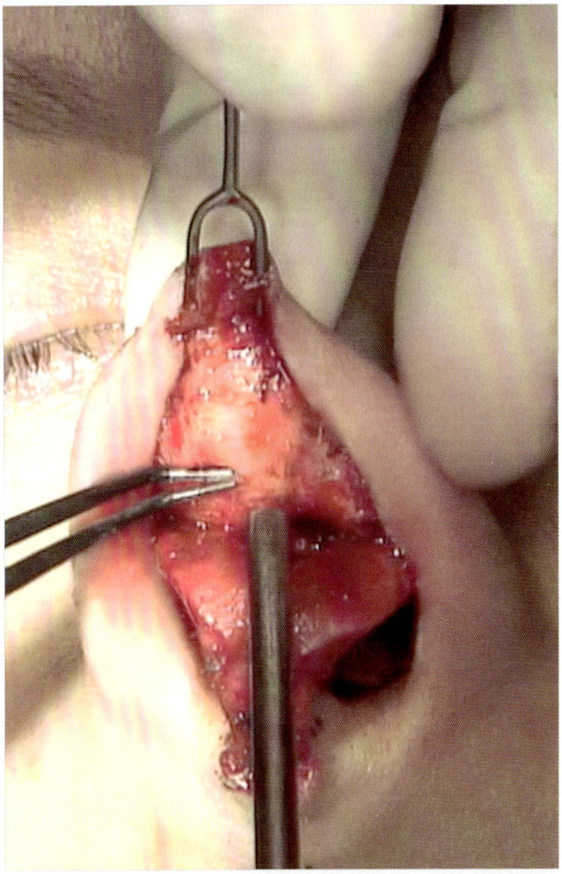

Fig. 13.4 Hemostasis of subcutaneous tissue: Fine, angled forceps; low energy.

A cautious approach allows uniform thinning of this subcutaneous layer without the risk of subsequent skin lesions. This in turn allows better adaptation of the skin to the new cartilaginous framework of the nasal tip, and thus a better overall outcome. A pollybeak deformity due to persistent skin thickening is effectively anticipated.

Thinning of subcutaneous tissue traumatizes soft tissues and may prompt initial swelling in some cases. The contour of the nasal tip thus may only be visible in the medium-term postoperative period after rhinoplasty (▶ Fig. 13.5a, b).

This procedure is usually easily performed during primary rhinoplasty, but indurated subcutaneous tissue due to postoperative scarring in revision cases cannot be thinned in the same manner. Fine superficial incisions into the scarred fibroadipose tissue may be helpful in such circumstances, before these scars are carefully removed in layers along the incisions, with the scissors laid flat.

If overly thickened subcutaneous tissue, with or without scarring, is not thinned out (perhaps if the surgeon prefers to forego this step), an alternative that may be considered is moderate lowering of the cartilaginous dorsum above the tip, to avoid unintentional elevation of the supratip region.

✓

To counteract swelling above the tip, it is worthwhile for an absorbable subcutaneous suture to connect the hypodermis to the supratip area at the level of the W-point, to close possible dead space when the skin flap is moved back at the end of the operation.

Particularly when there is no thinning of subcutaneous tissue, marked postoperative swelling in the supratip region or the entire tip may occur, which regresses over the course of weeks to months.

Persistent, residual thickening may give rise to an elevated supratip with a pollybeak abnormality; this can be treated with local steroid injections. Triamcinolone as a crystalline suspension (e.g., Kenalog, Kenacort, Volon A) is suitable for this purpose; rarely, it may lead to atrophy of the skin, as well as development of telangiectasias (facial erythrosis), inflammation, and pigmentary disorders skin, but I have never seen these side effects. The treatment can be repeated at 4–6-week intervals.

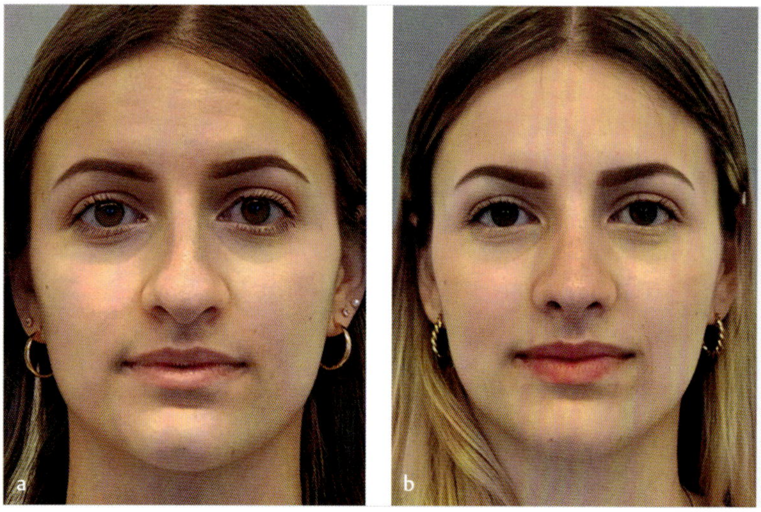

Fig. 13.5 Rhinoplasty with thinning of subcutaneous tissue; case study. (a) Voluminous tip and broad nasal base with thick skin. **(b)** Post rhinoplasty, with thinning of the fibroadipose subcutaneous tissue as well as wedge and sill resections (see also Chapter 14).

It is advantageous to be able to offer a treatment to patients who are concerned about swelling over the tip of the nose postoperatively. The affected patients feel significantly better when action is taken. Whether the subsequent decrease in swelling is due to the cortisone applied, or whether it would have occurred spontaneously, cannot be proven in individual cases. In any case, the goal is achieved and the patients have been helped.

If the skin is thick and oily (sebaceous), then repeated pretreatment with isotretinoin has been recommended (e.g. two to three times a week for a few weeks). While some studies appear to confirm the effectiveness of such pretreatment, others have concluded that after a longer period of time there is no difference between pretreated and non-pretreated noses in the postoperative results. The author has no findings of his own on this issue.

13.3 Thin Skin

While reshaped cartilage at the nasal tip may not be clearly discernable through thick skin, the opposite is true if the skin is too thin: every detail stands out, and every edge or asymmetry is prominent and troublesome.

Critical areas can be padded with fat, fascia, or connective tissue to reinforce thin skin after correction of the osseocartilaginous vault. It has been observed that placement of one or two layers of TachoSil (see section 17.2.3) stabilizes atrophic skin or subcutaneous tissue to some extent in appropriate cases and can be used when other tissues are not available.

Care should be taken to avoid sharp bony or cartilaginous edges in patients with noticeably thin skin, as these may later become visible. It has been repeatedly pointed out that the Goldman technique should not be used on the nasal tip in such cases (see section 12.2.1). This method of achieving an accentuated nasal tip by division of the domes is associated with a higher risk of a pinched nasal tip ("pinched nose"), even in patients with normal skin. The risk is significantly greater in those with thin or atrophic skin.

13.4 Excessive Skin

Surgeons are rarely required to deal with excessive skin during rhinoplasty. A skin coat that appears to be too large after a conventional reduction rhinoplasty usually reattaches itself to the new structure, due to the elasticity of the skin. To explain this better during discussions with patients, the process can be compared to the abdominal skin in pregnant women, which also returns to its original size after pregnancy. True primary excess skin is occasionally seen in older noses with drooping nasal tips and transverse folds of the skin, especially in the upper third. A narrow skin resection along a skin fold in the area of the radix may help stretch the skin tight ("nose lift") in these rare cases.

In patients with a drooping tip, especially with a hanging columella, after tip rotation and correction of the columella projection, there may be vertical folds of excess vestibular skin within the nostrils on both sides of the columella. These plications can be narrowly excised, followed by primary wound closure, to avoid visible excess skin after healing. In addition, excessive skin may be relevant if the framework of a very large nose has been reduced too much; it may then envelop the significantly reduced nasal scaffold like an incompletely filled bag. Such noses are soft and unstable on palpation, and may even tilt from one side to the other when the patient changes sides on lying down, in addition to being cosmetically very unappealing. The tip appears to sag, lacks definition, and is usually rounded in appearance. Such patients are offered revision surgery with reconstructive

13

augmentation using costal cartilage, if necessary – thus providing the sagging skin with a new scaffolding. This problem can be prevented by avoiding excessive ablation of the cartilaginous structure in patients with large noses and reducing it only slightly to optimize the nasal profile.

✔

In selected cases I therefore occasionally undertake reduction in two separate steps and in consultation with patients with very large noses who expressly insist on a significant reduction in nasal size.

The intervals between the interventions in these rare cases are about a year. Avoiding the drastic reduction in a single step allows the skin to adapt to the moderate reduction and gradual correction of the cartilaginous framework. This approach requires particularly close patient management. Patients have to understand why corrective surgery is undertaken in more than one session and over a prolonged period, to ensure their cooperation and prevent them turning away in disappointment after the initial procedure.

13.5 Scars and Other Lesions

Patients with posttraumatic or postoperative nasal skin scars may wish to have scar correction alongside rhinoplasty. Usually, wound healing proceeds normally in such cases even if combined with the typical open-approach rhinoplasty, provided that the scars are small and are correctable by simple excision of thin, ovoid strips along relaxed skin tension lines (RSTLs) or skin folds. The resulting defect is closed using primary tension-free adaptation of mobilized wound edges.

To prevent wound irritation by postoperative splints, it is useful to cut a recess in the foam pad that is glued as a cushion under the aluminum splint over the nasal dorsum (see Chapter 15) in the area of the skin excision and suture. The dressing over the nose is removed as usual after 5–6 days, with removal of scar revision sutures simultaneously or a few days later.

However, I prefer to carry out scar revision and rhinoplasty as separate procedures if a more complex skin flap is required for correction of a larger scar – such as a bilobed flap, Z-plasty, or melolabial skin flap – since healing after these procedures may be problematic when the two interventions are combined. Unless there are arguments to the contrary in the individual case, rhinoplasty is performed first and scar correction follows after an interval of at least 9 months.

These recommendations for scar revision apply equally to small and large benign nasal skin lesions that require treatment in addition to rhinoplasty.

Bibliography

Chu E, Davis RE. SMAS debulking for management of the thick-skinned nose. JAMA Facial Plast Surg. 2015; 17(4):305–306

Cobo R, Vitery L. Isotretinoin use in thick-skinned rhinoplasty patients. Facial Plast Surg. 2016; 32(6):656–661

Cobo R, Camacho JG, Orrego J. Integrated management of the thick-skinned rhinoplasty patient. Facial Plast Surg. 2018; 34(1):3–8

Davis RE, Hrisomalos EN. Surgical management of the thick-skinned nose. Facial Plast Surg. 2018; 34(1):22–28

Saadoun R, Riedel F, D'Souza A, Veit JA. Surgical and nonsurgical management of the nasal skin-soft tissue envelope. Facial Plast Surg. 2021; 37(6):790–800

Sazgar AA, Majlesi A, Shooshtari S, Sadeghi M, Sazgar AK, Amali A. Oral isotretinoin in the treatment of postoperative edema in thick-skinned rhinoplasty: a randomized placebo-controlled clinical trial. Aesthetic Plast Surg. 2019; 43(1):189–195

14 Correction of the Nasal Base

The nasal base is occasionally neglected during assessment of the nose, and accordingly also in rhinoplasty. However, the proportions of the nasal base – i.e., the nostrils, width, and lateral projection of the alar base – are of considerable importance for the overall appearance of the nose and face (▶ Fig. 14.1).

> Abnormalities of the nasal base cannot be corrected by interventions on the cartilaginous vault and may require resection of skin at the alar base or the nostrils.

The longitudinal axis of the nostril in a "western" White nose forms a relatively acute angle to the vertical (i.e., a vertical line through the columella), while this longitudinal axis is more horizontal and the angle to the vertical midline is wider in East Asian, South Asian, and Black noses (▶ Fig. 14.2).

Widely flared nasal alae with more or less horizontal nostrils, even in noses of White people, frequently produce an aggressive, grim facial expression, which can be significantly improved by appropriate surgical correction. The patient first has to be carefully examined to assess whether the width of the nostril or that of the nasal alae, or both, require correction before a decision is made on nasal base resection (▶ Fig. 14.3).

It should be noted that surgical measures at the tip of the nose have an influence on relationships at the base of the nose. Rotating the tip can stretch the front of the nose and appear to narrow the nasal base. Reducing the tip, on the other hand, can make the base of the nose appear wider. For this reason, after a rhinoplasty, the base of the nose has to be reevaluated before a final decision is made on measures to be taken at the base of the nose.

> In general, corrections of the nasal base are only carried out after completion of rhinoplasty and wound closure.

14.1 Alar Wedge Resection

Wedge resection of the alar attachment reduces the volume of wide and protruding nasal alae. However, it first needs to be assessed whether the lower thirds of the alae appear too wide (too thick), whether the lateral convexity significantly projects beyond the vertical through the medial canthus (▶ Fig. 14.4), or whether a combination of both abnormalities is present.

Excessive lateral projection may be due to overly broad, fleshy nasal alae; however, long, thin alae may also extend too far laterally, similarly resulting in a wide nasal base.

> The surgeon must assess the width of the nostrils, alar width, and the entire width of the nasal base.

A wide alar attachment is narrowed by wedge resection of the lateral surface of the alar base. The exact site and extent of the resection depend on individual findings (▶ Fig. 14.5a–d).

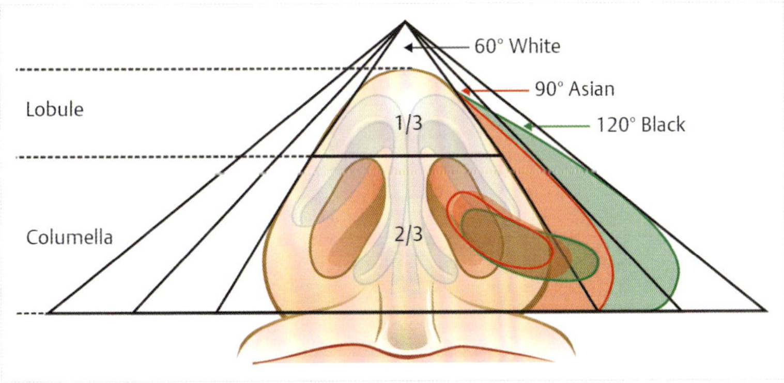

Fig. 14.1 Proportions of the nasal base. The anatomy and proportions of the nasal base, with ethnic variations in the angles formed by the nasal alae.

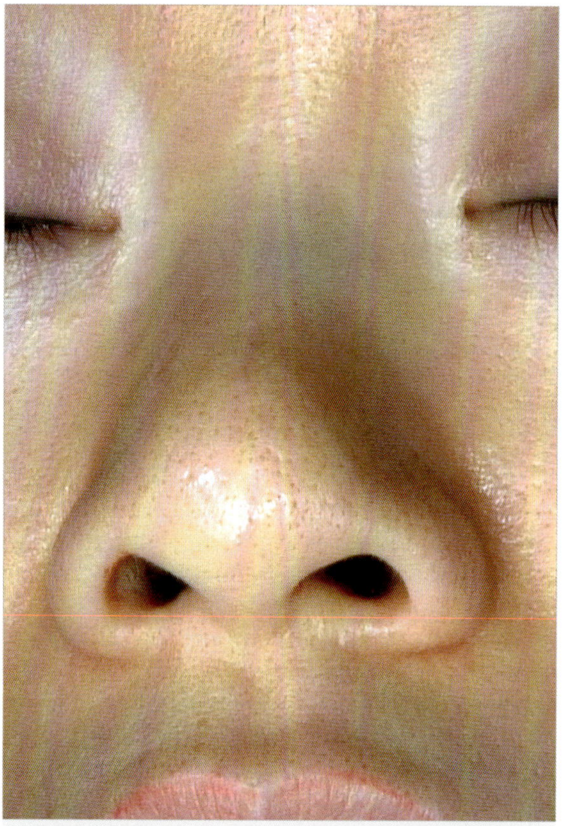

Fig. 14.2 Nasal base in an Asian patient. The nasal base is flattened, and the axis of the nostril is horizontally aligned.

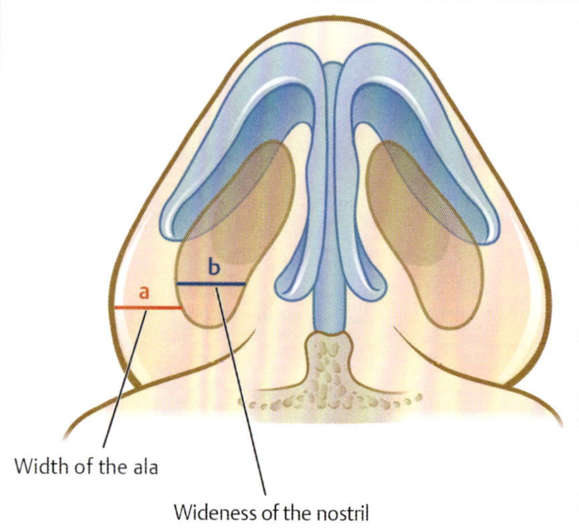

Fig. 14.3 Proportions of the nasal base. The alar width **(a)** and the horizontal width of the nostril **(b)** are particularly important for assessing the nasal base.

Overcorrection due to excessive resection must be avoided at all costs; this carries a risk of the nose appearing "surgically corrected," or it may even appear amputated and disfigured. The natural arch formed by the alar attachment must not be entirely eliminated. If this happens, the resultant vertically oriented contact of the ala to the skin of the cheek results in a most unnatural appearance and is difficult to correct.

14

Resection does usually not exceed a width of 2–4 mm. The required dimensions are first measured on either side with a millimeter scale, and the planned incision (and thus the extent of the resection) is then drawn in with a fine pen (see ▸ Fig. 14.12). This also makes it easier to imagine whether the planned cut-out has the right dimensions. Symmetry must be ensured; a mildly asymmetrical resection can be carried out if structural asymmetry is present to start with.

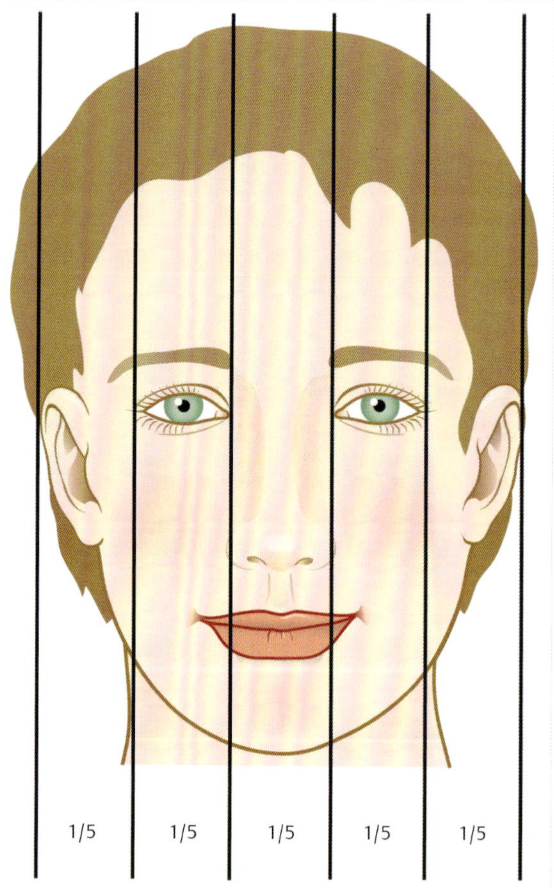

Fig. 14.4 Width of the nasal base. The lateral edge of the nasal alae usually extends only slightly beyond a vertical line through the medial canthus.

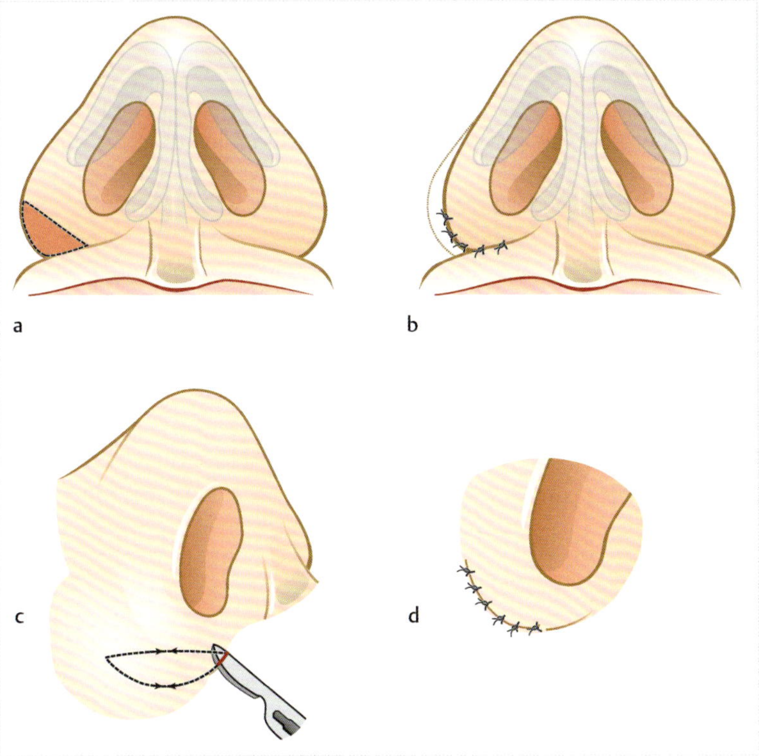

Fig. 14.5 Wedge resection of wide alae. **(a)** Caudal view before resection. **(b)** After resection and suturing. **(c, d)** As viewed from the side. The lower incision lies exactly in the alar crease **(c)**, as does the resultant suture **(d)**.

> It is very important to ensure that the lateral boundary of the resected wedge (and thus the resultant scar) lies exactly within the alar crease and is neither offset toward the nose nor toward the cheek.

Caudally, the incision usually does not exceed half the width of the nostril (▶ Fig. 14.5a). The medial incision is arcuate, with a slightly upward convexity (▶ Fig. 14.5c). Cranially, the incision and the resected wedge should not extend beyond the clearly visible alar crease, to ensure that the resultant scar is as inconspicuous as possible. Tissue is excised using two smooth incisions with a no. 15 blade. The resected wedge usually contains only skin and alar subcutaneous tissue, with usually no or little attached muscle. Heavy bleeding may occur after excision — best controlled with fine bipolar forceps angled at the tip, without injuring the cut edges of the skin (▶ Fig. 14.6).

In my experience, scars are less noticeable and have less retraction if I mobilize the wound edges a few millimeters in the subcutaneous plane with the blade before closing them.

The wound is closed in two layers: a deep-seated suture (5–0 polyglactin 210; e.g., Vicryl Rapide) brings together the cut surfaces approximately in the middle of

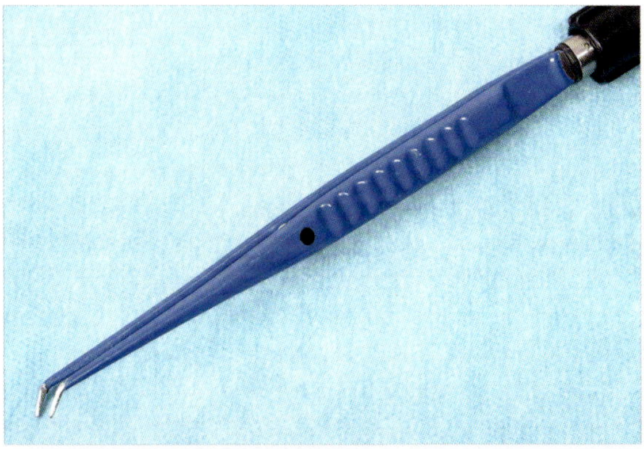

Fig. 14.6 Fine bipolar forceps. Although it provides effective hemostasis, care needs to be taken to avoid injury of the skin edges with the fine, angled bipolar forceps (Erbe Elektromedizin GmbH, Tübingen, Germany).

the wound. Ideally, the skin edges are adapted to align precisely after knot fixation of this suture. To prevent continued wicking, the thread ends have to be shortened in such a way that they do not protrude through the wounds. The skin is subsequently closed with delicate, well-adapted, nonconstricting single button sutures (6–0 polypropylene, e.g., Prolene).

It is often recommended in the literature for these sutures to be removed in the early postoperative period — i.e., after 4–5 days — to prevent the dreaded "ladder" suture marks within the scar. However, early suture removal may cause gaping of the wound due to mobility of the alar base consequent to movements of the mouth and cheek, with resultant traction at the wound edges. I only remove these delicate sutures, which do not carry a risk of suture marks, after the sixth postoperative day. Botulinum toxin (e.g., Botox) may be injected into the affected region lateral to the nasal alae in order to temporarily reduce the unfavorable effects of muscle traction on the wound. But normally it is not necessary to use it, and possible side effects also need to be borne in mind, particularly motor disorders of the upper lip.

After the stitches have been pulled, the suture line can be coated with cyanoacrylate skin adhesive (e.g., Dermabond, Liquiband) to prevent the wound from gaping after suture removal. This colorless, invisible coating also provides protection against contact with dirt, soap, or nasal secretions. Patients do not find the application problematic; the face can be washed as usual, and the transparent coating falls off spontaneously a few days later.

With the procedure described here, I have only seen small visible disturbances on scars in rare individual cases, and neither the doctor nor the patient need be overly apprehensive about this type of wedge resection. Nevertheless, every patient has to be informed about the risk of visible postoperative scars if an incision is planned on the outer skin of the nose.

If a slight dehiscence of the wound is visible after the sutures have been removed, then careful cleaning, disinfection, and keeping the wound dry are recommended. The wound will then slowly and secondarily also completely close. A secondary suture is only required extremely rarely.

Scar correction using dermabrasion or secondary resection should be considered in patients with hypertrophic scarring that is unresponsive to medical treatment with scar ointments and cortisone.

If the ala is unusually thick and fleshy, it can be thinned by partially removing some of the soft tissue in the nasal wing, starting from the incision for the wedge resection – i.e., fat, muscle, or the tough fibrous connective tissue that supports the lateral nostril instead of cartilage.

14.2 Resection at the Nostril Sill (Sill Resection)

Sill resection, or resection of the posterior (i.e., inferior) margin of the nares, may be considered in patients with wide, flaring nostrils (see ▶ Fig. 14.3). It is of course not possible to correct a nostril that is too large in the vertical longitudinal axis using this procedure. The preoperative analysis needs to be very precise here in order to avoid any misjudgment, which can very quickly lead to unsightly results. As is the case with lateral alar resection (see section 14.1), the planned sill resection is first drawn in with a fine pen. The midline is first identified to ensure symmetry, followed by marking of the area lateral to the midline, which should never be resected; this segment usually extends beyond the medial footplates of the alar cartilages. The resection itself rarely exceeds 2–3 mm in width. Laterally, it does not affect the arch of the alar base attachment, which must be preserved at all costs to ensure a natural appearance. A narrow wedge is then excised along the longitudinal axis, which does not extend beyond the nasal entrance threshold anteriorly – i.e., does not extend to the lip (▶ Fig. 14.7). The posterior extension into the nasal cavity depends on the depth to which the nostril appears too wide, with the longitudinal axis of the incision curving dorsally in a slightly lateral arc.

Careful hemostasis is ensured after resection, and the wound is closed with single button sutures using 6–0 polypropylene (e.g., Prolene). Case studies are shown in ▶ Fig. 14.8a–e and ▶ Fig. 14.9a, b.

> ✓
>
> Excessive excision must be avoided at all costs. Overcorrection during sill resection is not only associated with a cosmetically unsightly outcome, but also with the risk of a functional disorder with nostril stenosis, which is not easily amenable to correction.

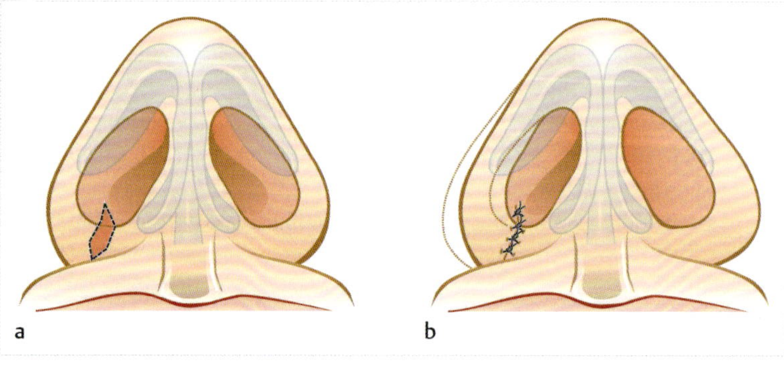

Fig. 14.7 Sill resection (schematic diagram). **(a)** Excessive resection of skin must be avoided, especially of the width; it should rarely exceed 2–3 mm. The length of resected tissue is variable, but never extends to the lip. **(b)** After suturing.

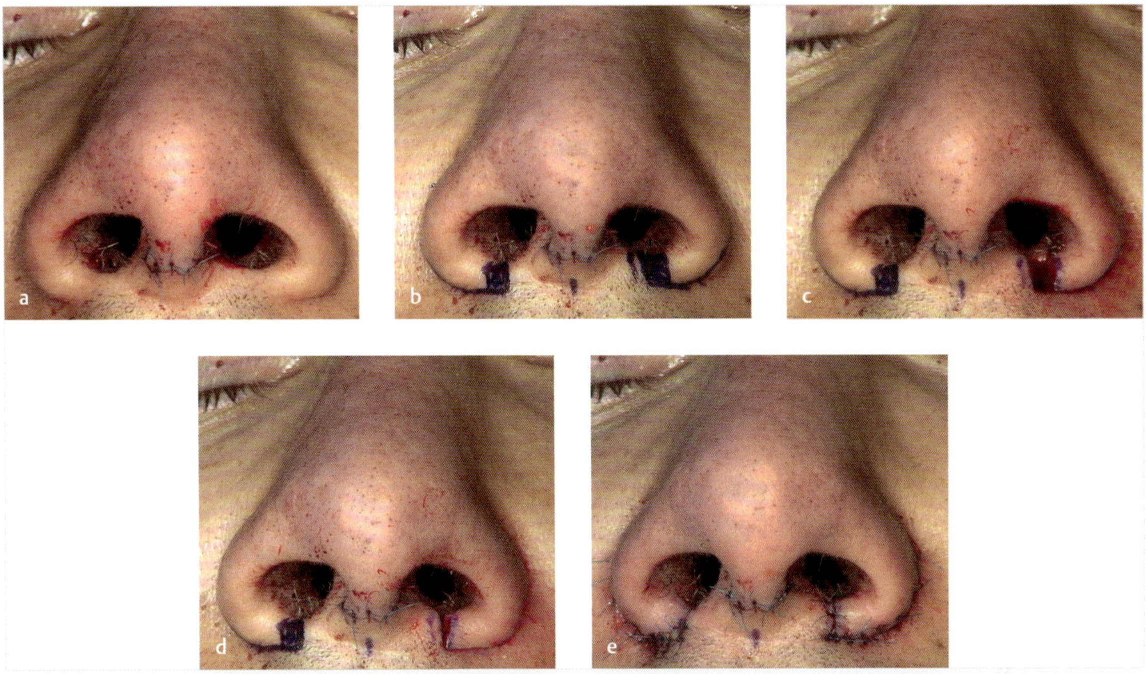

Fig. 14.8 **Nostril sill resections.** **(a)** Wide nostrils: condition after wound closure on the columella immediately after rhinoplasty. **(b)** After measurement, the slightly asymmetrical extent of the planned sill resection is drawn. **(c)** The condition after sill resection on the left. **(d)** The wound on the left has been approximated with a subcutaneous suture. **(e)** Condition after bilateral sill resection and skin suture. Even a moderate sill resection leads to significant improvement in the overall impression, without the risk of overcorrection.

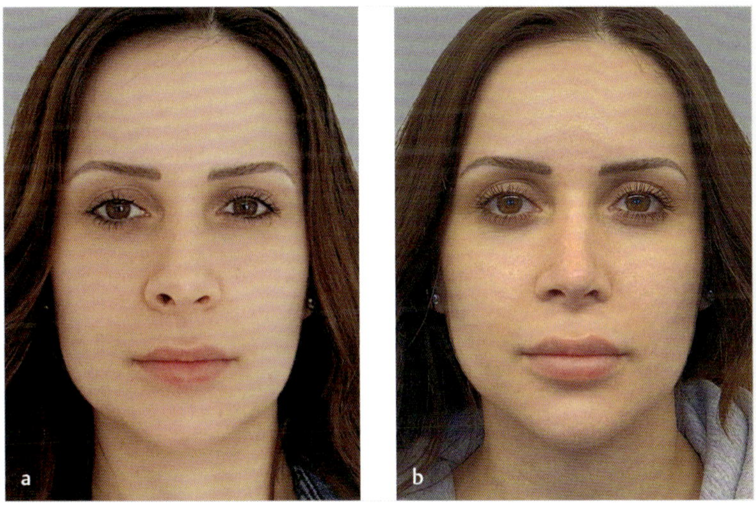

Fig. 14.9 **Sill resection in a revision case.** **(a)** Asymmetrical nostrils in a patient with a history of rhinoplasty elsewhere, including base resections. **(b)** Surgical correction with revision rhinoplasty, with an asymmetrical revision of the nostril sill resections, and asymmetric rim grafts.

14.3 Combination of Wedge Resections at the Nasal Base

Wedge resections at the nostril and the alar base can be combined if the nostrils and nasal alae are too wide. The procedural steps do not differ from those described for each excision separately (▶ Fig. 14.10a–c, ▶ Fig. 14.11a, b).

▶ Fig. 14.12a–c shows an intraoperative case study of combined alar wedge and nostril sill resections in an Asian patient.

It is possible, but not mandatory, for the areas of the alar wedge and nostril sill resections to meet to form a coherent excision field. Inadequate or asymmetrical resections can be corrected by revision as long as this does

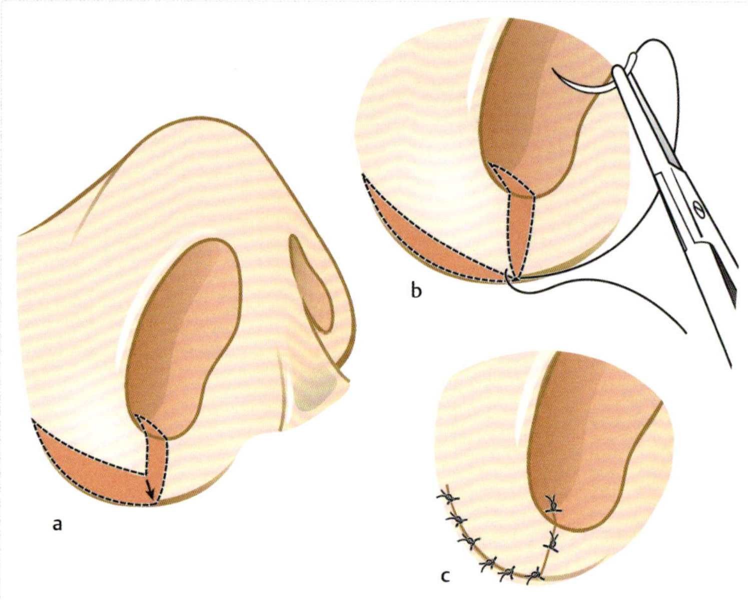

Fig. 14.10 Combined alar wedge and nostril sill resections. (a) Alar wedge and nostril sill resections are carried out simultaneously in most cases. **(b)** The first suture is the one at the concourse of the alar wedge and nostril sill resections. **(c)** Fine and precise suturing is indispensable for an aesthetically appealing outcome.

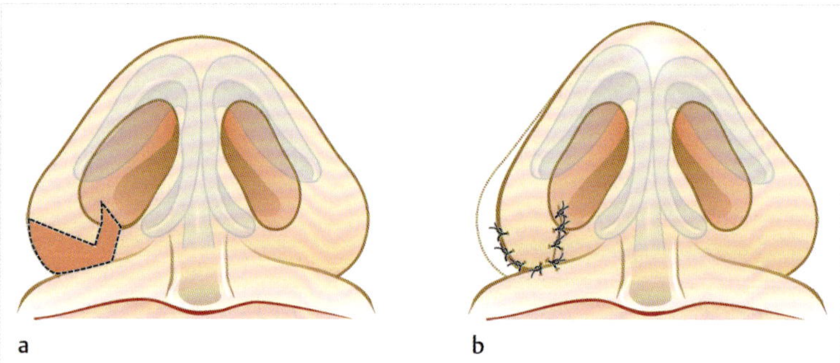

Fig. 14.11 Combined alar wedge and nostril sill resections. Combining the two excisions **(a)** results in narrowing of the alae and also of the nostrils **(b)**.

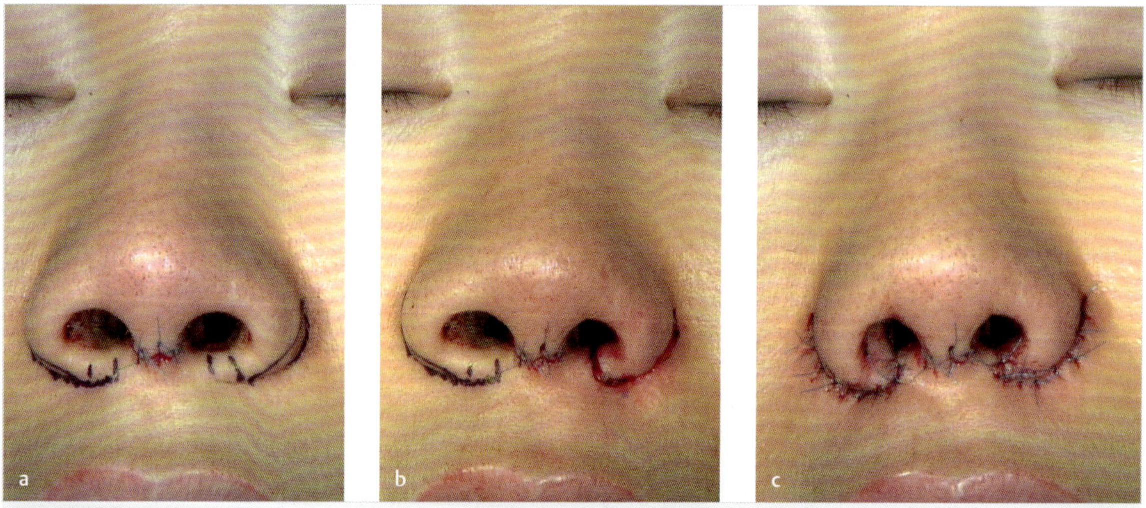

Fig. 14.12 Combined alar wedge and nostril sill resections, intraoperatively in an Asian patient. **(a)** Measurement and marking. **(b)** After left-sided resection. **(c)** Completed suture on both sides.

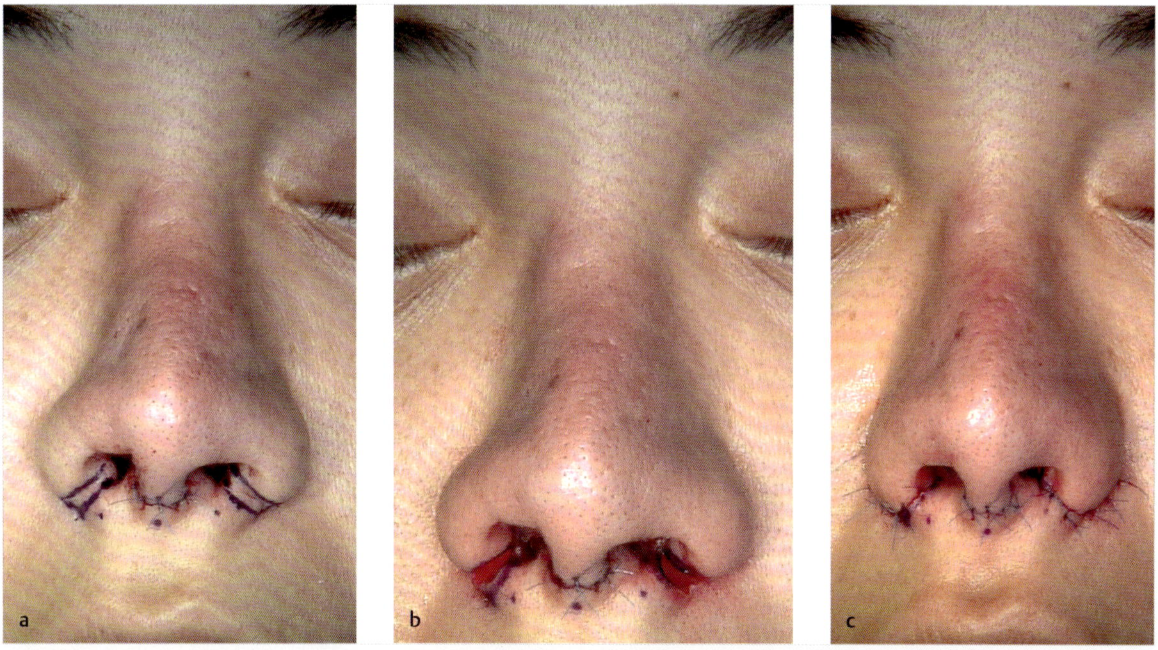

Fig. 14.13 Revision of alar wedge and nostril sill resections. Condition after a first operation elsewhere. (a) Measurement and marking. **(b)** Asymmetrical resection. **(c)** The completed suture.

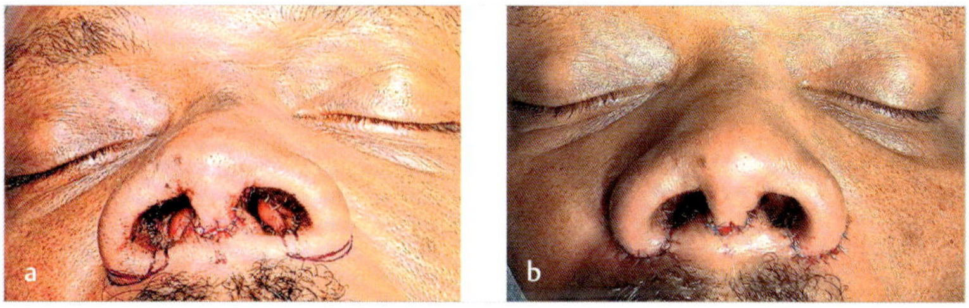

Fig. 14.14 Alar wedge and nostril sill resections in a Black patient. (a) The resections are measured and marked. **(b)** State after suturing.

not cause overcorrection (▶ Fig. 14.13a–c). If a sill resection is combined with the use of rim grafts, a reduction in the size of the nasal opening in the horizontal and vertical axes can be achieved (▶ Fig. 14.14a, b, ▶ Fig. 14.15a–h). These alar wedge and nostril sill resections can help reduce the occasionally somewhat grim facial expression that may be seen in patients with a broad nasal base.

I tend to be cautious about these resections at the base of the nose, because even a slight overcorrection quickly becomes noticeable and is difficult to correct. On the other hand, even a moderate, minor resection in suitable cases has a positive effect on the result, which those affected also notice. In any case, the surgeon should train his or her eye to recognize the indication for such resections at the base of the nose, since in suitable cases they can make a significant contribution to the overall result (compare also with ▶ Video 8.8).

> ✔
>
> Preoperatively planned alar wedge or nostril sill resections may not be required intraoperatively once rhinoplasty is complete. Resection may be unnecessary if an increase in nasal tip rotation or projection causes stretching of the alae, which then appear narrower than preoperatively (▶ Fig. 14.16a, b; see also ▶ Fig. 12.19a, b). It is advisable to bear this in mind and explain to the patient preoperatively that a definitive decision regarding an intervention on the base can only be taken at the close of surgery.

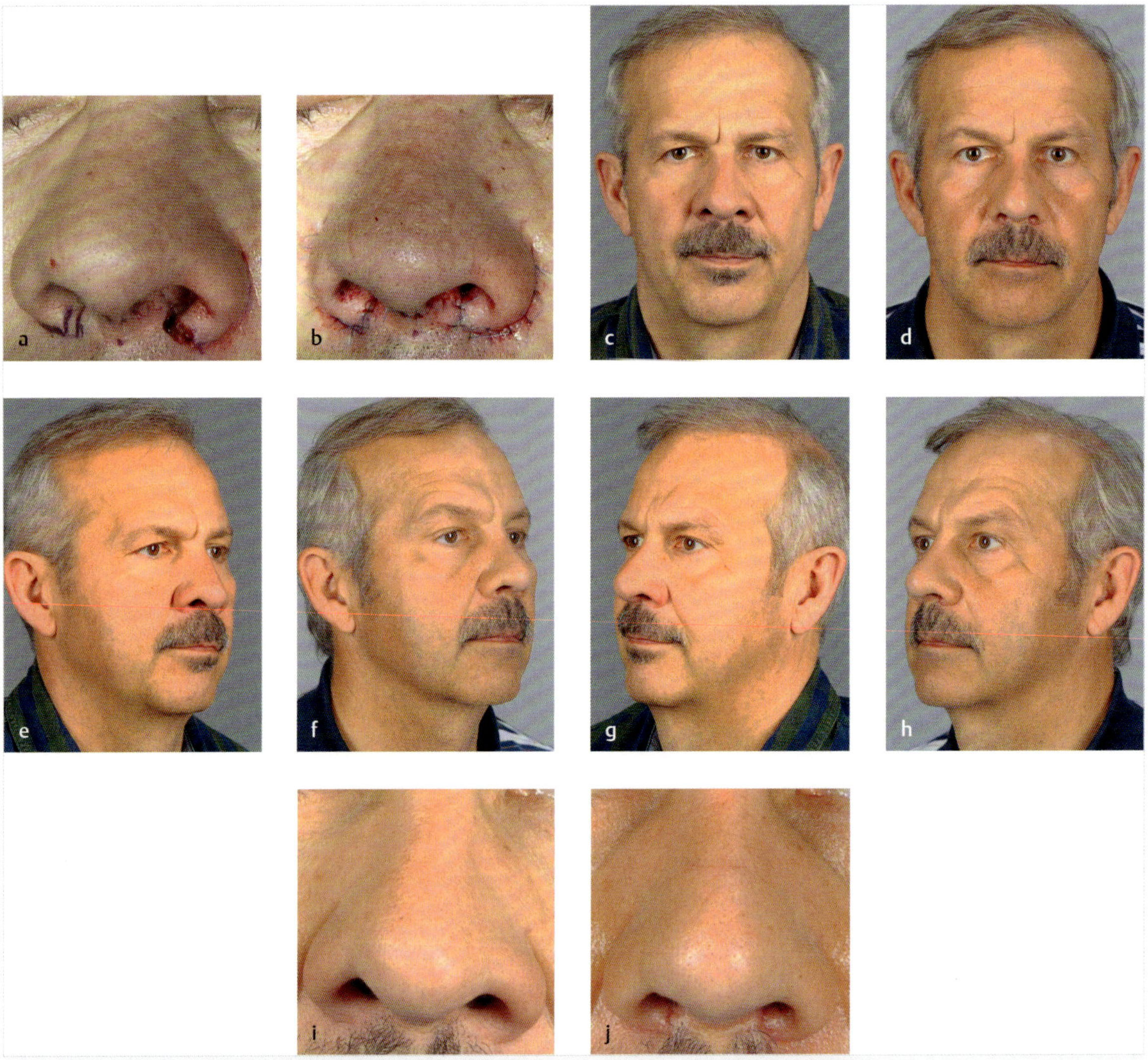

Fig. 14.15 The effect of rim grafts, small alar wedge, and nostril sill resections in combination; revision case study. (a) Large nostrils, with a wide nasal base. Nostril sill and small alar wedge resections immediately after rhinoplasty using rim grafts; marked on the right, left after resection. **(b)** After the suture on both sides. **(c, e, g) Clinical images before the operation:** frontal view **(c)**, oblique side view from the right **(e)**, oblique side view from the left **(g)**. **(d, f, h) Result**: frontal view **(d)**, oblique side view from the right **(f)**, oblique side view from the left **(h)**. Close-up, same patient **(i, j)**. Comparison of the preoperative **(i)** and postoperative **(j)** findings suggests that these alar wedge and nostril sill resections can help reduce the slightly grim facial expression that is sometimes found in patients with a broad nasal base.

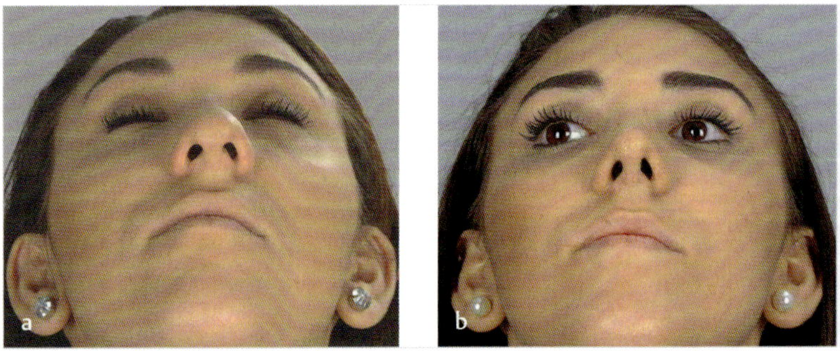

Fig. 14.16 Narrowing of the nasal base without wedge resection. (a) Wide tip and nasal base. **(b)** Alar wedge and nostril sill resections have been omitted after tip correction and narrowing of the medial footplates of the alar cartilages.

14

Bibliography

Cerkes N. Alar base reduction: nuances and techniques. Clin Plast Surg. 2022; 49(1):161–178

Foda HM. Nasal base narrowing: the combined alar base excision technique. Arch Facial Plast Surg. 2007; 9(1):30–34

Foda HM. Alar base reduction: the boomerang-shaped excision. Facial Plast Surg. 2011; 27(2):225–233

15 Wound Closure, Dressing, Postoperative Care, and Follow-up

The open and closed approaches differ little with regard to wound closure, dressing, and postoperative care.

15.1 Wound Closure and Dressing

The wound is closed when the surgeon is satisfied with all the details of his or her operation and the result of the rhinoplasty, and when there is no more bleeding.

> ✓
>
> Corrections of the nasal base (alar wedge and nostril sill resections; see Chapter 14) are generally performed only *after* closure of the open or closed access incisions, but prior to placement of Doyle splints and application of plaster with aluminum splint.
>
> To counteract swelling above the tip, it is worthwhile for an absorbable subcutaneous suture to connect the hypodermis to the supratip area at the level of the W-point, to close possible dead space when the skin flap is moved back at the end of the operation.

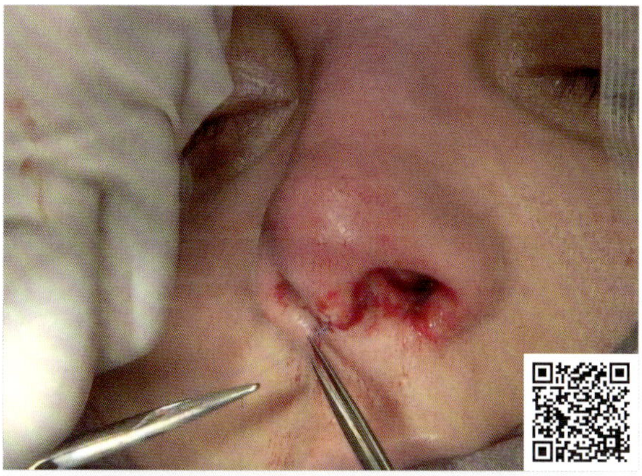

Video 15.1 Inner and outer wound closure (clinical case).

With the endonasal approach (see Chapter 16), the intranasal incisions are closed with a series of interrupted sutures made of rapidly absorbable material (Polyglactin 910; e.g., Vicryl Rapide) with a thread size of 5–0 or 6–0. In the open technique, the skin flap is put back. The columellar incision is closed first using 6–0 skin sutures (polypropylene, e.g., Prolene). The W-shaped incision facilitates precise adaptation of the wound edges for skin closure, with the first suture lying in the midline, followed by the lateral sutures. Five, or rarely up to seven, single button sutures are usually required on the columella (▶ Video 15.1, see Video 6.1; ▶ Fig. 15.1a, b). The columellar and marginal incisions are then closed on either side with 6–0 rapidly absorbable sutures (e.g., Vicryl Rapide) (▶ Fig. 15.2).

> ✓
>
> Single button sutures applied to the upper circumference of the nostril immediately below the alar domes may occasionally give rise to a small retraction ("notching") of the alar rim. When this undesirable phenomenon occurs, the suture responsible is immediately removed without being replaced.

Supporting endonasal silicone tubes may be used, depending on the extent of corrective measures on the septum (Doyle splints; ▶ Video 15.2; ▶ Fig. 15.3).

In a common case, after septoplasty the septal mucosa is reattached on either side with a continuous, absorbable mattress suture (5–0 polyglactin 910; e.g., Vicryl Rapide) in a zigzag pattern, and these silicone tubes are dispensable. However, endonasal supports may be beneficial for a few days after reconstruction of an unstable septum from multiple cartilage fragments. Doyle splints are fixed to the anterior septum with a transfixing, rapidly absorbable suture. Insertion may be facilitated by moistening these splints with saline solution. A long, slender speculum

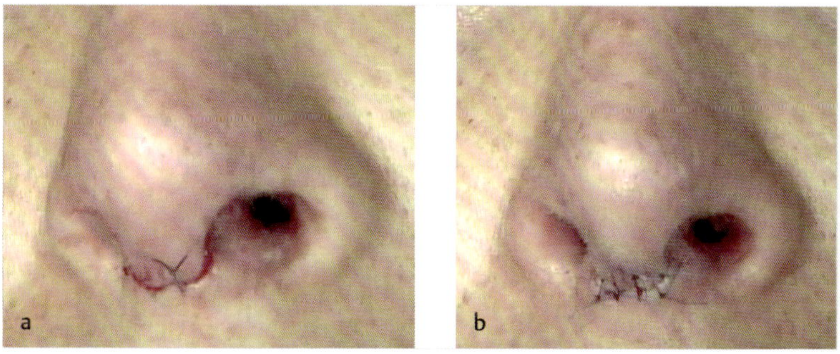

Fig. 15.1 Wound closure after open rhinoplasty. (a) The first suture (6–0 Prolene) is in the midline, at the tip of the "inverted V." **(b)** This is followed by four to six more sutures.

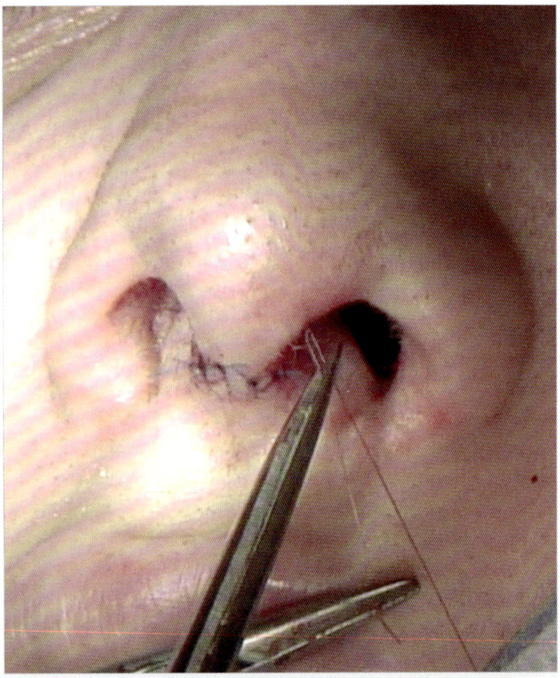

Fig. 15.2 Endonasal wound closure. 6–0 rapidly absorbable sutures are used.

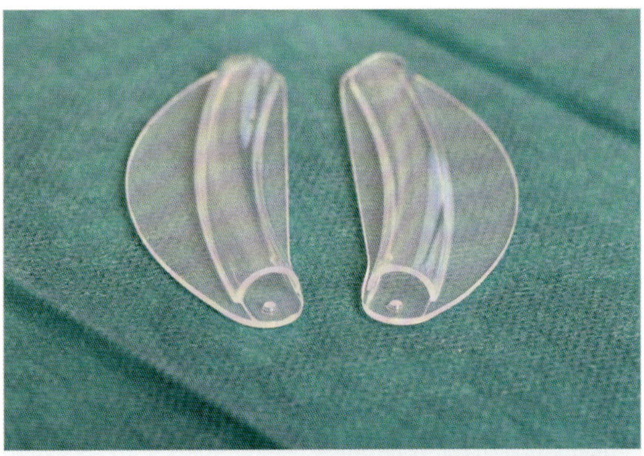

Fig. 15.3 Doyle splints. A tube keeps the airway patent, while the attached plate supports the septum (SPIGGLE & THEIS Medizintechnik GmbH, Overath, Germany).

opens up the depth of the nasal cavity, while a bayonet forceps grasps the tube (▶ Fig. 15.4a–d).

Doyle splints are usually removed from the second to fourth postoperative days, depending on the complexity of surgical procedures on the septum, but should be retained for a longer duration following closure of a septal perforation (see section 19.5). A nasal tampon can be placed lateral to the Doyle splint in the inferior nasal meatus to support hemostasis only in exceptional

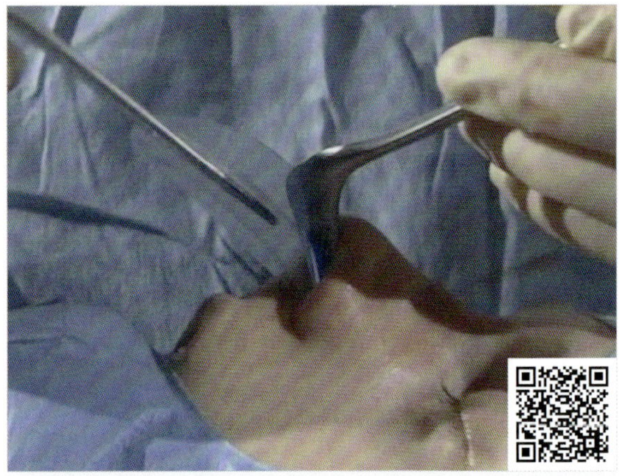

Video 15.2 Doyle splints; external aluminum splint.

circumstances, and should be removed the next day at the latest (▶ Fig. 15.5).

> ✔
>
> As long as Doyle splints or any kind of packing are in place, antibiotic protection is required, as the tubes obstruct the ostia of the sinuses and sinusitis can quickly develop.

Placement of the classic long-term packing nasal tamponade strips after septoplasty or rhinoplasty is obsolete, but it may be indicated for emergency management of uncontrollable nosebleeds (see section 23.4).

The nose is cleaned at the end of the operation. Adhesive tapes (such as Steri-Strip or Omnistrip patches) are attached to the nasal bridge, whether or not an osteotomy has been performed (▶ Fig. 15.6) and are retained until the sixth (fifth to seventh) postoperative day, provided they do not come off on their own beforehand.

Before application of the adhesive tape, the skin can be treated with tincture of benzoin for better adhesiveness (e.g., 90% tincture of benzoin 1 : 5, Siam benzoin tincture; Caesar & Loretz GmbH, Hilden, Germany) after it has been cleaned with water or saline solution and then dabbed dry, or it can be coated with some spray plaster (compare with ▶ Fig. 18.3f). A commercially available, well-fitting, and self-adhesive foam sheet with a feathered aluminum splint is placed on the nose in addition to the adhesive tapes if osteotomies have been performed on the bony nasal dorsum (▶ Video 15.2, ▶ Video 15.3; ▶ Fig. 15.7a–d). The aluminum splint is fixed with mild compression to allow stable positioning without undue pressure, and its feathered structure

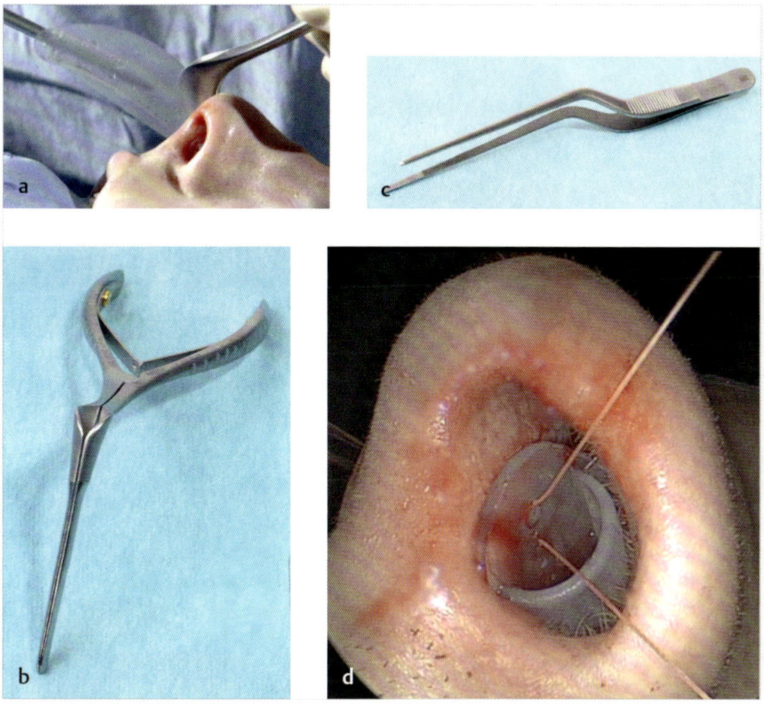

Fig. 15.4 Insertion of Doyle splints. Insertion of a Doyle splint **(a)** with a long speculum **(b)** (KARL STORZ SE & Co. KG, Tuttlingen, Germany) and bayonet forceps **(c)** (KARL STORZ SE & Co. KG, Tuttlingen, Germany). Fixation of the Doyle splints to the septum with a mattress suture (**d**, before knotting).

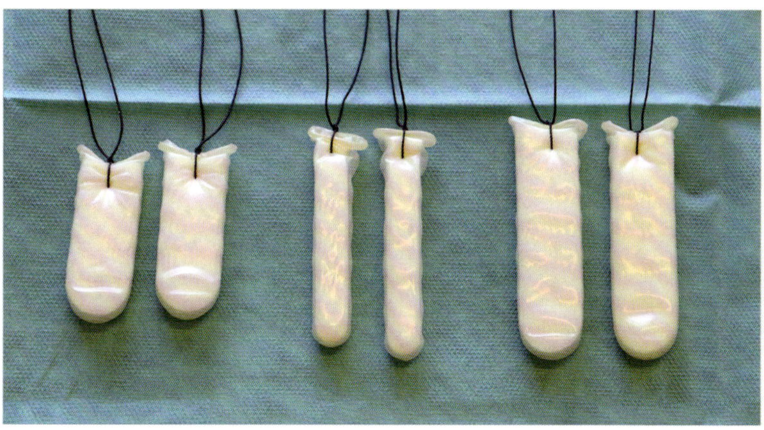

Fig. 15.5 Nasal tampons. These are available in three sizes for the nasal cavity (SPIGGLE & THEIS GmbH, Overath, Germany).

makes individual customization possible. These splints, together with appropriate foam sheets, come complete in three different sizes.

Soft-tissue swelling can be effectively treated by cooling the cheeks with cooling pads only in the first 2–3 days after the procedure. An automatically operated cooling system with a face mask (e.g., Hilotherm) should be used as soon as possible postoperatively on the day of the procedure, if available (▶ Fig. 15.8a, b). Cooling is achieved by allowing tempered distilled water to flow through a suitable mask. The temperature of the device should not exceed a maximum of 16–18 °C.

✔

"Ice cooling" has no advantages over these moderate temperatures.

The aluminum splint is placed on the nose for approximately 6 days (▶ Fig. 15.9). A second external splint can be placed after a week exceptionally, e.g. in patients who are undergoing extensive, complete hammer and chisel osteotomies (structure rhinoplasty), or if a let-down or push-down procedure has been performed, and retained

15

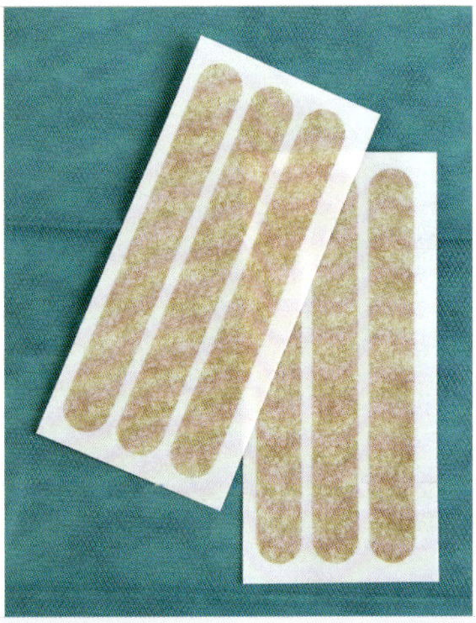

Fig. 15.6 **Adhesive strips.** Omnistrip reinforced adhesive skin closure strips, skin-colored. The strips are available in different widths and can be shortened as required (Paul Hartmann AG, Heidenheim, Germany).

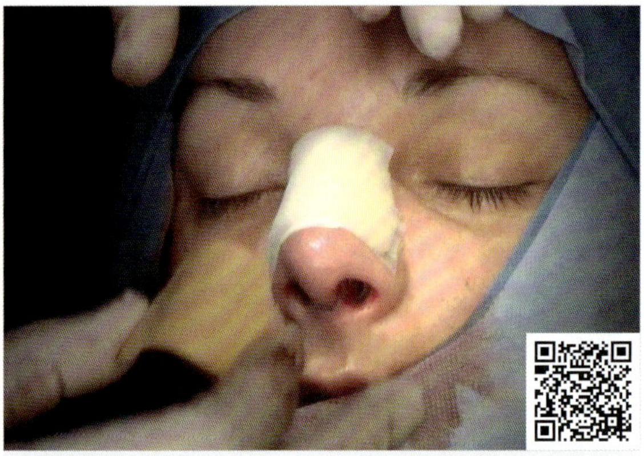

Video 15.3 Handling of plaster, foam, splint.

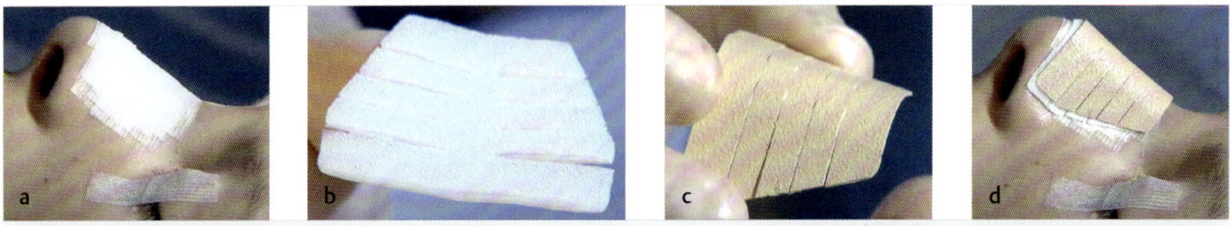

Fig. 15.7 **External nasal splint. (a)** Adhesive strips. **(b)** Foam pad. **(c)** A feathered aluminum splint (Audio Technologies SRL, Gossolengo, Italy). **(d)** A customized nasal splint, after fixation on the nasal bridge.

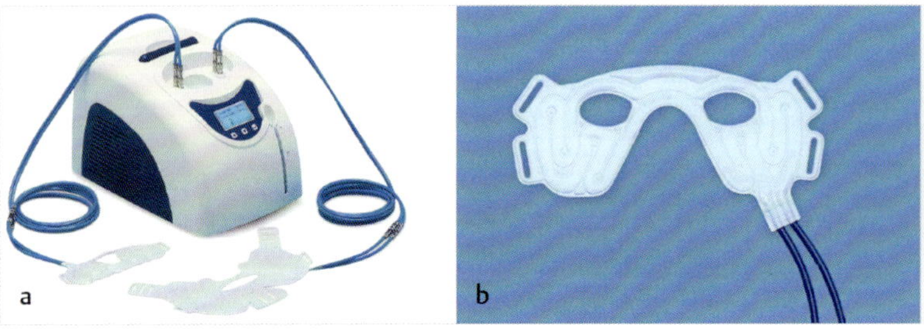

Fig. 15.8 **Hilotherm cooling. (a)** Control unit. **(b)** Nasal mask (Hilotherm GmbH, Argenbühl-Eisenharz, Germany).

for another week. The use of aluminum splints can be omitted, or suffices for a week, in patients undergoing surface rhinoplasty procedures, or lateral osteotomies only, as described with the piezoelectric technique (see section 8.3).

15.2 Postoperative Care and Follow-up

The physician's support and guidance in the first few days after surgery is crucial for the patients. They are then in a new situation characterized by the immediate physical consequences of the operation, but often also with concerns that the operation may not have been successful. Patients repeatedly view themselves in the mirror from their first waking moments in the recovery phase after the procedure. It is quite normal for surgeons not to be able to appreciate the final surgical outcome at this point – especially with a nose splint. However, patients often have different expectations in this regard and are sometimes completely appalled by their reflection in the mirror during the initial postoperative period,

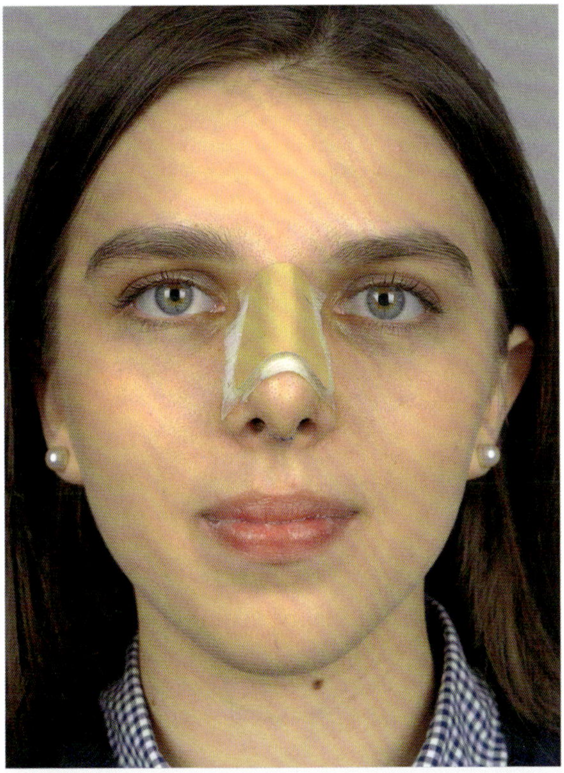

Fig. 15.9 Aluminum splint after rhinoplasty; clinical case. A patient with a large hump nose, 5 days after structure rhinoplasty with an external splint. See ▶ Fig. 12.8 for the surgical outcome.

during which the surgeon needs to comfort and reassure them.

15.2.1 Postoperative Care

Soft-tissue swelling of the face is usually most pronounced on the second to fourth postoperative days. Cooling with appropriate pads may be helpful, but in general does not have any appreciable effect after the third day.

Patients can clean their nostrils postoperatively on their own using water (without soap), and a nonspecific nasal ointment (dexpanthenol) or oil to loosen crusted blood. Secretions and encrustations in the nasal cavities are either suctioned off or removed by the surgeon using instruments from the second or third postoperative days, as far as necessary. The patients are not able to blow the nose in the early postoperative phase, but have to "sniff up" the secretion if necessary.

A decongestant nasal spray (e.g., xylometazoline or naphazoline, such as Privin or similar) can also be used up to three times daily in the short term if the interior of the nose is markedly swollen. The pediatric version is usually sufficient, while many patients find the adult preparation too potent. The condition with obstructed nasal breathing is uncomfortable but transient, and improves after a short period of time.

> ✔
>
> Some patients lack confidence with regard to self-treatment and care of the nose, or may underestimate the importance of cleaning for normal wound healing. The surgeon then has to take over wound care, since heavy encrustations over the suture may lead to impaired wound healing and unsightly scars.

The columella may occasionally develop painful, moderately severe reddening and swelling, indicating a circumscribed bacterial infection, which enters the tissue through the suture line. This inflammation usually recedes rapidly after suture removal (including in such cases the absorbable suture material at the nostrils). Cortisone and antibiotic-containing combination ointments (e.g., fluocinolone–neomycin; e.g., Jellin-Neomycin or Neo-Synalar ointment) are also beneficial and help with quick regression of symptoms.

15.2.2 Follow-up

The aluminum splint is placed on the nose for approximately 6 days. A second external splint may optionally be placed after a week in patients who are undergoing extensive, complete hammer and chisel osteotomies, or let-down and push-down procedures, and retained for another week.

> ✔
>
> The outer splint and plaster are not replaced if they come off prematurely after surface rhinoplasty even with lateral osteotomies, since bony stability is preserved. After a classic, complete hammer and chisel osteotomy, however, it is safer to replace a an untimely loosened aluminum splint with a new one, which ensures splinting until about the eighth to the twelfth day.

Columellar sutures are removed around the sixth postoperative day after open rhinoplasty, together with the aluminum splint. Using a microscope and a pair of microscissors with fine forceps (commercially available as disposable instruments) is very useful with the delicate suture material (▶ Fig. 15.10a, b). These instruments

15

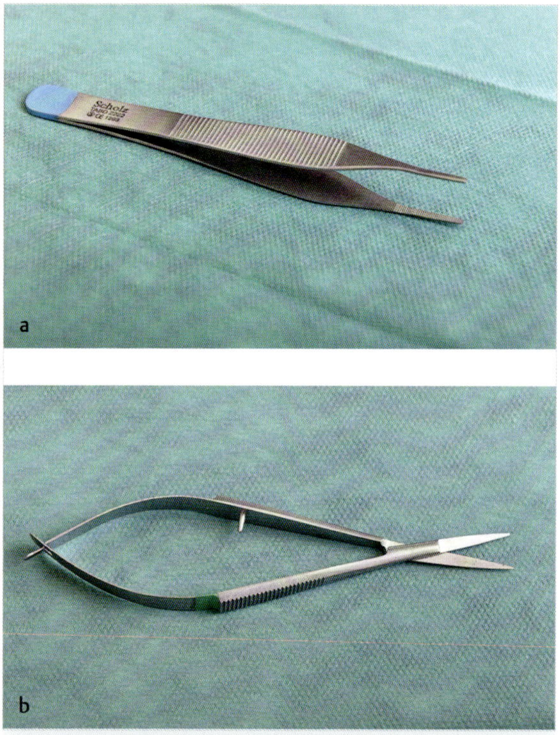

Fig. 15.10 Disposable micro instruments. Disposable microforceps **(a)** and microspring scissors **(b)** facilitate suture removal from the columella after rhinoplasty (Paul Hartmann AG, Heidenheim, Germany).

under high magnification avoid unnecessary and painful columellar trauma and reliably exclude the possibility of any residual delicate 6–0 suture remaining in the wound. Magnifying glasses are less effective than a microscope for the purpose.

Apart from the immediate postoperative care on day 1 and 2 after the operation, as a rule, I examine the patient roughly after 5-6 days postoperatively at the latest, for suture and splint removal, with follow-up after 2 weeks and 4 weeks. The early postoperative appearance of the nose is discussed in detail during these appointments. It must be reiterated to the patient that the final surgical outcome in the nose is by no means evident at this stage. Patients are typically concerned that the swelling, irregularity, and asymmetry in the early postoperative stage may be permanent features, and they examine the nose in the mirror several times a day. The surgeon needs to be patient and empathetic during this period.

In my experience, postoperative taping of the skin of the nose by the patients over a longer period of time does not have a significant effect on the outcome of the operation, although some studies seem to confirm this, at least in the case of thick skin. I am not comfortable with the idea that patients may be constantly manipulating the freshly operated nose.

Further follow-up appointments are arranged in consultation with the patient – e.g., after 3, 6, and 12 months. Most patients gladly return for these appointments to analyze the observable changes in the nose together with the surgeon. Follow-up is important for the surgeon to assess the medium-term and long-term postoperative changes in the nose and how patients are coping with them. Follow-up appointments also provide an opportunity for photo documentation and allow comparison of preoperative and postoperative findings.

> Some patients involve their surgeons in the postoperative evolution of their appearance by frequently sending photos and describing their findings. Such reports should be taken serious note of and commented on by the surgeon, since patients expect competent comments and feedback to interpret their own observations.

Last but not least – especially in cases that are not going optimally – contact with the patient must be maintained so that, if necessary, after a reasonable waiting period of 9–12 months, the option of a subsequent surgical correction can be discussed. If one loses touch with the patient, then there is a risk that he or she may turn to other consultants with no knowledge of the details of the treatment case, who may give inappropriate advice or information.

> Negligence or lack of follow-up, possibly even impolite treatment, must be avoided, as it may push an unsatisfied patient into taking recourse to legal action, or involving the media against the surgeon.

Bibliography

Cochran CS, Ducic Y, DeFatta RJ. Current concepts in the postoperative care of the rhinoplasty patient. South Med J. 2008; 101(9):935–939

Kenny H, Jonas RH, Oyer S. Columellar scar following open rhinoplasty using absorbable suture versus nonabsorbable suture: a meta-analysis. Facial Plast Surg Aesthet Med. 2023; 25(1):54–60

Özücer B, Yildirim YS, Veyseller B, et al. Effect of postrhinoplasty taping on postoperative edema and nasal draping: a randomized clinical trial. JAMA Facial Plast Surg. 2016; 18(3):157–163

16 Closed (Endonasal) Techniques

16.1 Preliminary Remarks

The debate around various surgical approaches keeps rhinoplasty surgeons busy at meetings and round tables worldwide, with the discussion becoming unnecessarily heated at times. When selecting incisions, it is only a matter of reaching and working on the cartilage and skeleton of the nose. However, it cannot be assumed that fundamentally different or better results will be achieved with an open or closed approach, although some studies claim to have demonstrated specific differences in the outcome. Cartilage and bone may be reshaped as desired – barring a few exceptions – with both the open and closed procedures. The factor of primary importance is not the technique per se, but rather the surgeon's ability to perform important maneuvers in order to reliably achieve a particular result using the selected approach.

At first glance, the closed approach appears to be more suitable if the goal being pursued is "preservation rhinoplasty." However, the layers of the skin and subcutaneous tissue, muscles, bones, cartilage, and mucous membrane can also be "preserved" with open access – in addition to the ligaments of the nose, which in turn can be more easily reconstructed with sutures with the open technique if they have been severed.

The most obvious difference between the two approaches is the small skin incision on the columella required for the open technique. This incision – with the minimal risk of a visible scar – is usually the key argument against "open rhinoplasty." I was also therefore an advocate of the closed technique for many years. In fact, however, there is only little risk of an unsightly scar if the columella is carefully incised and then closed again with fine sutures just as carefully.

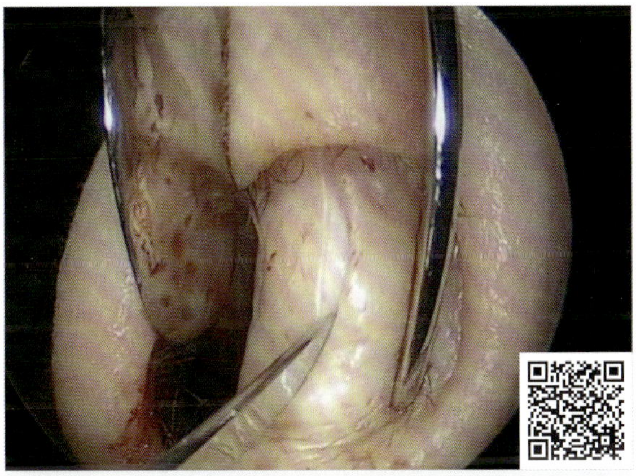

Video 16.1 Hemitransfixion incision (clinical case).

Nevertheless, closed procedures are justified, since open access is not always required for nasal surgery. It can also happen that a patient resolutely declines an open incision. Even in these cases, an experienced surgeon should in general be able to offer the desired nose correction.

16.2 Closed-Approach Incisions

Several different incisions can be used for closed rhinoplasty. They are selected on the basis of the individually intended surgical procedures. There is no such thing as a single "closed technique" in this respect, but rather a variety of endonasal access routes.

Preparation for a closed rhinoplasty does not differ significantly from the procedure for the open technique. Trimming of nostril hair is important, to improve visibility. A powerful head light is also recommended for optimal illumination.

16.2.1 Hemitransfixion Incision

The hemitransfixion incision is the classic approach to the nasal septum. The surgeon uses a slender nasal speculum to visualize the caudal edge of the septum and follows it while making the incision with the scalpel (▶ Video 16.1; ▶ Fig. 16.1, ▶ Fig. 16.2a). Depending on

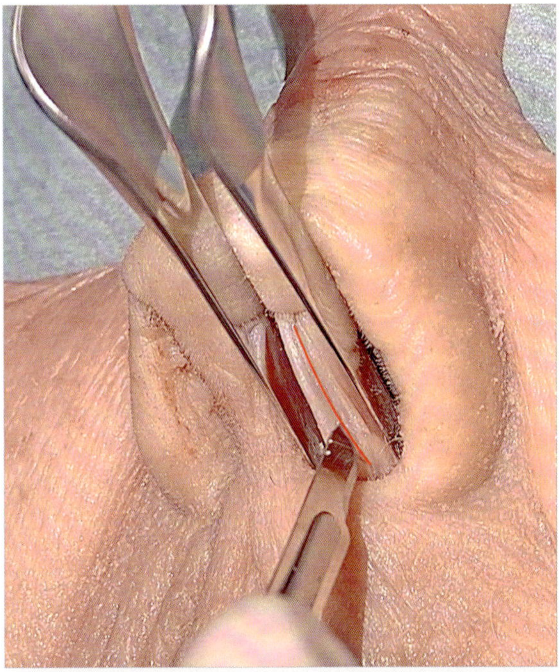

Fig. 16.1 Hemitransfixion incision. A left-sided hemitransfixion incision is shown; some surgeons prefer the right side (cadaver head).

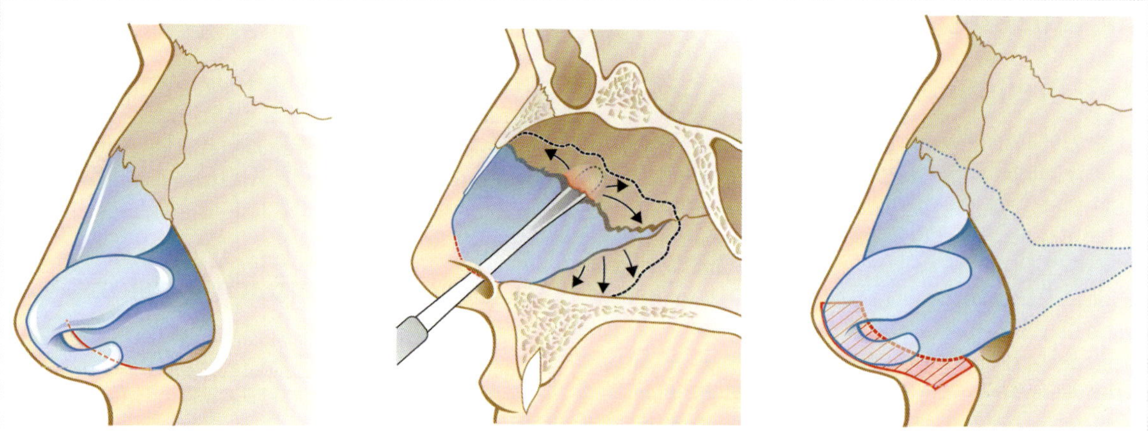

Fig. 16.2 Hemitransfixion incision. (a) The hemitransfixion incision follows the caudal edge of the septum on one side. **(b)**This incision provides access to the cartilaginous and bony septum and the vomer, maxillary crest, and anterior nasal spine. **(c)** It also allows retrograde access between the medial crura of the alar cartilages.

individual needs, this incision provides access to the cartilaginous and bony septum, as well as the vomer, the maxillary crest, and the anterior nasal spine (▶ Fig. 16.2b) A right-sided incision is often recommended, but surgeons may choose the side they are most comfortable with; I prefer using a left-sided incision. The surgical steps for cartilaginous and bony septoplasty are further described in Chapter 7.

If needed, the space between the medial crura of the alar cartilages or the premaxillary space in front of the anterior nasal spine can be opened via the hemitransfixion incision, using a retrograde approach (▶ Fig. 16.2c). This allows placement of grafts for correction of the columellar profile or nasolabial angle. This option may be important if, for instance, the deviated caudal edge of the septum ("septal subluxation") is to be straightened using an endonasal technique, with positioning and suturing in the midline between the medial crura of the alar cartilages, or for placement and fixation of an endonasal septal extension graft in the midline (see section 11.1.2).

Combining hemitransfixion incisions on either side results in complete "transfixion," in which both medial crura of the alar cartilages are separated from the septum by a continuous incision anterior to its caudal edge.

16.2.2 Marginal Incision

The marginal incision follows the caudal edge of the alar cartilage and is identical here to the incision for the open access (▶ Video 16.2; ▶ Fig. 16.3a, b, ▶ Fig. 16.4). The Kilner double hook is a valuable aid with this procedure (▶ Fig. 16.4, ▶ Fig. 16.5; see ▶ Fig. 6.8). The surface of the ipsilateral lower lateral cartilage and the upper lateral

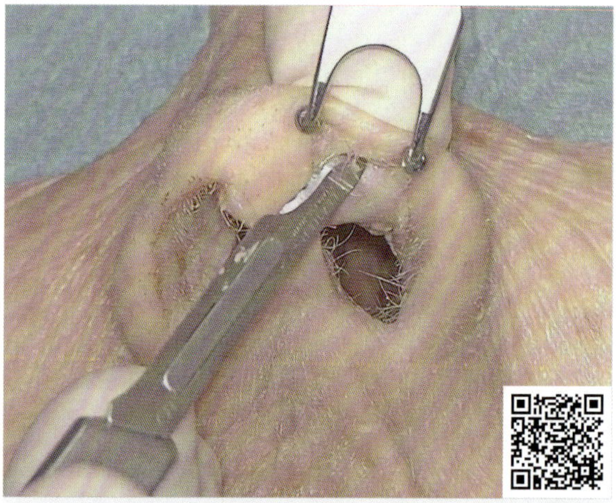

Video 16.2 Marginal incision (cadaver head).

cartilage can be accessed via this endonasal route (▶ Fig. 16.3c, ▶ Fig. 16.5), but further cranial visualization is restricted. The medial course of the marginal incision is identical to a columellar rim incision.

A unilateral incision of this kind already provides access between the medial crura of the alar cartilages and up to the caudal edge of the septum and beyond (see ▶ Fig. 16.3c). This approach facilitates minor corrections, resection, or augmentation in this region, without the need for an open procedure ("pocket surgery").

16.2.3 Alar Rim Incision

A variant of the marginal incision is the rim incision, which runs on the inner surface parallel to the alar rim at

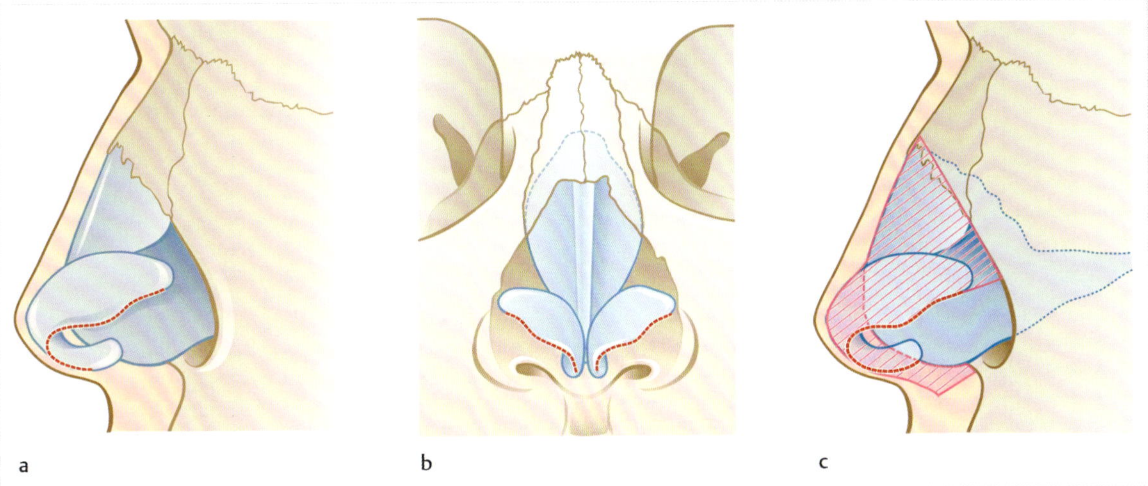

Fig. 16.3 Marginal incision (schematic diagram). The marginal incision follows the caudal edge of the alar cartilage (**a**, lateral view; **b**, frontal view), providing access to the lower lateral and upper lateral cartilages (**c**, hatched in red).

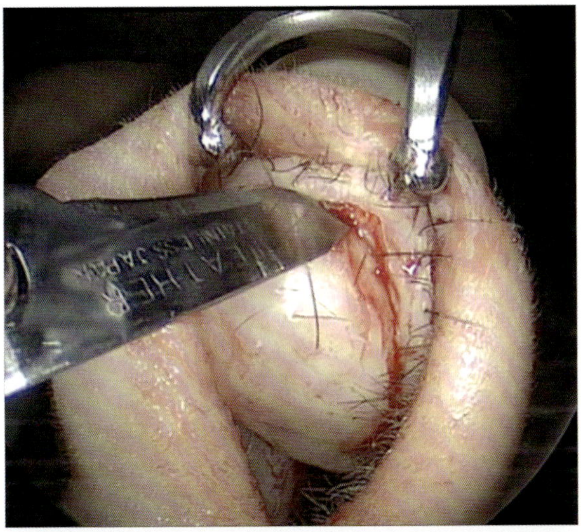

Fig. 16.4 Marginal incision. The incision precisely follows the caudal edge of the alar cartilage, which is exposed with the middle finger while the alar rim is retracted with the Kilner hook.

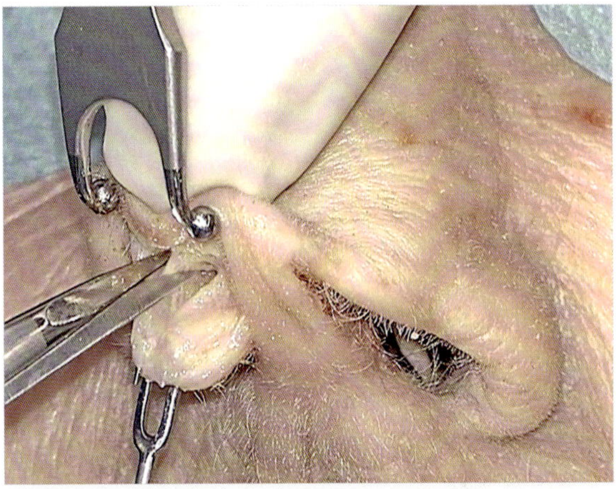

Fig. 16.5 Dissection of the alar cartilage through the marginal incision (shown in a cadaver specimen). The alar cartilage is mobilized via the marginal incision, with cutting and spreading movements using a pair of fine, pointed scissors. A small two-pronged hook exerts traction against the Kilner hook at the alar rim.

a distance of about 1–2 mm and merges with the classic marginal incision at its medial aspect (▶ Fig. 16.6a). This incision opens up the lateral soft-tissue space between the caudal rim of the alar cartilage and the cutaneous edge of the nasal ala, allowing easier placement of rim grafts (▶ Fig. 16.6b). Otherwise, for placement of a rim graft starting from the marginal incision, a soft-tissue pocket has to be prepared as a graft bed in the same area.

16.2.4 Intercartilaginous Incision

The intercartilaginous incision, which runs between the caudal edge of the upper lateral cartilage and the cephalic edge of the lower lateral cartilage, is extremely important in endonasal rhinoplasty (▶ Video 16.3; ▶ Fig. 16.7a–c, ▶ Fig. 16.8). It usually begins at the caudal edge of the septum, starting from the upper (anterior) section of a hemitransfixion or transfixion incision.

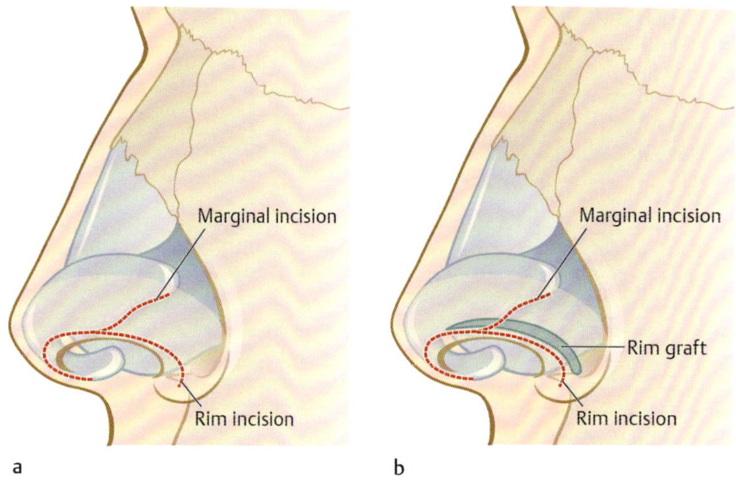

Fig. 16.6 Rim incision. The rim incision follows the inner skin edge of the nasal ala rather than the alar cartilage rim **(a)**, which facilitates placement of a rim graft **(b)**.

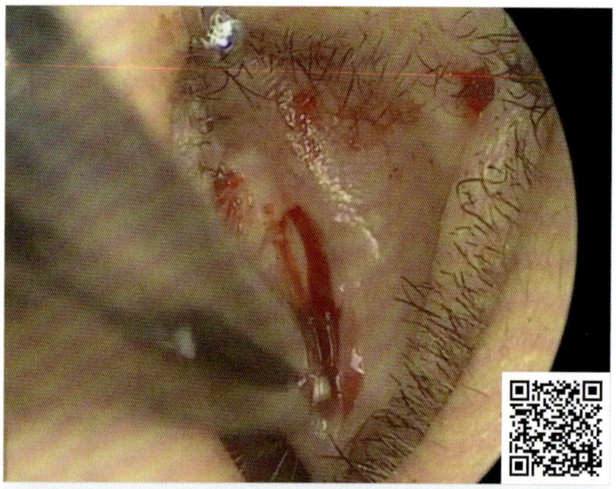

Video 16.3 Intercartilaginous incision.

Separation of the nasal skin allows visualization of the upper two-thirds of the nasal vault, with a variety of options for surgical correction being available, as has been described in other sections here. While this incision severs the horizontal (longitudinal) scroll ligaments, the vertical scroll ligaments can be spared by staying directly on the upper lateral cartilage, under the perichondrium (see also section 1.7). This incision severs the vestibular skin of the inner nose along the scroll area at the level of the nasal valve, as well as the cartilaginous bridge between the upper lateral and lower lateral cartilages (see ▶ Fig. 1.8). Critics of this incision fear negative effects on the nasal valve due to weakening of the cartilage or postoperative scar contraction. However, such complications are infrequent with careful handling of tissue and clean suturing for wound closure.

16.2.5 Transcartilaginous Incision

The transcartilaginous incision may be considered if a cephalic segment of the lateral crus of the alar cartilage is to be resected (▶ Video 16.4; ▶ Fig. 16.9a, b, ▶ Fig. 16.10a, b). The transcartilaginous incision ("cartilage-splitting approach") allows direct exposure and removal of this cephalic segment, using an endonasal approach. Otherwise, from the intercartilaginous incision, this cephalic resection would require a retrograde approach and would be technically more demanding.

The nasal dorsum may be further dissected as needed after cephalic resection, and the procedure then is no different from the procedure after the intercartilaginous incision. Simple cephalic resection of the lateral crus of the alar cartilage as a sole measure — only indicated in very few cases — may be undertaken comparatively easy via this endonasal incision (▶ Fig. 16.11a, b). In contrast, for example, creating a lateral crural turn-in flap through the transcartilaginous incision or through any other endonasal access route is distinctly challenging. A delivery approach or an open technique is therefore preferable for this purpose (see section 10.2.2).

16.2.6 Delivery Approach (Luxation)

In comparison with the types of endonasal approach listed above, the delivery approach with a closed technique allows a complete overview and provides several options for reshaping the alar cartilages (▶ Video 16.5, ▶ Video 16.6; ▶ Fig. 16.12a–d, ▶ Fig. 16.13a–c).

An intercartilaginous incision is combined with a marginal incision and transfixion to facilitate delivery. The alar cartilage is then separated from its skin cover and can be "luxated" outward through the nostril, exposing it

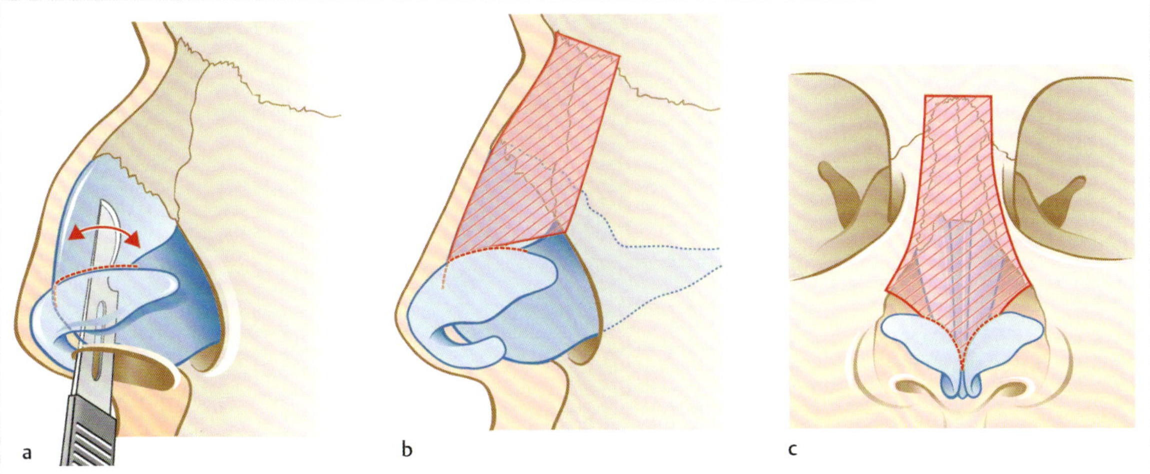

Fig. 16.7 **Intercartilaginous incision. (a)** The intercartilaginous incision runs exactly between the upper lateral cartilage and the cephalic rim of the lower lateral cartilage. **(b, c)** It allows access to the upper two-thirds of the nasal vault bilaterally (hatched in red).

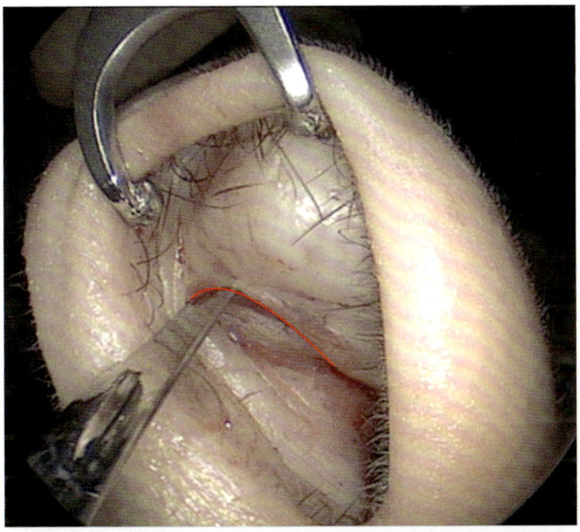

Fig. 16.8 **Intercartilaginous incision; intraoperative example.** Left intercartilaginous incision. The incision is made in the fold between the cephalic rim of the lower lateral cartilage and the upper lateral cartilage. Medially, it merges into a hemitransfixion incision or, if the incision is bilateral, into a transfixion incision.

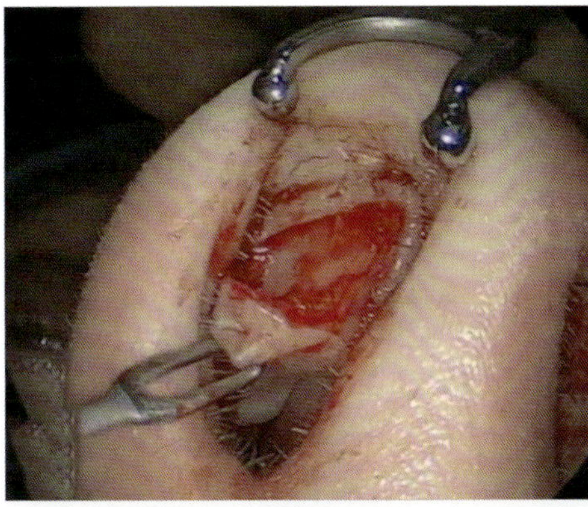

Video 16.4 Transcartilaginous incision and exposure of the cephalic edge of the alar cartilage.

for surgical correction. The double-pronged nasal hook (Kilner hook; see ▶ Fig. 6.8) is typically held at the alar rim with the thumb and index finger during mobilization of the alar cartilage, while the middle finger stabilizes the ala from the outside, supporting it during dissection with a pair of fine, pointed scissors. The alar cartilage is extracted caudally and outward with increasing mobilization using a fine double-pronged hook held by an assistant (▶ Fig. 16.13a). The alar cartilages delivered can be supported by alar splints to ensure symmetry; these are provided with millimeter markings and also serve as a support for the scalpel (▶ Fig. 16.13b, c).

The incisions should be long enough to provide a complete overview of the cartilage and allow freedom of movement for further surgical procedures. The lateral crus of the alar cartilage can be released entirely at its lateral aspect, if required, and extracted for processing. In contrast to exposure of the alar cartilage with the open approach, the lateral crus of the alar cartilage is inevitably wholly separated from the upper lateral cartilage during delivery. Thus, the alar and upper lateral cartilages cannot be viewed together in their entirety using this method.

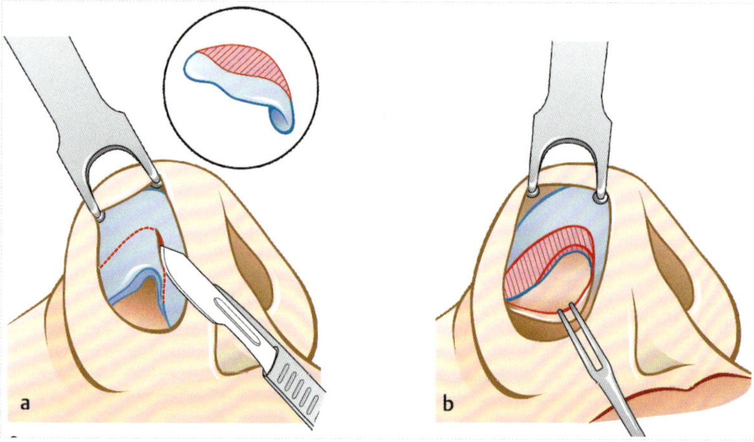

Fig. 16.9 Transcartilaginous incision. **(a)** The transcartilaginous incision severs the vestibular skin and lower lateral cartilage along a line parallel to the cephalic rim of the lateral crus. **(b)** A small flap of vestibular skin is formed endonasally over the cephalic portion of the alar cartilage.

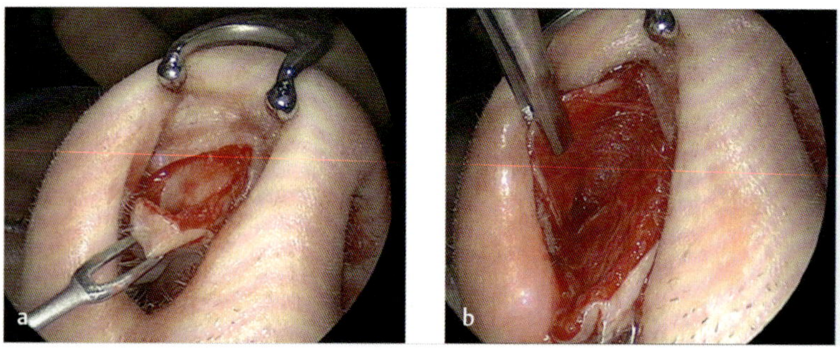

Fig. 16.10 Transcartilaginous incision; intraoperative example. (a) Transcartilaginous incision on the right. The incision runs roughly across the center of the lateral crus of the alar cartilage and exposes the cephalic edge of the cartilage; the vestibular skin is elevated with a small two-pronged hook. **(b)** The cephalic edge is grasped with Adson–Brown forceps and can now be cut as needed.

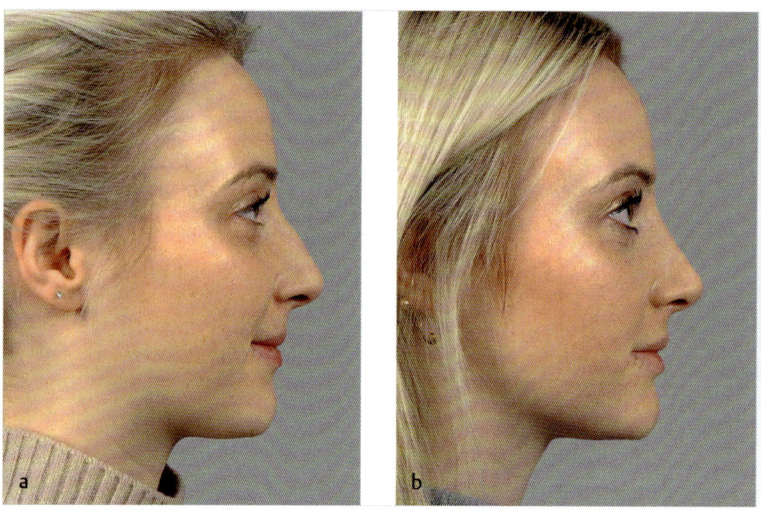

Fig. 16.11 Cephalic resection using the endonasal approach; clinical case. **(a)** Hump nose. **(b)** After endonasal hump removal with cephalic resection using the transcartilaginous approach.

> ✔
>
> The intercartilaginous incision also opens up the nasal cavity at the intercartilaginous fold, which is not the case with the open technique. Some rhinoplasty surgeons therefore consider that this type of closed rhinoplasty is even more "aggressive" than the open access route.

Handling of the delivered alar cartilages depends on the individual needs in a given case. In principle, the surgeon has a wide choice of sutures, excision techniques, or grafts (▶ Fig. 16.14a, b; for details, see Chapters 10–12).

Sutures between the two alar cartilages (e.g., interdomal sutures) can also be accurately placed using this endonasal approach, even if the columellar skin gets in the way. The needle is either passed behind this dermal

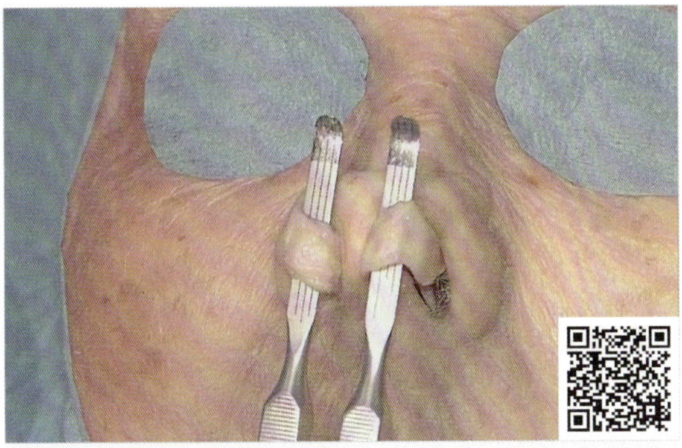

Video 16.5 Delivery technique (cadaver head).

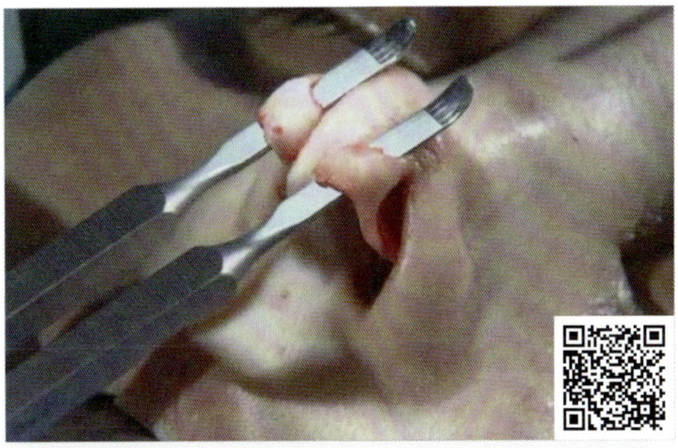

Video 16.6 Delivery technique (clinical case).

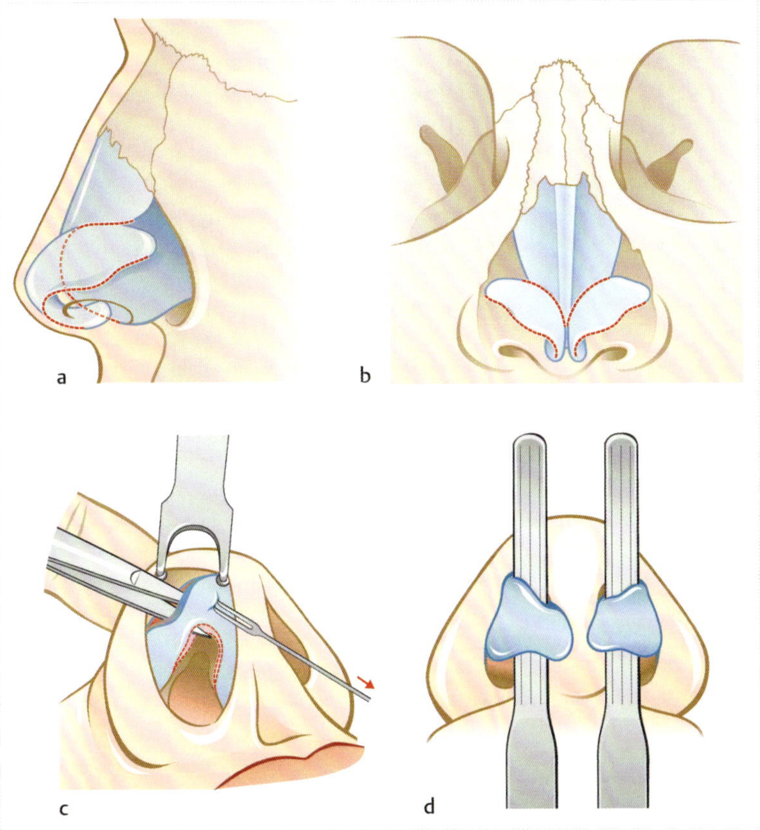

Fig. 16.12 Delivery approach (luxation; schematic diagram). **(a, b)** An intercartilaginous incision is combined with a marginal incision and transfixion for cartilage delivery. **(c, d)** The alar cartilages can be "luxated" bilaterally from their anatomical positions through the nostrils once they have been separated from the overlying skin. With support from alar guiding instruments, the cartilages are then exposed for manipulation of any kind.

bridge, or both alar cartilages are extracted together through one nostril (▶ Fig. 16.15a, b).

> Rhinoplasty surgeons may require more skill and practice to achieve a successful outcome with the closed technique than with an open one.

The surgeon can also use cartilage grafts of choice using closed procedures; the only thing missing is the overall view of the nasal structures provided by the open approach. The "luxated," delivered cartilages are intermittently replaced in their original positions under intact skin so that the effects of these surgical maneuvers on the appearance of the nose are visible immediately and more clearly than with an open access route.

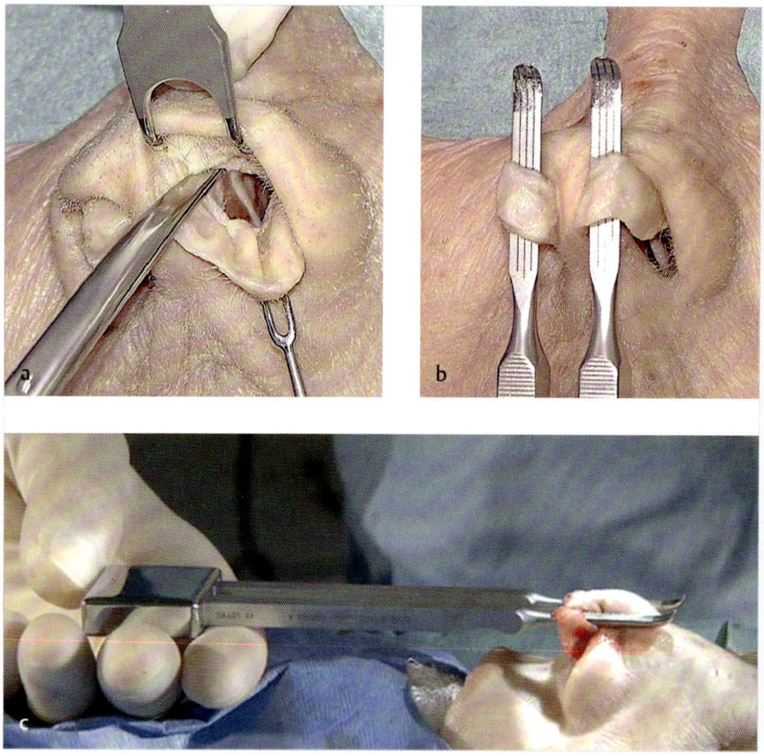

Fig. 16.13 Delivery approach. (a) The alar cartilage is "luxated" from its anatomical position, and the skin is dissected with scissors from the marginal to the intercartilaginous incision, in close contact with the cartilage (cadaver specimen). **(b)** The alar cartilages are placed onto alar guiding instruments on either side after complete "luxation" (KARL STORZ SE & Co. KG, Tuttlingen, Germany). **(c)** Optionally, the two splints of the instrument unit can be fixed and stabilized with a connecting block (clinical case).

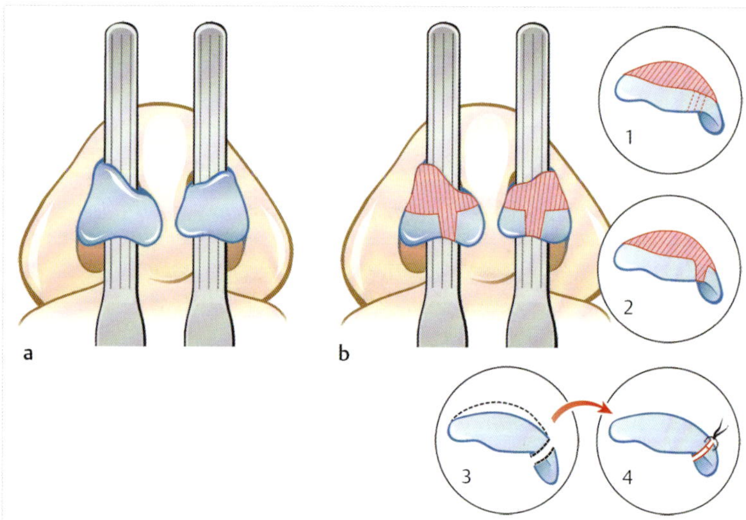

Fig. 16.14 Delivered alar cartilages (schematic diagram). **(a)** The interventions on the exposed alar cartilages depend on requirements in the individual case. **(b)** The examples in the graphic show scoring (1) and wedge resection (2) of the dome, domal strip resection (3), and dome suture (4).

All intranasal incisions are carefully closed at the end using fine, rapidly absorbable sutures (6–0 or 5–0 polyglactin 910; e.g., Vicryl Rapide). Tamponades are just as unnecessary as with the open technique; surgical dressing is similarly performed in much the same manner and is dependent on the surgical procedure undertaken on the cartilaginous and bony vaults. Placement of an external aluminum splint depends on whether and which osteotomies have been required, and not on the choice of open or closed approach for rhinoplasty.

The endonasal osteotomy technique is described in section 8.2.

16.3 Open or Closed Approach?

As described in this chapter, endonasal approaches provide a wide range of surgical options with the closed technique (► Video 16.7, ► Video 16.8, ► Video 16.9, ► Video 16.10, ► Video 16.11, ► Video 16.12, ► Video 16.13, ► Video 16.14). For decision-making on whether an open

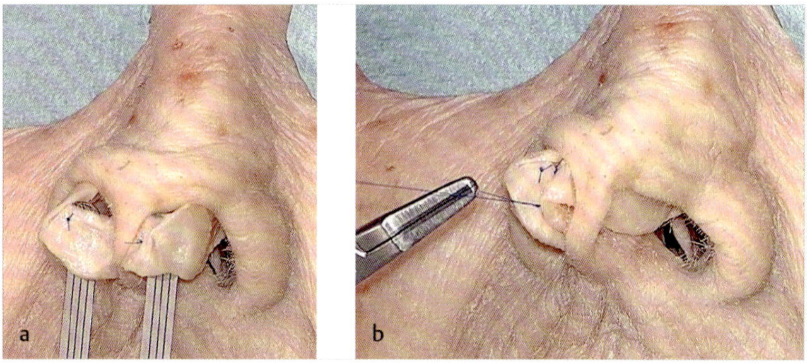

Fig. 16.15 Suturing techniques at the nasal tip during delivery (shown in a cadaver specimen). **(a)** Domal sutures after wedge resections at the domes. **(b)** Interdomal suture; both alar cartilages are delivered through one nostril. The intact columella skin should be noted.

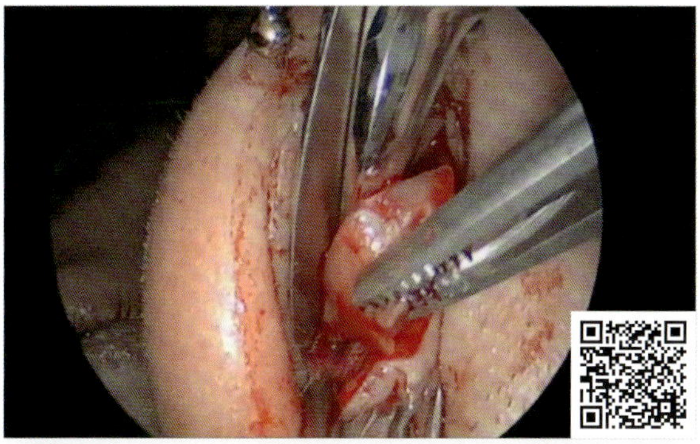

Video 16.7 Endonasal cephalic resection (clinical case).

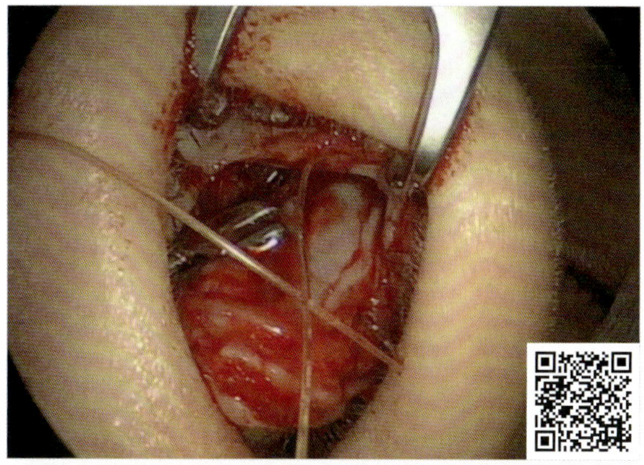

Video 16.8 Endonasal crura suspension suture (clinical case).

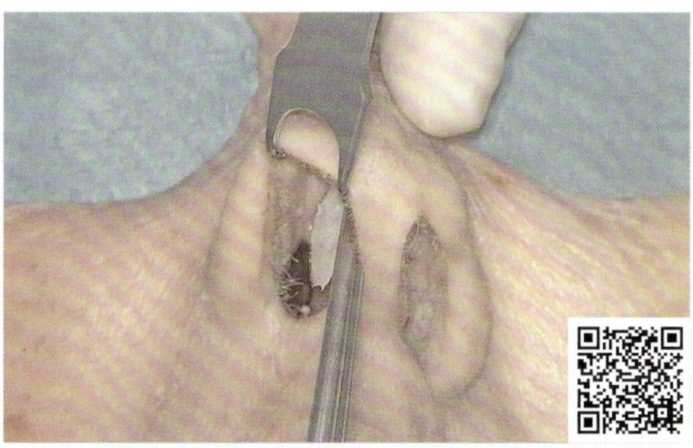

Video 16.9 Intercartilaginous incision and dorsal onlay graft (cadaver head).

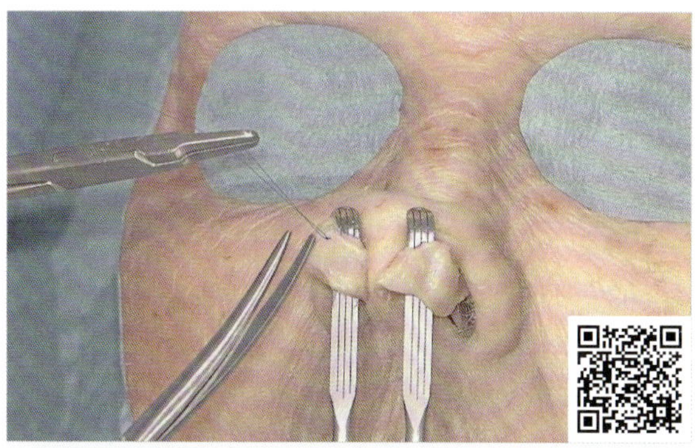

Video 16.10 Delivery with alar scoring, domal wedge resection, and tip sutures (cadaver head).

or a closed procedure is preferable in a given case, it is helpful to consider the respective advantages of the methods (▶ Table 16.1). Endonasal incisions allow rapid access to circumscribed areas of the nose that require isolated correction ("pocket surgery"). This advantage over the more complex open approach should be used in suitable cases for narrowly defined indications. A closed endonasal approach offers a less complicated, rapid access route when the nasal dorsum or the upper two-thirds of the nasal vault alone require correction and the nasal tip is not the primary area of interest (▶ Fig. 16.16a–d). On the other hand, the open procedure provides simplified access, a

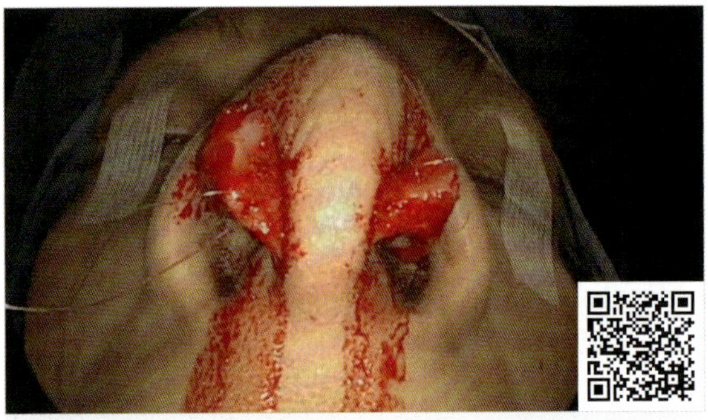

Video 16.11 Endonasal interdomal suture (clinical case).

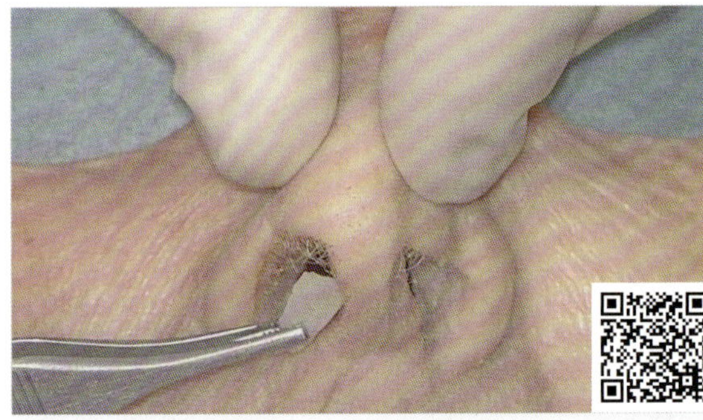

Video 16.12 Endonasal tip graft (cadaver head).

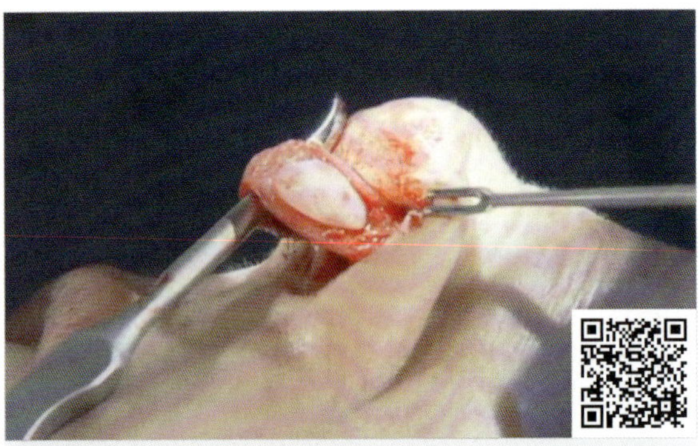

Video 16.13 Complex endonasal correction of a tip with a convexity control suture, batten graft, strut, and button graft (clinical case).

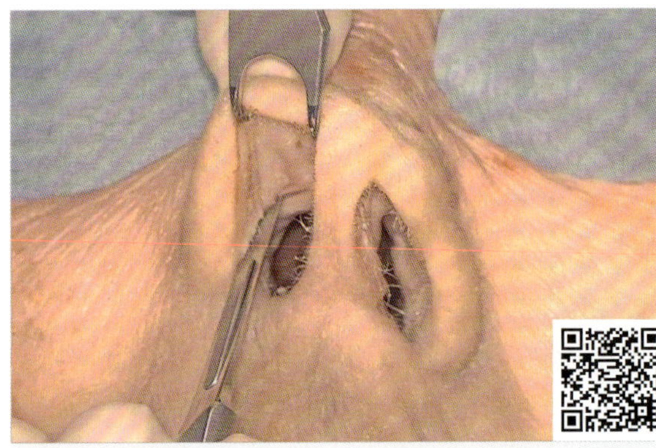

Video 16.14 Intercartilaginous incision and dorsal onlay graft (cadaver head).

Table 16.1 Comparison of preferred applications of the open and closed approaches

Indications for a closed approach
• Corrections/revisions of the upper two-thirds/on the nasal dorsum
• Circumscribed corrections of the columella / nasal alae / tip (pocket surgery)
• Patient declines the open technique
Indications for an open approach
• Major asymmetry/scars/complex corrections of the tip, supratip, and middle third
• Short columella/small nostrils
• Reconstruction of a stable framework (with costal cartilage)
• Closure of large septal perforations
• Piezoelectric surgery

better overview, and greater latitude, if the aim is correction of complex deformities or revision of severely scarred noses, especially in the region of the tip and supratip (▸ Fig. 16.17a–h). The same also applies to a particularly short columella or small nostrils, which make closed access too narrow. The open approach is superior to an endonasal procedure if it is necessary to insert complex supporting structures consisting of interconnected costal cartilage transplants. This also applies to the treatment of large septal perforations and the use of the piezoelectric technique.

Advocates of the closed technique and supporters of the open approach are no longer openly hostile to each other – unlike in the past – since it is now well known that these surgical techniques complement each other and that each may be indicated in a given case. Surgeons select one method over the other on the basis of their individual experience and skill.

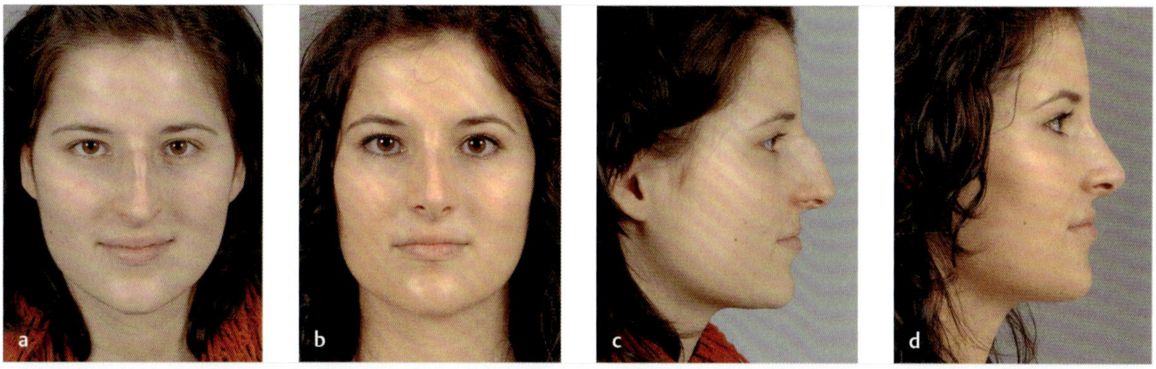

Fig. 16.16 Endonasal rhinoplasty; clinical case. (a, c) Crooked hump nose. **(b, d)** After endonasal rhinoplasty with conventional instruments; luxation technique.

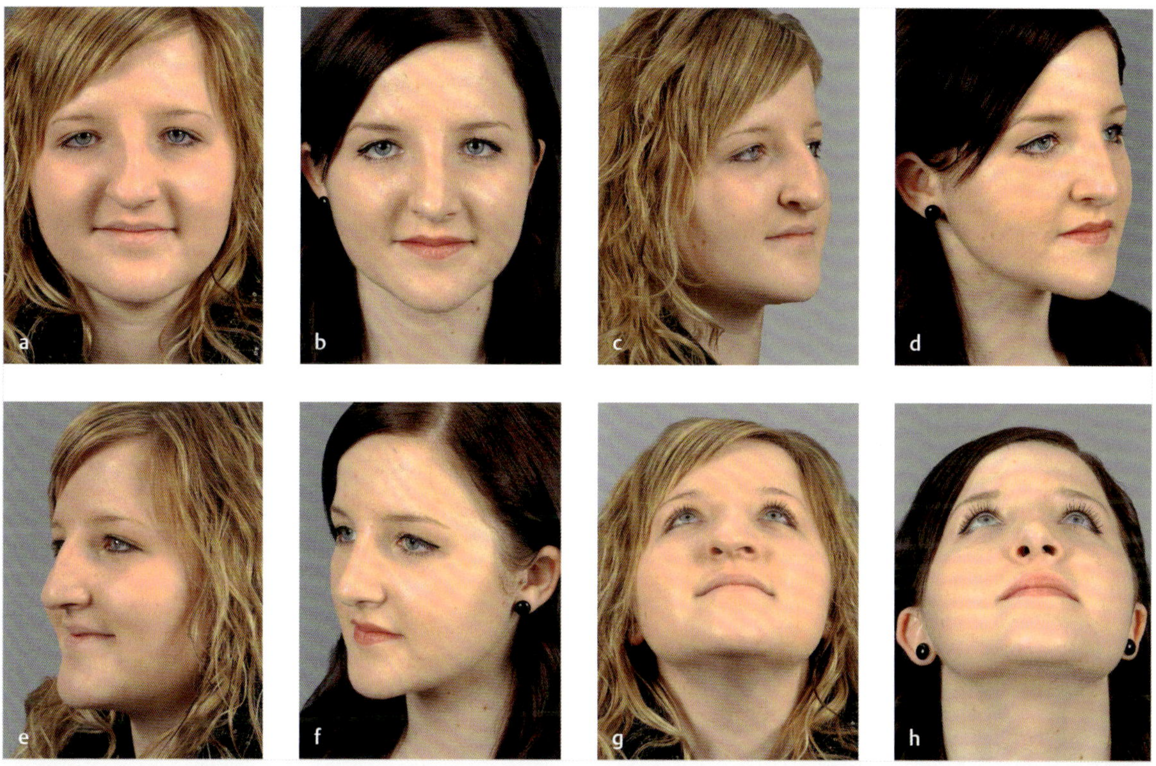

Fig. 16.17 Hump, asymmetry, and complex deformities of the nasal tip as indications for an open technique. **(a, c, e, g)** An open approach is recommended in patients with complex deformities such as these – asymmetric crooked hump nose with tip drop and wide, asymmetric tip. **(b, d, f, h)** After open access rhinoplasty. The result shown was achieved in two operative steps.

Bibliography

Aiach G. Atlas of rhinoplasty: open and endonasal approaches. Vol. 2. St. Louis: Quality Medical Publishing; 2003

Albert MG, Constantian MB. The principles and practice of primary endonasal rhinoplasty. Ann Plast Surg. 2022; 88(1):7–13

Berghaus A. New instruments for rhinoplasty: operating mirror and alar guiding set. Plast Reconstr Surg. 2006; 117(7):2224–2225

Berghaus A. Modern rhinoplasty: is there a place for the closed approach? Facial Plast Surg. 2016; 32(4):402–408

Cafferty A, Becker DG. Open and closed rhinoplasty. Clin Plast Surg. 2016; 43(1):17–27

Joseph J. Nasenplastik und sonstige Gesichtsplastik. Leipzig: Curt Kabitzsch; 1931 [Reprint; Kaden, Heidelberg:2004]

Pastorek N, Ham J. The underprojecting nasal tip: an endonasal approach. Facial Plast Surg Clin North Am. 2004; 12(1):93–106

Sheen JH. Closed versus open rhinoplasty – and the debate goes on. Plast Reconstr Surg. 1997; 99(3):859–862

Tardy ME. Rhinoplasty: the art and the science. Philadelphia: Saunders; 1997

17 Reconstruction of the Nasal Framework

Revision surgery after rhinoplasty or corrective surgery for trauma sometimes entails several reconstructive procedures, which may be more like a nasal reconstruction rather than a typical rhinoplasty. Surgeons who wish to achieve good results with revision rhinoplasty also need to be familiar with nasal reconstruction procedures. This is particularly true for restoration of the supporting framework, including the septum, lateral walls, and nasal dorsum.

17.1 Reconstruction of the L-strut

As mentioned under septoplasty in section 7.4, an L-shaped frame of septal cartilage (L-strut) has to be preserved over the nasal dorsum and the caudal edge of the septum in all procedures on the cartilaginous septum, in order to prevent the collapse of the middle and anterior nasal vault (▶ Fig. 17.1).

This functional supporting framework has to be reconstructed if it is defective, as in patients after prior rhinoplasty or trauma. The L-strut should be at least 8–10 mm wide. Intentional or unintentional intraoperative elimination of this cartilaginous angle requires immediate reconstruction and restabilization with cartilaginous strips or delicate bony lamellae, such as those obtained from the perpendicular plate, and must be securely fixed with sutures (see section 7.4 for surgical principles).

The L-strut may be unavailable in patients with a severe saddle deformity of the anterior nose with retracted columella following trauma, tumor surgery, previous septoplasty, or rhinoplasty, and it has to be reconstructed in such cases ("foundation graft"). Auricular cartilage alone is very often not sufficient for reconstruction, and augmentation using costal cartilage is required in order to ensure stability.

The costal cartilage transplant must not be too large, despite the required stability; a voluminous graft may heal poorly, as cartilage is nourished by diffusion. Ideally, intact graft material should be used for replacement of the septum, and it must be of the same thickness as the deficient cartilage, with a maximum thickness of 2 mm.

Although a costal cartilage graft can be shaped into a one-piece L-strut, like many colleagues I prefer to combine two separate grafts (▶ Fig. 17.2): an anterior septal replacement graft and another replacement graft for the nasal dorsum. There are several arguments in favor of this approach:

- This construction provides several configuration options.
- It is easier to obtain two shorter pieces from one rib than a longer, angular one.
- In case the cartilage bends later, this will have less of an effect on shorter grafts than on longer ones.

First, a septal replacement graft is inserted (see section 11.1.2), supplemented by a dorsal foundation graft, which has a small recess in the front edge for central attachment to the septal replacement graft. Both grafts have to have the appropriate shape and size, and they are securely sutured together using 5–0 PDS. The anterior septal replacement graft should be sutured firmly to the anterior nasal spine, if possible, and the dorsal graft to the bony nasal dorsum.

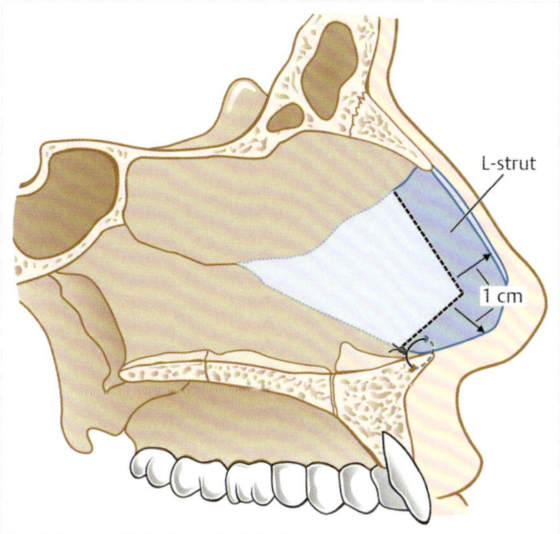

Fig. 17.1 L-strut. The L-strut of the septum has to be retained or reconstructed as a stable functional component of the nasal framework.

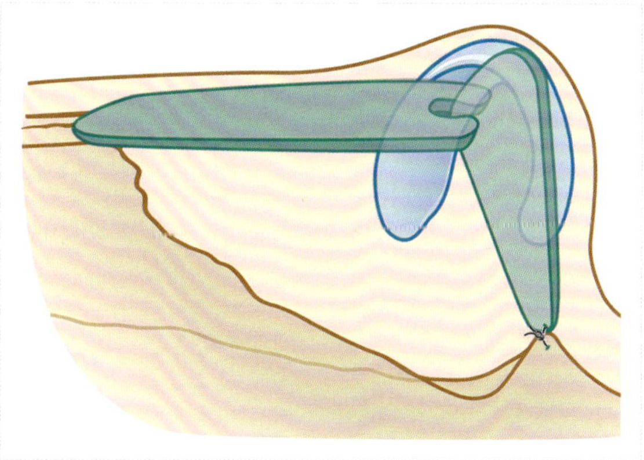

Fig. 17.2 Two-piece L-strut. A two-piece L-strut can be used, with the two parts securely held together.

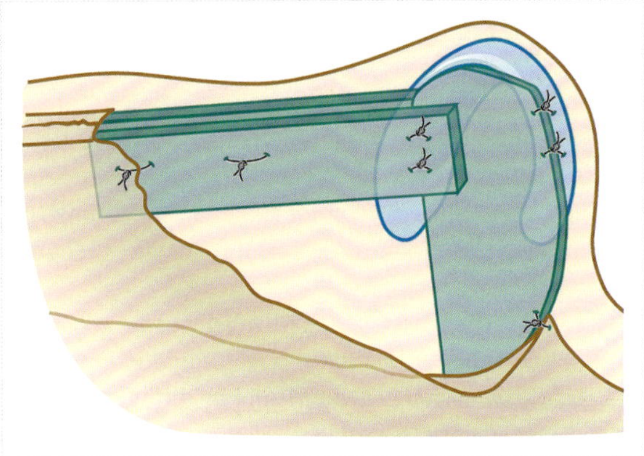

Fig. 17.3 Replacement of the septum with a septal graft and two spreader grafts. The new framework is securely attached to the nasal bone, the anterior nasal spine, and the lateral cartilages. Additional cartilage grafts can be used to replace the upper lateral cartilages in patients with collapsed lateral walls.

Two lateral spreader grafts (▶ Fig. 17.3) can also be used as an alternative to a single piece of cartilage for the nasal dorsum.

✓

Intraoperative fabrication of sterile models — e.g., from cardboard or aluminum suture packaging — is highly recommended before trimming of costal cartilage grafts (▶ Fig. 17.4), for the following reasons:

- The need for repeated tentative insertion of the graft into the graft bed is largely eliminated.
- The time required for graft remodeling is significantly reduced.
- The risk of bacterial infection of cartilage is also significantly reduced.
- Errors in trimming suitable transplants to the appropriate size, and thus material losses, are largely avoided.

Additional grafts can then be affixed to this basic framework (functional structure; foundation graft) as needed, such as replacements for the upper or lower lateral cartilages, and onlay grafts for further elevation of the nasal dorsum (the aesthetic structure), if required (see section 17.2).

This form of nasal vault reconstruction can also be used in cases of septal perforations that cannot be simultaneously closed due to their sheer size (▶ Fig. 17.5a–d; ▶ Video 17.1). The cartilage grafts are then placed between the mucosal layers on each side — without opening up the edges of the perforation, which would

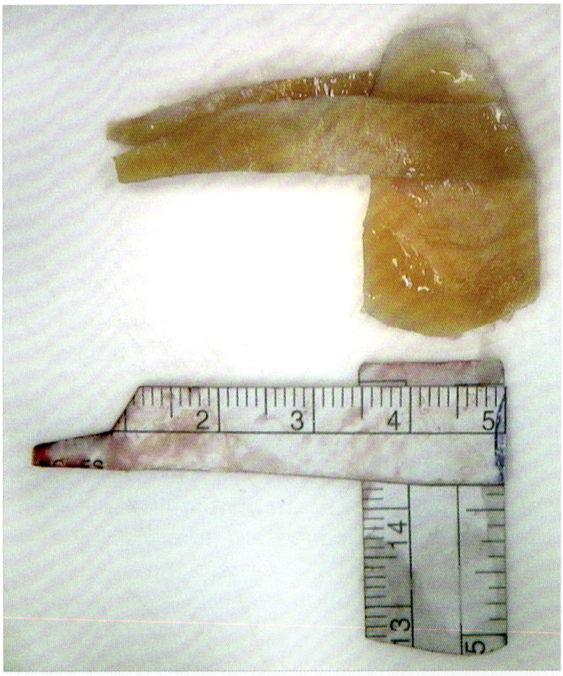

Fig. 17.4 L-strut and a paper model. A composite rib graft for the septum and nasal dorsum, with a prefabricated model made of paper.

facilitate bacterial infection of the reconstructed nasal vault, thereby compromising the surgical outcome.

✓

Intraoperative and postoperative antibiotic therapy is strongly recommended (e.g., with ampicillin/sulbactam; e.g., Unasyn), since purulent infection can rapidly destroy costal cartilage and the reconstructed nasal vault.

Costal cartilage is practically always used for constructs of this size, and it inevitably gives rise to a relatively rugged framework. Its contours can then be rounded off and irregularities corrected by coating with diced cartilage (▶ Fig. 17.6a–g; see section 17.2.3).

17.2 Reconstruction and Augmentation of the Nasal Dorsum

17.2.1 Onlay Grafts

An excessively depressed nasal dorsum is elevated using cartilage grafts, including onlay grafts as compact transplants (▶ Fig. 17.7, ▶ Fig. 17.8a, b), or diced, fragmented

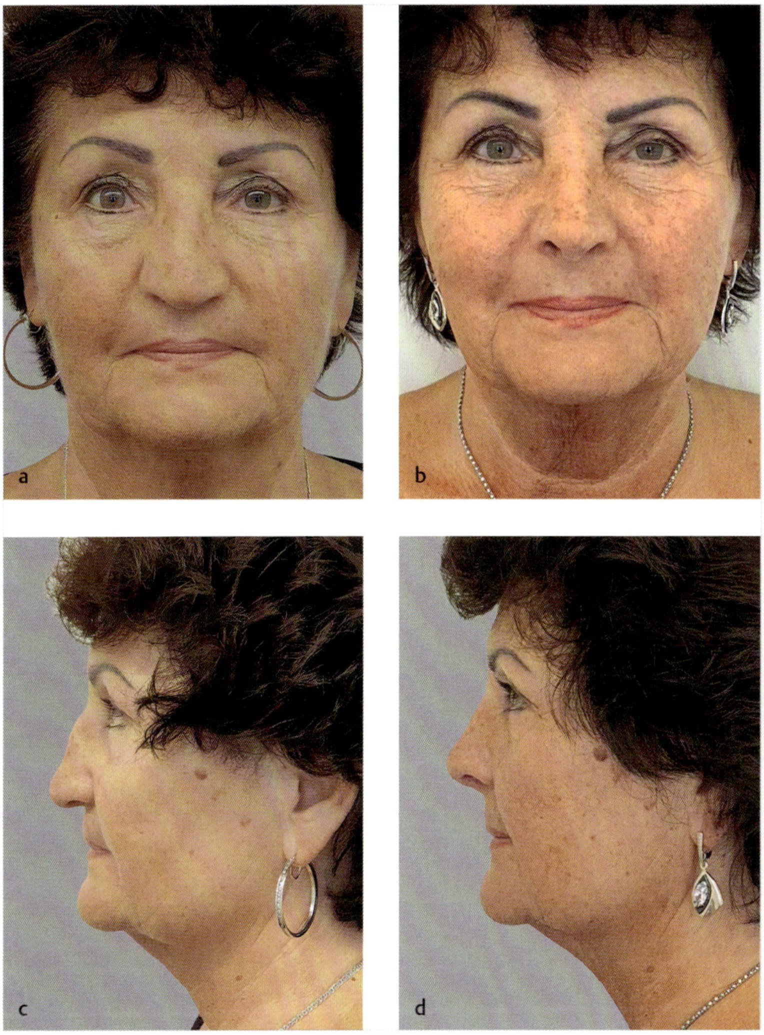

Fig. 17.5 Reconstruction of the nasal framework in a patient with a large septal perforation; case study. (a, c) Drooping nasal tip with unstable nasal framework and large septal perforation consequent to nasal trauma in infancy. **(b, d)** The nasal framework has been reconstructed using costal cartilage transplants, as shown in ▶ Fig. 17.3. The reconstruction was performed around the perforation between the preserved mucous membranes, without opening the perforation.

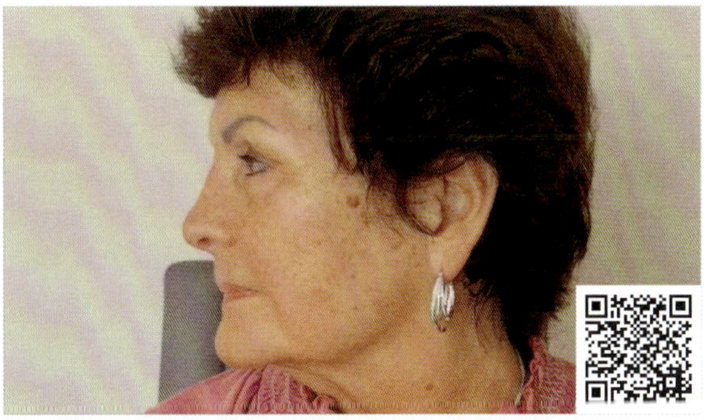

Video 17.1 Reconstruction of the L-strut in a patient with a large septal perforation.

cartilage (aesthetic structure; see ▶ Fig. 17.6). The edges of onlay grafts should not become visible through the skin over time ("contouring") and must therefore be thinned with the scalpel or manually softened with a squeezing forceps (compare with ▶ Fig. 12.27, ▶ Fig. 12.28). A depressed nasal dorsum in patients with a saddle nose can usually be corrected using an onlay graft harvested from conchal cartilage (▶ Fig. 17.8a,b).

Small irregularities can be corrected by endonasal insertion of tiny onlay grafts through an intercartilaginous incision into a narrow graft bed under the dorsal nasal skin (pocket surgery). This procedure carries a low risk of subsequent dislocation (migration). Larger transplanted cartilage can be sutured to the graft bed (see ▶ Fig. 17.7). Very delicate grafts or fragile cartilage (especially from the rib) involve a risk of graft fracture through the suture, which can be reduced by passing 6–0 or 5–0 sutures through prefabricated perforations in the cartilage (▶ Fig. 17.9). These perforations into the cartilage can be made using a large cannula, diamond drill, or — particularly advantageously — a piezoelectric device. The graft

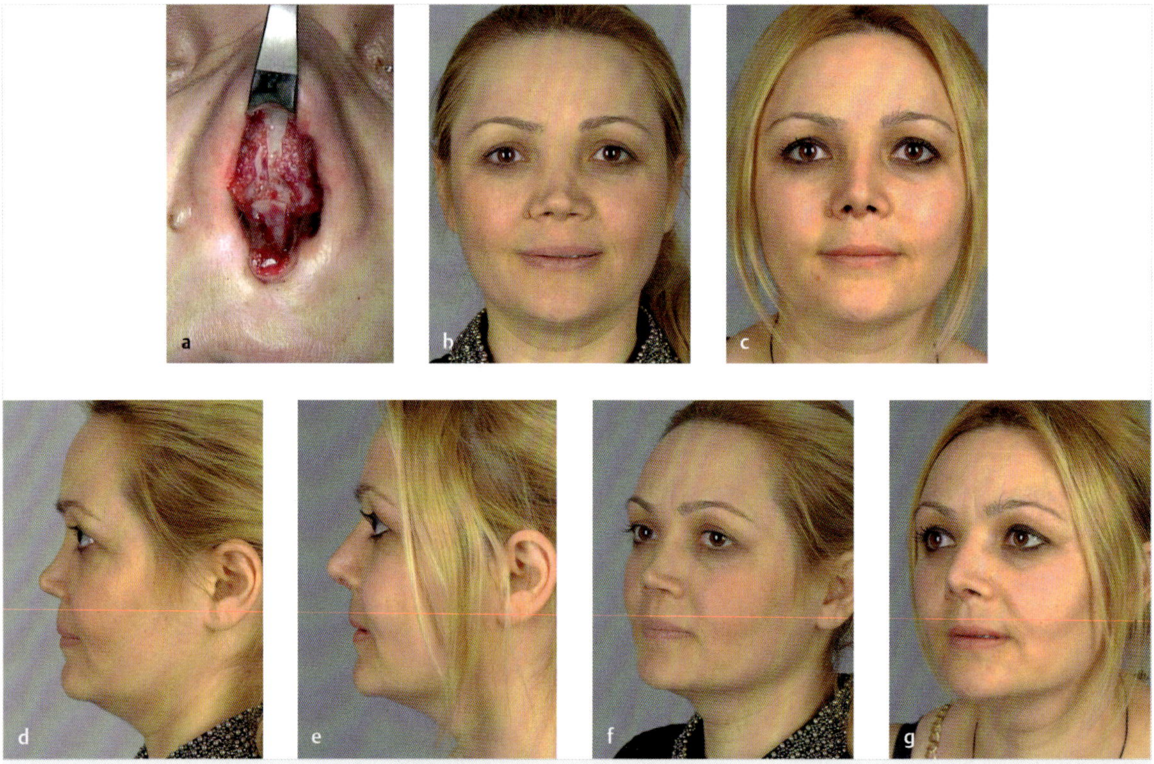

Fig. 17.6 Rib cartilage frame and diced cartilage. (a) The intraoperative situation after reconstruction of the nasal framework with costal cartilage and contour correction with diced cartilage. The diced cartilage allows rounding and volume replenishment of the new cartilaginous vault. **(b, d, f)** Preoperative views of the severely saddled nose. **(c, e, g)** The result after reconstruction of the nasal framework with solid and diced costal cartilage.

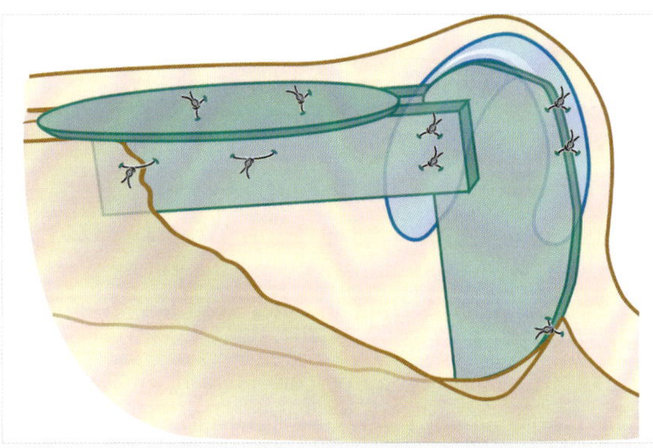

Fig. 17.7 Onlay graft. Augmentation of the nasal dorsum with an onlay aesthetic structure graft, placed on two functional foundation grafts using costal cartilage. A graft of this size is held in place with sutures.

can also be affixed using fibrin glue or TachoSil, if necessary (▶ Video 17.2; ▶ Fig. 17.10a, b; see below and section 17.2.3). The risk of migration is slightly higher with conchal grafts than with grafts harvested from septal or rib cartilage.

> If at all possible, a graft should be sutured in such a way that fine corrections of the graft edges can still be carried out with a scalpel, without cutting the suture.

To avoid some of the risks associated with solid rib segments and diced cartilage fascia constructs – such as edge visibility, potential warping, distortion, junction irregularity, and asymmetries in the dorsal contour – E. Robotti has proposed a promising technique using a sandwich of perichondrium and rectus fascia (SPF) or a sandwich of perichondrium, rib lamination, and rectus fascia (SPLF) as a single unit over the entire dorsum.

17.2.2 Radix Graft

A deep radix lies below the dorsal line of the nose and is comparable to a saddle nose, which is also characterized by a depressed nasal dorsum. A deep radix is frequently associated with a narrow nasofrontal angle, with the radix and medial canthus lying close together, as seen on the

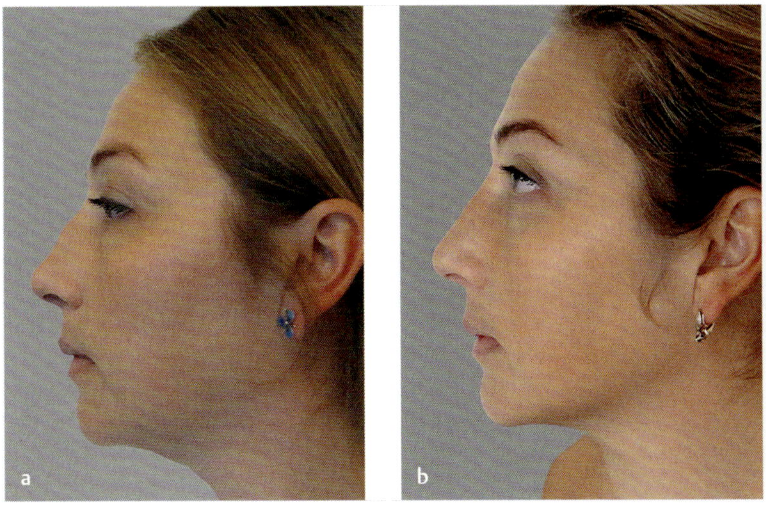

Fig. 17.8 Correction of a saddle nose with conchal cartilage. (a) Saddle deformity of the cartilaginous framework after septoplasty elsewhere. **(b)** After endonasal correction using a conchal cartilage graft.

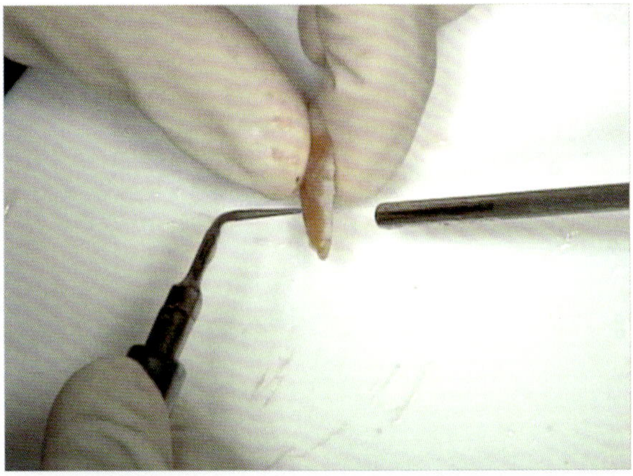

Fig. 17.9 Making holes in a graft. The piezoelectric technique is ideally suited for perforating a cartilage transplant, even if there is some calcification in it.

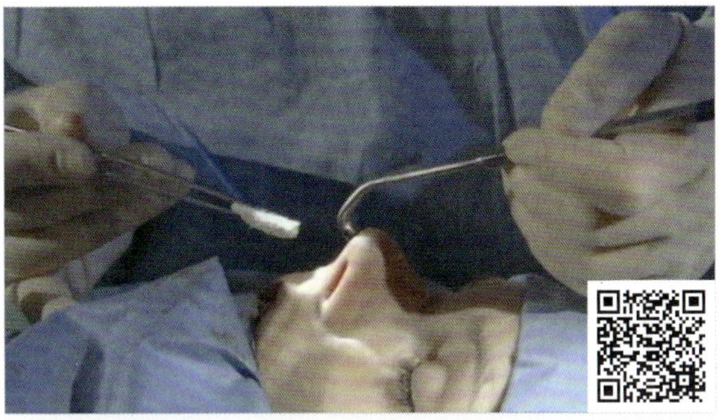

Video 17.2 Correction of a saddle nose using conchal cartilage and TachoSil (clinical case).

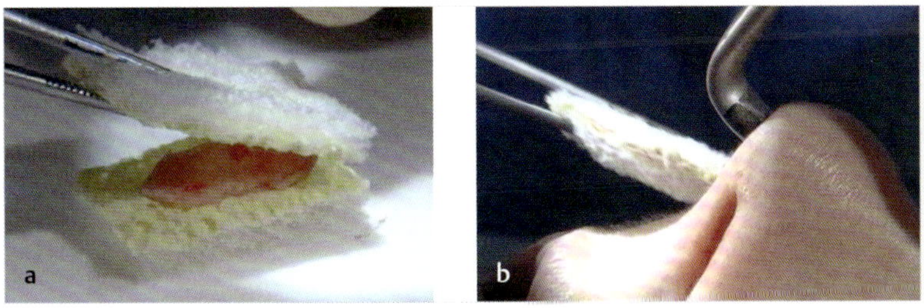

Fig. 17.10 Fixation of a solid cartilage graft with TachoSil. (a) The cartilage graft is inserted between two layers of TachoSil, creating a compound "sandwich" in the example shown. **(b)** Introduction into the nasal dorsum via an endonasal approach.

lateral view (see section 2.9). This may necessitate augmentation only in this circumscribed, cranial segment of the nasal dorsum. A radix graft is used in such instances (▸ Fig. 17.11a,b).

Compact pieces of cartilage cut to size are ideal for this purpose. These are firmly fixed in a narrow graft bed (usually easily prepared in this region, unlike the middle third of the nasal dorsum) to prevent graft dislocation (▸ Fig. 17.12a,b). Suture fixation of a radix graft, on the other hand, is much more difficult. The radix can also be augmented using finely fragmented, diced cartilage, if a compact transplant is not available.

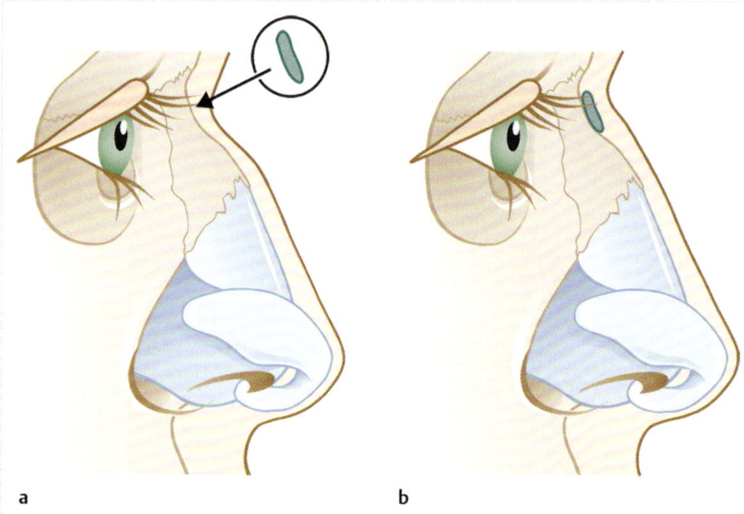

Fig. 17.11 Radix graft. A low radix **(a)** is elevated using a radix graft **(b)**.

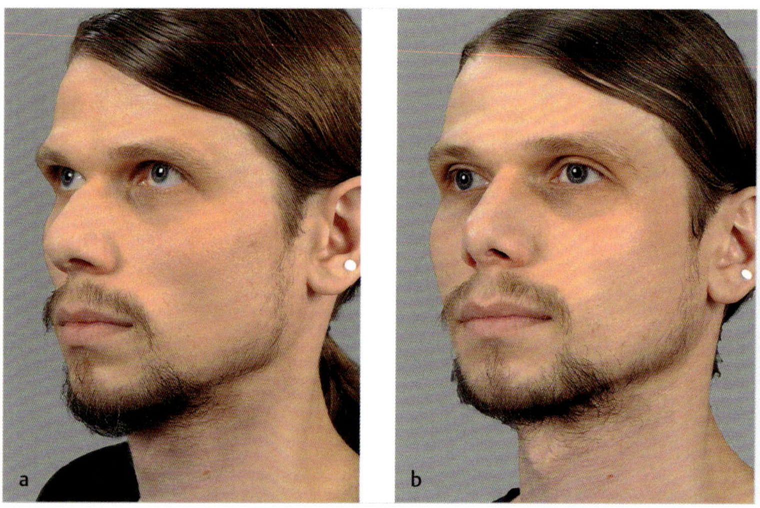

Fig. 17.12 Correction of a low radix with a radix graft; clinical case. (a) Low radix, with a narrow nasofrontal angle. **(b)** After rhinoplasty, with a compact radix graft.

Not every low-seeming radix requires correction using a radix graft. Careful preoperative analysis helps determine whether lowering the nasal dorsum by hump reduction will adequately correct this appearance in a given case (▶ Fig. 17.13a, b).

17.2.3 Diced Cartilage

Finely diced cartilage has proven useful in many types of reconstructive plastic surgery. Cartilage can be used in the form of coarse or fine cubes, fine flakes, in finely diced form, or even as a paste during rhinoplasty, depending on individual needs. All graft cartilage – whether it is from the nasal septum, the ear, or the rib – can be diced as required.

Cartilage is diced on a stable, flat, metallic, or hard plastic worktop, ideally using a large, sterile dermatome blade gripped with both hands. The process of chopping into progressively smaller pieces is similar to chopping onions in the kitchen.

> ✓
>
> Preparing the cartilage in this manner is time-consuming and may take 30 minutes or more, depending on the amount and fineness of the cartilage to be diced. A surgical nurse or an assistant can take over this procedure to save time, while the surgeon continues with the operation.

Moisture released from the cartilage during this process should be absorbed by dabbing with a dry compress, so that the material is largely dry before it is used for transplantation.

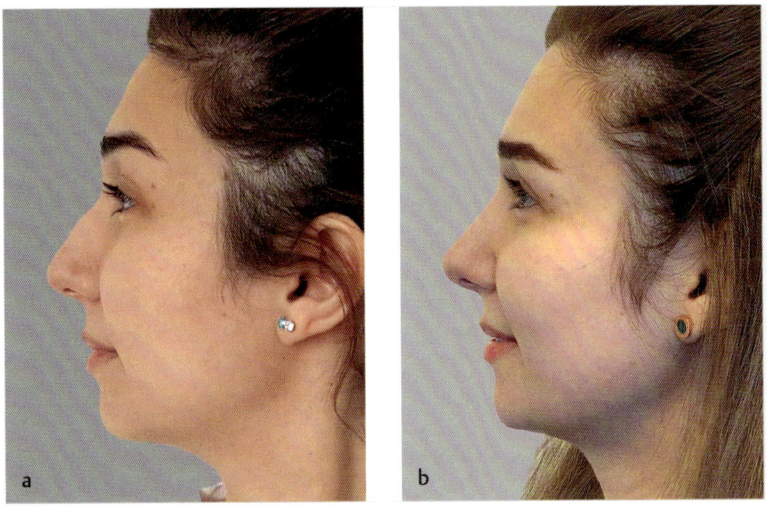

Fig. 17.13 Correction of a relatively deep radix by hump removal; clinical case. (a) A relatively low radix in a patient with hump nose. **(b)** Corrective rhinoplasty with hump removal, without a radix graft.

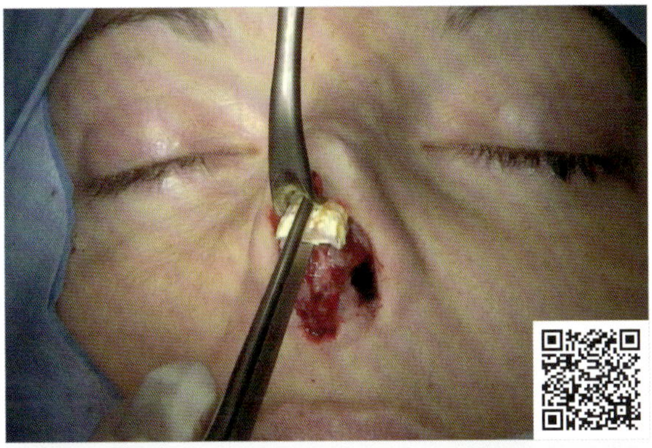

Video 17.3 Diced cartilage and TachoSil for correction of the nasal dorsum (clinical case).

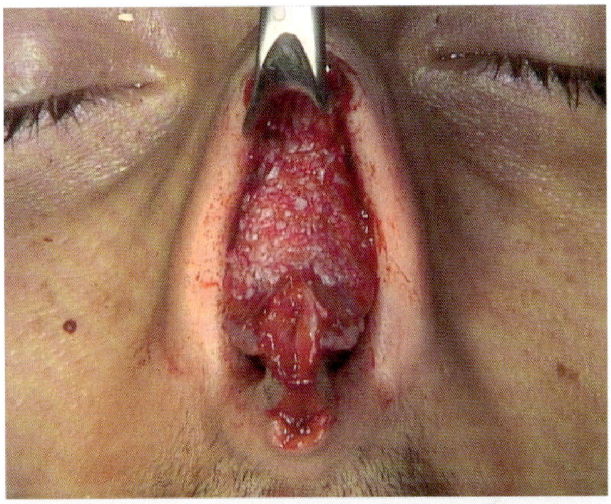

Fig. 17.14 Diced cartilage to correct the profile of the nasal dorsum.

Diced cartilage is ideally suited for correcting minor defects and irregularities, especially on the nasal dorsum (▶ Video 17.3; ▶ Fig. 17.14), lateral walls, or nasal tip. If a comprehensive reconstruction of the nasal framework is carried out with costal cartilage, the material provides support for the precision work, rounding off the framework structure like a filling material at the end. Tiny pieces of diced cartilage have been found to undergo more rapid absorption than compact pieces. Nevertheless, the use of overly large diced cubes should be avoided, especially in patients with thin skin, since their contours begin to show through over time (known as the "cobblestone" effect; ▶ Fig. 17.15a, b). The edges of the diced fragments should not exceed 0.5 mm in length; the smaller they are, the lower the risk of contouring.

Based on experience, diced septal cartilage does not undergo significant absorption, but one must generally expect a certain degree of absorption of auricular and especially costal cartilage, regardless of the size of the fragments used.

Fixation of Diced Cartilage

The extent to which diced cartilage can be left in situ without any fixation remains unclear. Application of a few drops of the patient's blood is sufficient for small volumes. When in doubt, I prefer securing larger quantities of diced cartilage using a layer of TachoSil.

Diced Cartilage and TachoSil

TachoSil is a ready-to-use collagen foam or sponge, coated with a layer of human fibrinogen and thrombin, mimicking the final steps of physiological blood clotting in vivo. The material is used for intraoperative hemostasis, and

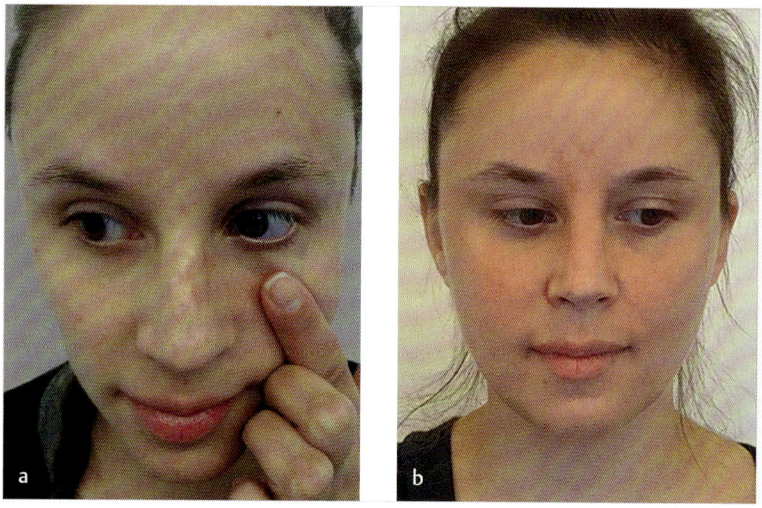

Fig. 17.15 Cobblestone deformity. **(a)** Cobblestone deformity due to inadequately crushed diced cartilage in a patient with thin skin. **(b)** Nine months after revision of the nasal dorsum and covering with TachoSil.

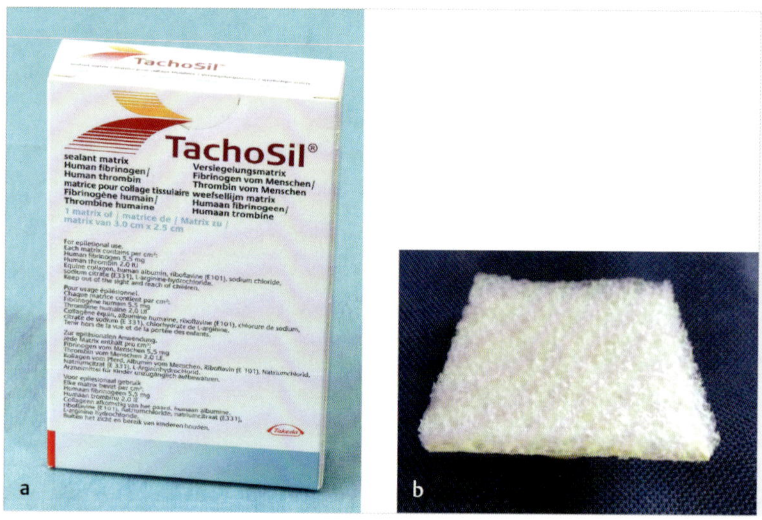

Fig. 17.16 TachoSil. **(a)** TachoSil sealant matrix. **(b)** Before moistening. The yellowish area containing the active pharmaceuticals is on the underside (Corza Medical, Inc., Westwood, MA, USA).

also for sealing and bonding anatomical structures. The dry foam has a honeycomb structure, attributable to the type I collagen it contains (▶ Fig. 17.16a, b). Both coagulation factors and the local antibiotic riboflavin are present as a coating on the yellow aspect of the foam. The material is dry-processed as far as possible and applied at the required site – e.g., to cover or wrap diced cartilage. Moisture produced by the addition of water or blood results in a reaction of the active substances and rapid clot formation. The TachoSil layer rapidly becomes soft and very sticky, resulting in a paper-thin sealant patch, which is about 2 mm thick when dry (▶ Fig. 17.17). Hemostasis or tissue fixation can thus be achieved within 3–5 minutes.

The resultant collagen patch with fibrin clot creates an airtight and liquid-tight tissue seal. Enzymatic resorption of TachoSil takes about 12 weeks. Histological studies have shown complete absorption with fibrinolysis of the clot, followed by the invasion of fibrovascular granulation tissue containing fibroblasts, neutrophils, lymphocytes, and giant cells.

TachoSil is available in three different sizes; for rhinoplasty, the smallest size of 3.0 × 2.5 cm is appropriate. A layer of this biological adhesive can be placed on cartilage in situ before the skin flap is repositioned (▶ Fig. 17.14, ▶ Fig. 17.17). Alternatively, diced cartilage can be applied extracorporeally to a layer of TachoSil or sandwiched between two TachoSil layers and then used in this stabilized form in the operating field (▶ Fig. 17.18a–d).

TachoSil is particularly easy to use in comparison with platelet-rich fibrin, as well as liquid fibrin adhesives such as Tisseel or Tissucol. It does not need to be refrigerated or frozen and is available in ready-to-use packaging. TachoSil can be trimmed exactly to the required size with simple scissors.

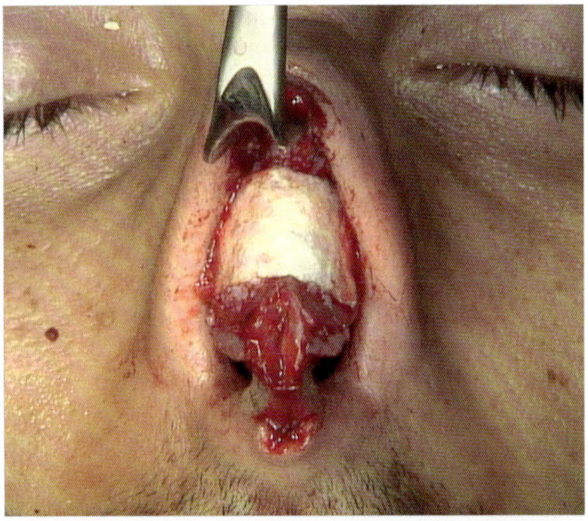

Fig. 17.17 Fixation of diced cartilage with a layer of TachoSil.

The patient should be informed about the use of TachoSil during the preoperative briefing, as it is a blood product. The surgeon should always clarify whether using TachoSil represents an off-label use in the given case, and this may need to be communicated to the patient.

Diced Cartilage and Platelet-Rich Fibrin

Platelet-rich fibrin (PRF) is obtained by first drawing venous blood from the patient and centrifuging it in a special centrifuge for about 8 minutes, depending on individual needs. This procedure produces a clot, which can be used as desired by the surgeon. The product is also believed to have a beneficial effect on wound healing.

PRF is thus an autologous blood product and provides an elegant method of fixing the smallest pieces of cartilage or

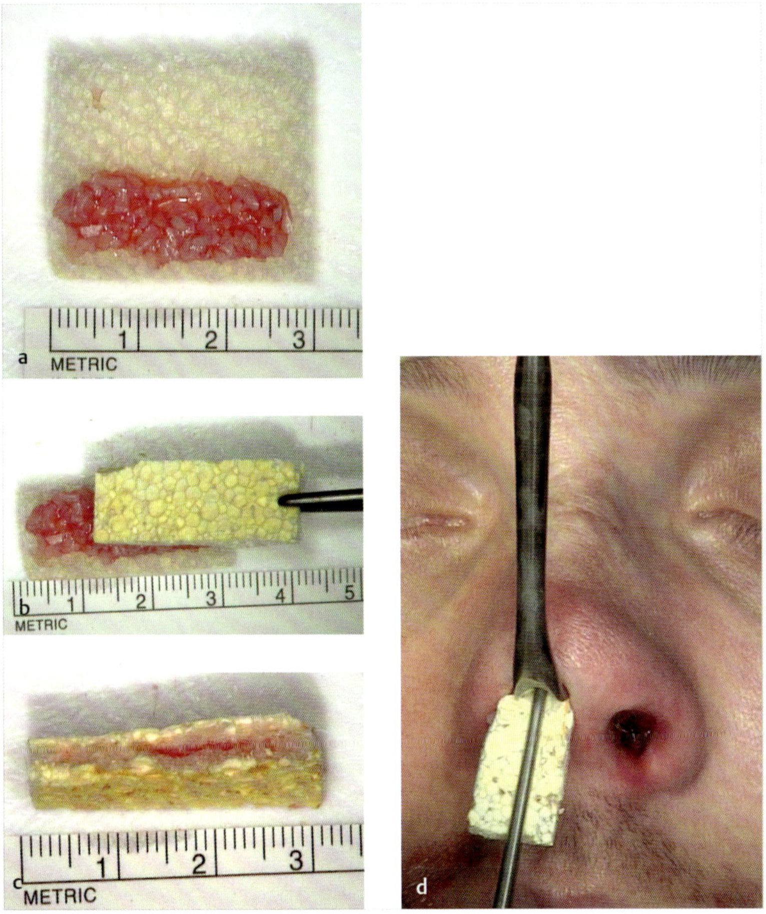

Fig. 17.18 A diced cartilage–TachoSil "sandwich." (a) Diced cartilage (DC) on a layer of TachoSil. **(b)** Covered with another layer of TachoSil. **(c)** The resulting "sandwich" comprised of DC and TachoSil. **(d)** The DC–TachoSil sandwich in this example was placed on the nasal dorsum via an endonasal approach (pocket surgery).

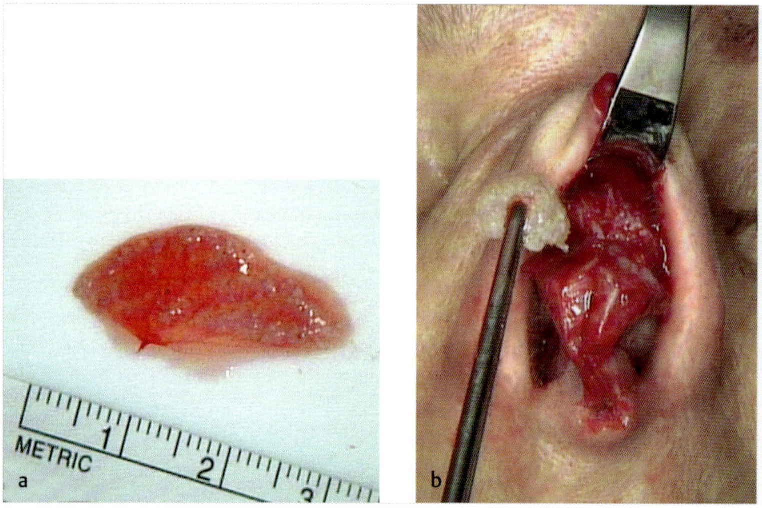

Fig. 17.19 Diced cartilage and platelet-rich fibrin. (a) Diced cartilage embedded in platelet-rich fibrin. **(b)** Intraoperative application.

diced cartilage. Cartilage material placed in situ can be coated with PRF, which adheres to and secures it at the intended site. PRF can also be mixed with diced cartilage on the instrument table. Relatively stable graft material is obtained after clot formation, and it can be inserted into the surgical field as needed, either as a whole piece or sliced into smaller fragments with a scalpel (▶ Fig. 17.19a, b).

In my own experience, tissue bonding with PRF is not always as reliable as with TachoSil. Classic fibrin glue (e.g., Tissucol) can be used in a similar fashion.

Diced Cartilage and Patient Blood

Using the patient's own blood, which clots and provides physiological fixation, is the simplest method of stabilizing diced cartilage. Unfortunately, this method is not nearly as reliable as the other methods described above, and fixation with blood is therefore generally only used as an emergency measure on a very small scale.

Diced Cartilage and Fascia

A commonly recommended procedure for using diced cartilage is encasement with autologous temporal fascia obtained from the temporal region via a separate approach. Diced cartilage is inserted into a small fascial tube or bag and sutured, and the composite graft is then used for augmentation.

Although the good results reported by other authors using diced cartilage in autogenous fascia are not to be disputed, I have achieved satisfactory results with TachoSil over the years and have never considered it necessary to turn to the rather laborious and cumbersome processing of autogenous fascia for this indication. The disadvantage of this is that it requires another operating field and is significantly time-consuming. In addition, when temporal fascia is used, it cannot be clearly predicted whether and to what extent it will be resorbed, or whether scarred nodules or dislocation are to be expected – such influences can, however, significantly affect the result on the bridge of the nose.

Bibliography

Berghaus A, San Nicoló M, Jacobi C. Use of a fibrinogen-thrombin sponge in rhinoplasty. HNO. 2018; 66(2):103–110

Branham GH, Ed. Nasal reconstruction. Facial Plast Surg. 2017 Feb;33(1) ISSN 0736–6825

Burget GC, Menick FJ. Aesthetic reconstruction of the nose. St. Louis: Mosby; 1994

Daniel RK, Calvert JW. Diced cartilage grafts in rhinoplasty surgery. Plast Reconstr Surg. 2004; 113(7):2156–2171

Daniel RK. Diced cartilage grafts in rhinoplasty surgery: current techniques and applications. Plast Reconstr Surg. 2008; 122(6):1883–1891

Erol OO. The Turkish delight: a pliable graft for rhinoplasty. Plast Reconstr Surg. 2000; 105(6):2229–2241, discussion 2242–2243

Fedok FG. Costal cartilage grafts in rhinoplasty. Clin Plast Surg. 2016; 43(1): 201–212

Gantous A, Fernández-Pellón Garcia RF. Nasal reconstruction in granulomatosis with polyangiitis: a two decade review. Facial Plast Surg Aesthet Med. 2023; 25(1):61–67

Hoehne J, Gubisch W, Kreutzer C, Haack S. Refining the nasal dorsum with free diced cartilage. Facial Plast Surg. 2016; 32(4):345–350

Li J, Sang C, Fu R, et al. Long-term complications from diced cartilage in rhinoplasty: a meta-analysis. Facial Plast Surg Aesthet Med. 2022; 24(3): 221–227

Menick F. Nasal reconstruction. Saunders/Mosby, Elsevier; 2009

Miller MQ, Dighe A, Cui Q, Park SS, Christophel JJ. Regenerative medicine in facial plastic and reconstructive surgery: a review. JAMA Facial Plast Surg. 2016; 18(5):391–394

Peer LA. Diced cartilage grafts. J Int Coll Surg. 1954; 22(3 Pt 1):283–291

Robotti E, Leone F. The SPF-SPLF Graft: building the ideal dorsum in revision rhinoplasty. Plast Reconstr Surg. 2020; 145(6):1420–1424

Sheen JH. Spreader graft: a method of reconstructing the roof of the middle nasal vault following rhinoplasty. Plast Reconstr Surg. 1984; 73(2):230–239

Tasman A-J, Suárez GA. The diced cartilage glue graft for radix augmentation in rhinoplasty. JAMA Facial Plast Surg. 2015; 17(4):303–304

Toriumi DM. Subdorsal cantilever graft for elevating the dorsum in ethnic rhinoplasty. Facial Plast Surg Aesthet Med. 2022; 24(3):143–159

Zelken J, Chang CS, Hsiao YC. The pi graft for correction of severe saddle nose deformity. Facial Plast Surg. 2016; 32(4):452–459

18 Grafts and Implants

In nasal surgery, grafts are transplants that are indicated for functional, cosmetic, or reconstructive purposes. Grafts made of cartilage are mainly used in rhinoplasty, and bone is rarely required. In contrast, implants involve foreign materials, which (in addition to metals, ceramics, etc.) can include plastics in particular (see ▶ Table 18.1 for an overview).

18.1 Cartilage or Plastics?

Like many of my colleagues, I prefer to use **autogenous cartilage transplants** in rhinoplasty – i.e., grafts obtained from the same patient in whom they are used.

Allogeneic grafts – i.e., cartilage or fascia derived from human donors and not from the patients themselves, and preserved using chemicals or irradiation – appear to be associated with a higher risk of absorption or infection. However, **cryopreserved** human rib cartilage transplants that have been chemically treated and then deep-frozen have recently become available. They are reported to be better tolerated and more durable (personal communication from F. Herrlinger, Institute of Transfusion Medicine and Tissue Bank, Charité Medical University, Berlin, Germany). My initial experience with some of these transplants has been consistently positive (▶ Fig. 18.1a, b). It remains to be seen whether this will be confirmed over a longer observation period. If so, it would mean a significant simplification for rhinoplasty, as harvesting of costal cartilage could be replaced by such transplants.

Constant movements and micromovements in the lower half of the nose result in eventual rejection of even tissue-compatible **plastic implants**; implants consisting of such foreign materials are therefore associated with a high incidence of failure.

Although the results with plastic implants are initially satisfactory in patients undergoing primary surgery and may well remain stable for a long period in intact tissue, the failure rate is too high to justify their use. This is all

Table 18.1 Various transplants and implants, with their advantages and disadvantages

Material	Advantages	Disadvantages / risks
Autogenous cartilage		
• Septal cartilage	Stability Handling Permanency	Small volume
• Auricular cartilage	Availability	Small volume Poor stability Possible contouring Possible dislocation
• Costal cartilage	Availability Volume Stability	Possible absorption or warping Complex handling if calcified
Preserved allogeneic materials		
• Cartilage, fascia	Availability	Possible risk of infection, absorption, and foreign body reaction
Plastics		
• Porous polyethylene (PE; Medpor) • Gore-Tex • Silicone	Availability Stability Volume No second intervention Durability	Higher risk of infection and rejection; generally not recommended in nasal surgery
Fillers (injectable; absorbable)		
• Hyaluronic acid and others	No surgery, no general anesthesia Rapid effect with suitable indication	Limited range of indications No supportive function Duration of effect limited Risk of serious subsequent damage

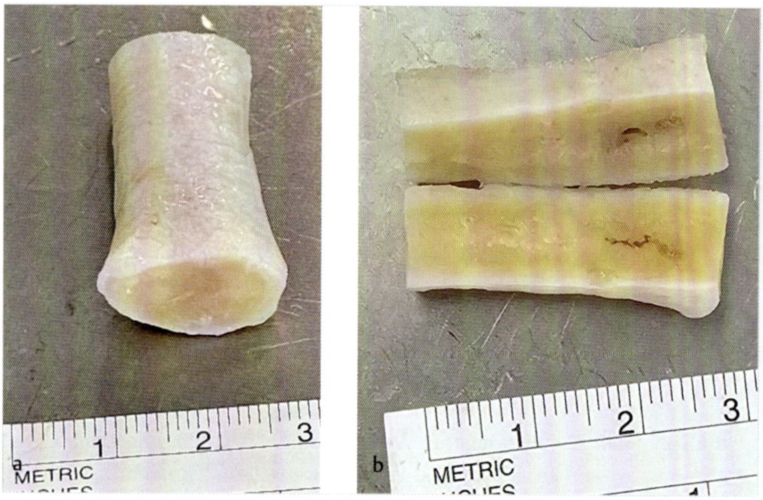

Fig. 18.1 Cryopreserved costal cartilage. **(a)** Human cryopreserved costal cartilage, from the Institute of Transfusion Medicine and Tissue Bank, Charité Medical University, Berlin, Germany. **(b)** Visually and qualitatively, the material hardly differs at all from autogenous costal cartilage in a young patient. The cut surface is comparatively soft and contains only very few zones of low calcification.

the more so since in patients with "healthy" noses who have not previously undergone surgery, there is usually still enough cartilage available from the nasal septum, or if necessary from the cavity of the ear concha, for there to be no need for synthetic materials.

A need for foreign material only arises in cases in which both the septal and auricular cartilage has already been "used up" for reconstructive measures during revision surgery. However, especially in these patients, in whom replacement material is particularly desirable given the lack of cartilage after multiple previous operations, plastic implants are associated with a particularly high incidence of infection and rejection due to severe scarring of atrophic skin and mucosa. Autogenous cartilage is therefore recommended in patients who might theoretically specifically benefit from a plastic implant. Cartilage can be harvested from the rib if septal and auricular cartilage are unavailable in such cases.

It follows from the above that – given the current state of research and development – only autogenous cartilage that comes from the patient can really be regarded as safe augmentation material in nasal surgery. This includes septal, auricular, and costal cartilage. The value of cryopreserved cartilage as graft material still needs to be confirmed through long-term follow-up.

Any reference to "grafts" primarily implies autogenous cartilage material; above all, septal cartilage, auricular cartilage in patients undergoing revisions, or costal cartilage in those requiring more extensive reconstruction. Cartilage material obtained using "tissue engineering" has not yet found its way into routine nasal surgery.

18.2 Harvesting Cartilage Transplants

The selection of the donor organ – nose, ear, or rib – depends on the availability, volume, and quality of cartilage required.

18.2.1 The Nose as a Cartilage Donor

Nose surgeons are fortunate in that they are able to take the best transplant material from the same organ on which they are working anyway.

Septal Cartilage

Cartilage harvested from the nasal septum is ideal for grafting in rhinoplasty in many respects (▶ Table 18.1). Septal cartilage is stable and is not absorbed; adequate amounts are available for most interventions in primary rhinoplasty, and it can be easily accessed for nasal correction without any need to open up another surgical site. Septal cartilage harvesting can be combined with septoplasty, which serves to improve nasal breathing. The two procedures are often very similar, and reference may also be made to Chapter 7 here.

The septal cartilage is easily harvested, with a particularly good overview using the open technique once the quadrangular plate has been exposed, starting from the caudal edge of the septum. Cartilage can also be well harvested via an endonasal hemitransfixion incision, traditionally used for septoplasty (▶ Video 18.1).

The mucoperichondrium must be separated in as intact a state as possible before a cartilage graft is harvested, preventing the development of large tears or defects in this soft-tissue layer. A sharp Freer elevator is ideally used for excision of the graft and separation from the nasal crest of the maxilla and the edge of the perpendicular plate (▶ Fig. 18.2a–c; see also ▶ Fig. 7.7).

✔

It is essential to ensure that the L-strut, approximately 1 cm wide, is preserved as a framework for the septum while cutting out the cartilage.

As there is no further layer of tissue between the mucosal layers after the cartilage has been removed, there is a risk of a resulting septal perforation, particularly if there are corresponding lesions on both sides and/or poorly perfused, atrophic mucosa. Any mucosal perforations are therefore treated with rapidly absorbable 5–0 single interrupted sutures. A septal hematoma can be effectively prevented by multiple side-changing, horizontal mattress sutures placed in a zigzag manner that reattach the mucous membranes to each other and to the septum on either side (see ▶ Fig. 7.19). With this kind of suture, splinting of the nasal septum with silicone plates or Doyle splints is usually unnecessary after the harvesting of a septal cartilage graft.

✓

Once harvested, all cartilage grafts, regardless of their origin, are stored in a moist compress in a safe place, preferably in a separate container, on the instrument table to prevent them from being accidentally disposed of.

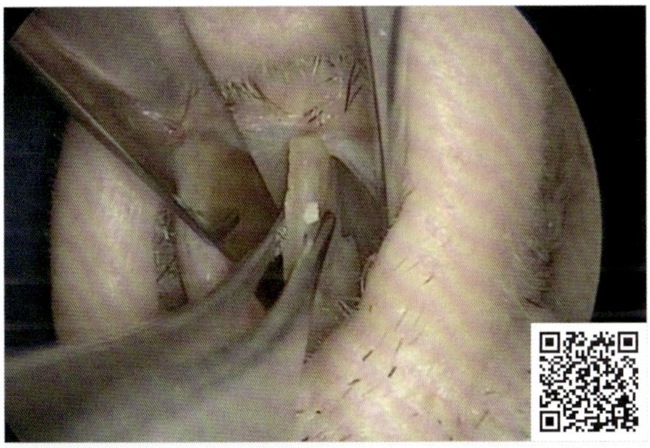

Video 18.1 Endonasal harvesting of septal cartilage (cadaver head).

Alar Cartilage

The more or less narrow resection of cephalic alar cartilage edges is often part of a nasal tip correction (see section 10.2). Cartilage obtained in this way from the edges of the lateral crura should be preserved, like all material removed during rhinoplasty.

The delicate alar cartilage is generally unsuitable for supportive functions; nor can one expect any significant augmentation using this material. However, the fine strips obtained from the crura of the alar cartilages may well be used to compensate for minor irregularities or to add to the cartilaginous mass available for dicing.

18.2.2 The Ear as a Cartilage Donor

Auricular cartilage is the most common alternative when septal cartilage is unavailable.

Conchal Cartilage

In principle, all posteriorly convex regions of auricular cartilage can be resected without significant loss of shape (Gorney et al.; see Bibliography), but cartilage from the cavity of the concha is the most suitable graft material. However, conchal cartilage is not really equivalent to septal cartilage, as it is softer, less malleable, and more brittle. The dimensions, volume, and firmness of auricular cartilage can vary greatly from person to person; the patient's ears therefore have to be examined by palpation before the cartilage is used as graft material. Bilateral harvesting of conchal cartilage can be considered in consultation with the patient, if it is foreseeable that cartilage harvested from one ear may not be sufficient — unless costal cartilage is preferred.

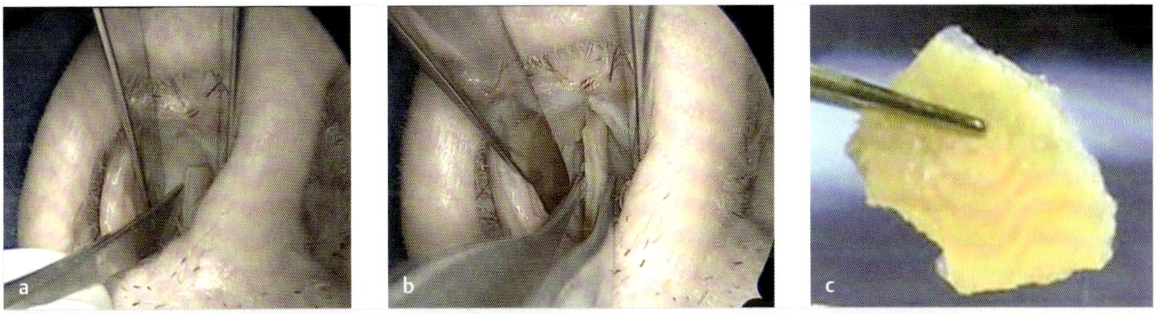

Fig. 18.2 Harvesting a septal cartilage graft (shown in a cadaver specimen). **(a)** Harvesting a cartilage transplant from the septum (endonasal procedure). **(b)** Taking the graft out using Adson–Brown forceps. **(c)** The harvested graft.

18

Patients should be advised about the possible harvesting of auricular cartilage prior to rhinoplasty, even if there is only a remote possibility that such a transplant may be required. Complex forensic choices (is it permissible to harvest auricular cartilage without the patient's consent?) may have to be made if the surgeon is faced with this situation intraoperatively without the patient having been previously informed.

If it is clear that conchal cartilage will be required for rhinoplasty, then for practical reasons harvesting of the transplant should be carried out before the rhinoplasty. The fact that the auricle is regarded as sterile, in contrast to the nose, argues in favor of this sequence. In addition, the surgeon does not need to interrupt the rhinoplasty later to harvest auricular cartilage. If possible, therefore, it is advisable to measure the correct size of cartilage needed on the nose beforehand, so as not to rely on estimates and ensure that the harvested graft is sufficiently large.

It is quite likely that only very little usable septal cartilage will be available during revision surgery in a patient who has previously undergone surgery on the nose, including septoplasty. It is recommended that the presence and amount of available cartilage should be assessed once the local anesthetic has been infiltrated into the septum at the start of revision surgery. It can then be decided with greater certainty whether auricular cartilage is required, or whether available septal cartilage alone will be sufficient.

If there is any doubt whether ear cartilage will be needed during the operation, it has proved useful to disinfect the ear region as well when preparing for the rhinoplasty, so that the ear cartilage can be accessed quickly if necessary.

In contrast to rhinoplasty, I move to a sitting position to harvest auricular cartilage, just as in any ear operation. After local infiltration, a skin incision approximately 1.5–2.0 cm long is made over the posterior aspect of the cavum conchae, along the convexity of the cavity of the concha (the incision thus differs from that used for otoplasty, which requires an incision parallel to the helical rim at a distance of 1 cm). The cartilage of the cavity of the concha is exposed at the posterior aspect following division of the overlying soft tissues (▸ Video 18.2, ▸ Video 18.3; ▸ Fig. 18.3a–g).

During cutting around the area to be lifted, one should be guided by the expected need, which should be measured precisely beforehand on the nose, as far as possible. In case of doubt, not less, but more than can be expected should be taken. However, only cartilage that has a dorsal curve is taken.

I first use the scalpel to cut around the entire cartilaginous segment, without injuring the anterior auricular skin. I then grasp the cartilage at one edge with the Adson–Brown forceps, elevate it slightly, and detach it from the anterior skin covering with fine, pointed scissors using partly cutting and partly spreading movements. Any bleeding is controlled with fine bipolar forceps using low, but adequate thermal energy.

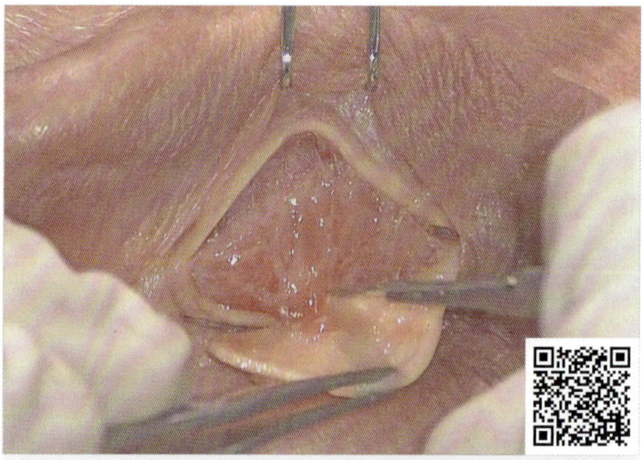

Video 18.2 Harvesting of conchal cartilage (cadaver head).

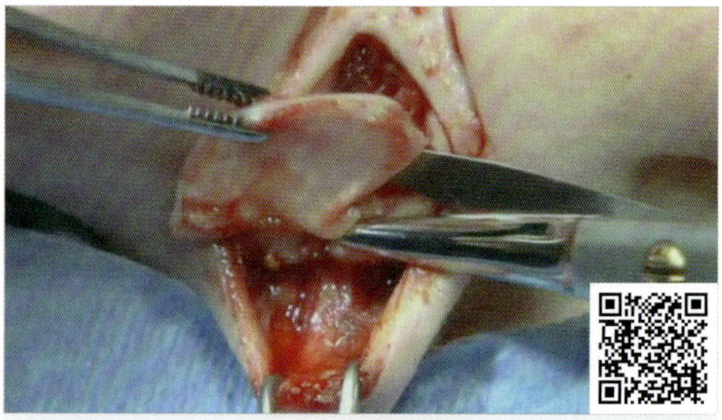

Video 18.3 Harvesting of conchal cartilage (clinical case).

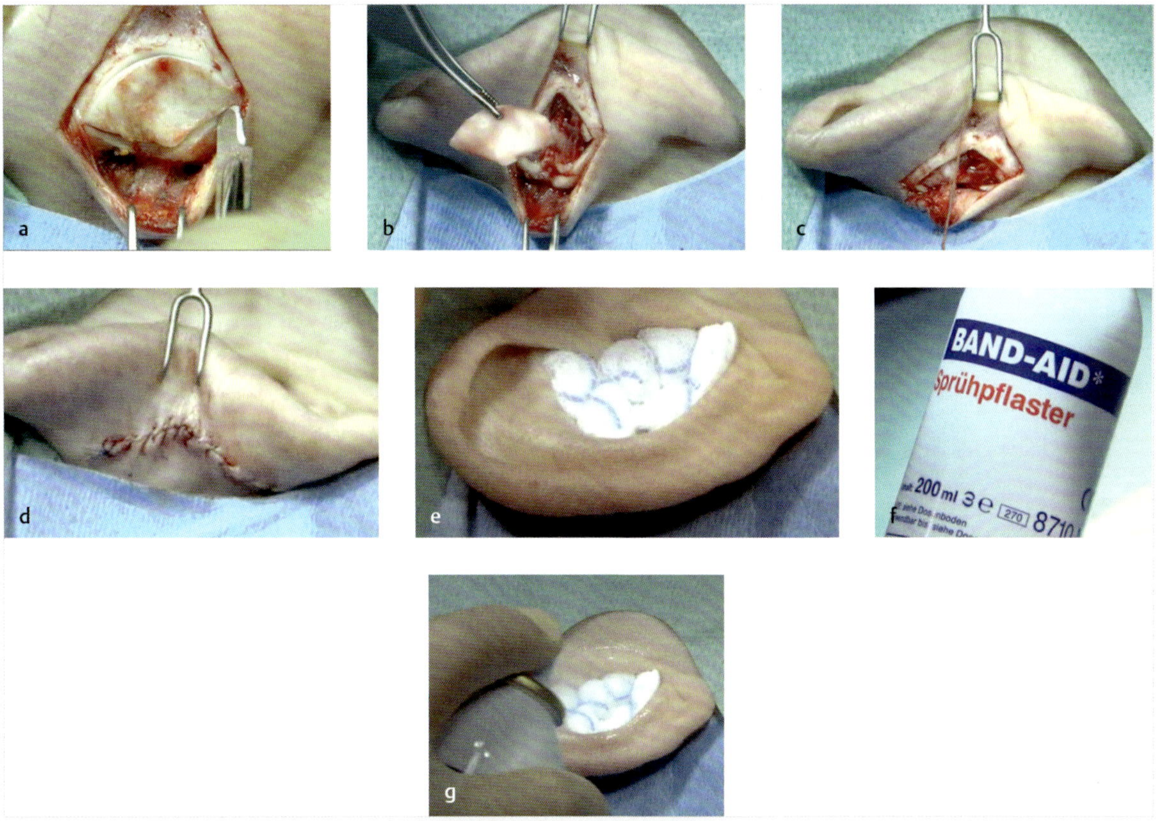

Fig. 18.3 Harvesting a conchal cartilage transplant. (a) Postauricular incision and cutting around the cartilage of the cavity of the concha. **(b)** Elevation and harvesting of the graft. **(c)** Wound closure, with a subcutaneous suture for hematoma prophylaxis. **(d)** Skin closure. As an alternative to the overcast suture shown here, a rapidly absorbable intracutaneous suture, which does not require removal, is most suitable). **(e)** Dressing: packing the cavity of the concha with small spherical swabs for hematoma prophylaxis. **(f, g)** Fixation of the swabs with a plaster spray.

> ✔
>
> Thermal skin lesions at the front side have to be avoided at all costs; postoperative bleeding is also undesirable, since it may result in hematomas, potentially leading to abscess and ear deformity.

The two-layer wound closure supports bleeding control. First, the subcutis of the ventral skin is firmly connected to the subcutaneous tissue of the dorsal skin covering using a quickly absorbable suture. This tight adaptation eliminates the dead space after cartilage harvesting and effectively counteracts hematomas and seromas. This is followed by a continuous intracutaneous suture, usually also with rapidly absorbable 5–0 suture material. After this wound closure, no subsequent suture removal is required on the ear.

Surgical dressing should also prevent hematoma formation. The cavity of the concha is packed with a few small spherical swabs under slight pressure, held in place by applying spray plaster. This is followed by the application of compresses and a light head bandage. All dressing material can be removed 1–2 days postoperatively.

The surgeon needs to bear in mind that conchal cartilage is more prone to dislocation than septal cartilage, and the edges of these grafts tend to become visible under the skin (contouring). Adequate fixation and flattening of the transplant margins must therefore be ensured. Unwanted bulging of the conchal cartilage – e.g., when it is used as a septal replacement graft – can be eliminated by placing two strips of conchal cartilage together with their concave side and suturing them tightly together (▶ Fig. 18.4a–d). On the other hand, the elastic curvature of these auricular cartilage transplants is

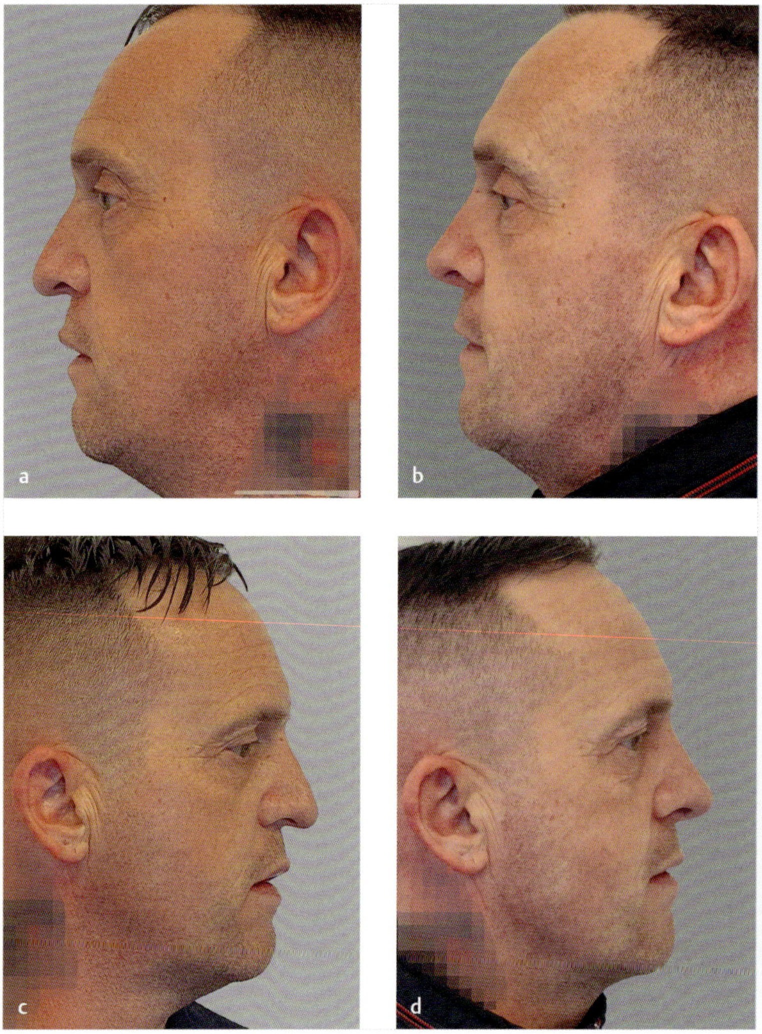

Fig. 18.4 Conchal cartilage as a septal extension graft; clinical example. Correction of a narrow nasolabial angle using a septal extension graft consisting of two strips of concha cartilage adapted to each other. **(a, c)** Preoperative side views. **(b, d)** The result. The reconstruction was carried out around a large septal perforation between the preserved mucous membranes, without opening them. Cartilage removal from the ear left no visible consequences.

particularly useful for replacement or reinforcement of alar cartilages. In general, auricular cartilage is more suitable than costal cartilage for use at the nasal tip (▶ Fig. 18.5a–f, ▶ Fig. 18.6a–f).

Composite Grafts

The ear is the only organ from which cartilage grafts can be harvested together with the delicate overlying skin ("composite grafts"), especially in the cymba conchae, where thin skin is tightly adherent to curved cartilage (▶ Fig. 18.7). Grafts of this type are used to correct two-layer nasal defects during rhinoplasty.

The natural curvature of the furrow in the cymba conchae allows harvesting of a suitable composite graft from this site for transplantation into the nostrils – for example, to correct nostril stenoses (▶ Fig. 18.8a–d). The resultant skin defect in the cymba conchae is covered by generously detaching the surrounding skin from the cartilage and moving it over the defect, which generally allows tension-free closure (▶ Fig. 18.9a–c). Composite grafts of this type may be useful when the (cutaneous) edge of the nasal ala is to be lowered (see section 10.9.2), or for reconstruction of the nasal alae. The curvature of the cartilage graft helps restore the arcuate attachment of the alar base to the cheek (▶ Fig. 18.10a, b).

Similarly, smaller composite grafts can also be harvested from the triangular fossa, or from the scapha between the helical rim and the antihelix (see ▶ Fig. 18.7). Small cartilage grafts can of course also be taken without skin from the same regions if a larger volume is not needed.

18.2.3 The Rib as Cartilage Donor Site

Rib cartilage can be used as graft material when septal or auricular cartilage is inadequate, or when the conchal

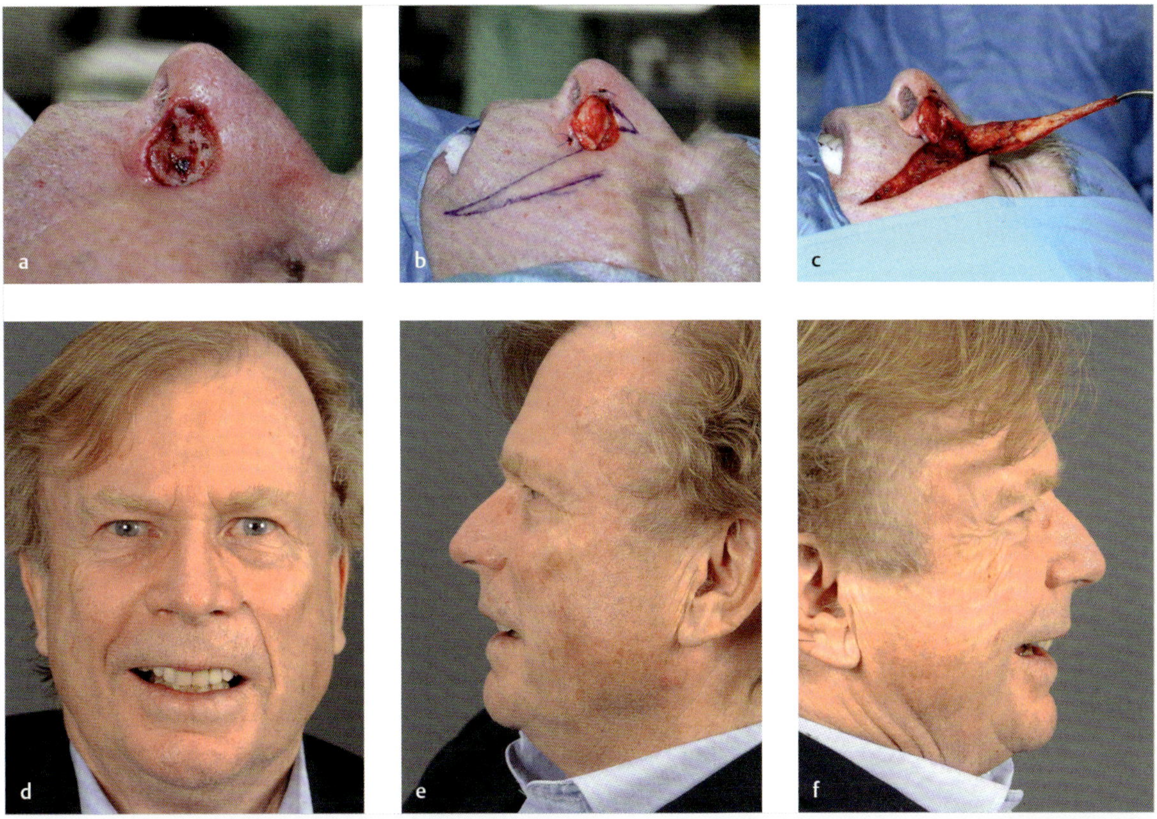

Fig. 18.5 Nasal alar reconstruction with conchal cartilage and a melolabial flap. (a) A nasal alar defect, with partial loss of alar cartilage after resection of a basal cell carcinoma. **(b)** Stabilization and reconstruction of the nasal ala using conchal cartilage. The planned melolabial flap has been marked. **(c)** The melolabial flap before incorporation into the defect. **(d, e)** Frontal and lateral views after stable healing of the cartilage and skin. **(f)** View of the opposite side for comparison.

cartilage is too soft for the intended use in the absence of septal cartilage (▶ Fig. 18.11a–d). Indications for rib transplants include total or subtotal nasal reconstruction, although the transition between reconstructive and cosmetic surgery is indistinct.

In the case of a nose that has collapsed due to loss of structure and with preserved skin, the surgical techniques for reconstructing the framework do not differ significantly from those required for the reconstruction of a (partly) missing nose. As stated above for the harvesting of ear cartilage with rhinoplasty, it is also the case with removal of costal cartilage that this surgical step should be carried out before the nasal surgery, for practical reasons. The volume of cartilage required can only be roughly estimated at this point. The surgeon should make a generous estimate and harvest sufficient material to avoid a lack of cartilage at a later point. A graft approximately 4 cm long from an average-sized rib is sufficient in most cases, even for more extensive reconstructions.

> ✓
>
> It is advisable to work simultaneously on the nose while the rib is being harvested, with two teams if possible. The rhinoplasty surgeon usually stands to the right of the patient's head; costal cartilage is therefore best harvested by the second team working simultaneously on the left thorax. Ideally, the nasal surgeon would have already prepared the nose for placement of the cartilage graft at the appropriate time, just as the costal cartilage becomes available. This is much less time-consuming than having one surgeon performing both procedures consecutively.

Rib cartilage may show patchy calcification in parts – especially in patients over the age of 50 years, but certainly in younger ones as well – which may either impede its use or interfere with precise shaping of grafts. Extensive induration due to calcification may be present in exceptional cases, making the costal cartilage practically unusable for

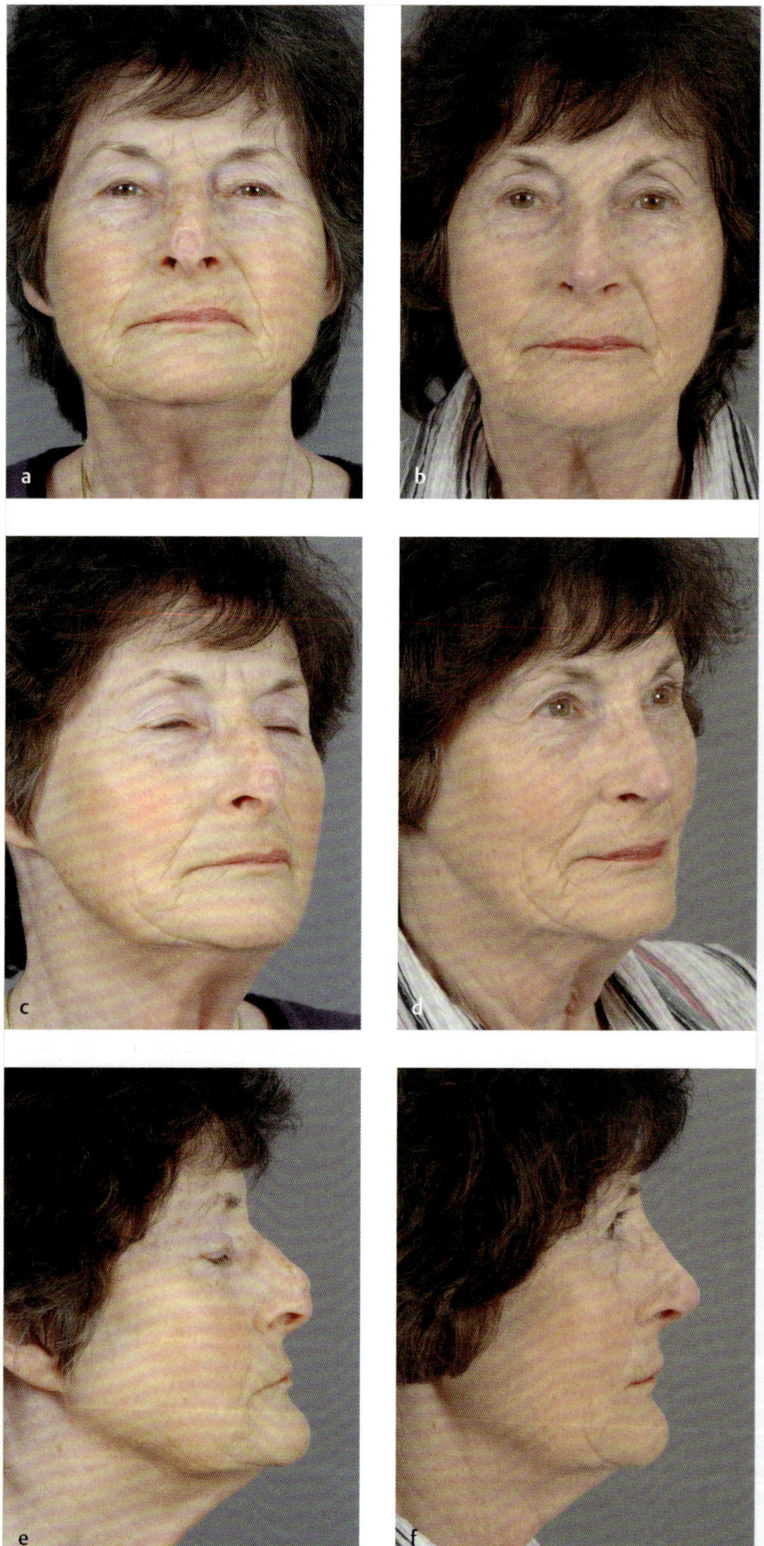

Fig. 18.6 Reconstruction of the nasal tip with conchal cartilage and a paramedian forehead flap. (a, c, e) A nasal tip defect after tumor resection with a simple skin graft cover carried out elsewhere. **(b, d, f)** After nasal tip reconstruction with conchal cartilage and a paramedian forehead flap. The nasal framework was reduced at the same time, using classic rhinoplasty techniques.

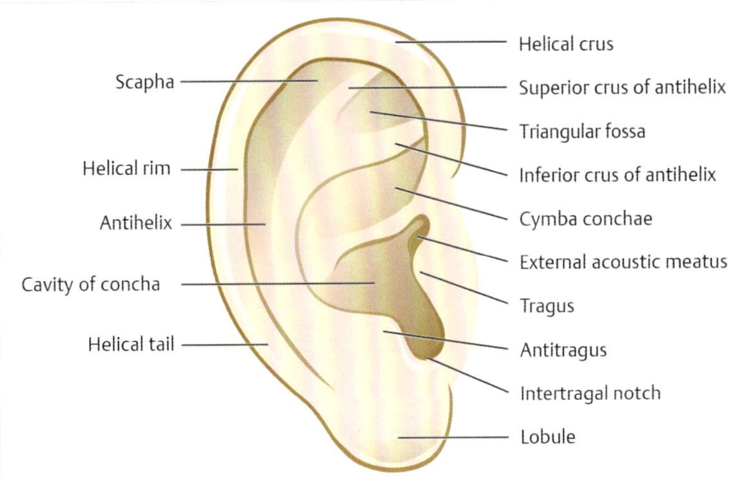

Fig. 18.7 Anatomy of the auricle. The cavity of the concha and the cymba are particularly suitable as donor regions for auricular cartilage transplants.

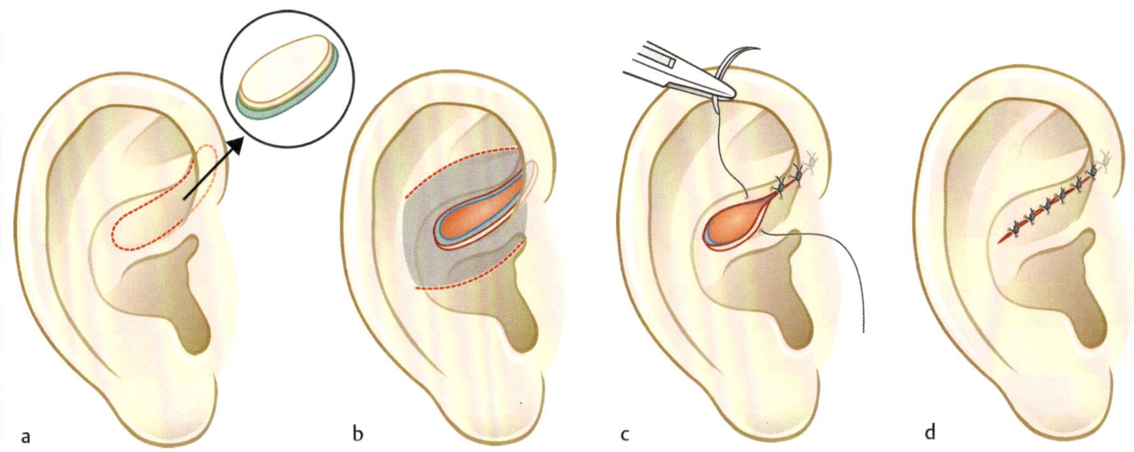

Fig. 18.8 Composite graft from the cymba conchae; schematic diagram. **(a)** The cartilaginous disk is usually slightly larger than the attached skin. **(b)** After extensive mobilization of the surrounding skin, primary wound closure is carried out **(c, d)**.

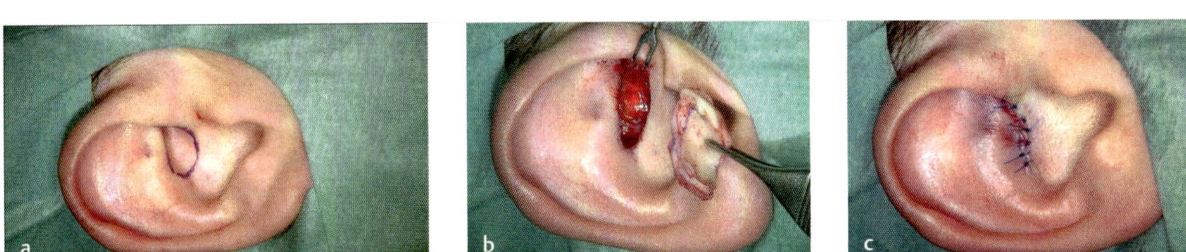

Fig. 18.9 Harvesting a composite graft from the ear. (a) Marking the required size in the cymba conchae. **(b)** Graft harvesting. **(c)** After wound closure.

reconstructive nasal surgery. Preoperative **ultrasonography** of the cartilaginous ribs, which allows optimal assessment of the extent of calcification, is recommended for timely identification of such cases. If calcified zones are present, rib cartilage can still be processed by using a piezo technique for cutting (see p. 234).

A segment of costal cartilage 3–4 cm long is usually harvested from the seventh to the tenth ribs for reconstructive

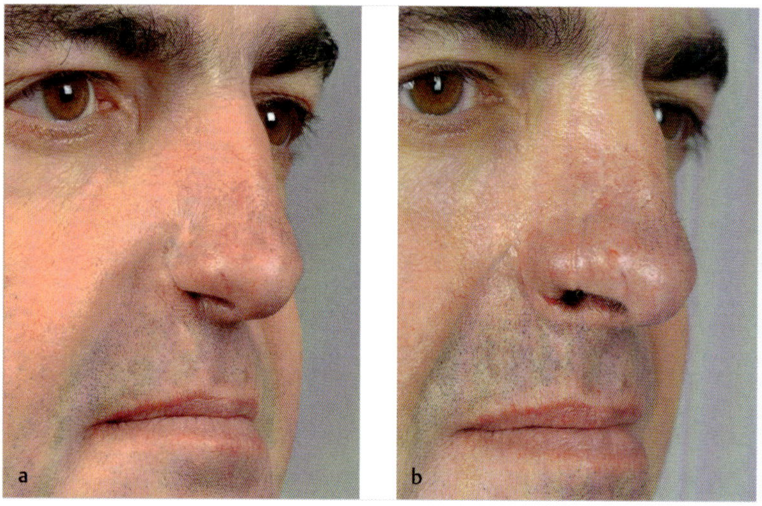

Fig. 18.10 Alar reconstruction with a composite graft. (a) A defect in the right nasal ala after tumor resection. **(b)** After ala reconstruction with a composite auricular graft on the inside and a melolabial cheek flap on the outside.

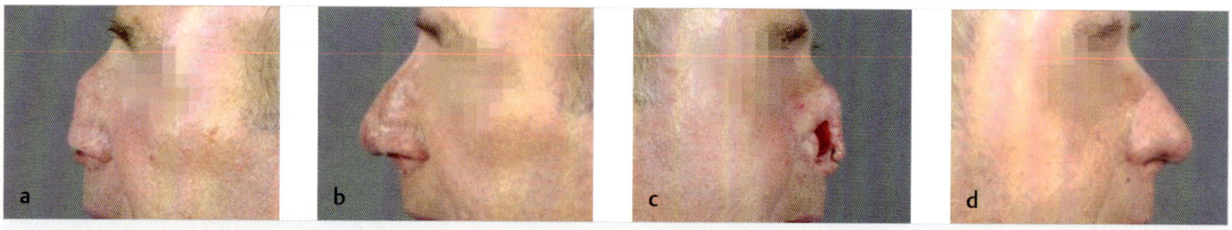

Fig. 18.11 Partial nasal reconstruction. (a, c) A partial defect in the nose after tumor resection. **(b, d)** After reconstruction with rib grafts and a paramedian forehead flap.

nasal surgery. However, rib selection may depend on various factors, such as anatomical conditions, findings on palpation, and ultrasound images, if necessary. The site of the skin incision should also be considered, and the incision itself should be as short as possible to minimize the visible scar.

The incision does not need to be as long as the desired cartilage graft, due to the mobility of the overlying skin and soft tissues, allowing the incision to be moved around as needed. The skin incision approximately 2 cm long is best placed at the point of intersection of the **midclavicular line** with the **submammary fold**, which is frequently visible in both men and women (▶ Fig. 18.12). The mamillar line, occasionally recommended as an intersection point, is less suitable, since the position of the nipple often changes with patient position, not only in women. The skin incision in principle roughly follows the selected rib palpable directly under the incision, but should be placed along a skin fold, if present.

It is useful to precisely mark the submammary fold preoperatively when the patient is seated, as it may shift considerably after the patient has been positioned on the operating table — potentially leading to errors of judgment with incorrect positioning of the scar. If the surgeon is experienced in dealing with endoscopic procedures, he or she can also use a 30° telescope during harvesting of costal cartilage. This allows the skin incision to be kept a few millimeters shorter.

The surgeon may need to penetrate a thick layer of subcutaneous fat after incising the skin, to be able to access the external oblique muscle (▶ Fig. 18.13). The muscle can be easily divided using an electric knife or with the radiofrequency technique to minimize bleeding. Instead of cutting through, longitudinal splitting and separation of muscle fibers is an elegant method of dividing the muscle. This ensures better wound healing in the postoperative period and reduces postoperative pain for the patient.

✔

If the surgeon wishes to use muscle fascia for nasal surgery, the fascia of the rectus abdominis can be exposed while removing rib cartilage, and a piece of it that has the required size can be removed (▶ Fig. 18.13).

The rib is identified by palpation, and the incision is held open by the assistant with appropriately sized retractors and moved over the rib as needed (▶ Video 18.4). Once an adequately long rib segment has been visualized, the presence of sufficient cartilaginous rib should first be confirmed by identifying the osseocartilaginous junction, which is located in the lateral aspect of the presenting rib. The bony rib is harder and reddish-gray–brownish in color, while the cartilaginous rib is softer and yellowish-whitish. The perichondrium is then opened through a longitudinal incision and two or three transverse incisions, to detach it from the rib using suitable raspatories. The feared complication of a pleural lesion is a rarity if one proceeds cautiously, and I have fortunately never encountered this complication in countless cases of rib graft harvesting over many years. The perichondrium is always

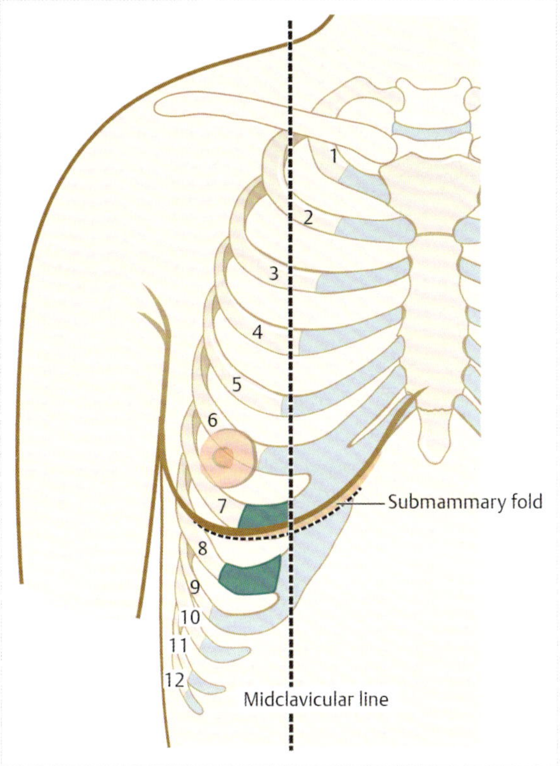

Fig. 18.12 Harvesting of costal cartilage. The incision for harvesting of costal cartilage is placed in the submammary fold, at the crossing point with the midclavicular line.

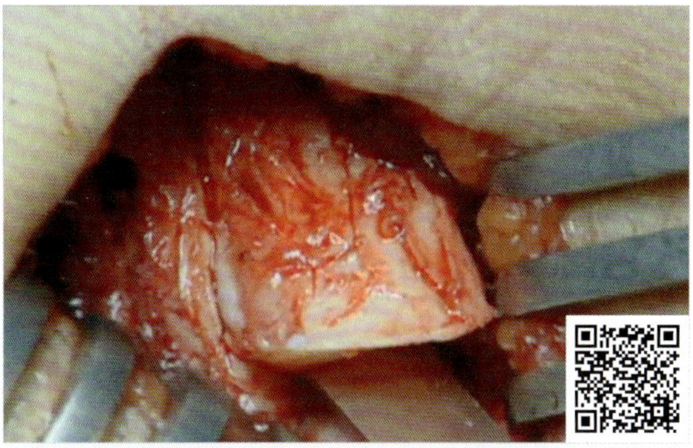

Video 18.4 Harvesting of costal cartilage (clinical case).

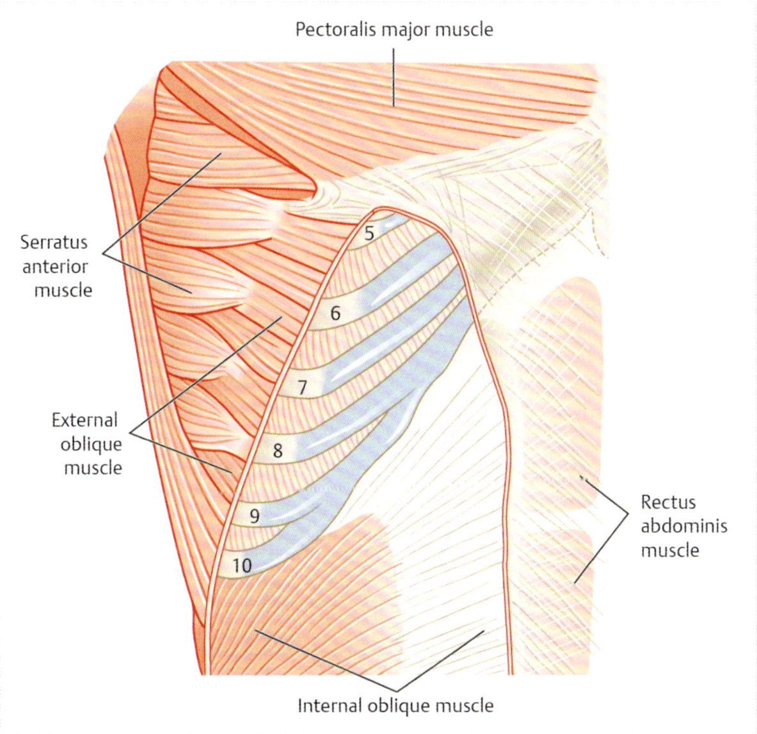

Fig. 18.13 Anatomy of the costal arch and chest wall muscles. The external oblique muscle covers the costal arch.

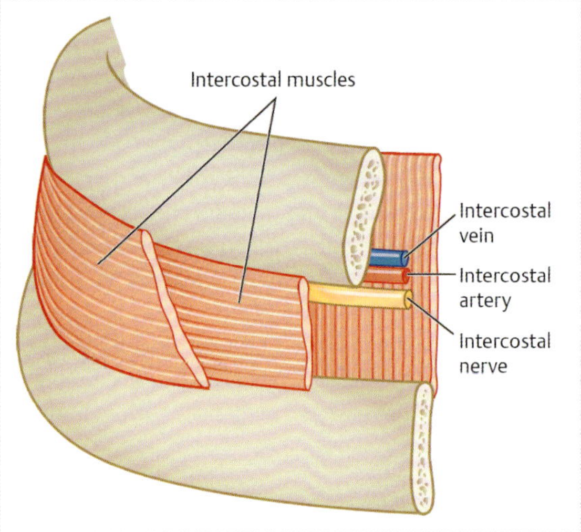

Fig. 18.14 Intercostal vessels and nerves. Vascular injuries should be avoided as far as possible while harvesting costal cartilage.

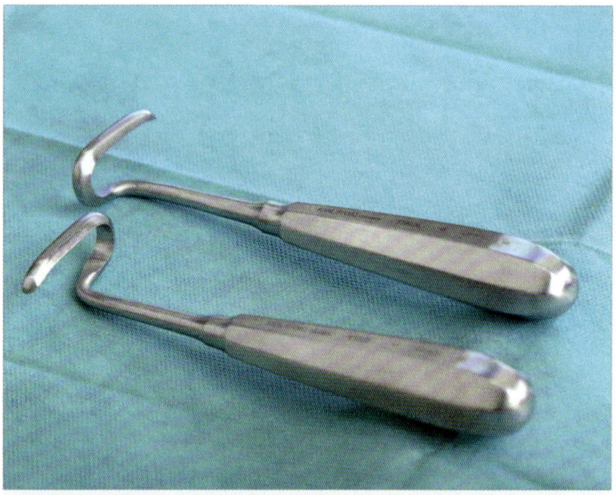

Fig. 18.15 Doyen raspatory. The Doyen raspatory is ideal for passing under the rib (KARL STORZ SE & Co. KG, Tuttlingen, Germany).

dissected with the instrument in strictly direct contact to the cartilage. This procedure also reduces the risk of injuring the intercostal vessels running along the inner and inferior margin of the rib (▶ Fig. 18.14).

A curved Doyen raspatory (▶ Fig. 18.15) can be used to pass completely under the rib, to detach the entire circumference of the cartilaginous rib from the perichondrium. The rib is then first severed near the osseocartilaginous junction immediately above the undermining raspatory, to prevent accidental injury to deeper tissues and the pleura. A sharp Freer instrument (see ▶ Fig. 7.7) may be safer than a scalpel for this cut.

The graft is lifted at the site of separation with a one-pronged hook; any adherent perichondrium can usually be pushed off from the inner aspect under vision until the entire cartilaginous segment is exposed. Another medial incision finally separates the cartilage transplant, which is then removed and secured on the instrument table (▶ Fig. 18.16a–g).

An indispensable "water test" is performed subsequently, in which the surgical site is filled with saline solution and the patient is subjected to positive-pressure ventilation (positive end-expiratory pressure, PEEP). Rising air bubbles signify pleural injury. Smaller isolated bubbles occasionally seen during this test arise from tissue gaps containing small amounts of air, usually cease to appear after a short period of time, and do not indicate an underlying complication.

The wound is closed in multiple layers after placement of a Redon drain. The skin can be sutured with intracutaneous sutures of the appropriate size (such as 3–0 polypropylene – e.g., Prolene). Especially with a longer cut, it is useful to exit the intracutaneous plane for one or two oversewn sutures approximately in the center of the incision to facilitate removing them later, after which intracutaneous suturing can be continued. The visible thread in the center of the suture line can be severed after 6–8 days, and the two short intracutaneous sutures are then removed (▶ Fig. 18.17). Otherwise, a long continuous intradermal suture may be tightly adherent to the rough skin of the chest wall and may be difficult to remove completely.

This suture modification can be omitted when using absorbable suture material (such as 3–0 poliglecaprone 25 – e.g., Monocryl), with only the knots at the wound edges being severed later.

Processing of Harvested Costal Cartilage

Various devices are available for cutting the harvested rib to size. Size 15, 10 and 20 blades (depending on the size of the cartilaginous segment to be reshaped) are the most useful. A piezoelectric device, if available, is ideally suited for fine surface processing, thinning, and perforation of cartilage grafts – especially if the cartilage is partly calcified and offers considerable resistance to processing with a scalpel (▶ Video 18.5, ▶ Video 18.6; ▶ Fig. 18.18a, b).

The piezo technique makes it possible to use calcified costal cartilage transplants for reconstructive nasal surgery in older patients (▶ Fig. 18.19a, b).

Warping and Resorption of Rib Cartilage Shavings

Intraoperative and postoperative warping of harvested costal cartilage grafts is a feared complication. It is

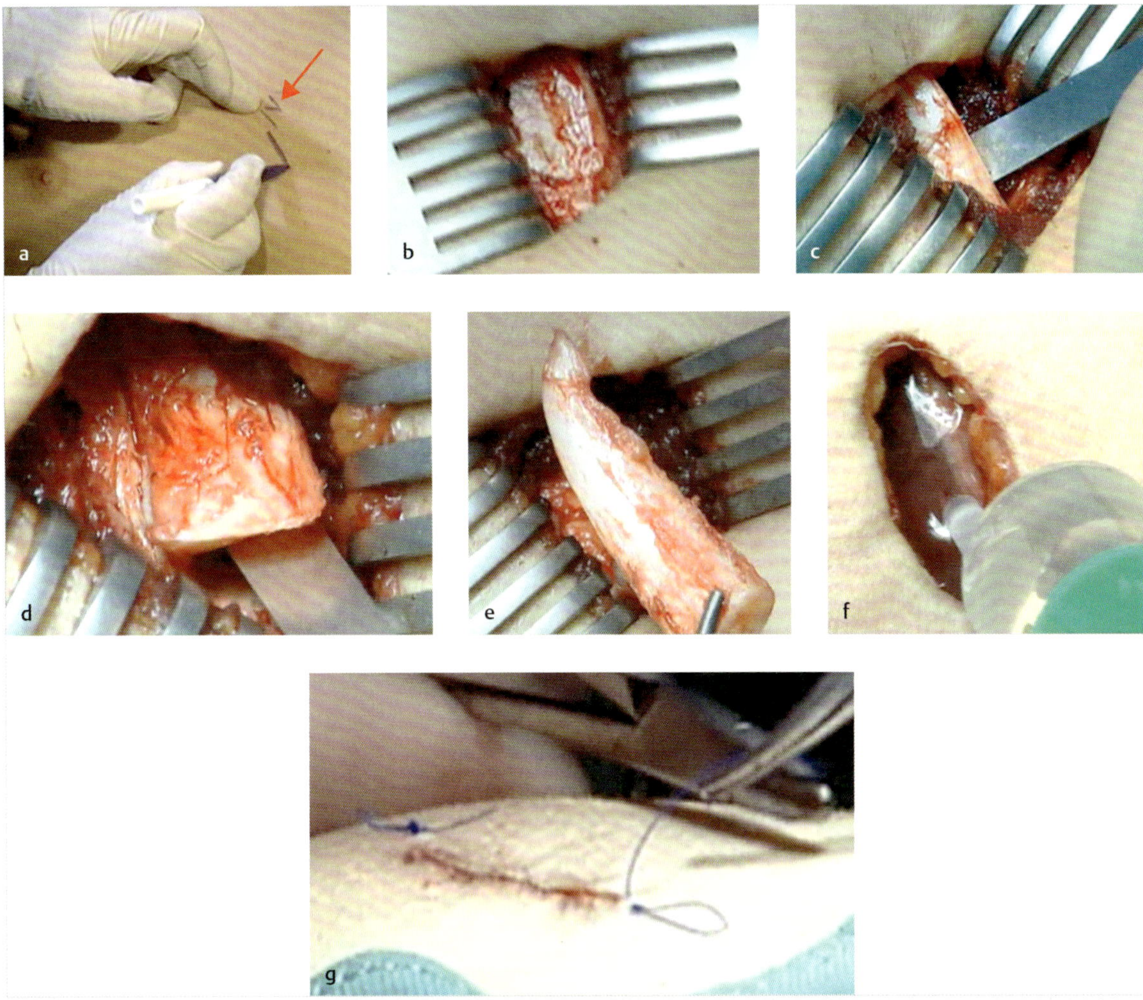

Fig. 18.16 Harvesting of a costal cartilage graft. (a) Marking the incision. The xiphoid (red arrow) is used for orientation. **(b)** Splitting of muscles to expose the rib. **(c)** Complete removal of the perichondrium with a raspatory. **(d)** Lateral division at the osseocartilaginous junction, and medial elevation of the rib. **(e)** Removal after complete medial transection. **(f)** Water test. **(g)** Wound closure in multiple layers, with an intracutaneous skin suture.

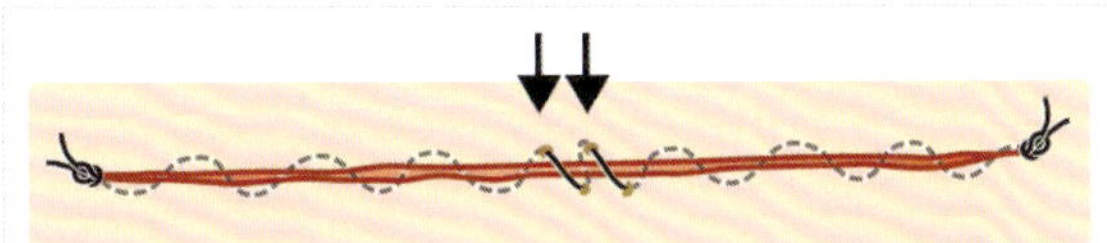

Fig. 18.17 Interrupted intracutaneous suture after costal cartilage harvesting. The overcast suture in the middle of the wound makes it easier to pull the threads later.

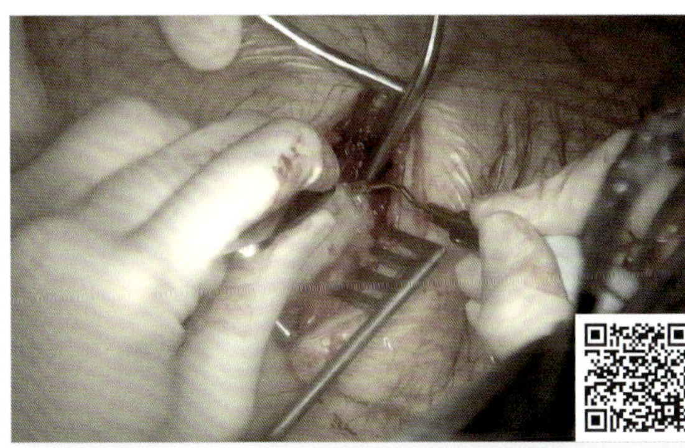

Video 18.5 Rib harvesting using the piezo technique (clinical case).

important to bear in mind that excised and trimmed pieces of cartilage that lie on the instrument table for a while may have a tendency to warp, and this needs to be taken into account during further processing. Early studies showed that strips obtained from the central axis of a cartilaginous rib warp to a lesser extent than those obtained from its edges (according to Davis and Gibson, 1956). Unfortunately, however, even central segments from the core of the rib are susceptible to warping. In addition, extensive reconstructive surgery usually requires every piece of excised rib, and the periphery of it (which is more prone to warping) inevitably also has to be used. These lateral graft strips are handled in such a way as to ensure that warping does not matter – e.g., by dicing them into tiny pieces or using them as grafts in areas where warping is irrelevant.

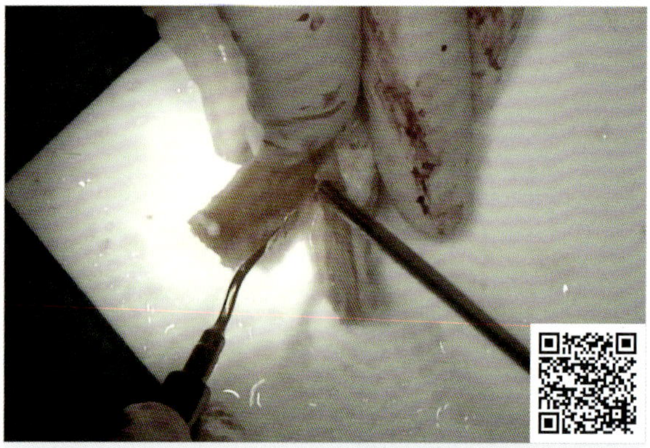

Video 18.6 Rib processing using piezo instruments.

Parallel placement of two thin slices of cartilage, each with opposite bending tendencies, can stabilize the transplant as a whole in one plane. However, a 100% guarantee against long-term warping of cartilage cannot be assured. This needs to be clearly communicated to the patient during the preoperative briefing. Marked warping of cartilage eventually requires revision surgery (▶ Fig. 18.20a, b).

In addition, any costal cartilage graft may undergo postoperative absorption. Both undesirable sequelae – warping and resorption – occur in about 25% of transplanted costal cartilage pieces in the long term, as has been observed in various studies. The extent of absorption may range from an insignificant volume loss to complete loss of the transplanted material, and is unpredictable. All affected patients therefore have to be briefed about both warping and cartilage loss due to partial or complete resorption of the rib grafts.

An unusual and extremely rare complication following transplantation of a rib is continued growth of the graft. A few published cases have reported an excessive increase in the length of the nose ("Pinocchio nose"), probably due to the unintentional transplantation of growth zones.

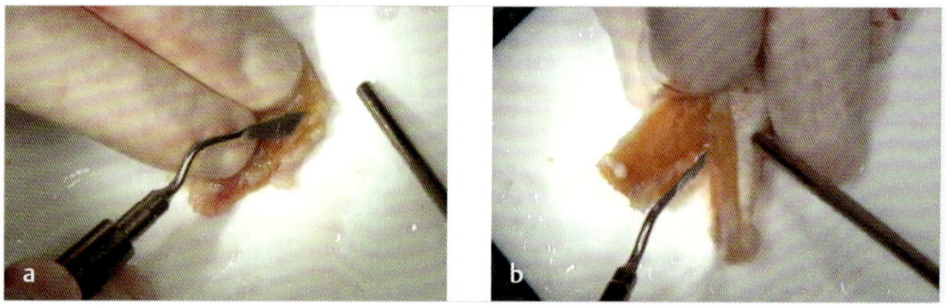

Fig. 18.18 Rib graft and piezo technique. (a) Processing a rib graft using the piezo technique: trimming the edge. (b) Splitting the rib.

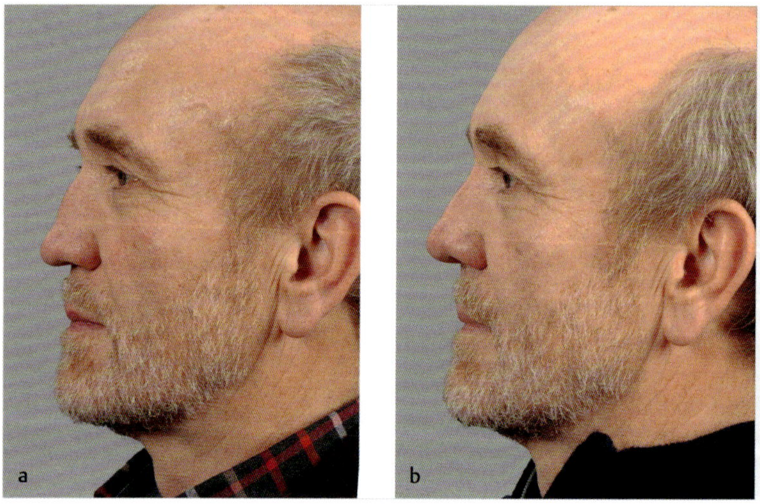

Fig. 18.19 Partly calcified costal cartilage graft; case example. (a) Saddle nose, with an unstable anterior nose and tip drop. (b) After reconstruction with a two-part L-strut from moderately calcified costal cartilage.

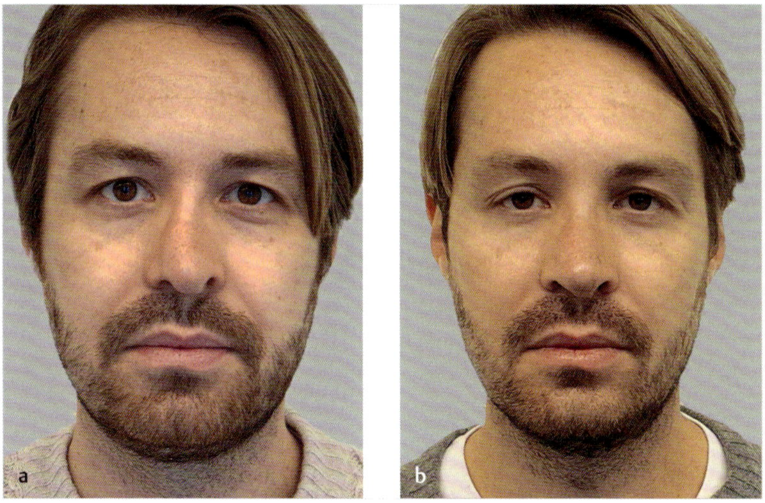

Fig. 18.20 Warping of costal cartilage; case study. (a) A warped costal cartilage transplant, approximately 15 years after reconstruction of the nasal vault performed elsewhere following trauma. **(b)** After revision surgery, with correction of the graft shape using the open technique.

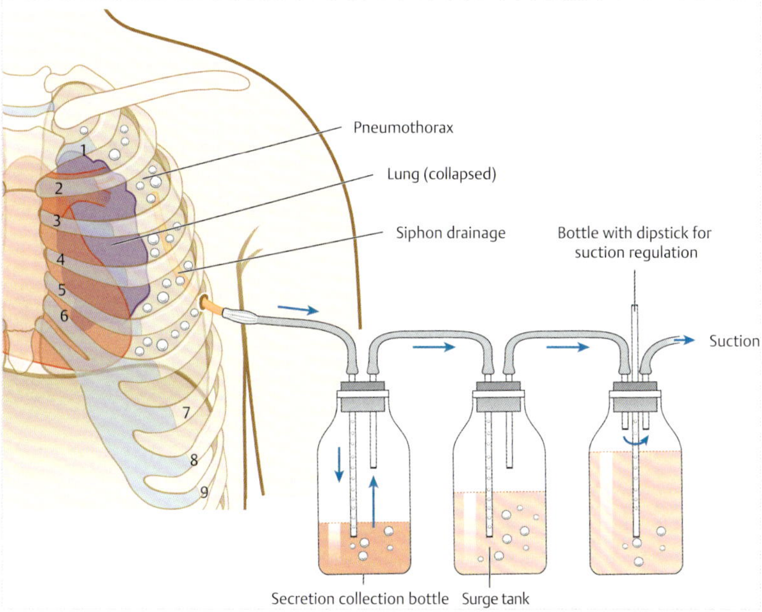

Fig. 18.21 Bülau chest drain (schematic diagram). Intrapleural air (which enters through the pleural defect) is suctioned away in a controlled manner to allow reexpansion of the lungs.

Infection of Rib Transplants

Rib grafts are usually required during rhinoplasty in complex revision cases after one or more previous operations. The risk of infection is higher in such patients due to the concomitant presence of several risk factors: previously injured, scarred tissue, prolonged surgery time, and grafts from another part of the body. The use of diced cartilage can further increase the risk of infection.

These conditions justify the administration of intraoperative and prolonged postoperative antibiotics, particularly because a purulent infection on the reconstructed nose can quickly lead to complete loss of the rib cartilage structure that has been built up, and thus to total failure of the operation.

Treatment of a Pleural Lesion

A pleural lesion with pneumothorax identified during the water test is treated in consultation with the anesthetist and a surgeon, if available. The treatment consists of suturing the lesion and/or placing a chest drain (▸ Fig. 18.21).

Despite the rarity of this complication, rib cartilage must only be harvested in a well-equipped environment in which provisions for competent handling of pneumothorax are available.

18

Bibliography

Berghaus A, Stelter K. Alloplastic materials in rhinoplasty. Curr Opin Otolaryngol Head Neck Surg. 2006; 14(4):270–277

Cochran CS. Harvesting rib cartilage in primary and secondary rhinoplasty. Clin Plast Surg. 2016; 43(1):195–200

Davis SJ, Landeen KC, Sowder JC, et al. Complications associated with use of porous high-density polyethylene in rhinoplasty. Facial Plast Surg Aesthet Med. 2022; 24(5):337–343

Davis WB, Gibson T. Absorption of autogenous cartilage grafts in man. Br J Plast Surg. 1956; 9(3):177–185

Falces E, Gorney M. Use of ear cartilage grafts for nasal tip reconstruction. Plast Reconstr Surg. 1972; 50(2):147–152

Genther DJ, Papel ID. Surgical nasal implants: indications and risks. Facial Plast Surg. 2016; 32(5):488–499

Gorney M, Murphy S, Falces E. Spliced autogenous conchal cartilage in secondary ear reconstruction. Plast Reconstr Surg. 1971; 47(5):432–437

Jovanovic S, Berghaus A. Autogenous auricular concha cartilage transplant in corrective rhinoplasty. Practical hints and critical remarks. Rhinology. 1991; 29(4):273–279

Kowalski HR, von Sneidern M, Wang RS, et al. Complications of Nasal Tip Stabilizing Grafts with Autologous Versus Irradiated Homologous Costal Cartilage in Septorhinoplasty: A Systematic Review. Facial Plast Surg Aesthet Med. 2024 Nov-Dec;26(6):775–781

Maring VP, Landecker A, Gunter JP. Harvesting rib cartilage grafts for secondary rhinoplasty. In: Gunter JP, Rohrich RJ, Adams WP, eds. Dallas rhinoplasty. 2nd ed. St. Louis: Quality Medical Publishing; 2007

Mohan R, Shanmuga Krishnan RR, Rohrich RJ. Role of fresh frozen cartilage in revision rhinoplasty. Plast Reconstr Surg. 2019; 144(3):614–622

Stelter K, Strieth S, Berghaus A. Porous polyethylene implants in revision rhinoplasty: chances and risks. Rhinology. 2007; 45(4):325–331

Toriumi DM, Kao R, Vandenberg T, Cristel R, Caniglia AJ. Auricular composite graft survival in rhinoplasty. Facial Plast Surg Aesthet Med. 2023; 25(1): 6–15

19 Special Issues

A few specific topics are dealt with in this chapter, each of which has recurring special, typical aspects in nasal surgery.

19.1 The Crooked Nose

It is important to distinguish between crooked noses resulting from trauma and those with congenital causes. Careful clinical examination is also essential to evaluate whether the bony skeleton, the cartilage, or both are involved.

19.1.1 Crooked Nose Following Trauma

The simplest case is the acute situation of a crooked nose presented after fresh trauma, such as after an accident during sports or at home, or after a physical conflict. The clinical examination includes palpation to identify crepitation and dislocation of fracture fragments, and nasal endoscopy to diagnose a fractured septum. Computed tomography (CT) of the paranasal sinuses is recommended, in order to rule out fractures of other structures in addition to the nasal bones, as well as to document the fracture for legal or insurance queries (▸ Fig. 19.1). The findings should also be photographed for documentation.

Immediate straightening with repositioning of fracture fragments can be undertaken in some cases with unequivocal findings and minimal soft-tissue swelling.

A fractured septum, which usually results in obstructed nasal breathing that is distinctly perceived by the patient, or preexistent and symptomatic septal deviation should not be ignored, and the patient should be advised to undergo simultaneous septoplasty.

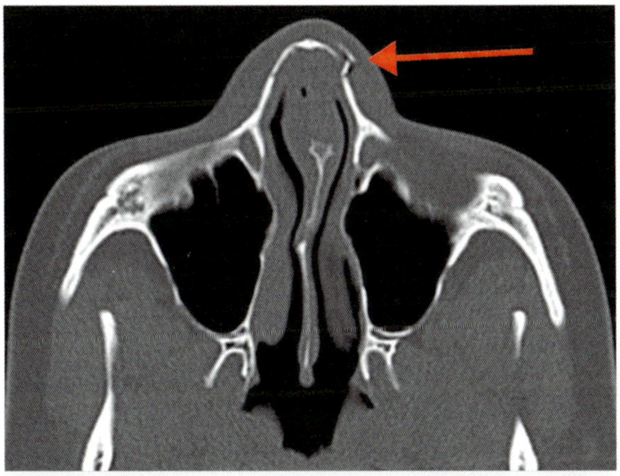

Fig. 19.1 **Axial computed tomography scan in a patient with nasal bone fractures.** Multiple nasal bone fractures (arrow).

After repositioning, bone fragments that have been propelled into the nasal cavity can be held in place for a few days after fracture reduction using a nasal tamponade (see ▸ Fig. 15.5) in combination with Doyle splints (see ▸ Fig. 7.20, ▸ Fig. 15.3). The outer aluminum splint applied to prevent further dislocation has to be lightly placed without any pressure, to prevent displacement of repositioned bone into the nasal cavity.

Soft-tissue edema or hematomas often preclude careful clinical evaluation and fracture reduction in the early posttraumatic phase. One can then wait about 8–10 days until the edema regresses and the findings can be better assessed before the fracture is reduced.

Although special elevators are available for repositioning fracture fragments, the blunt end of a Freer elevator (see ▸ Fig. 7.7), Joseph raspatory (see ▸ Fig. 8.5), or comparable instruments may also come in handy.

> ✔
>
> Reduction of a nasal bone fracture using the closed technique (i.e., predominantly by elevation or digital reduction) does not always restore the original nasal shape. The patient has to be informed that deformities may persist even after a correctly performed intervention, and surgical correction with a revision septoplasty or rhinoplasty may be required at a later time.

Failure to recognize or treat a dislocated nasal bone fracture may result in permanent deformity, with or without functional impairment, which can be treated at a later date with cosmetic and/or functional septorhinoplasty. A waiting period of 9–12 months is recommended in these cases to allow evaluation and treatment once the soft-tissue swelling has abated significantly and tissues have healed completely.

Repeat osteotomy of fracture lines using a closed technique may suffice if secondary posttraumatic reduction is required for repositioning of dislocated fracture fragments alone. It is not uncommon for the bone to break along the old fracture line during osteotomy, and subsequent elevation or digital repositioning into the correct position, as with immediate posttraumatic reduction, may produce the desired result (▸ Fig. 19.2a, b).

Regardless of the actual consequences of trauma, a typical septorhinoplasty is required if other deformities should be simultaneously corrected, such as a hump nose, size of the nose, tip abnormality, etc.

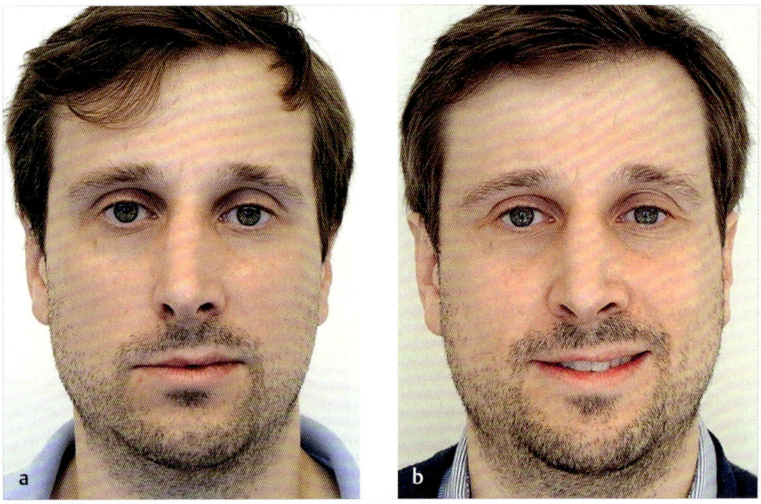

Fig. 19.2 Crooked nose after sports trauma. 18 years after a nasal trauma during sports, the patient suffers from significant nasal breathing obstruction. There is a pronounced deviation of the septum to the left, corresponding to the deviation of the nose to the right **(a)**. After functional septorhinoplasty, including the use of a spreader graft on the left, nasal breathing is free **(b)**.

Patients frequently attribute a nasal hump to a previous nasal trauma, even though a fracture line cannot be demonstrated. Typically, an association between the hump nose and injury cannot be established on clinical examination and imaging. These are mostly congenital humps, or they have developed and progressed independently of an accident over the years but have attracted the patient's attention only after a nasal injury. Patients with a hump nose also initially notice swelling after blunt nasal trauma, with persistence of the hump once the swelling subsides. A sympathetic explanation by the surgeon suggesting that the hump was probably present before the nasal injury may quickly help resolve the matter. It is rare for a patient's description of the origin of a nasal hump to be used to obtain a rhinoplasty under medical insurance cover.

19.1.2 Nontraumatic Crooked Nose

> ✔
>
> Individuals with asymmetry of the facial skeleton also have a congenital predisposition to develop a crooked nose. The patients may not always be aware of such asymmetries, even if they are pronounced. It is of prime importance to point out facial asymmetry before surgical correction; patients look at themselves much more closely in the mirror postoperatively, and any noticeable asymmetry may be falsely attributed to the operation.

A preoperative examination has to be carried out to assess whether the bony or cartilaginous component of the nose is crooked, or whether a combination of the two is present. **Cartilaginous** crooked noses are commonly present in patients with septal deviation, since the position of the septum may determine the alignment of the entire nose ("where the septum goes, the nose goes too") (▶ Fig. 19.3a, b). The surgeon then has to ensure that the cartilaginous nasal dorsum and the nasal septum are repositioned in the midline. This may require spreader grafts, stabilizing cartilage, or bone slivers to support an unstable cartilaginous septum on either side. Extracorporeal septoplasty to reconstruct an L-strut also needs to be considered in cases of marked warping that cannot be corrected by other means (see Chapter 7). Slippage of the caudal septum from a midline anterior nasal spine is best prevented using a suture that passes through the septum and a drill hole in the nasal spine.

A crooked nose due to deviation of the **bony framework** from the midline can only be corrected by osteotomy of the nasal bones. Slightly asymmetrical osteotomies can be performed if asymmetry of the nasal skeleton is present (▶ Fig. 19.4a–d). Assuming that the nasal bone is wider on the side opposite to the deviation (i.e., on the left in patients with a crooked nose to the right), the nasal framework can be straightened in severe cases using either a double osteotomy on the side of the wider nasal bone, or removal of a narrow strip of bone along the osteotomy line. Minor asymmetry of the bony nasal dorsum, with one edge slightly higher than the other, can be specifically corrected with precise superficial ablation of that edge using the piezoelectric technique.

If the surgeon uses the push-down or let-down preservation techniques, a bony crooked nose can be corrected by moving the entire mobilized nasal framework from the deviated position to a midline position (see section 8.4).

Nasal tip asymmetry that results in a crooked nose due to unevenly shaped nasal domes requires appropriate corrective surgery of the alar cartilages.

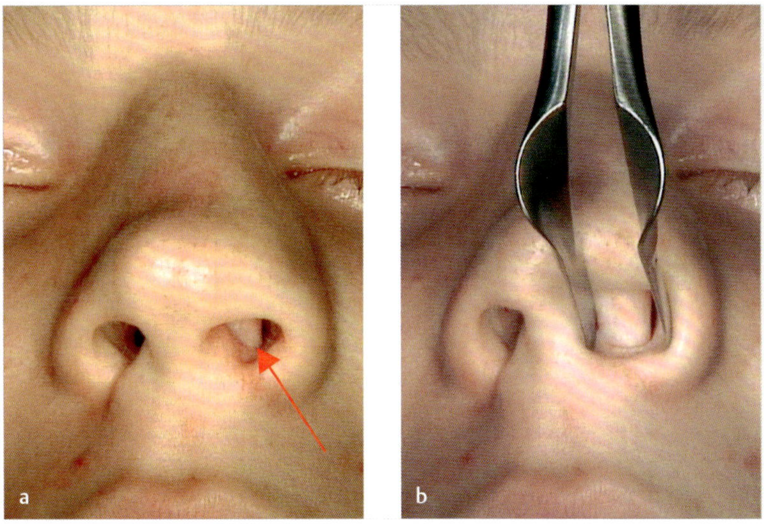

Fig. 19.3 Crooked nose with septal deviation. (a) Crooked nose with septal deviation (arrow). **(b)** Deviated caudal edge of the septum (septal subluxation).

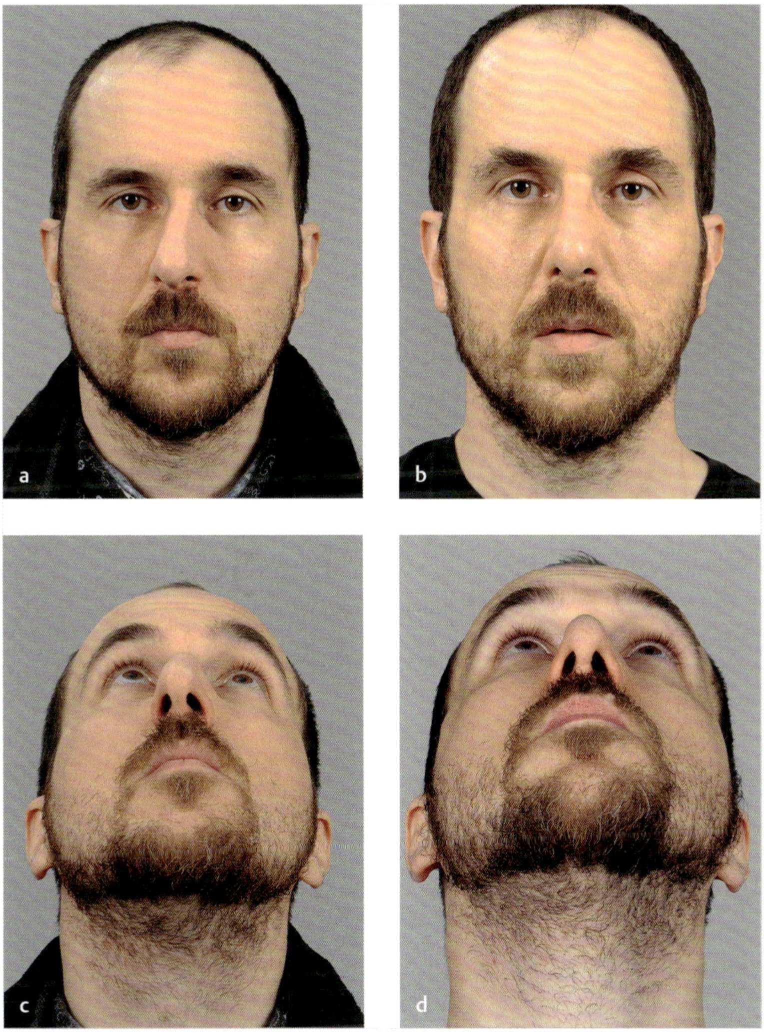

Fig. 19.4 Crooked nose. Bony and cartilaginous nasal deviation and hump **(a, c)**. After correction **(b, d)**.

Crooked noses often have to do with a combination of functional and aesthetic demands. The exact aim of the procedure needs to be discussed very carefully with the patient. It must be made clear that functional improvement does not automatically lead to beautification of the nose and that a cosmetic correction usually requires further, possibly very complex, surgical steps. It may also be necessary to address the fact that this separate effort is not covered by possible insurance cover that may be claimed for the functional correction (▶ Fig. 19.5a–d).

19.2 The Saddle Nose

A saddle nose is present when the nasal dorsum, or part of it, lies significantly lower than a straight line drawn between the radix and the nasal tip (see section 2.8) and is most commonly observed after complicated septoplasty or trauma. The saddle usually affects the cartilaginous part of the dorsum, but the bony vault may also be involved (▶ Fig. 19.6a, b).

Methods for augmenting a saddle nose are described in Chapters 17 and 18. Correction of saddle nose should not be confined to elevation of the depressed nasal dorsum; a concomitant hump does not have to remain untreated (▶ Fig. 19.6a, b). In addition, a saddle nose is frequently very wide, and narrowing of the bony vault using osteotomies should be considered.

Care must be taken not to ignore abnormalities of the columellar profile in patients with a saddle nose due to loss of septal cartilage – e.g., due to a septal abscess – and deficient cartilaginous support for the anterior nose. A retracted or "hidden" columella and a narrow nasolabial angle are frequently associated with a saddle nose. Correction of these deformities may be beneficial from a cosmetic point of view, but also from a functional point of view as well, as this also results in straightening and stabilization of the anterior nose (▶ Fig. 19.7a, b).

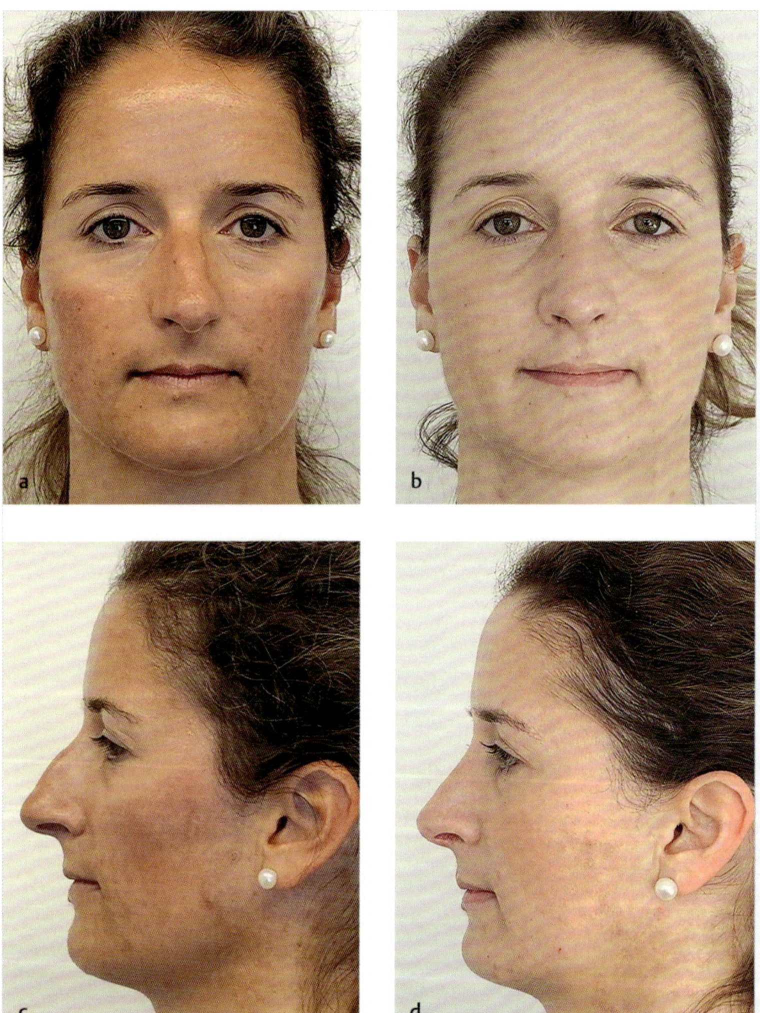

Fig. 19.5 Crooked nose with functional and cosmetic demands; case study. (a, c) Deviated nose with a hump. The patient requested a comprehensive functional and cosmetic correction. **(b, d)** Status after rhinoplasty. In these cases, fulfilling the cosmetic requirement is considerably more complex than improving the function. This needs to be explained to patients, who often do not realize that cosmetic corrections are usually much more difficult to achieve than a functional improvement of nasal breathing.

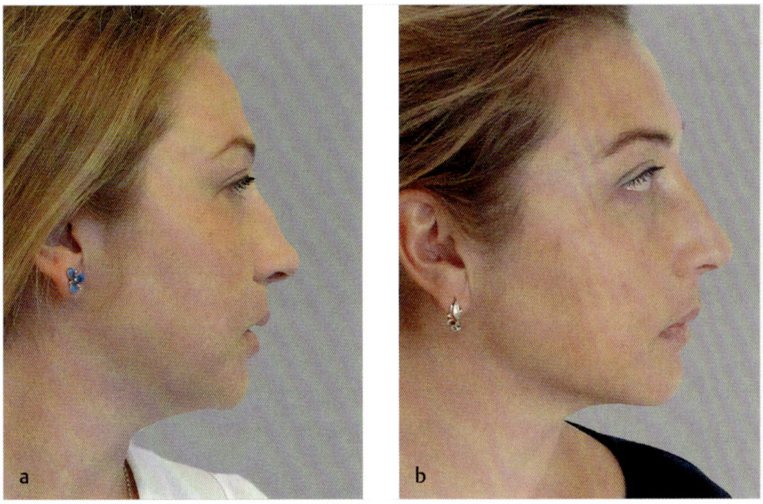

Fig. 19.6 Saddle nose. (a) Anterior saddle nose following septoplasty. **(b)** After correction of the saddle nose using conchal cartilage graft, with concomitant minimal hump reduction.

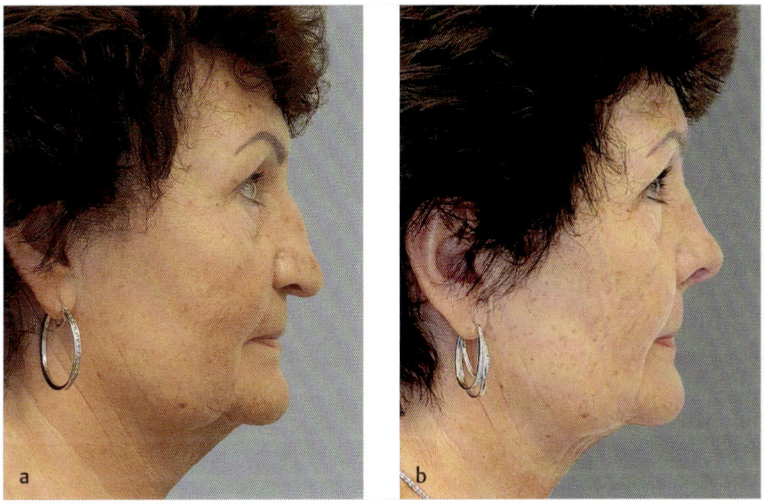

Fig. 19.7 Saddle nose with involvement of the anterior nose. (a) Saddle nose with a depressed, weak anterior nose. **(b)** After reconstructive rhinoplasty with costal cartilage grafts.

A disproportionately large, bulbous, or boxy tip can be simultaneously corrected along with a saddle nose in some cases in order to achieve an aesthetically appealing surgical outcome, provided this has been discussed with and agreed to by the patient.

> ✔
>
> It is advisable to discuss any additional abnormalities and the available corrective options with the patient before operating on a saddle nose, to ensure an overall satisfactory result.

It was suggested that a reversed preservation technique can also be used to correct a saddle nose. In this case, the bony and cartilaginous dorsum is mobilized with incisions similar to those for the preservation procedure (see Chapter 8.4), raised overall, and underlaid with a graft (in the “reverse spare roof technique,” after Ferreira and Santos; see the Bibliography below).

19.3 Nasal Deformity with Cleft Lip and Palate (“Cleft Nose”)

A “cleft nose” is the typical nasal deformity in patients with a cleft lip and palate. The deformity is predominantly unilateral, but bilateral clefts also occur. Cleft lip and palate, which cause severe functional impairment, are typically corrected by oral and maxillofacial surgeons and orthodontists during the patient’s early childhood. The nasal deformity, on the other hand, generally becomes important only in the adolescent or adult patient, when – in addition to breathing problems – cosmetic aspects play an increasingly important role. Significant septal deviation causing considerable functional impairment is frequently associated with this condition, and it should be corrected together with the external shape of the nose.

Certain typical features are present to a variable extent on the side of the cleft lip and palate in patients with a cleft nose deformity:

- Flattening and ptosis of the nasal dome and alar cartilage on the affected side in comparison with the contralateral side
- Wide but flat, short, and attenuated alar cartilage
- Frequently marked septal deviation, with a wide maxillary crest
- Reduced bony substructure of the maxilla at the level of the alar base on the side of the cleft

Surgical correction should take all of these aspects into account to ensure the most symmetrical outcome possible.

The open technique provides the best options for achieving the desired change in shape. The septum has to be straightened, while the shape and dimensions of the alar cartilage on the side of the cleft are adapted to the healthy opposite side to ensure symmetry. The healthy alar cartilage can also be reshaped to adapt to the contralateral, abnormal side.

The alar dome on the side of the cleft can be rotated and adapted to the opposite side using the lateral crural steal procedure, supplemented by narrowing of the cephalic edge of the lower lateral cartilage with a turn-in flap. The attenuated alar cartilage usually has to be reinforced and extended laterally with a robust lateral crural strut or lateral crural extension graft (▸ Fig. 19.8a, b).

Narrowing of the lateral crus of the alar cartilage on the healthy side may facilitate adaptation to the abnormal side. The reshaped nasal domes are secured in their new, symmetrical position using domal and interdomal sutures. Additional rim grafts help stabilize and symmetrically configure the nasal alar rims, while a tip graft ensures a symmetrical nasal tip. The weak attachment of the alar base to the cheek on the side of the cleft can be effectively reconstructed using an arcuate composite graft, as described in section 18.2.2.

The nostril on the side of the cleft may occasionally require widening with a small skin flap. This can be achieved with a V–Y plasty, in which a strip of skin is moved from the floor of the nostril to the lateral aspect of the columella. A cranially pedicled skin flap derived from the scarred upper lip, following previous closure of the cleft lip, can also be used in some cases. This procedure simultaneously allows correction of the lip scar. As a rule, however, I prefer to undertake revision surgery for a lip scar in a separate session, independently of the rhinoplasty, if the patient wishes this.

A sufficiently large cartilage graft is applied to the maxilla lateral to the piriform aperture through an incision at the nostril floor, or alternatively via a sublabial approach (▸ Fig. 19.9a, b), to elevate the "socket" under the alar base on the side of the cleft.

Many patients with a cleft deformity and significant septal deviation have an abundance of septal cartilage, which can be harvested to augment the lateral crus of the alar cartilage on the affected side. Conchal cartilage can also be used if a larger amount of cartilage is required. However, the surgeon should not hesitate to harvest a costal cartilage graft if it is foreseeable that even larger amounts of cartilage may be needed. This may be the case if a septal extension graft and cartilage material are required for maxillary augmentation in addition to the grafts for the alar cartilages.

Both cartilaginous and bony septal deviation may often coexist with a cleft nose, and surgical correction places

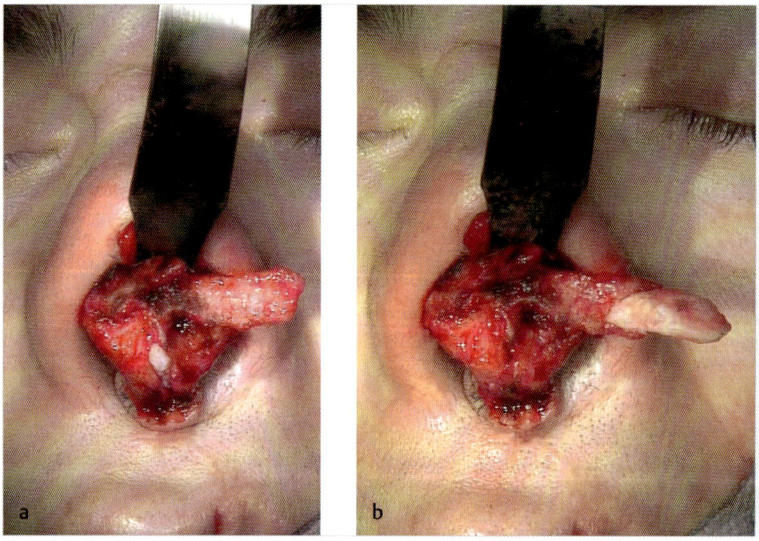

Fig. 19.8 Lateral crural extension graft for cleft nose deformity. (a) The mobilized lateral crus of alar cartilage. **(b)** Elongation with a lateral extension graft (from conchal cartilage in this case).

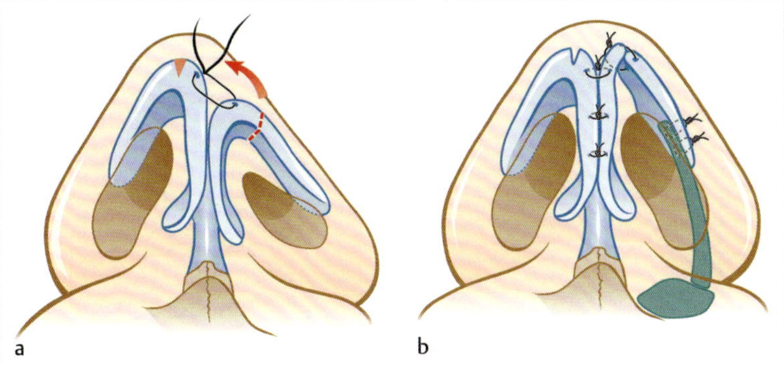

Fig. 19.9 Socket graft for cleft nose. **(a)** Asymmetrical shaping of the alar cartilages using standard techniques is aimed at aligning the two sides. **(b)** Frequently, the alar cartilage on the side of the cleft has to be supported using a lateral extension graft, which sits on a socket graft over the maxilla.

greater demands on the surgeon than septoplasty without cleft lip and palate deformity (▶ Fig. 19.10a–j).

A preoperative CT of the paranasal sinuses clearly depicts these findings. The surgeon typically encounters scarred tissue on the affected side during dissection of the nasal floor, due to previous surgical closure of the palate cleft. Reopening this scar and thus the cleft must be avoided at all costs, to prevent the development of a fistula between the nasal and oral cavities.

> ✔
>
> The surgeon should obtain a careful patient history before operating on a cleft nose (does fluid drip from the nose when the patient is drinking?) and thoroughly examine the patient (with probing if required) to exclude the presence of a residual oronasal fistula in the scarred nasal floor. If an oronasal fistula is present, it may well be closed during rhinoplasty by freshening its edges and inserting cartilage or bone.

The surgeon must be aware that achieving structural symmetry during correction of a cleft nose, especially in patients with marked deformity, may be very challenging despite surgical expertise and all possible surgical maneuvers (▶ Fig. 19.11a–h, ▶ Fig. 19.12a–f, ▶ Fig. 19.13a–f). More than one operation may often be necessary. The patient should also be briefed preoperatively about realistic prospects regarding the surgical outcome. Experience has shown that such patients usually do not have unrealistic expectations and are pleased with every distinctly visible improvement. It is therefore neither necessary nor useful to raise false expectations.

19.4 Binder Deformity

Binder syndrome (maxillonasal dysplasia) is primarily a developmental disorder of the anterior maxilla and nose. A flat, underdeveloped midface (midface hypoplasia), as well as an abnormally short nose with a flat radix and flattened nasal tip with a short columella, are typically present, frequently with small nostrils, an underdeveloped maxilla, and mandibular abnormalities.

Open rhinoplasty is the procedure of choice, since endonasal access through the small nostrils is extremely difficult in typical cases. The methods described in Chapters 11 and 12 are used for augmentation, rotation, and projection of the tip.

Sources in the literature frequently recommend moving skin from the philtrum of the upper lip to the columella with the help of a V–Y plasty to lengthen a short columella. However, this technique results in scarring of the nasolabial junction, which precludes correction and is likely to give the nose a permanent "operated" appearance. I therefore avoid using advancement flaps of this type. The skin of the columella that has not been pretreated is usually sufficiently elastic to cover the columella even after marked nasal tip rotation with elongation of supporting cartilaginous structures. The results obtained in this way in my patients confirm the usefulness of this approach (▶ Fig. 19.14a–f).

19.5 Septal Perforation

The most frequent causes of septal perforation include complicated **septoplasty** and persistent digital manipulation of the nasal septum (the "**piercing finger**"). **Cocaine abuse** is a much less common cause, but may lead to particularly extensive defects. Typical symptoms include crust formation, recurrent bleeding, and obstructed nasal breathing due to abnormal, irregular airflow. In addition, small perforations are often associated with a whistling sound during nasal breathing. Very small perforations, especially those located more dorsally, may remain asymptomatic and untreated.

A common approach to the closure of such perforations involves extensive bilateral mobilization of the septal and nasal floor mucosa in the vicinity of the perforation, extending from a hemitransfixion incision on either side, or an open approach – especially for perforations larger

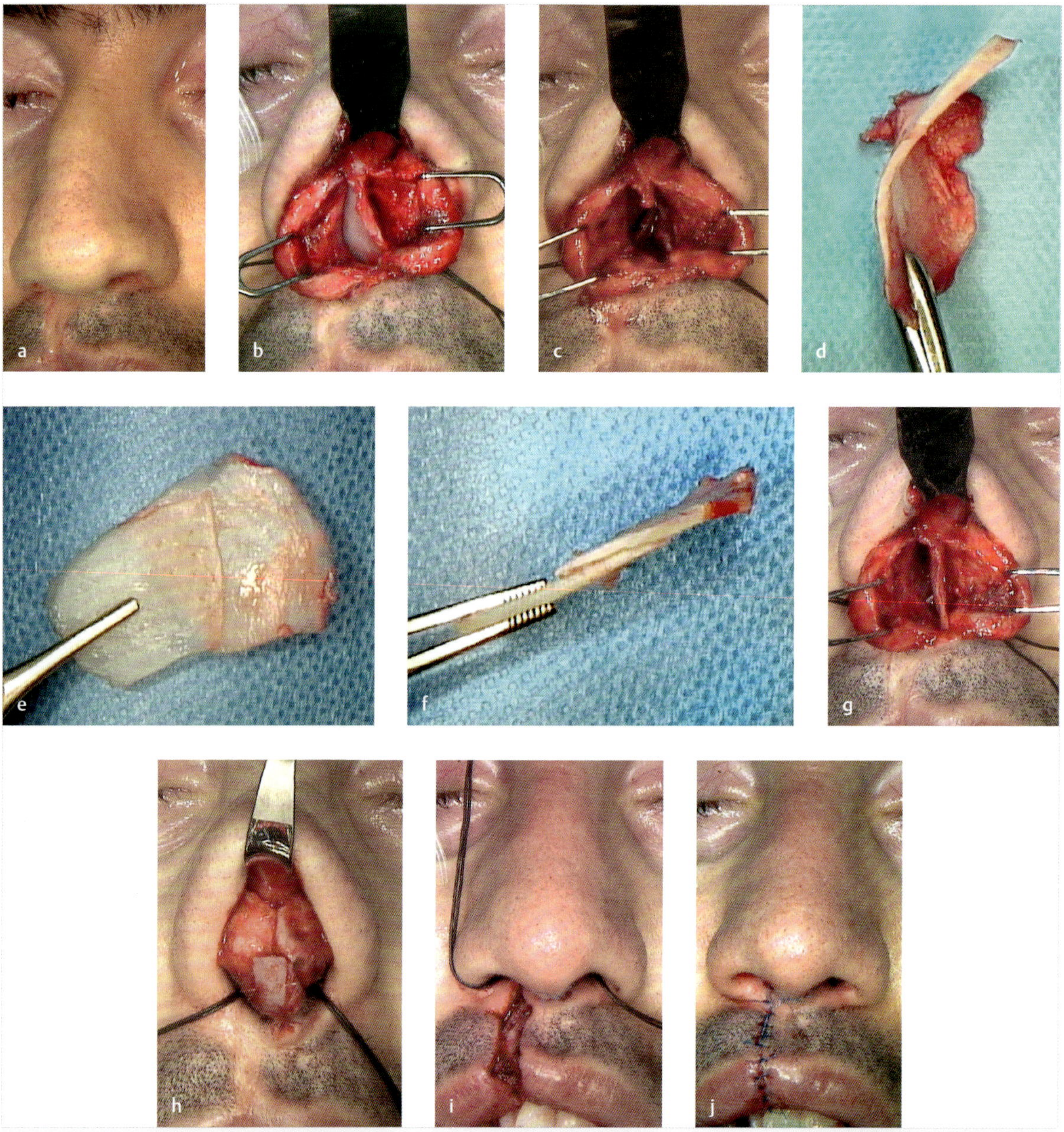

Fig. 19.10 Cleft nose deformity on the right; intraoperative view. (a) Cleft nose deformity, with deviation and hump. **(b)** Marked septal deviation and subluxation. **(c)** Empty septal site after subtotal removal of the septum for extracorporeal correction. **(d)** Septal deviation visualized after removal of the septum. **(e)** The septum was reconstructed extracorporeally from two elements: lateral view; **(f)** top view. **(g)** Reimplantation of the reconstructed septum between the mucosal layers. **(h)** Correction of the alar cartilages, tip graft. **(i)** Lip scar revision: scar excision. **(j)** After additional work on the bone and suture.

than 1.5 cm in diameter – which significantly improves visualization in these cases. Once the mucosa has been mobilized, a longitudinal mucosal incision is made under the nasal dorsum and another on the nasal floor in the lateral nasal wall under the inferior turbinate (▶ Fig. 19.15a).

This results in large, bilateral, dorsally pedicled mucosal flaps, which can then be mobilized over the nasal septal defect. The perforation defect in the mucous membranes is then closed with a few interrupted sutures (▶ Fig. 19.15b). Complete suturing on both sides closes the septal perforation. The cartilaginous defect can be filled with a delicate cartilage or fascial graft. This technique can be used to close perforations up to a vertical diameter of approximately 1.5 cm (▶ Fig. 19.16a, b).

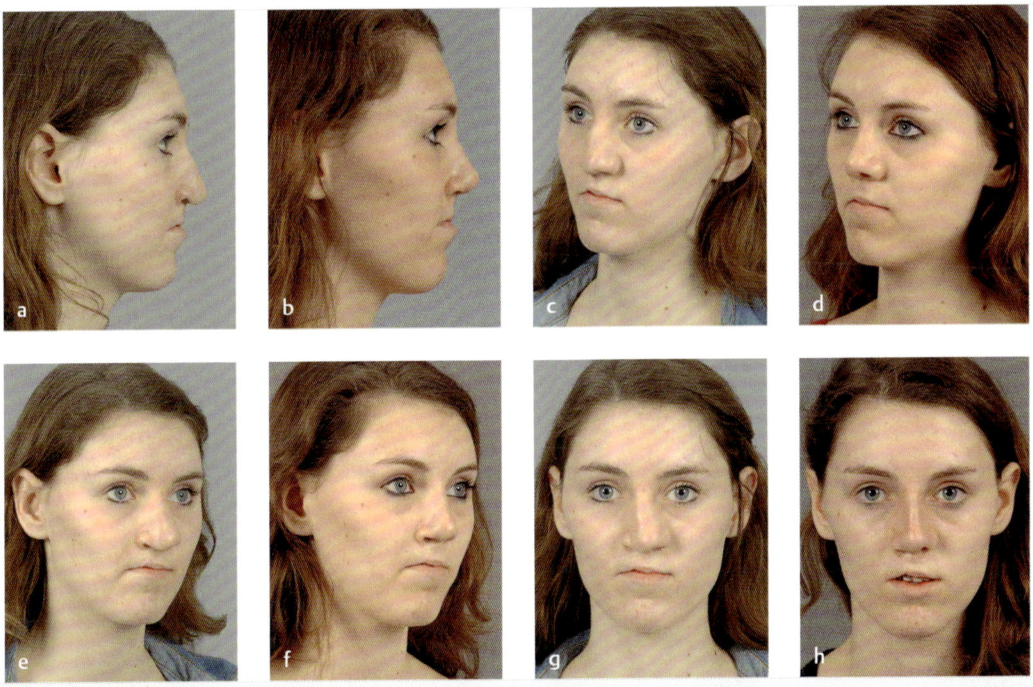

Fig. 19.11 Cleft nose deformity on the right; case study. Before surgery: lateral view **(a)**; **(c)** three-quarters view, left; **(e)** three-quarters view, right; **(g)** frontal view. After septorhinoplasty: **(b)** lateral view; **(d)** three-quarters view, left; **(f)** three-quarters view, right; **(h)** frontal view.

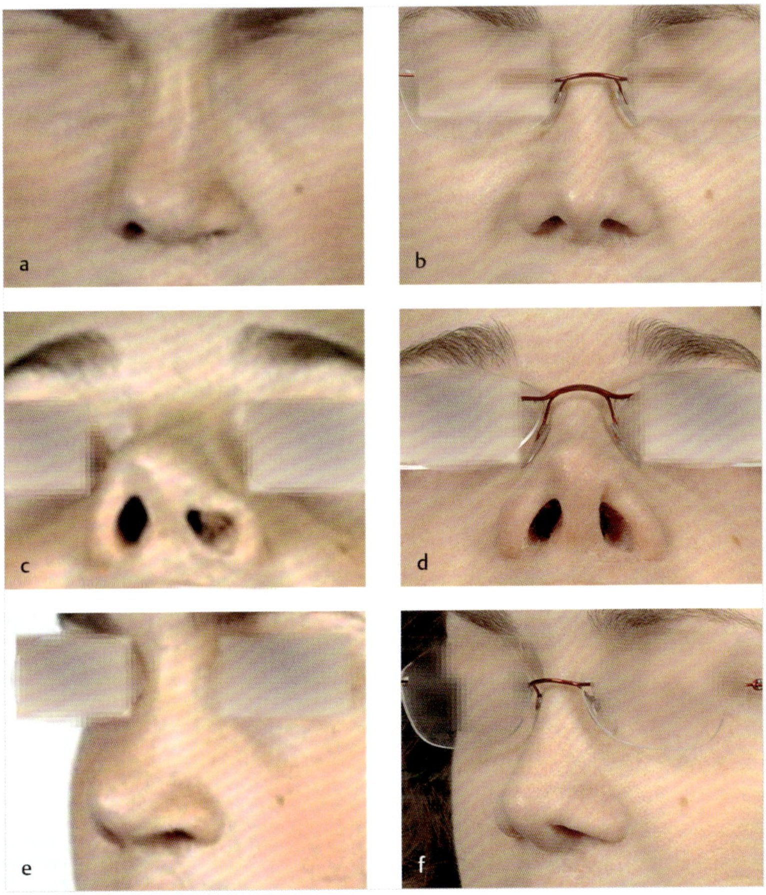

Fig. 19.12 Cleft nose deformity on the left; case study. (a, c, e) Typical findings with a left-sided cleft nose deformity. **(b, d, f)** Six years after correction with endonasal rhinoplasty.

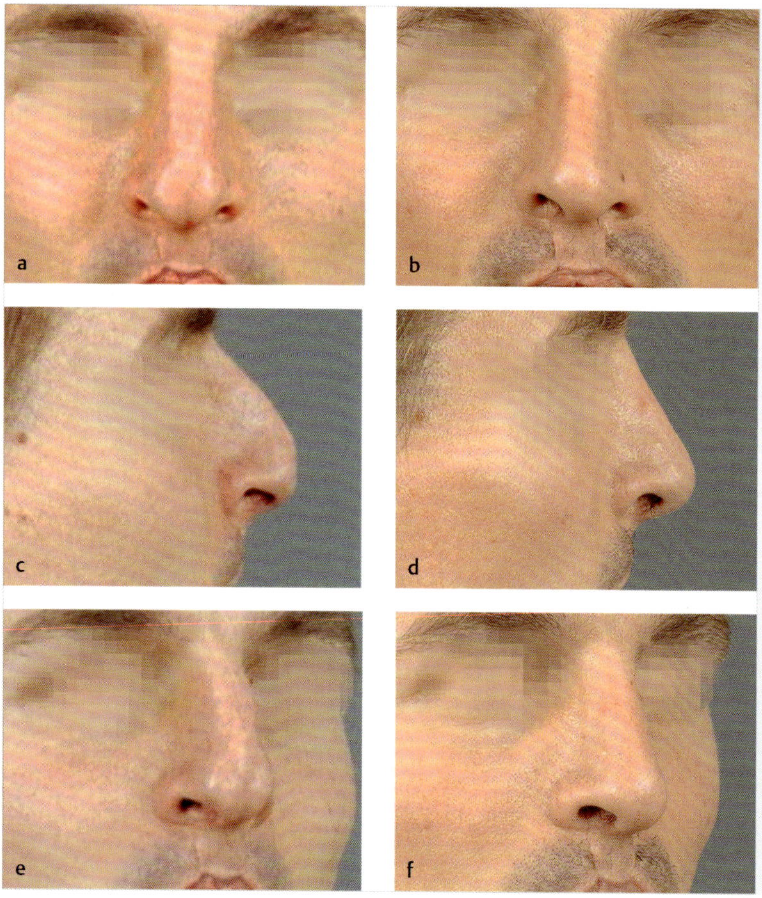

Fig. 19.13 Bilateral cleft nose deformity; case study. (a, c, e) Findings in a patient with a bilateral cleft nose deformity. **(b, d, f)** After correction with rhinoplasty.

If it occurs in individual cases, any minor residual defect visualized in the postoperative period after closure can generally be closed with a similar procedure during revision surgery, after a waiting period of 9–12 months.

An alternative procedure for larger perforations, which omits the use of these mucosal advancement flaps, involves closure of the perforation using a "sandwich," consisting of a stabilizing plate of conchal cartilage or resorbable biomaterial (such as polydioxanone – e.g., PDS), covered on each side with temporalis fascia and sutured within it. This "sandwich graft" is inserted into the perforation after mobilization of the surrounding mucosa on each side, and is then fixed to the septum using resorbable mattress sutures (▶ Fig. 19.17a–c). The septum is splinted on both sides with fixed silicone plates until healing is complete, which may take 6–8 weeks; consistent nasal care is required during this period.

Temporal fascia is obtained by incising along the hairline behind the ear, and the resultant scar is barely visible. The stabilizing PDS plate can be covered with the **superficial** temporal fascia on one side if it is robust enough, and with the **deep** temporal fascia on the contralateral side. This procedure reduces the temporal fascia defect by half in comparison with bilateral coverage with deep temporal fascia.

✓

Even under good conditions and with perfect surgical technique, the success of a closure technique for septal perforations is never guaranteed. Therefore, patients must be clearly informed that the procedure may be unsuccessful, with persistence of the defect.

Finally, **obturators** can be used for closure, which are inserted as silicone buttons into the perforation to seal the defect. They can be precisely adapted to the defect in a given patient using magnetic resonance imaging (MRI) or CT data. Unfortunately, I have not personally seen a satisfactory repair of a septal perforation using an obturator, although the procedure may be useful in certain cases. Over the longer term, chafing due to the contact between the plastic button and the edges of the perforation may, however, result in enlargement of the defect.

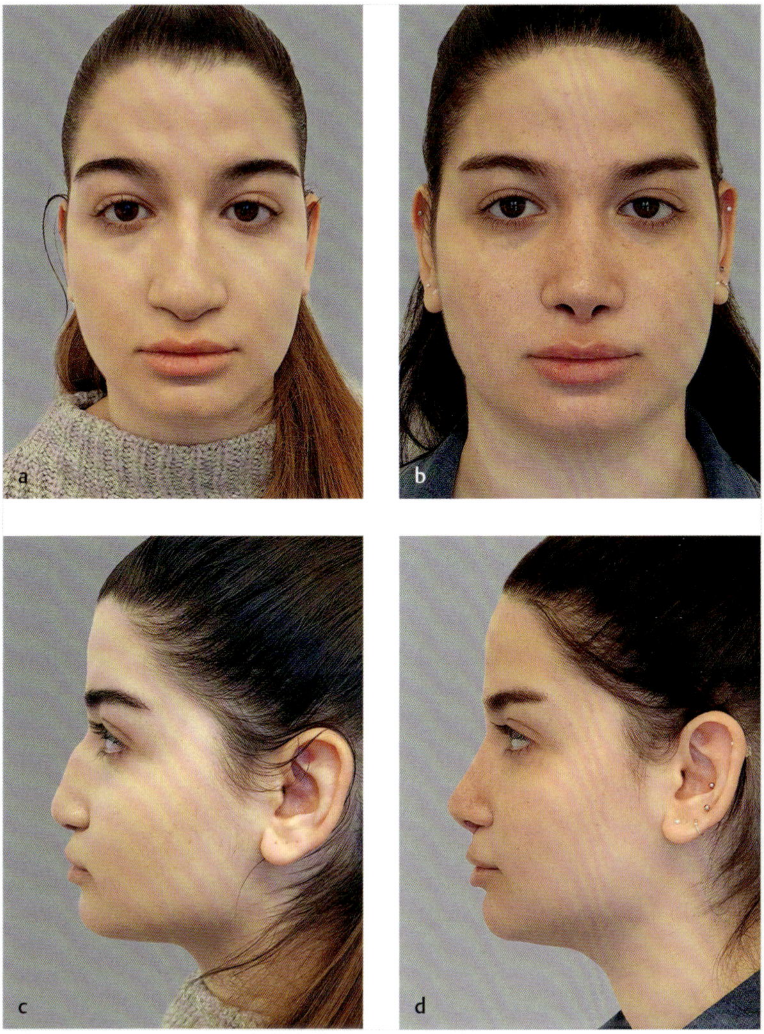

Fig. 19.14 Binder deformity. (a) Nasal deformity in Binder syndrome: frontal view. **(c)** Lateral view. After rhinoplasty: frontal view **(b)**; lateral view **(d)**.

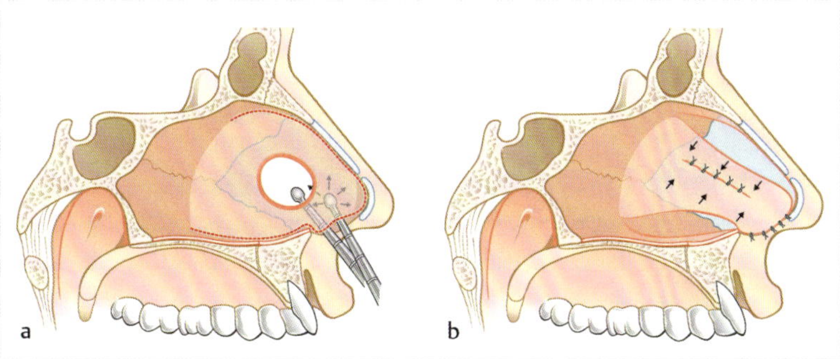

Fig. 19.15 Septal perforation: closure with a mucosal advancement flap. (a) Starting from a hemitransfixion, an incision under the nasal roof and over the nasal floor gives rise to a large, dorsally pedicled mucosal flap bilaterally after extensive mobilization of septal mucosa. **(b)** The perforation is closed by advancing the mucosa bilaterally and suturing over the defect. Anteriorly, the mucosa is reattached lateral to the columella at the caudal edge of the septum.

19.6 Rhinophyma

Rhinophyma (rosacea) consists of growths of connective tissue and sebaceous glands (phyma), and represents a severe, progressive form of rosacea of the skin ("hammer nose," "pug nose," "conk"; ▸ Fig. 19.18). An association with excessive alcohol consumption that was previously often assumed has not been confirmed; nor has the presumed tendency of the lesion toward malignant degeneration been confirmed.

I prefer to remove the nodular thickenings with a commercially available mechanical razor, and larger volumes can first be removed with a scalpel (▸ Fig. 19.19a, b). A fingertip inserted into the nostril makes it easier to work

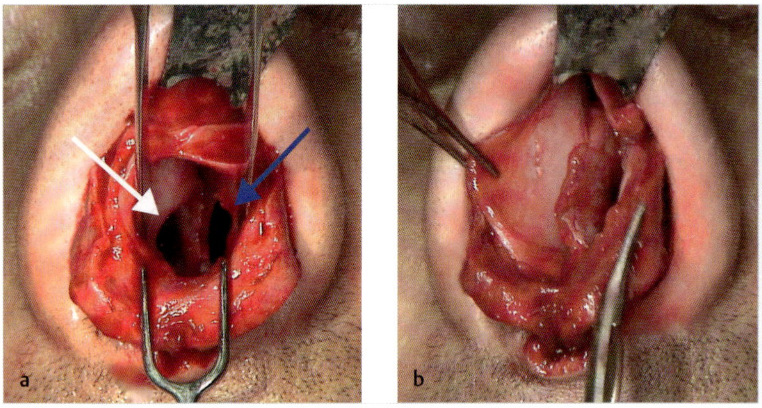

Fig. 19.16 Septal perforation closure; intraoperative view. (a) Visualization of the defect using the open technique; defect in the cartilage (white arrow) and in the mucous membrane (blue arrow). **(b)** Closure of the perforation using a left-sided mucosal flap.

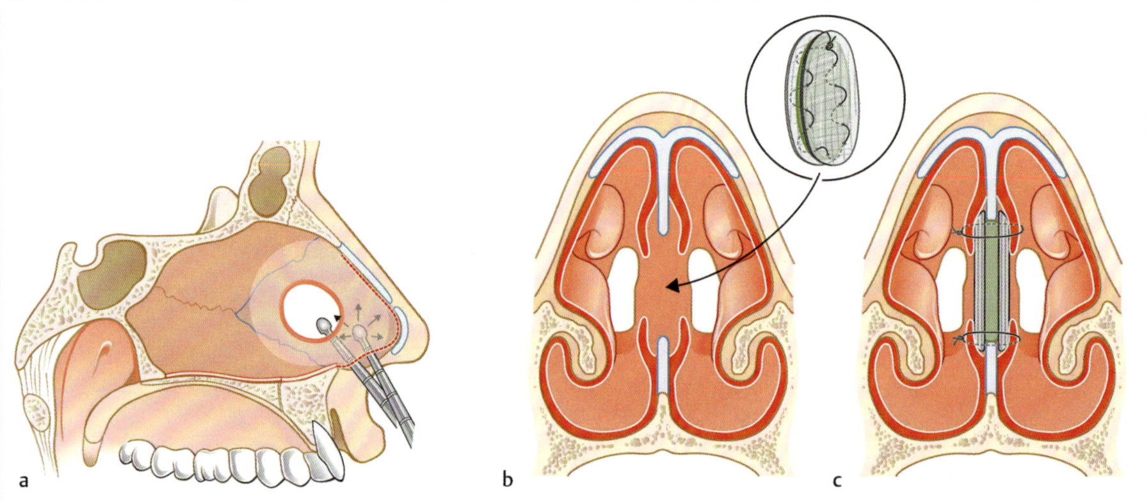

Fig. 19.17 Closure of septal perforation with a "sandwich patch." (a) The mucosa around the perforation is mobilized bilaterally using the closed or open approach. **(b)** The perforation is closed using a "composite graft" consisting of two layers of fascia with a stabilizing core. **(c)** After suture fixation.

on the tissue at the nasal alae. It is imperative for the surgeon to avoid excessive tissue removal and exposure of nasal cartilage during ablation. This may lead to unsightly scar contractures on the new skin cover, which are difficult to correct.

> ✓
>
> When removing rhinophyma, it is not important to create a perfectly proportioned nose at all costs. The patients are usually happy if it is possible to remove the excess volume without scarring, so that they have their "old nose" back.

The procedure usually results in excessive bleeding, best controlled by intermittent cooling and compression rather than aggressive coagulation, since associated thermal injury may result in undesirable scars. Any residual bleeding at the close of the procedure is controlled by applying fibrin glue or TachoSil. Ointment gauze is applied as a bandage at the end of the procedure; it is changed repeatedly during the following days until healing is complete (▶ Fig. 19.19c). New epithelialization of the treated surface usually takes place surprisingly quickly, starting from the ducts of the incised sebaceous glands (▶ Fig. 19.20a–d).

19.7 Tumorous Skin Lesions

Any nasal or facial skin lesions that are noticed by the surgeon in a patient who is undergoing rhinoplasty must be discussed with the patient. A detailed description of the pathology and treatment of skin tumors is beyond the scope of this book. The more common skin lesions include **benign lesions** (verruca vulgaris, nevus, etc.), **precancerous lesions**, and suspected malignancies or **malignant tumors** (keratoacanthoma, basalioma, squamous cell carcinoma, malignant melanoma, etc.). Excision and histological examination must be performed in every suspected case, in keeping with applicable oncological criteria. Lesions of this type may also involve the nostrils and the nasal cavities, and must never be ignored. This is especially true for tumors in which there is a suspicion of malignancy, which have to be evaluated further. Clear agreement has to be reached with the patient, even for obviously benign lesions, on whether a given lesion should be removed for cosmetic reasons or – as is frequently the case – should remain intact, as in patients who are very particular about a "birthmark" or "beauty spot" remaining untouched (▶ Fig. 19.21a, b, ▶ Fig. 19.22a–d).

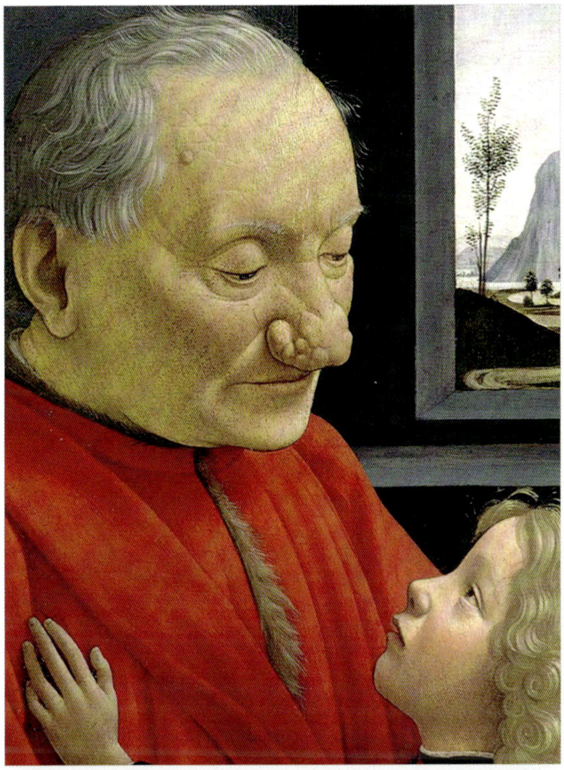

Fig. 19.18 Rhinophyma. The most famous rhinophyma in art history: Domenico Ghirlandaio (1448–1494), *Ritratto di vecchio con nipote* ("An Old Man with His Grandson"; Florence, *ca.* 1488). The absence of the typical reddening of the skin is probably explained by the fact that the portrait was made posthumously.

19.8 Lip Lift

Patients occasionally wish to combine a lip lift with rhinoplasty. Analysis is carried out to start with to determine whether the patient's upper lip is actually too long. The average distance between the columella and the vermilion border of the lip is 15–18 mm, as mentioned in the literature, but there are marked interindividual variations.

The most widespread technique for shortening or lifting the upper lip is the "bullhorn" lip lift, in which a segment of skin is excised between the base of the nose and the upper lip; the term is derived from the shape of the subnasal incision. The disadvantage of this procedure is that the resultant scar is largely concealed, but does lie in a visible region of the face. This incision is not identical to the W incision on the columella for open rhinoplasty. It is reasonably recommended that lip elevation should be deferred and undertaken after rhinoplasty, to avoid risking skin necrosis between the bullhorn and columellar inverted-V incisions.

A more elegant method involves using the open technique to expose the space anterior to the anterior nasal spine and anterior to the lower circumference of the piriform aperture bilaterally, followed by even reduction of the soft tissues of the upper lip to a small extent and subsequent suturing of the lip in an elevated position at the

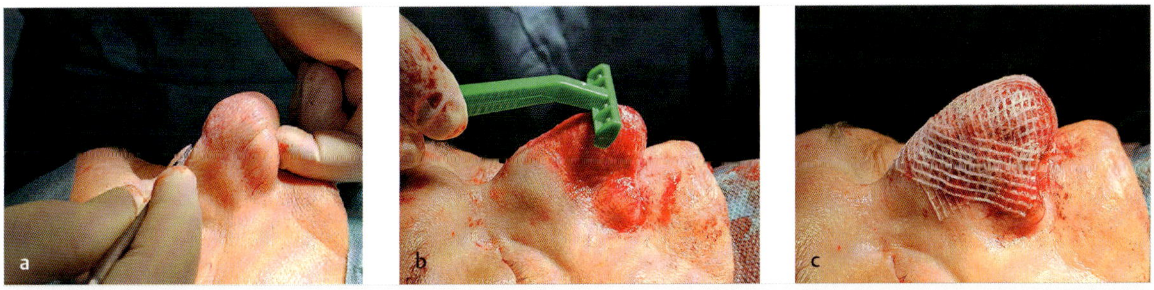

Fig. 19.19 Removal of a rhinophyma. (a) Larger volumes can first be removed with a flat blade. Placing a finger in the nostril is very helpful for controlling the process. **(b)** Using a commercially available mechanical razor, the removal of the rhinophyma can be controlled very well and the danger of penetrating too deeply into healthy tissue can be minimized. **(c)** Dressing. Bleeding at the end of the procedure is best stopped using a layer of TachoSil foam, followed by a layer of ointment gauze.

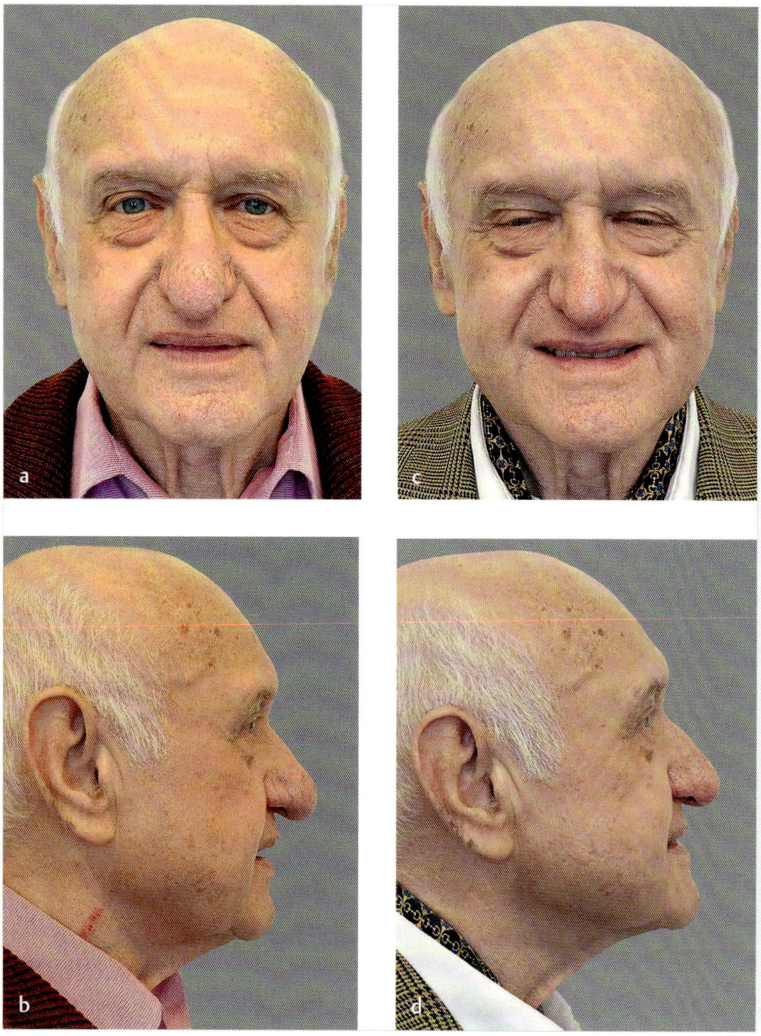

Fig. 19.20 Removal of a rhinophyma; case study (in the same patient as in ▶ Fig. 19.19a–c). **(a, b)** Preoperative. **(c, d)** Just 2–3 weeks later, epithelialization is practically complete, and a bandage is not necessary. The patient was very happy that the nose had returned to its original shape.

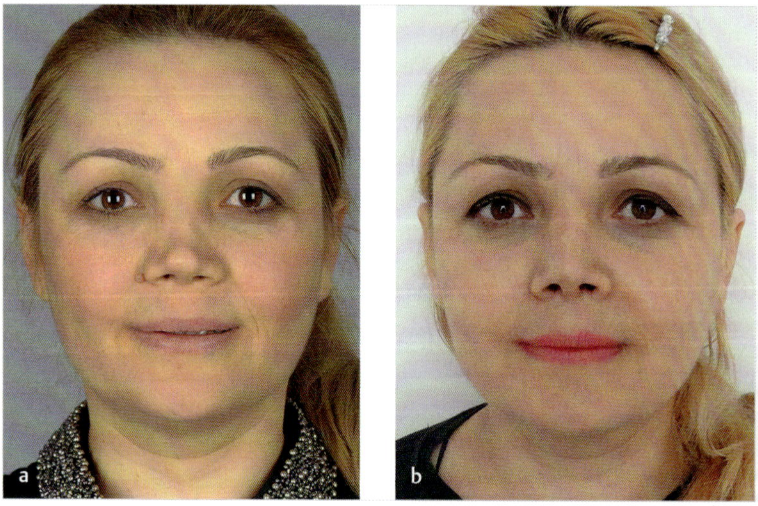

Fig. 19.21 Epidermal nevus as a secondary finding. (a) Nevus in the right nasal alar crease as a secondary finding in a patient with saddle nose. **(b)** After rhinoplasty using costal cartilage and removal of the verrucous lesion.

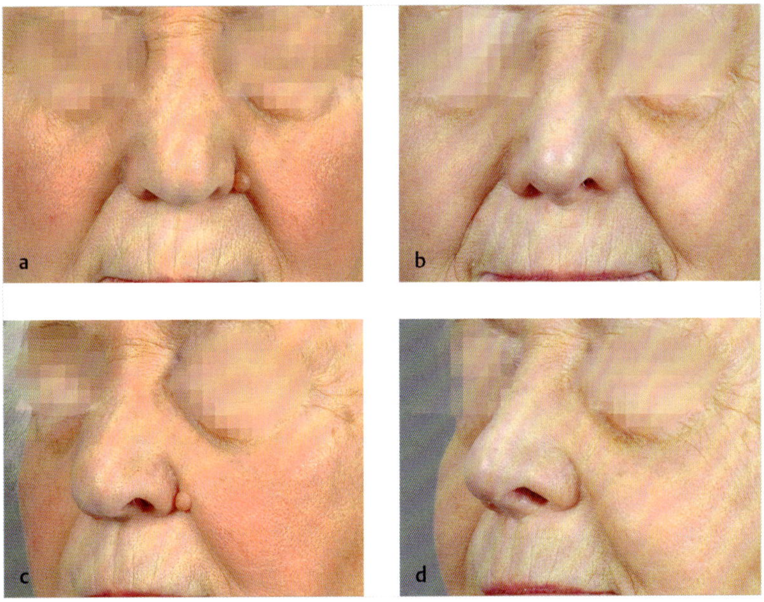

Fig. 19.22 Rhinoplasty and epidermal nevus. (a, c) Disproportionate nose, with a hanging tip and an epidermal nevus on the left. **(b, d)** Condition after rhinoplasty and resection of the nevus. It is noteworthy that the patient decided to have rhinoplasty and removal of the nevus at the age of 84 years. She was very happy with the result.

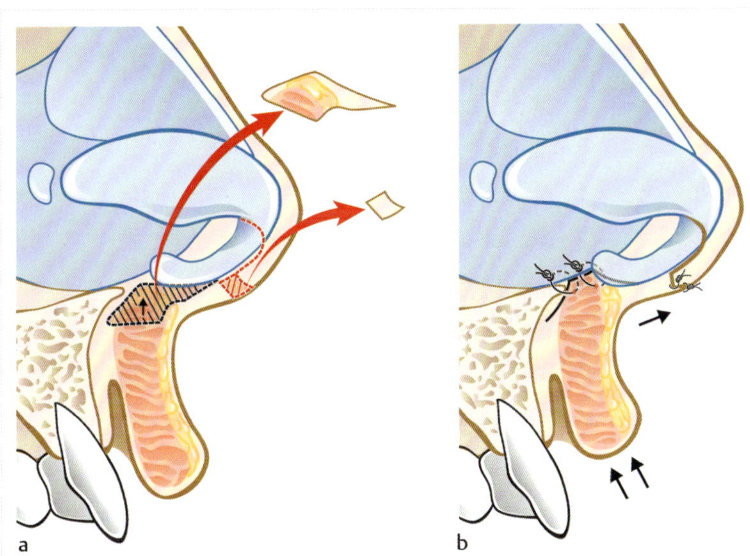

Fig. 19.23 Lip lift with open rhinoplasty; schematic diagram. **(a)** The lip is lifted after excision of a small amount of premaxillary soft tissue and a narrow strip of skin on the columella, without an additional incision. **(b)** After suturing.

caudal edge of the septum or the anterior nasal spine (▶ Fig. 19.23a, b). This procedure is particularly useful if the central segment of the lip is to be raised by a maximum of approximately 2 mm (▶ Fig. 19.24a, b).

The caudal edge of the septum and/or the spine may also be recessed slightly in some cases, to make room for the soft tissues of the lip. Elevation on both sides of the columella may give rise to excessive folds of skin, which can be reduced at the lateral edges of the columella. A narrow, 1-mm strip of skin can also be resected at the site of the inverted-V incision (see ▶ Fig. 19.23). Patients must be advised that lip mobility may be restricted due to surgical manipulation in the early postoperative period.

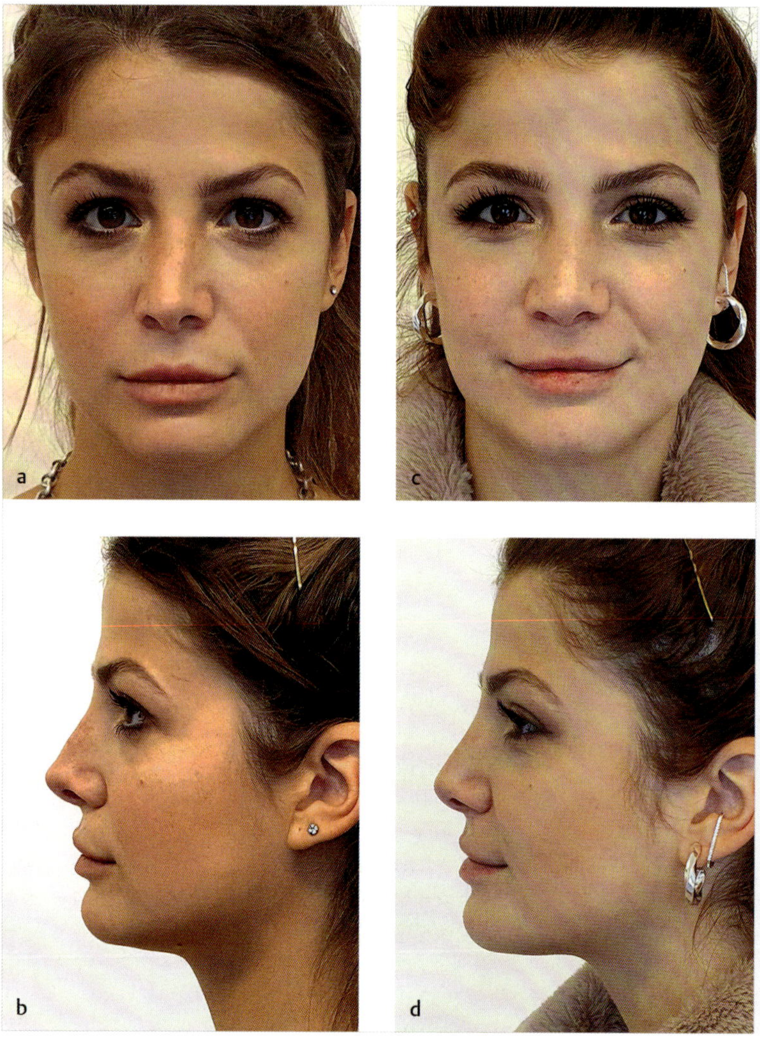

Fig. 19.24 Lip lift with open access rhinoplasty; case study. (a, b) A deviated nose with a small hump, prior to revision rhinoplasty. The patient wished to have a concurrent lip lift. **(c, d)** After revision rhinoplasty with a lip lift using the open technique. The technique described here allows moderate lifting of the lip, particularly in the central segment. In comparison with the more common bullhorn technique, a larger, potentially visible scar is avoided.

Bibliography

Akkina SR, Most SP. Treatment of the crooked nose. Clin Plast Surg. 2022; 49(1):111–121

Bloom JD, Immerman SB, Constantinides M. Osteotomies in the crooked nose. Facial Plast Surg. 2011; 27(5):456–466

Davis SJ, Rossi Meyer M, Misch E, et al. Septal perforation repair using a temporoparietal fascia and polydioxanone plate construct: a multi-institutional analysis. Facial Plast Surg Aesthet Med. 2023; 25(3):212–219

East C. Preservation rhinoplasty and the crooked nose. Facial Plast Surg Clin North Am. 2021; 29(1):123–130

Echo A, Momoh AO, Yuksel E. The no-scar lip-lift: upper lip suspension technique. Aesthetic Plast Surg. 2011; 35(4):617–623

Ferreira MG, Santos M. Preservation rhinoplasty in the saddle nose: the reverse spare roof technique. Facial Plast Surg Aesthet Med. 2022; 24(3): 168–170

Fink C, Lackey J, Grande DJ. Rhinophyma: a treatment review. Dermatol Surg. 2018; 44(2):275–282

Foda HMT. [The crooked nose: correction of dorsal and caudal septal deviations]. HNO. 2010; 58(9):899–906

Kim SW, Rhee CS. Nasal septal perforation repair: predictive factors and systematic review of the literature. Curr Opin Otolaryngol Head Neck Surg. 2012; 20(1):58–65

Kosins AM, Daniel RK, Nguyen DP. Rhinoplasty: the asymmetric crooked nose—an overview. Facial Plast Surg. 2016; 32(4):361–373

Meyer R, Berghaus A. Closure of perforations of the septum including a single-session method for large defects. Head Neck Surg. 1983; 5(5): 390–400

Olds CE, Sykes JM. Cleft rhinoplasty. Clin Plast Surg. 2022; 49(1):123–136

Romo T, III, Sclafani AP, Falk AN, Toffel PH. A graduated approach to the repair of nasal septal perforations. Plast Reconstr Surg. 1999; 103(1):66–75

Sykes JM, Kim JE, Shaye D, Boccieri A. The importance of the nasal septum in the deviated nose. Facial Plast Surg. 2011; 27(5):413–421

Vuyk HD. A review of practical guidelines for correction of the deviated, asymmetric nose. Rhinology. 2000; 38(2):72–78

Young K, Rowe-Jones J. Current approaches to septal saddle nose reconstruction using autografts. Curr Opin Otolaryngol Head Neck Surg. 2011; 19(4):276–282

20 Complications, Undesirable Results

20.1 Preliminary Remarks

Many surgeons rightly consider rhinoplasty to be the most challenging procedure in facial aesthetic plastic surgery, if not in aesthetic surgery in general, for a variety of reasons:

- Several types of tissue – skin, subcutaneous tissue, fat, connective tissue, perichondrium, periosteum, cartilage, bone, mucosa, muscles and tendons, nerves and vessels – contribute to the shape, structure, and function of the nose. It is a complex and essential sensory organ, all of which has to be appropriately and perfectly worked on during rhinoplasty to achieve a satisfactory outcome.
- The dimensions and anatomical position of these structures have specific, closely defined relationships to one another, which need to be surgically established to ensure a good result.
- In addition to the cosmetic requirements, functional concerns have to be taken into account. This occasionally requires measures that are actually contrary to the goal that would be desirable from a cosmetic point of view.
- And in addition to all of that, it is not possible in the middle of the face to conceal the nose, so that even small deviations from the ideal surgical result are noticeable.

Against this background, it would be presumptuous and unrealistic to assume that one can become an experienced rhinosurgeon, producing excellent results one after another, without ever having any undesirable results. But it is not only the surgeon's awareness of this that is important. It is just as important to let the patient participate in these considerations – i.e., to make the prospects of success and the risk of possible complications seriously clear to him or her before the operation. Even if patients are severely burdened by the appearance of their nose and urgently want to have it corrected, the operation is still a cosmetic procedure that is not medically indicated. Any complication that occurs, which may then become medically relevant, is therefore all the more serious.

When patients say, "It couldn't look any worse than this!" before rhinoplasty, the statement has to be contradicted as a matter of principle – since every surgical procedure carries a risk of a worse and undesirable outcome, which the patient needs to be aware of.

> ✔
>
> An experienced rhinoplasty surgeon is not required to emphasize the risk of complications during the preoperative briefing to the point of alarming the patient. However, it must be emphasized that the risks mentioned in this context are real, and the patient needs to make an informed decision in favor of or against the operation.

Some of the more common undesirable outcomes and complications are described below, and ways of preventing them or treating them are outlined.

20.2 Inverted-V Deformity

An inverted-V deformity develops when the middle cartilage framework (the upper lateral cartilages and septum) is completely separated from the nasal bones without subsequently being sutured to the bony vault or otherwise stabilized to form a stable unit. The cartilaginous vault may then sink relative to the bony framework, giving rise to an unsightly step deformity – an inverted V – between the cartilaginous and bony vault during healing. This undesirable configuration can also be regarded as a variant of saddle nose.

Corrective surgery usually consists of elevating and widening the lateral cartilaginous walls using spreader grafts, possibly augmented by cartilaginous overlays over the lateral walls and/or dorsum of the middle third of the nose. The extent of bony remodeling required, with the aim of narrowing the anatomical structures, depends on the individual case (▶ Fig. 20.1, see also case study in ▶ Fig. 19.21).

20.3 Pollybeak Deformity

Pollybeak deformity is an alteration of the nasal shape that typically occurs as a complication of rhinoplasty, but may also be due to congenital malformations or trauma. It is characterized by the typical appearance of a dorsal nasal convexity located in the supratip region of the nose, which is particularly annoying in the side profile, while at the same time the nasal tip droops downward. The appearance vaguely recalls the shape of a parrot's beak (▶ Fig. 20.2a, b, ▶ Fig. 20.3a, b, c), and is due to a disproportion between the height of the supratip region and the nasal tip. The elevated supratip may be due to an inadequately reduced anterior septal angle, or the presence of scarred, voluminous fibroadipose subcutaneous tissue in this region. The surgeon can prevent pollybeak deformity by ensuring that the nasal tip lies higher than the supratip, both visually and on palpation, before ending the surgical procedure. It may be necessary to check whether reduction in the height of the anterior septum and the anterior septal angle is required, or the underlying fibroadipose subcutaneous tissue requires thinning, or whether greater rotation of the nasal tip complex is desirable – for example, with a tip graft.

Even if the anatomical relationships are correct at the close of surgery, postoperative swelling of the fibroadipose subcutaneous tissue and/or derotation of the tip may also give rise to a pollybeak deformity, which does not regress or regresses only very slowly.

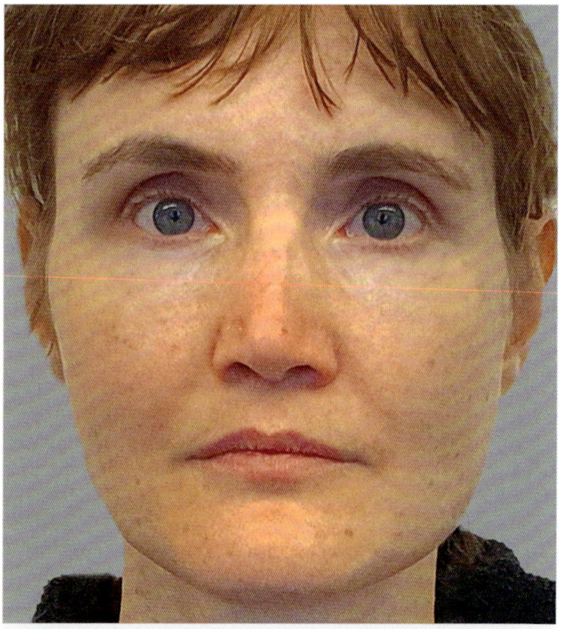

Fig. 20.1 Inverted-V deformity. A step is both palpable and visible between the bony and cartilaginous frames of the nose after rhinoplasty, with an inverted-V appearance.

✓

As a measure for preventing pollybeak deformity, I thin out hyperplastic subcutaneous adipose connective tissue in the supratip region (see section 13.2).

In cases of early postoperative deformity resembling pollybeak that is due to swollen soft tissue or scars above the tip, an intralesional injection of triamcinolone crystal suspension may be helpful. If this procedure is used repeatedly, a pause of several weeks should be left between applications. This treatment does not, of course, have any effect on a high anterior septal angle.

Pollybeak deformity is distinctly rare if the surgeon's attention and operative skills during primary rhinoplasty are geared toward achieving an optimal relationship between the nasal dorsum and the nasal tip, as explained above. This spares both the surgeon and the patient the need for unpleasant follow-up treatment with corticosteroid injections and revision surgery, which may be unavoidable in patients with a persistent pollybeak deformity (▶ Fig. 20.3 a-c).

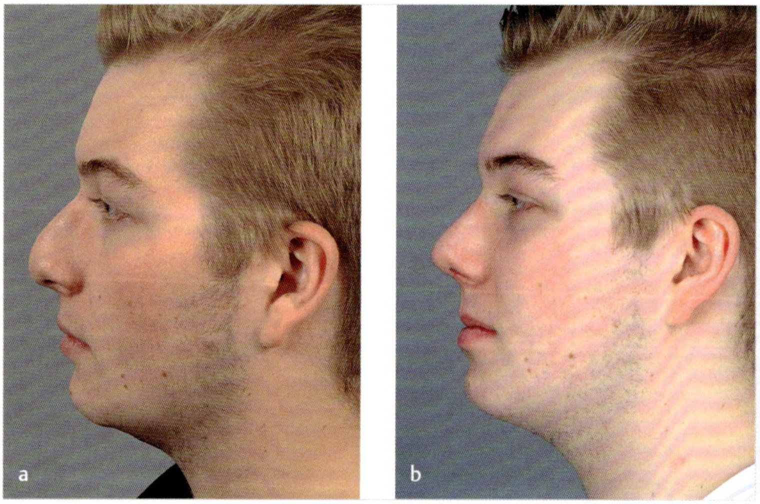

Fig. 20.2 Pollybeak after trauma. (a) Pollybeak after a road traffic accident. **(b)** After corrective rhinoplasty (see also ▶ Fig. 12.31a–d; section 12.2.2).

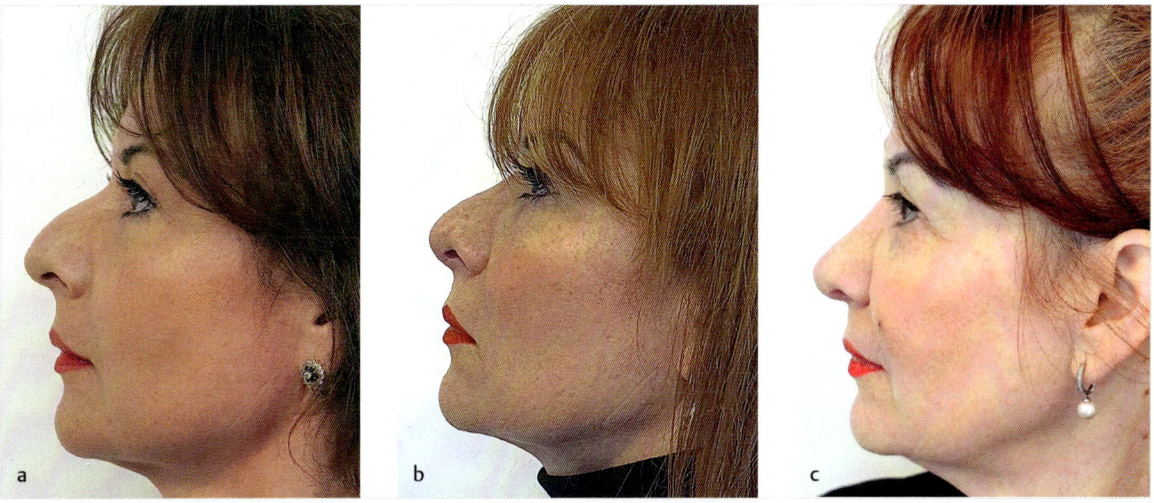

Fig. 20.3 Pollybeak after rhinoplasty. (a) The patient presented to rhinoplasty already with a supratip elevation. **(b)** Postoperatively, a pollybeak deformity developed over time due to a callous scar in the subcutaneous tissue. Cortisone injections did little to help. **(c)** Acceptable result from the patient's perspective after 2 years, achieved only after surgical removal of the scar in combination with raising the tip using a tip graft and subsequent repeated cortisone injections.

20.4 Nasal Telangiectasia (Couperose)

Redness occasionally occurs on the nasal dorsum postoperatively, particularly in the region of the rhinion and bony dorsum, even with careful dissection of the skin flap. This postoperative complication occurs much more often and is more severe after second or multiple nasal procedures than after primary rhinoplasty. Under a magnifying glass or microscope, increased vascularity can be seen in these cases, with a network of dilated veins (nasal telangiectasia [couperose]). This appearance may have an adverse impact on the overall outcome of rhinoplasty, even if surgery is otherwise successful.

The lesions should be observed initially, and patients should be reassured and informed that the lesion is likely to fade away over weeks or even months, with or without skin care (rosacea cream). Patients can be offered laser therapy of the visible vascular network if the redness has not yet subsided even months later. A vascular laser with a suitable wavelength or a KTP laser that couples to the red color of vessels is best suited for this. The energy and spot size can be easily regulated, and conspicuous vessels are thus accurately targeted while the surrounding skin remains unaffected (▶ Fig. 20.4a,b). The treatment only requires surface anesthesia – for example, with a lidocaine/prilocaine cream (e.g., Emla) – and lasts no more than 10–15 minutes. One therapeutic session is usually sufficient, but the procedure may need to be repeated in severe cases. Using excessive energy during laser treatment may lead to thermal skin injury, which must be avoided at all costs.

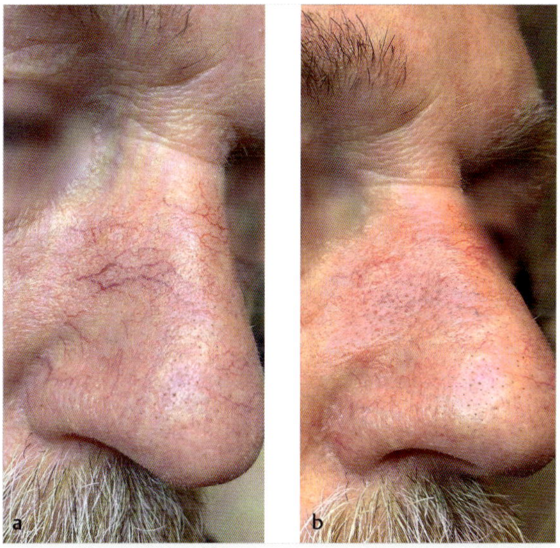

Fig. 20.4 Nasal telangiectasia (couperose). (a) Noticeable vascular pattern in the nasal skin. **(b)** Condition after laser treatment. (With permission of Diedejan ter Horst [Bachelor of Science, Dermal Clinical], Berg Clinic, Zeewolde, The Netherlands. Indication: Teleangiectasia. Laser system: QuadroStarPRO YELLOW. Thank you to Prof. Gerd Gauglitz, Haut- und Laserzentrum Glockenbach, Munich, Germany, for his support in obtaining this figure.)

20.5 Infection

The nostrils and nasal cavities are often considered to be contaminated with bacteria, which carry a high risk of infection. However, postoperative suppuration after rhinoplasty is rare as long as there are no unusual circumstances.

The patient receives a single-dose antibiotic perioperatively for infection prophylaxis, since rhinoplasty operations usually last 2 hours or longer. A cephalosporin is administered intravenously on the day of the operation; ampicillin/sulbactam (e.g., Unasyn) is a good alternative, in view of its better efficacy following oral administration in case the antibiotic needs to be continued postoperatively.

Long-term antibiotics can be continued in the postoperative period in the following circumstances:

- Revision surgery, especially with severe scarring after multiple previous operations, or following severe trauma
- Use of cartilage grafts or diced cartilage from the ear or from the rib
- Tendency to develop infection or history of recurrent purulent nasal infections
- Known immunodeficiency or immune defect

Smaller, isolated erythematous areas over the columella or nasal base, possibly with punctiform pus discharge from a suture channel in the early postoperative phase, are disinfected and treated initially with local antibiotic (and cortisone) ointments alone (such as Jellin-Neomycin ointment) after suture removal. The condition then regresses within a short period of time, provided the suture has been completely removed.

More extensive local postoperative suppuration has to be investigated further using a smear. The treatment consists of wound irrigation with disinfectant solution and/or H_2O_2, and local antibiotic ointment in combination with systemic antibiotic therapy – as appropriate, depending on the pathogen identified on microbiological examination.

In addition to the treatment outlined above, an affected graft bed has to be opened and infected cartilage removed if suppuration occurs after costal cartilage transplantation or after large amounts of diced cartilage have been used. The chances of saving these infected fragments from disintegration through conservative treatment and irrigation alone are small. The infection generally spreads to other structures in the nasal vault and eventually to the subcutaneous tissue and skin, possibly resulting in difficult-to-treat lesions.

20.6 Septal Perforation

Bilateral tears or mucosal defects with a concomitant absence of cartilage give rise to continuous, triple-layer septal defects. These defects usually develop as a complication of septoplasty, especially after correction of severe septal deformities with traumatized, poorly vascularized mucosa. Patients have to be informed about the risk of perforation, since the septum is often being operated on for cartilage harvesting during rhinoplasty, especially in revision surgery. Studies have shown that a permanent septal defect can often be avoided if mucosal tears are identified and promptly sutured during dissection.

Patients must not be left in the dark if a nasal septal defect is identified during the postoperative follow-up, particularly since they will probably soon be suffering from the typical symptoms of such a lesion: whistling sounds during nasal breathing, recurrent epistaxis, crust formation, and obstructed nasal breathing.

> ✓
>
> The situation may become worse with a progressive increase in the size of the defect and the development of a saddle nose and/or columellar retraction. Closure of the defect is recommended at an early stage for this reason alone. As with all revision surgery procedures after septorhinoplasty, however, a waiting period of approximately 9–12 months is recommended to allow tissue healing before closure of the perforation.

The techniques for closing septal perforations are discussed in section 19.5.

20.7 Crooked Nose, Asymmetry

It is not uncommon to observe that the nose is not precisely symmetrical in the middle in the early postoperative stages after rhinoplasty. During this phase, patients examine the nose and face particularly carefully in the mirror several times a day. A deviated or asymmetrical nose and nostrils of unequal size are then quickly interpreted as a sign of a failed operation with a poor outcome. It is imperative for the patient to be informed that findings of this type in the early postoperative period are not necessarily permanent and will probably improve during the subsequent weeks and months, with every chance that the abnormalities will eventually regress completely. It is important not to overlook or belittle an imperfect surgical outcome, but rather to calm patients down and avoid panic. It may be useful to briefly explain how the problem could be solved at a later time if it persists. Temporary correction of circumscribed asymmetry with filler injections may also be considered in some cases (see Chapter 22).

Permanently deviated noses should only undergo repeat surgery after the usual waiting period of approximately 12 months. Some patients regard asymmetry of

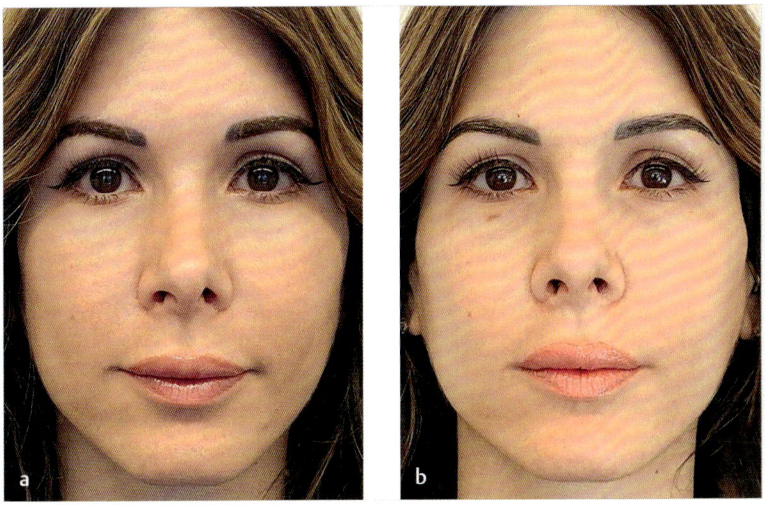

Fig. 20.5 Asymmetric alar rims and asymmetry of the columella post rhinoplasty. (a) After rhinoplasty, the patient complained of the asymmetrical elevation of the left nasal rim and an asymmetrical projection of the right foot of the medial crus. **(b)** Condition after endonasal revision with rim graft on the left and correction of the position of the caudal septum, which led to symmetry at the columella.

the nostrils as a particularly serious postoperative flaw and fussily observe it for months. It is helpful in such cases to point out that after a reasonable waiting time, if there is no improvement, small rim grafts, possibly inserted endonasally, can be used to remedy the situation (▶ Fig. 20.5a, b, see also section 10.3). Asymmetrical alar wedge and nostril sill resections may also be considered, depending on the needs in the individual case (see Chapter 14; ▶ Fig. 14.9a, b).

20.8 Saddle Nose

Saddle nose deformity usually results from excessive resection during septoplasty, but may also be due to excessive reduction of the dorsum. Due to overlying tissue swelling, the saddle deformity is frequently not evident during the early postoperative period and only becomes fully visible in the medium to longer term once the edema has abated. As mentioned earlier, revision surgery should not be performed too early, to ensure correction of the full extent of the deformity. A filler can be applied in the interim, but augmentation with grafts is the best long-term solution (see section 17.2).

✔

A conchal cartilage graft is often used for corrective surgery, as the available septal cartilage may be inadequate in patients undergoing revision surgery, especially in those with a saddle nose after septoplasty (see the case study in ▶ Fig. 19.6 a,b). A rib cartilage graft is only required in very severe cases (see the case study in ▶ Fig. 19.7 a,b).

20.9 Undercorrection, Persistent Hump

As with an undesirable saddle nose, inadequate correction of a hump may not be noticeable at first due to postoperative swelling. It becomes visible only later when the soft-tissue swelling has receded. Patients may occasionally say that the hump was initially removed during the procedure but then “grew back.” This is of course not correct, since the incompletely removed hump was only being obscured by edematous soft tissue.

This form of undercorrection, with persistence of a slightly raised nasal dorsum, is certainly not consistent with the desired outcome, but is often not problematic for the patient. Moderate elevation of the nasal dorsum due solely to soft-tissue and periosteal swelling still has a good chance of improving during the postoperative phase, and this can be easily explained to the patient. If the swelling then recedes, the person affected will also notice this positively; at the same time, over the course of months, the patient's initially overprecise self-observation often, but not always changes to a more relaxed attitude, and along with this a residual finding of dorsal elevation is sometimes accepted.

A residual hump is particularly feared when preservation rhinoplasty is used (compare with section 8.4). If the surgeon has the impression that a push-down or let-down alone is not sufficient to safely correct a hump, then a combination with additional processing of the surface of the dorsum, as in a surface rhinoplasty, should definitely be considered. This “hybrid technique” significantly increases the safety of controlling a hump.

If surgical revision is necessary, then a small residual hump (in contrast to overcorrection) can be corrected

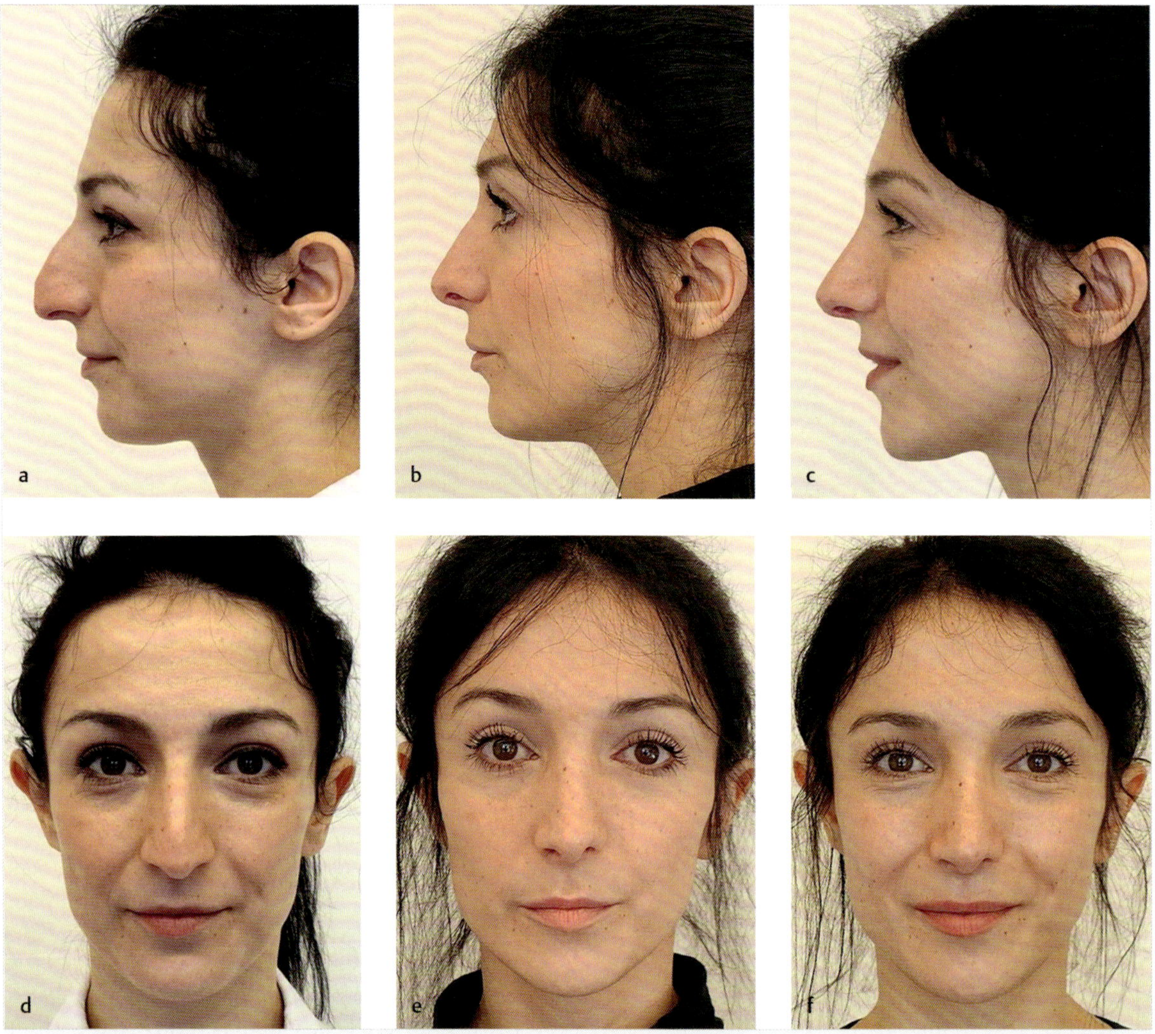

Fig. 20.6 Recurrence of a hump after preservation rhinoplasty. (a,b,c) side view; **(d,e,f)** frontal view. 30-year-old patient with a large hump and under-rotated nasal tip **(a, d)**. One year after preservation rhinoplasty with the let-down technique, a partial recurrence of the hump could be seen, which is why the patient was very dissatisfied despite the reduction achieved **(b, e)**. Only the revision with conventional instruments, including lateral and paramedian osteotomies, satisfied the patient. At the same time, the definition of the tip was enhanced with a tip graft, in accordance with the patient's wishes.

with relatively little effort, and an endonasal approach often suffices. If only the height of the nasal bridge is to be reduced, subsequent processing with piezo technology or conventional instruments may be sufficient. If additional narrowing is also desired, lateral and possibly paramedian osteotomies cannot be avoided during the revision operation, i.e. the revision is then carried out as a structural rhinoplasty (▸ Fig. 20.6**a-f**).

✓

In general, the surgeon is well advised to select a more conservative approach when deciding on the degree of reduction. Adequate material will thus be available if revision surgery is required in a dissatisfied patient, and this is far better than having to augment the nasal vault after overcorrection.

20.10 Obstructed Nasal Breathing

Every operation on the nose must address both cosmetic and also functional aspects. Patients find any worsening of nasal breathing after rhinoplasty stressful and disappointing. In the immediate postoperative period, it may be due to various easily treatable causes. These include endonasal soft-tissue swelling, secretions, and crusting, which are rapidly amenable to treatment with suction, mechanical cleansing, decongestant spray, or nasal irrigation. Tissue swelling in the postoperative period, with increased nasal secretions as in rhinitis, often leads patients to think they have a cold. At this stage, it is usually easy to assure them that the condition is short-lived and temporary.

Patients become justifiably concerned when nasal airway obstruction persists over the medium to long term, or has a delayed onset. The reasons behind the disorder then need to be carefully analyzed and appropriate management has to be considered.

> ✔
>
> Not all causes of obstructed nasal breathing may be visible with the speculum. Using a rigid endoscope is therefore helpful in arriving at a definitive diagnosis.

20.10.1 Nasal Valve Insufficiency and Nostril Stenosis

Collapse of the nostrils on inspiration may be due to persistent septal subluxation after surgery, which then has to be corrected by revision surgery. More often, however, the cause is nasal valve collapse. Surgery may make the alar cartilage too weak, or may excessively narrow the angle of the nasal valve.

Nasal Valve Insufficiency

Insufficiency of the nasal valves is investigated using the Cottle test and instrumental stabilization of the nasal alae to elucidate the cause (see section 3.2.2; ▶ Fig. 20.7, ▶ Fig. 20.8). Even in these cases, revision surgery has to be deferred until tissue healing is complete, and this may be unpleasant for both the patient and the surgeon. It is not entirely impossible that the situation may improve over a period of months as the alar scars consolidate. Patients with very severe nostril collapse (▶ Fig. 20.8) can be offered nasal stents to insert at night. These soft plastic tubes are commercially available as an anti-snoring remedy (e.g., RuneSol nasal dilators, ▶ Fig. 20.9).

Dilators are primarily intended as a temporary bridging device in the early postoperative period after rhinoplasty, but with consistent use they may adequately stabilize the nostril in such a way that operative correction may eventually no longer be necessary. A therapeutic trial of them is therefore worthwhile. However, inserting the stents during the day is not feasible in most cases, as they are visible externally.

A slightly more invasive method of stabilizing the nasal valve involves applying small, stabilizing rods comprised of absorbable, tissue-friendly material derived from lactic acid (Latera; Stryker Corporation). These stabilizers, which are not externally visible, are introduced subcutaneously into the affected area of the nasal valve using an applicator. The procedure is performed on an outpatient basis with the patient under local anesthesia (▶ Fig. 20.10).

The procedures described in section 10.3 for stabilizing the nasal valve can be implemented if the measures specified above are inadequate. Lateral crural strut and batten grafts (for the inner nasal valve) and rim grafts (for the outer valve) may be primarily considered, as well as spreader grafts to widen the inner nasal valve. In addition, attention needs to be given to possible concurrent weakness of the medial pillar comprising the

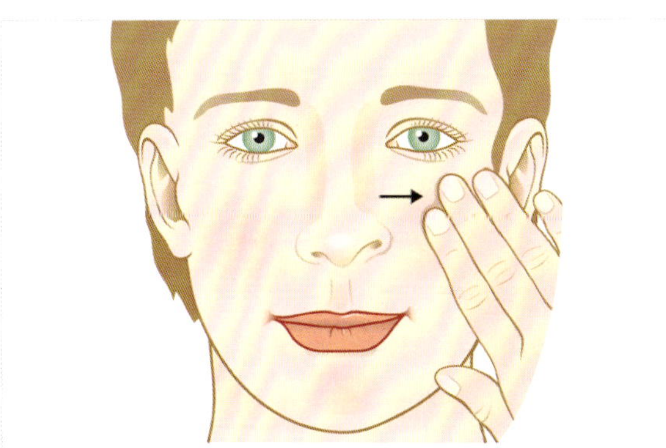

Fig. 20.7 Cottle test. Pulling the cheek and nasal alae laterally opens the nasal valve and improves nasal breathing.

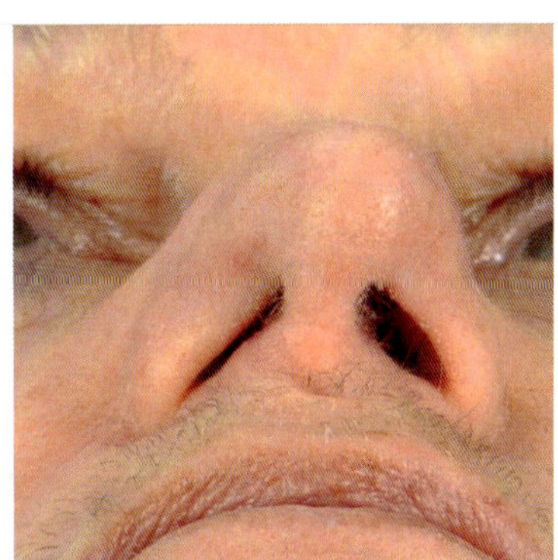

Fig. 20.8 Nostril collapse during inspiration. Nasal valve insufficiency on the right side after rhinoplasty.

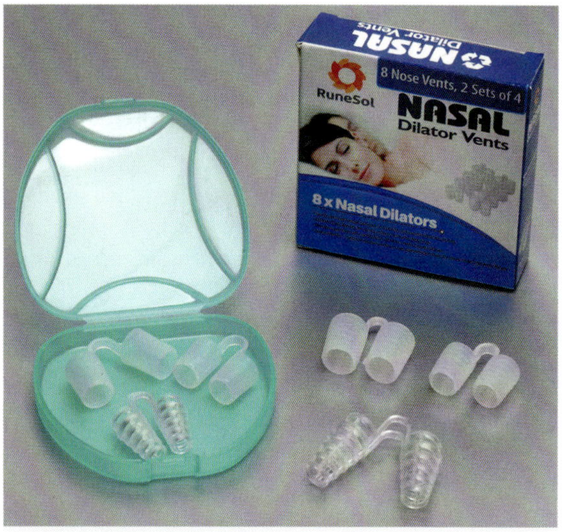

Fig. 20.9 Nostril dilators. The commercially available nasal dilators (RuneSol Ltd., Warrington, UK) are available in various forms from different suppliers.

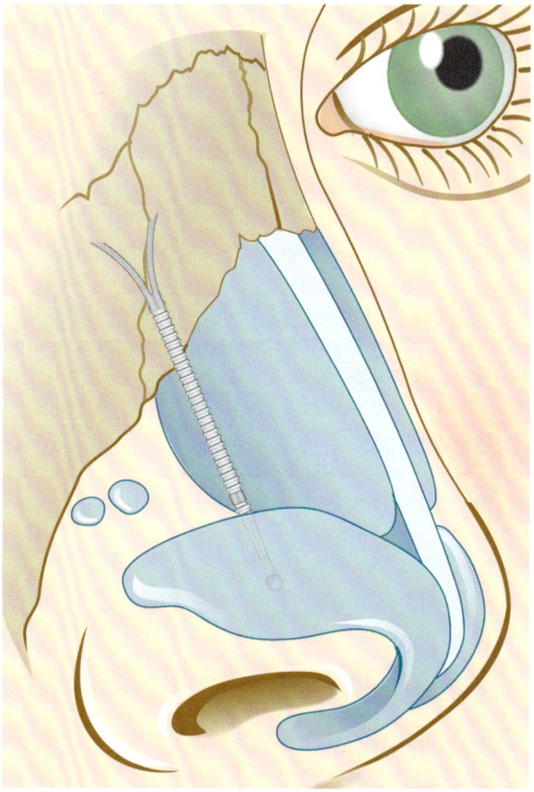

Fig. 20.10 Latera implants (Stryker Corporation). The Latera implant consists of an absorbable lactic acid derivative and is supplied with an applicator. For stabilizing the nasal valve, it is placed endonasally in the area of the valve, i. e., medial to the cephalic margin of the lower lateral cartilage, and lateral to the upper lateral cartilage.

caudal septum and medial crura, which will also have to be corrected if necessary (see section 11.1.2) (▸ Fig. 20.11a, b).

Nostril Stenosis

Correctly performed rhinoplasty should not give rise to nostril stenosis. Nevertheless, the condition is occasionally seen after (revision) sill resections and other procedures involving the nostrils. Inserting a skin graft into the stenosed region is not sufficient for correcting acquired or congenital nostril stenosis. Surgical enlargement of a nostril is only successful using a stabilizing cartilage transplant. Composite grafts from the cymba conchae, with their natural curvature and thin skin closely attached to the cartilage, are therefore particularly suitable for widening stenosed nostrils (▸ Fig. 20.12a, b; see section 18.2.2).

Depending on the individual situation and the site of the stenosis, an elongated composite auricular graft (see section 18.2.2) is inserted into a concealed incision running along the floor of the nostril or laterally at the alar base, immediately posterior to the nasal sill. A graft bed is prepared in the (frequently scarred) soft tissue. It must be large enough to accommodate the cartilaginous component of the composite graft. The skin edges of the composite graft are sutured to the edges of the incision in the nostril. The composite graft is then securely fixed to the graft bed with a deep mattress suture. This suture passes outward and back again exactly along the alar crease and can be removed after 6–8 days.

20.10.2 Synechiae

Extensive endonasal surgery during septorhinoplasty may injure large mucosal surfaces of the septum and lateral nasal walls and make them susceptible to adhesions and synechiae. Endonasal silicone splints such as Doyle splints (see ▸ Fig. 7.20) should be used in such high risk cases to avoid the development of synechiae and should be left in place for longer than the usual 2–3 days,

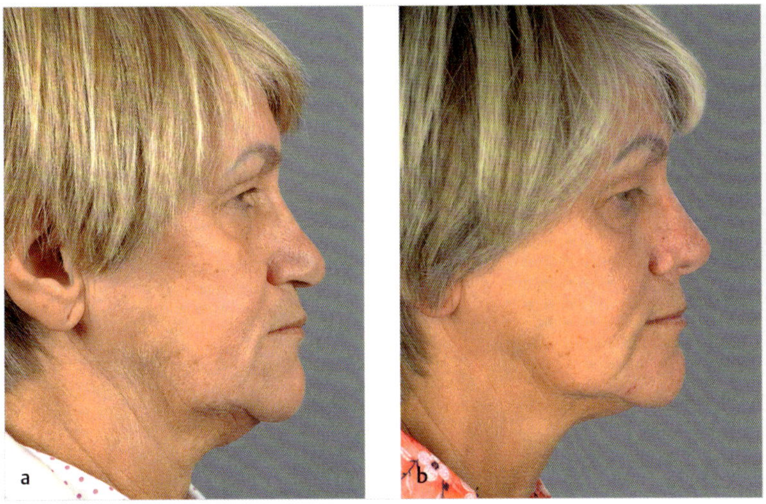

Fig. 20.11 Nasal valve insufficiency; clinical case. (a) Nasal valve insufficiency with weakness of the nasal alae, lack of support for the anterior septum, and drooping tip with a narrow nasolabial angle. **(b)** After correction with septal extension graft, repositioning of the upper lateral cartilages with suspension sutures, and lateral batten grafts.

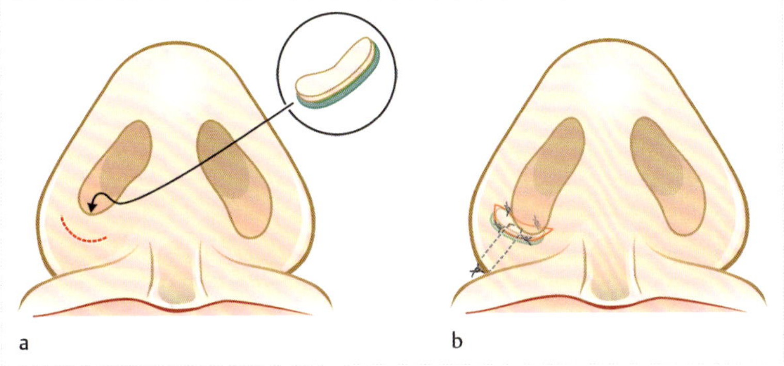

Fig. 20.12 Composite auricular graft for nostril stenosis. (a) An auricular skin–cartilage transplant is suitable for widening the nostril. **(b)** After suture fixation, including a temporary transalar mattress suture.

possibly up to 8-10 days. The nose has to be regularly examined with endoscopy even after removal of the endonasal splints, and any fibrin clots or fresh adhesions between mucous membranes need to be ablated as prophylaxis against synechiae.

Adhesions between the septum and the middle or inferior turbinate, between the middle turbinate and the lateral nasal wall, or between the septum and the lateral nasal wall, and at the angle of the nasal valve, may be functionally troublesome. An endoscope is usually required for diagnosis.

Endonasal synechiae are treated by transection and resection, and troublesome scars are ablated. Any concurrent residual or recurrent septal deviation (see Chapter 7) or turbinate hyperplasia (see Chapter 5) is also corrected or revised. Careful follow-up is required to prevent recurrent adhesions.

Bibliography

Eytan DF, Wang TD. Complications in rhinoplasty. Clin Plast Surg. 2022; 49 (1):179–189

Heilbronn C, Cragun D, Wong BJF. Complications in Rhinoplasty: A Literature Review and Comparison with a Survey of Consent Forms. Facial Plast Surg Aesthet Med. 2020 Jan/Feb;22(1):50–56

Hussein WK, Foda HM. Pollybeak deformity in Middle Eastern rhinoplasty: prevention and treatment. Facial Plast Surg. 2016; 32(4):398–401

Kiyohara N, Badger C, Tjoa T, Wong B. A comparison of over-the-counter mechanical nasal dilators: a systematic review. JAMA Facial Plast Surg. 2016; 18(5):385–389

San Nicoló M, Stelter K, Sadick H, Bas M, Berghaus A. Absorbable implant to treat nasal valve collapse. Facial Plast Surg. 2017; 33(2):233–240

San Nicoló M, Stelter K, Sadick H, Bas M, Berghaus A. 2-year follow-up study of an absorbable implant to treat nasal valve collapse. Facial Plast Surg. 2018; 34(5):545–550

21 Revision Surgery

There can be no generally approved treatment approach for revision cases. The problems that arise during revision surgery vary enormously and are difficult to classify into definitive categories. A distinction also has to be made between whether patients are undergoing the first revision or whether they have already had two or more previous operations.

21.1 The Revision Surgery Patient

However diverse the surgical issues may be, a common observation in patients who are candidates for revision surgery is that they are frequently subject to bias and tend to have lost trust in the surgeon or even medical practice in general. Some patients therefore return to a rhinoplasty surgeon only years later, although they may have been suffering from a deformity that they would not have imagined could be a possible outcome of the procedure before undergoing surgery. In contrast, other patients demand revision surgery very soon after the operation (but occasionally not with the first surgeon, whom they no longer trust). It can be particularly difficult and unpleasant to deal with patients who make severe accusations against their previous surgeons, rate them excessively negatively on the Internet, or are pursuing them legally.

It goes without saying that a dissatisfied patient has the right to complain and also to clarify through legal channels whether any avoidable mistakes have been made. However, the intended next surgeon in such cases may involuntarily wonder whether he or she is likely to be next in line to face the patient's ire.

21.2 Revision Surgery of the Nasal Framework

Revision surgery is most commonly undertaken to correct various asymmetries, irregularities, defects, and deformities in the cartilaginous or bony nasal framework. Either too much material may have been removed from vital areas during the previous operation (as is mostly the case), or too much may have been left behind (▶ Fig. 21.1a–d, ▶ Fig. 21.2a–d) or transplanted. Parts of the nasal vault may have been displaced, or various parts of the nose may be disproportionate (▶ Fig. 21.3a–d, ▶ Fig. 21.4a, b).

21.3 Grafts for Revision Surgery

In order to be successful, revision surgery must try to provide a cosmetically appealing and adequately stable nasal framework, which has usually been weakened by prior surgery. Material is frequently needed for the purpose, and the first decision is on the site from which graft material can be harvested before a revision procedure is undertaken.

Many rhinoplasty patients undergo more or less extensive septal surgery, possibly because graft material is already considered necessary for various purposes at the time of the initial procedure. Postoperative changes or defects in the septal cartilage are therefore frequently encountered during revision surgery. The examination before revision surgery thus includes endonasal palpation of the (former) quadrangular plate, which has often been replaced with scar tissue covered by mucosa, or fragmented, reimplanted cartilage material, which is no longer suitable for reshaping the external nose. Even if apparently stable cartilage is palpable after septoplasty, it is often found to be disappointing in terms of quality and volume following exposure using laborious dissection of scarred septal mucosa. In addition, the risk of inducing septal perforation should not be underestimated during extensive dissection of cartilage remnants between friable mucosal layers.

> ✓
>
> If sufficient material cannot be definitively obtained from the patient's septum, it is therefore advisable to carry out a quick search for other autogenous cartilage grafts early before the revision surgery.

Harvesting a conchal cartilage graft in such cases is usually considered first, as the ear is easily accessible to the surgeon during rhinoplasty and carries a low risk of complications. Significant consequences are not expected for the patient as a rule (see section 18.2.2). However, it should be noted that auricular cartilage is not the ideal graft material for every region of the nose, and the amount of conchal cartilage may be inadequate for revision rhinoplasty even when harvested from both ears.

The choice of graft material therefore has to take the requirements of revision surgery into account. Auricular cartilage in larger pieces is considered suboptimal for use on the nasal dorsum and the middle third of the nasal framework, given its curvature, elastic properties, and poor malleability. Conchal cartilage transplants, on the other hand, are ideal for partial or total reconstruction of the alar cartilages, in view of their curvature and elasticity (▶ Fig. 21.5a, b).

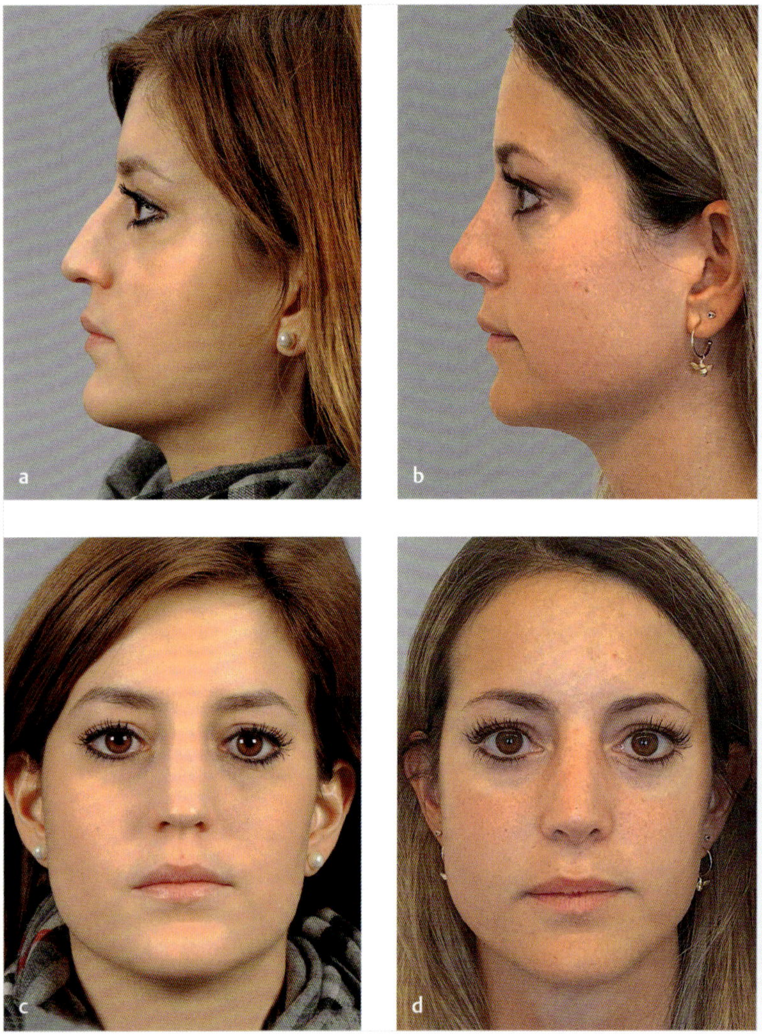

Fig. 21.1 Revision rhinoplasty, case study. Dissatisfied patient after rhinoplasty performed elsewhere. **(a)** The patient mainly complained about the hump that still existed on the side view, and the hanging tip. **(c)** In the front view, the width of the dorsum and the retracted columella were disturbing. **(b, d)** After revision rhinoplasty.

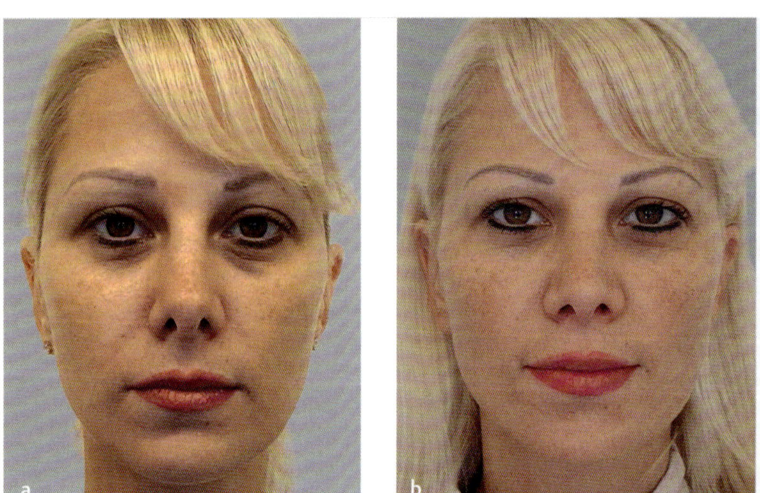

Fig. 21.2 Revision rhinoplasty, case study. Unhappy patient after rhinoplasty performed elsewhere. **(a)** In the first procedure, the tip remained overrotated; notching of the elongated, large nostrils. **(b)** Condition after revision, with reduction of tip rotation and lowering of the nasal alar edges with rim grafts from remnants of septal cartilage.

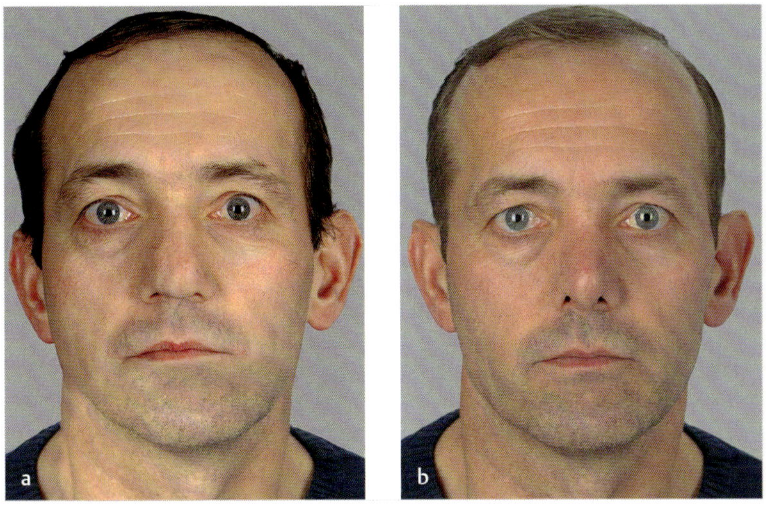

Fig. 21.3 Revision rhinoplasty, case study. (a) Nasal deformity as an unwanted result following rhinoplasty performed elsewhere. There is framework asymmetry, open roof, and deformity of the tip. **(b)** After revision rhinoplasty, including septal extension grafts, rim grafts, and tip grafts fashioned from residual septal cartilage.

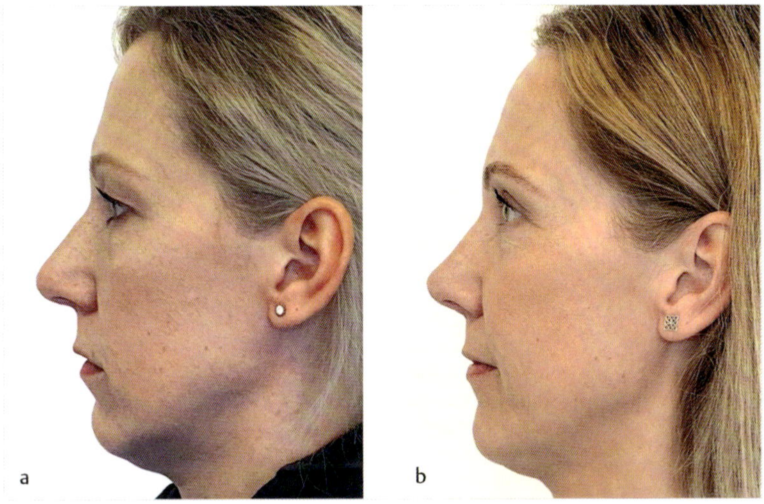

Fig. 21.4 Tip revision. After rhinoplasty performed elsewhere, the patient was not happy with the shapeless, round, and slightly drooping tip **(a)**. Satisfied patient after revision rhinoplasty, among other things using a tip graft **(b)**.

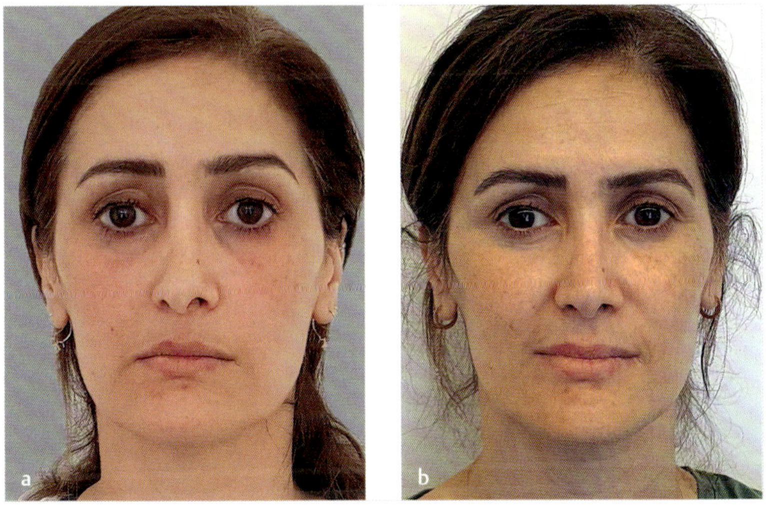

Fig. 21.5 Revision rhinoplasty using auricular cartilage. (a) Asymmetric nasal tip deformity after rhinoplasty performed elsewhere. The deviation was associated with a severe functional impairment in nasal breathing. The revision was complicated by a simultaneous septal perforation. **(b)** After revision using conchal cartilage transplants. The patient had undisturbed nasal breathing.

Auricular cartilage can also be used to a limited extent as a septal extension graft, although the curvature of the cartilage has to be corrected. This can be achieved by trimming the cartilage to size or by suturing two grafts curved in opposite directions. Section 18.2.2 provides further details on the use of auricular cartilage as graft material.

On the other hand, if a large amount of material is required for reconstruction of the middle and upper thirds of the nasal vault, the patient should be appropriately informed that costal cartilage may be needed for the purpose. Although harvesting rib cartilage does result in a scar on the chest wall, the incision need not be longer than 2–3 cm (experienced surgeons manage with even shorter incisions), and the scar is not particularly noticeable with careful positioning, meticulous suturing, and good healing. At least 3–4 cm of a cartilaginous rib is obtained as a rule, and this almost always meets the requirements of a standard revision rhinoplasty (see the case study in ▸ Fig. 17.5).

It should be noted that even in patients under the age of 50 years, costal cartilage may sometimes be partially calcified, which may significantly interfere with graft processing and reshaping. A preoperative ultrasound examination of the costal arch is recommended in order to estimate the extent of calcification. Heavily calcified ribs have been repeatedly discovered quite unexpectedly during harvesting of costal cartilage in the absence of a screening ultrasound examination. Unsuccessful transplantation then leads to serious problems both intraoperatively and during the postoperative discussion with the patient. The use of piezo instruments for processing of calcified rib cartilage grafts can be very helpful to overcome such problems. Section 18.2.3 provides more details on the use of costal cartilage as graft material.

As mentioned in section 18.1, human cryopreserved costal cartilage seems to be a real alternative to autogenous rib cartilage.

21.4 Revision Surgery Without a Graft

One occasionally encounters cases in which adequate graft material has been introduced from the septum, ear, or rib during a previous procedure, with failure to achieve a satisfactory result. Poorly defined contours with noticeable deformities are occasionally evident, especially when coarse costal cartilaginous grafts have been used during the first operation. Large amounts of inadequately processed or inappropriately placed material may have been transplanted in some cases, or the shape and position of the transplants may change over time. Reshaping of cartilage material already present in the nose is desirable in such cases (see the case study in ▸ Fig. 18.20; ▸ Fig. 21.6a, b). Depending on the extent of scarring, transplants may be (partially) removed, reworked, and reimplanted, or a preexisting scar–cartilage conglomerate can be reshaped in situ. This type of procedure is also suitable when reworking diced cartilage, with or without a fascial sheath.

21.5 The Skin in Revision Surgery

With adequate handling, the skin is not endangered in most patients with a previously operated nose, even in revision surgery. Reopening incisions for open access during a second procedure is also generally unproblematic, including very narrow resection of unsightly columella scars. However, subcutaneous scars are present in such cases, making separation of the skin flap and the cartilaginous structures during revision rhinoplasty quite difficult and time-consuming (▸ Video 21.1). Thinning of a thick fibroadipose subcutaneous layer may be desirable to correct a thickening above the tip, leading to pollybeak deformity. Due to associated scarring, however, this maneuver is usually much more challenging and also riskier during revision surgery than during the first intervention, when the tissue is still delicate and fine. During revision surgery, on the other hand, thinning of a dense subcutaneous scarry rind has to be preceded with a few longitudinal incisions to allow careful removal of fine strips of this dense tissue with a pair of scissors, without injuring the dermis (see Chapter 13).

> ✓
>
> When an unsightly scar from an inverted-V incision in the columella is being corrected by resection and resuturing, care needs to be taken to resect only the minimum amount necessary. Generous resection may lead to a wide gap between the cut edges in the columella skin, leading to tension on the new suture line — and thus to a visible scar again.

Some patients who have undergone multiple previous operations have visible changes in the overlying skin, including minor retractions, nasal telangiectasia (couperose), or even noticeable scars or skin defects in the most severe cases. The range of treatments for such lesions de-

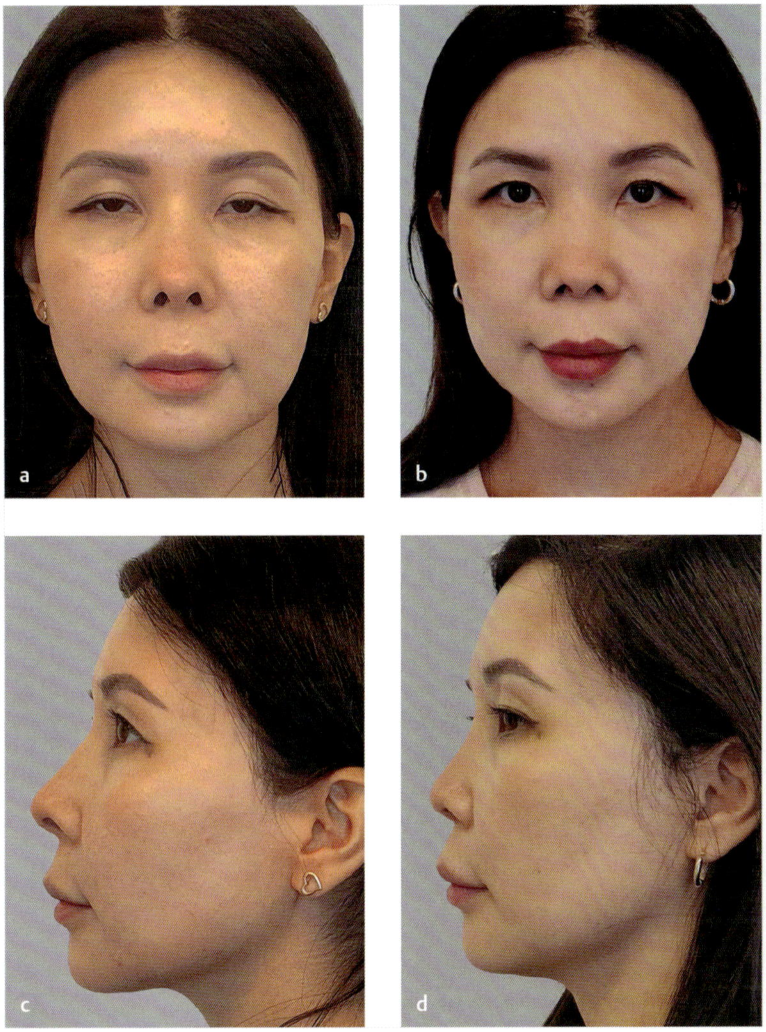

Fig. 21.6 **Revision after augmentation rhinoplasty.** Condition after an augmentation with costal cartilage carried out in South Korea (**a**, front view; **c**, side view). During the postoperative course, the patient became increasingly unhappy with the result, as she did not recognize herself with the new profile and felt a loss of identity. **(b, d)** After revision with extensive removal of the transplanted costal cartilage, including premaxillary "midface advancement grafts," the patient was more happy with her previous Asian nose and regained more self-confidence.

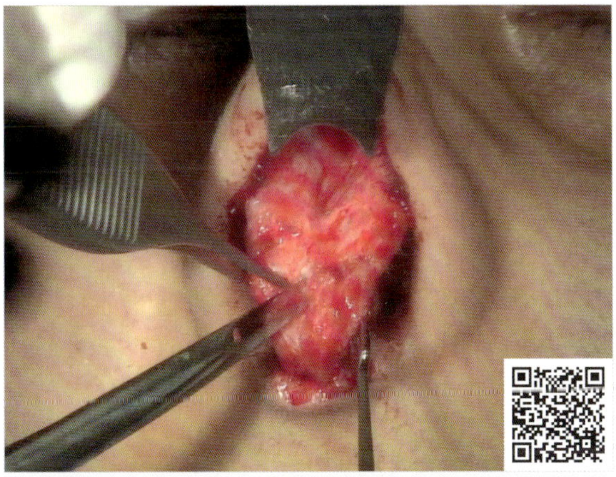

Video 21.1 Revision case, with scars on the alar cartilages.

pends on the individual case, and includes dermabrasion or laser therapy for regeneration of the surface epithelium and vascular or KTP laser for treatment of nasal telangiectasia (couperose, see ▶ Fig. 20.4a,b), correction of retracted scars with stabilizing cartilaginous discs, as well as scar excision and defect coverage with skin flaps in severe cases.

If the skin is severely affected over a large area and massive scars with contraction mean that a satisfactory result cannot be expected from a revision, even with the installation of a new cartilage framework, then resection of the damaged skin and replacement with a paramedian forehead flap may be necessary. Such interventions have more in common with nasal reconstruction procedures than with typical rhinoplasty (▶ Fig. 21.7a–f).

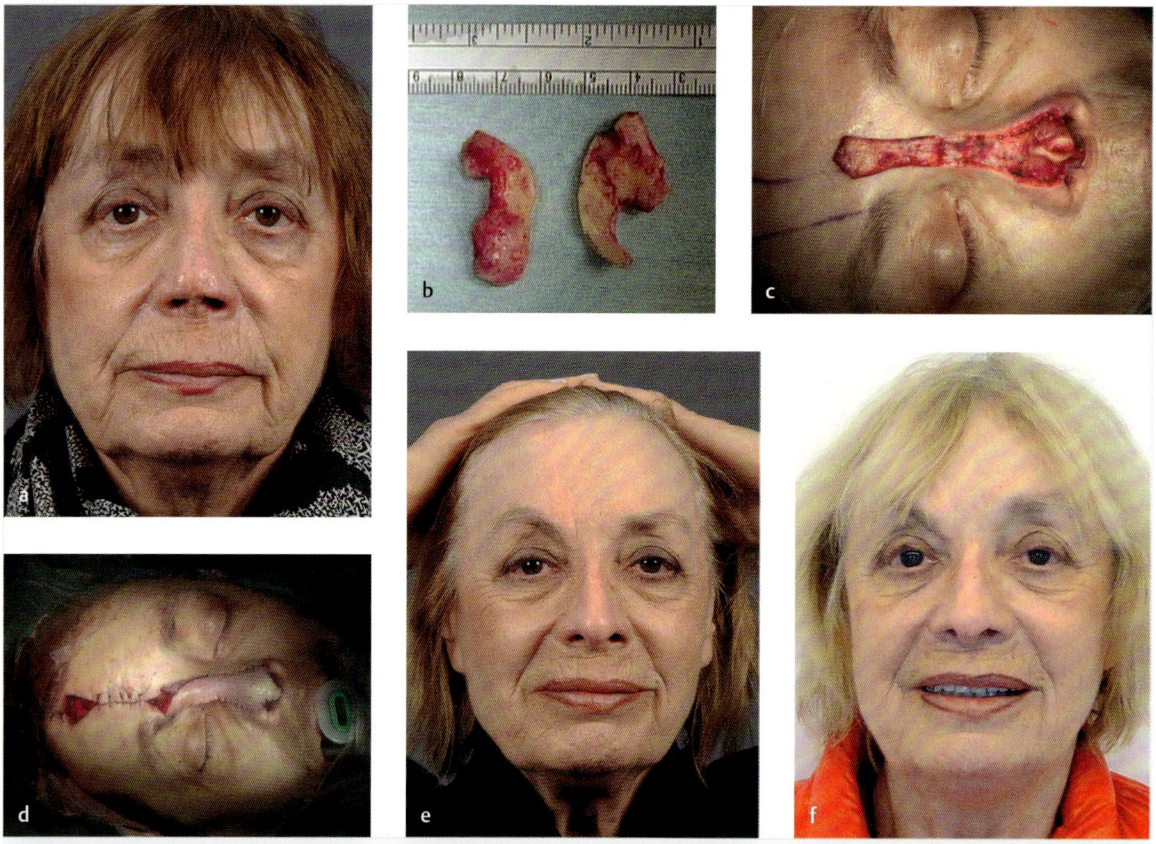

Fig. 21.7 Reconstruction of the nasal tip with conchal cartilage and paramedian forehead flap. **(a)** A 70-year-old patient with a nasal tip defect after resection of a hemangioma in early childhood. Attempts at reconstruction elsewhere at the ages of 21 and 45 years had not led to the desired success. **(b)** Conchal cartilage grafts from both sides used for reconstruction. **(c)** Cartilage transplants appropriately incorporated. A nasal dorsum skin flap has been dissected to temporarily cover the back of the paramedian forehead flap (marked on the forehead). **(d)** The paramedian forehead flap has been incorporated into the defect. **(e)** The patient 1 year after the operation. **(f)** Another 9 years later, when she was 79 years old; stable result.

Bibliography

Ballert JA, Park SS. Functional considerations in revision rhinoplasty. Facial Plast Surg. 2008; 24(3):348–357

Daniel RK, Sajadian A. Secondary rhinoplasty: management of the overresected dorsum. Facial Plast Surg. 2012; 28(4):417–426

Davis RE. Revision of the overresected nasal tip complex. Facial Plast Surg. 2012; 28(4):427–439

Davis RE. Revision rhinoplasty. In: Johnson JT, Rosen CA, eds. Bailey's head and neck surgery—otolaryngology. 5th ed. Philadelphia: Wolters Kluwer/ Lippincott, Williams & Wilkins; 2014:2989–3052

Davis RE, Bublik M. Common technical causes of the failed rhinoplasty. Facial Plast Surg. 2012; 28(4):380–389

Davis RE, Bublik M. Psychological considerations in the revision rhinoplasty patient. Facial Plast Surg. 2012; 28(4):374–379

Foda HMT. Rhinoplasty for the multiply revised nose. Am J Otolaryngol. 2005; 26(1):28–34

Loyo M, Wang TD. Revision rhinoplasty. Clin Plast Surg. 2016; 43(1):177–185

Meyer R. Secondary and functional rhinoplasty: the difficult nose. Orlando, FL: Grune & Stratton; 1988

Meyer R. Secondary rhinoplasty. Berlin: Springer; 2002

Paun SH, Nolst Trenité GJ. Revision rhinoplasty: an overview of deformities and techniques. Facial Plast Surg. 2008; 24(3):271–287

Spataro E, Piccirillo JF, Kallogjeri D, Branham GH, Desai SC. Revision rates and risk factors of 175 842 patients undergoing septorhinoplasty. JAMA Facial Plast Surg. 2016; 18(3):212–219

22 Use of Fillers

Classic surgical rhinoplasty, as described in this book, is likely to remain the long-term gold standard of treatment for most nasal deformities. However, smaller depressions, asymmetries, and irregularities can also be corrected with the help of injectable filler materials (known as "fillers"). This form of nonsurgical rhinoplasty (NSR), which seems to be the most appropriate term in this context, is also occasionally referred to as "injection rhinoplasty," "medical rhinoplasty," or "liquid rhinoplasty."

Patients may be considered candidates for NSR if they

- either cannot or do not wish to undergo typical surgical correction (e.g., due to the costs involved, or because they cannot afford to take a longer period of leave),
- have deformities that can generally be corrected using fillers,
- have a low radix, due to which the nose appears short,
- have a saddle nose.

> ✔
>
> A large, overprojected nose, large humps, and disproportionately large parts of the nose can only be treated with surgical therapy. Reduction rhinoplasty requires surgery (see the case study in ▶ Fig. 22.1a–f).

It is essential for surgeons using NSR to be well-versed in the regional anatomy and, in particular, the vascular anatomy of the nose, in order to avoid complications. Equally important is a thorough knowledge of the rules of normal nasofacial proportionality.

Fillers are usually not injected with the patient under general anesthesia, since one of the attractions of this form of treatment is that it can be used quickly and without substantial effort. Some users consider that local anesthetic should not be given either, as the anesthetic injection already leads to a change in shape, making the assessment of the filler volume difficult. Local anesthesia may also mask pain as a sign of vascular occlusion, resulting in delayed diagnosis of damage that has occurred.

Others prefer block anesthesia of the affected region before the filler is injected into the nose. The anesthetic is not injected at the same site as the filler, but peripherally, corresponding to the course of the afferent nerves. A good knowledge of the anatomy of the afferent sensory nerves is therefore required. Many fillers now come in a prefilled syringe that already contains a local anesthetic (such as lidocaine).

Surface anesthesia is yet another option. It can be achieved by administering lidocaine/prilocaine ointment (such as Emla) before the procedure.

22.1 Types of Filler for Nonsurgical Rhinoplasty (NSR)

The substances that are currently mainly in use for corrections of the nose are **hyaluronic acid, calcium hydroxyapatite**, and **agarose fillers**, among others. Their advantages are that these materials are degraded in tissue and in principle do not last permanently. Although absorption may take several months or even much longer in this way, particularly in the nose, the patients are better protected against undesirable results and late complications.

Hyaluronic acid also has the advantage that it is dissolved by hyaluronidase, which can be used as an antidote in the event of intra-arterial injection or other complications or undesirable outcomes.

Agarose fillers are biocompatible and of non hydrophillic nature, as they function as hydrocolloids. Through this property agarose can be expected to allow more precise and safer interventions in NSR by avoiding compression phenomena, as it does not absorb water from tissue. Another advantage using agarose lies in its ability to stimulate collagen production and other components of the extracellular matrix, so it functions also as a tool for hypotrophic scar treatments of the nasal skin. Similar to hyaluronic acid it can be dissolved by hyaluronidase and even by topical vitamin C injections.

Autologous fat is also available for injections after appropriate preparation, and is regarded as at least a partly permanent filling material.

Platelet-rich fibrin (PRF) and platelet-rich plasma (PRP) have been used increasingly in recent times. PRP is the patient's concentrated, enriched blood plasma, which contains growth factors and proteins in addition to platelets. Stem cells obtained from the patient's blood may allow regeneration of deficient or damaged tissue, in addition to functioning as a filler.

A product called Ellansé (polycaprolactone and carboxymethylcellulose) that has recently appeared on the market not only acts as a filler itself, but allegedly also supports its effectiveness by stimulating collagen production.

22.2 Risks of Nonsurgical Rhinoplasty (NSR)

Patients must be informed about the dangers when injectable materials are used in the nose. They may be

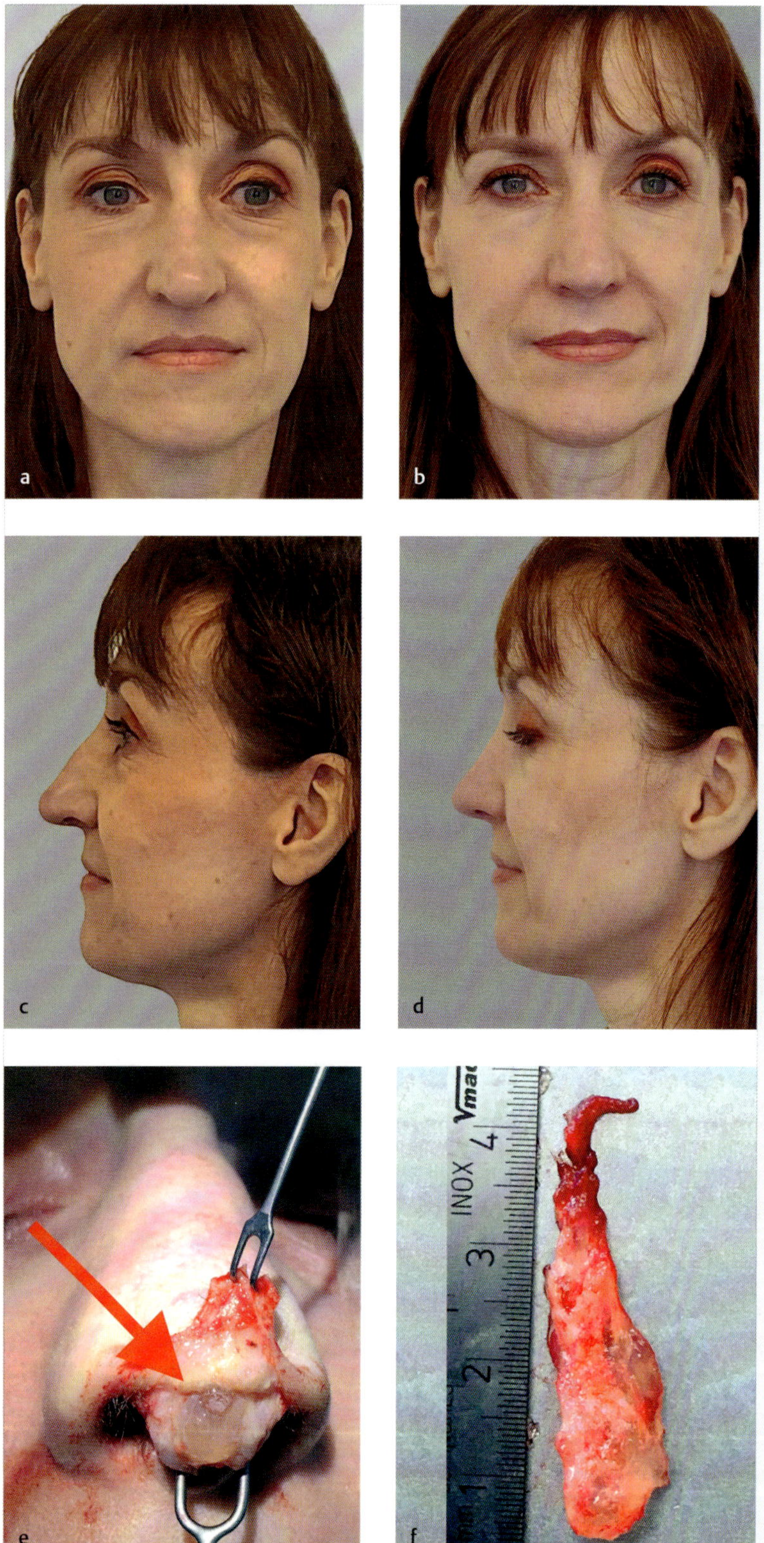

Fig. 22.1 Inappropriate use of a filler. The patient initially had a large, overprojecting nose with a hump. These findings were inappropriately intensified by filler injection (**a**, frontal view; **c**, side view). During revision rhinoplasty, all of the filler material was removed, in addition to several classic surgical steps (**b**, postoperative frontal view; **d**, postoperative side view). Due to the overstretched, excess skin with scarred subcutaneous tissue after the filler application, the tip of the nose could only be reduced to a limited extent. **(e)** The last injection of filler took place 6 months before the revision operation. Filler material is seen in the tip area intraoperatively (red arrow). **(f)** The resected tissue, with partly encapsulated filler.

associated with dramatic consequences in some cases, and this is an argument against the routine use of nasal fillers. Filler-induced vascular occlusion – with resultant tissue loss, especially skin necrosis, blindness, or even cerebral infarction – carries the highest risk. Complications such as these, some of which may be catastrophic, are rare but have been repeatedly described in the literature. Research has shown that blindness consequent to the use of facial fillers is most common when they are applied to the nose and glabella.

Other, less serious complications such as infection, edema, hematoma, pain, allergic reactions, foreign-body reactions, nodule formation, and migration of material may occur as delayed reactions even months or years later, and should not be ignored or underestimated. What is known as the "Tyndall effect" is a bluish discoloration of the skin, which is thought to be due to excessive amounts of superficially injected material.

Another condition described as "Avatar nose" refers to an unnaturally wide nasion area, secondary to local filler spread. A nasofrontal angle of 125–130° is perceived as the most attractive, but an overcorrection with injectables might disrupt facial harmony by the smoothing of this anatomical zone, leading to a "Greek nose" as seen in ancient Greek busts.

"Primary" filler injections differ from postsurgical "secondary" injections in that the latter have a higher risk of complications, consequent to a change in anatomical conditions that makes it difficult or impossible to work in defined layers. The altered anatomical course of vessels also increases the risk of vascular occlusion.

✔

Surgeons who intend to use fillers for nasal correction need to be thoroughly familiar with the properties of the various available filler materials. In particular, one must be aware of the effects, risks, and side effects, as well as ensuring that the agents have been approved for the intended use, as this information also has to be communicated to the patient before treatment.

In addition, everyone who administers such injections must be well versed in the treatment of dangerous (acute or delayed) complications, and the required medication must be available on site — such as hyaluronidase if a hyaluronic acid product is used.

There has been a marked upswing in recent years in the use of fillers for facial and nasal surgery. New products with new properties are constantly being developed and launched commercially. Current developments in this field cannot be fully reflected here, particularly since this textbook is primarily devoted to surgical rhinoplasty.

Bibliography

Bravo BSF, Bravo LG, Mariano Da Rocha C, De Souza SB, Lopes FL, Totti J. Evaluation and proportion in nasal filling with hyaluronic acid. J Clin Aesthet Dermatol. 2018; 11(4):36–40

Cotofana S. Commentary on: Decreased Filler Volumes with Repeat Micro-Liquid Nonsurgical Rhinoplasty Sessions. Facial Plast Surg Aesthet Med. 2024 Nov-Dec;26(6):762–763

Dayan SH, Bassichis BA. Facial dermal fillers: selection of appropriate products and techniques. Aesthet Surg J. 2008; 28(3):335–347

Fitzgerald R, Bertucci V, Sykes JM, Duplechain JK. Adverse reactions to injectable fillers. Facial Plast Surg. 2016; 32(5):532–555

Johnson ON, III, Kontis TC. Nonsurgical rhinoplasty. Facial Plast Surg. 2016; 32(5):500–506

Karapantzou C, Jakob M, Kinney B, et al. The use of algeness in the face and neck: a safe, alternative filler for cosmetics and reconstruction. Ann Transl Med. 2020 Mar; 8 (6):362

Marotta J. Nonsurgical rhinoplasty complicates surgical rhinoplasty. Facial Plast Surg Aesthet Med. 2022; 24(1):61–62

Mehta U, Fridirici Z. Advanced techniques in nonsurgical rhinoplasty. Facial Plast Surg Clin North Am. 2019; 27(3):355–365

Sung MS, Kim HG, Woo KI, Kim YD. Ocular ischemia and ischemic oculomotor nerve palsy after vascular embolization of injectable calcium hydroxylapatite filler. Ophthal Plast Reconstr Surg. 2010; 26 (4):289–291

23 Dealing with Unexpected Incidents

Surprising incidents can occur in any operation. They can jeopardize the process as well as the result, and always require highly individualized, spontaneous decisions by surgeons and their teams. In order not to react rashly in an emergency, the surgeon should be mentally prepared for problems that can be expected to a certain extent because in principle there is a known potential for them to occur.

23.1 What If Less Graft Material Than Initially Expected Is Available Intraoperatively for Rhinoplasty?

This is not really an exceptional situation. Even experienced surgeons encounter circumstances in which significantly smaller amounts of nasal or conchal cartilage are available during revision surgery than prior inspection and palpation suggested. One may consequently face a problematic situation in which only a small amount of conchal cartilage is available and a larger rib graft is required, but matters are complicated by a lack of preparation and patient briefing.

Recovery from this type of situation should not involve the use of plastic implants, particularly if this has not been discussed with the patient beforehand. Alloplastic materials of this type are frequently associated with implant failure, and extrusion and revision surgery must be expected sooner or later. Harvesting cartilage grafts from donor regions for which the patient has not provided prior consent cannot be recommended either.

It may be helpful to remember that malleable graft material can still be obtained from the perpendicular plate, for instance, which can be used to augment stable segments of the nasal vault. In addition, every little piece of available cartilage and bone needs to be collected in such cases. These fragments are easily stacked and wrapped in TachoSil (see section 17.2.3), so that one larger graft can be made out of many small ones.

✔

The surgeon can best avoid such situations by informing the patient beforehand on the slightest suspicion that conchal or costal cartilage may be required, and by preparing the appropriate surgical fields for the operation.

23.2 What If a Device Fails?

This problem needs to be reckoned with in every operation, since technical products cannot be guaranteed to last forever. Electrically powered equipment – such as suction devices, drills, saws, and piezoelectric instruments – plays a significant role in rhinoplasty.

While a second suction tool is usually available in the operating room, failure of a drill or piezo unit may be problematic. The surgeon should be able to carry on with the procedure using conventional instruments (chisel, hammer, rasp) if a spare device is not available.

✔

Even if the surgeon has become accustomed to working with electrically powered instruments or piezo technology, a sterile set of classic instruments must be available on site, ready for use when needed, and the surgeon must be appropriately trained in their use.

23.3 What If Harvested Cartilage Falls to the Floor?

Harvested cartilage grafts on the instrument table are "worth their weight in gold" for the surgeon. The importance of graft materials also needs to be communicated to assistants and nursing staff at the operating table, to prevent loss of these grafts at all costs. During a change in staff, newcomers must be informed about the site of placement of graft material on the table.

Cartilage stored in moist conditions has a smooth, slippery surface, and therefore particularly grippy Adson–Brown forceps or similar instruments are chosen to hold the grafts. The surgeon will try to work on the transplant material on a sufficiently large surface. It is best to avoid any gaps between the instrument table and the operating table, so that loose pieces of cartilage that become independent are prevented from leaving the sterile area. A piece of cartilage may nevertheless slip away and fall to the ground.

Surgeons must then decide whether they are willing to take responsibility for continued use of the cartilage after extensive disinfection in a suitable solution. Harvesting of a new graft, if possible, must be considered alternatively.

23.4 What If Uncontrollable Bleeding Occurs?

It goes without saying that the usual hemostatic measures form part of every surgical procedure. These include the use of bipolar or monopolar coagulation forceps and temporary compression, cooling, and irrigation of bleeding tissue; application of swabs or cotton wool with epinephrine-containing solutions may be extremely helpful. Appropriate blood pressure reduction by the anesthetist to achieve hemostasis is a matter of routine during general anesthesia.

Exceptionally heavy bleeding may occur from large vessels in the nose and the paranasal sinuses, such as the ethmoid, sphenoid, or sphenopalatine arteries. The nasal surgeon who is not familiar with endoscopic sinus surgery may have difficulty in identifying and appropriately targeting these deep-seated vessels, and suitable instruments and endoscopes may also not be available. Appropriate tamponade materials should be available in the operating room for such cases and can be used to pack the nasal cavity. These include strips for continuous tamponade or prefabricated "finger cots," consisting of foam strips with a latex-free rubber cover (see Chapter 15, ▶ Fig. 15.5). Experienced users may also stock special balloon catheters, which are inflated after insertion into the nasal cavity and control bleeding by compression.

✓

It is imperative for hemostasis to be ensured at the close of the procedure. If there is any doubt, the surgeon should examine the oral cavity to exclude posterior pharyngeal bleeding at the end of the operation.

Heavy and persistent bleeding is handled as an emergency. With professional attendance, the patient should be transferred for further investigations and treatment to an emergency unit or a center for otorhinolaryngology after the best possible tamponade and preparation, or initiation of blood transfusions if necessary.

Bibliography

Krulewitz NA, Fix ML. Epistaxis. Emerg Med Clin North Am. 2019; 37(1):29–39

24 FAQs, A–Z: Information for Patients

For patients, the operation represents a turning point in life, with effects and accompanying circumstances that they are far less able to assess than the surgeon, who experiences the same situation over and over again. All patients need to be given the opportunity to ask all relevant questions, which have to be answered credibly and competently, even though the surgeons may be under pressure in a busy hospital. The doctor–patient relationship may become strained if it becomes apparent postoperatively that aspects that are important from the patient's point of view were not communicated and discussed beforehand. It is advisable for the surgeon to address specific separate issues that may initially seem irrelevant to patients ("Are you planning to travel anywhere after the operation?"; "What sort of sports or exercise do you do?" etc. A sheet with relevant questions and answers to be handed out to the patients is helpful, see ▶ Table 24.1.

24.1 Air Travel

There are no objections if an overseas or long-distance patient wishes to travel home by air before the stitches are removed, with the stitches being removed by a physician in their home country. As a rule, however, patients who need to travel far remain on site until the stitches have been removed, around day 6. Air travel is not restricted after that. It should be borne in mind, however, that the risk of an impact on the nose is somewhat greater during travel in a cramped aircraft.

If there is concern that swelling in the nose could cause problems in the sinuses and middle ear during pressure equalization on flights, patients can be given a nasal decongestant spray to use before take-off and landing (xylometazoline).

24.2 Blowing the Nose

Blowing the nose involves digital compression of the nostrils and should therefore be avoided for about 2–3 weeks after the operation (or 3–4 weeks after alar wedge and nostril sill resections at the nasal base).

However, secretions accumulate in the nasal cavities after the procedure and have to be drained. The simplest alternative to blowing the nose is then "pulling up" the nose and spitting out the secretions. In addition, the doctor should offer every patient nasal suction and cleansing as often as required, but at least once or twice a week. The patient can also consult an otolaryngologist who is familiar with this treatment and closer to their home (see also sections 24.4 and 24.14 below).

24.3 Children, Pets

Young children may kick their feet, flail their arms, and bang their heads. Dogs can accidentally jump onto their owners. The nose should therefore be protected when dealing with young children and dogs, or kept out of reach for about at least 3 weeks, if possible.

24.4 Cleansing the Nose

The nostrils and freshly sutured wounds on the columella and alar bases can be cleansed with pure water. Commercially available oil (baby oil, skin care oils, etc.) and cotton swabs (Q-tips) available in pharmacies can help loosen wound crusts over the nostrils. If patients can keep the wounds free of incrustation by caring for the nasal openings, then they are making a valuable contribution to undisturbed wound healing. The surgeon should take over immediate postoperative care if patients do not feel confident in doing this on their own (see also section 24.14 below).

24.5 Cooling

Cooling of facial soft tissues may help reduce facial swelling only in the first 2–3 days, but is not mandatory. If available, cooling can be carried out using a Hilotherm device over a suitable mask on the day of the operation and the day after, with the temperature being adjusted to 15–18 °C (see Chapter 15). Alternatively, cooling pads can be used. It should be ensured that any manipulation in this early postoperative phase does not dislodge or loosen the bandage and splint.

24.6 Dream Nose

It is normal and understandable for patients to try to visualize their expectations regarding the upcoming operation by illustrating the noses they are hoping for in photographs of famous models and movie stars. The surgeon must not refuse to look at these images and discuss the options with the patient, even if it may be clearly impossible to achieve the "ideal" shape that the patient dreams of. Surgeons should carefully state that the presentation of these desired noses is helpful for understanding what kind of change in profile the patient is looking for, even if the results of the operation will not be the same. In addition, patients must understand that the nose of their dreams belongs to a totally different face and would probably not suit the patient's

Table 24.1 A–Z Information for patients about rhinoplasty

Ability to work	At a PC, in the home office: from the 2nd day after surgery; otherwise, load-dependent from the 2nd to 4th week.
Air travel	Allowed from the 3rd day after surgery. If nose is blocked, consider using decongestant.
Nose blowing	Avoid for 3 weeks after surgery and for 3 to 4 weeks after a base resection. Instead, pull up your nose or have it professionally cleaned.
Nose cleaning	Clean the nasal entrance with warm water; avoid soap on wounds for 2 to 3 weeks. Use panthenol if needed, and seek medical support if necessary.
Cooling	Possibly on day 1 and 2 after surgery, if needed; Hilotherm® cooling system may be used.
Eating, chewing	Restrictions are only required after a lip lift and extensive alar wedge or nostril sill resections.
Facial expressions, laughing	Limit extensive movements of the upper lip and cheeks for about 3 weeks after alar wedge or nostril sill resection.
Eyeglasses: includes safety and lab glasses, ski and diving goggles, etc.	Can be worn for short periods starting three weeks after surgery; extend wear time if problem-free. Consider using contact lenses.
Showering, hair washing	Wait 2 days before washing hair. Initially, avoid soap or shampoo in the wound area; from the 3rd week, it is allowed.
Homeopathic remedies	As per the patient's preference.
Infants, dogs, horses	Keep your distance for 2 to 4 weeks.
Internal nose after surgery	If blocked, use short-term decongestant spray (e.g., xylometazoline, Otriven); nasal cleaning by a doctor; nasal douche after 2 to 3 weeks; nasal oil
Mouth and nose protection (face mask)	No restriction, do not tie too tight.
Pain	Usually none; if there is pain, consider taking Ibuprofen® or similar.
Revision surgery	Not before (9 to) 12 months.
Public exposure after surgery (customers, stage, TV)	This can be considered starting from the third week after surgery.
Sick note	For 1 to 2 weeks, if there is a medical indication for surgery.
Sleeping position	Initially with the headboard raised; avoid sleeping on the stomach; side sleeping is possible.
Sports	Light activities (e.g., jogging) after 2 to 3 weeks, increase gradually; swimming after 4 weeks; ball sports, contact sports, high diving, etc. after 6 to 8 weeks. Professional athlete should wear a face mask
Sun, solarium	Avoid excessive exposure for 4 weeks; wear a baseball cap, seek shade, and use sunscreen with SPF 30+.
"Taping" the nose after surgery	Not mandatory.

individual physiognomy. It is therefore much more effective and helpful to do preoperative planning with the support of a simulation program using pictures of the patient's own face, instead of looking at photos of celebrities.

If patients find it difficult to understand that it is not possible to promise 1-µm precision in nasal surgery, then I like to try a comparison with a car-repair shop: "A human being is not a car." In a car, you can achieve exactly the shape that is intended – for example, by attaching a suitable fender. Surgery on biological tissue is much more difficult and follows different principles.

24.7 Eating, Chewing

Patients are occasionally misled by information available on the Internet or other sources suggesting that they should not chew or eat solids after the operation. This is not necessary, unless alar wedge resections or lip lift have been performed at the same time as the rhinoplasty (see section 24.9). In the latter cases only, intensive movements of the upper lip and cheeks should be avoided for about 2–3 weeks.

24.8 Face Mask

If a mask has to be worn in the postoperative period (e.g., during a pandemic, or for professional reasons, as with doctors) then it is not a fundamental obstacle for a rhinoplasty. Masks that can be appropriately tightened behind the head are preferable. Moderate contact pressure allows the mask to be optimally applied to the face and fulfill its function without affecting the nose or the aluminum splint.

24.9 Facial Movement, Laughing

The patient's facial expressions are not necessarily restricted after rhinoplasty, but immobilizing the perioral muscles for 2–3 weeks, as far as this is possible, is advisable only after alar wedge and nostril sill resection, or a simultaneous lip lift.

24.10 Follow-up Costs, Insurance

Opinions differ on whether the patient has to be billed for postoperative appointments. However, patients greatly appreciate not being charged for follow-up treatment, and this in itself is beneficial for the healing process.

Patients in whom surgical revision is being considered may be concerned about paying the same sum as for the initial operation with the same surgeon. The surgeon may have fixed rates for revision surgery, or may settle charges on a case-by-case basis. However, it is beneficial for the further doctor–patient relationship if the patient is informed in good time that corrective surgery, if at all necessary, would cost only a fraction of the initial operation (e.g., 10–30%).

Several companies now offer insurance cover for possible cosmetic correction following aesthetic operations. Patients who are interested should ideally contact the company concerned for details of costs, duration, and scope.

A special situation may arise if the patient develops a **medical** complication as a consequence of the cosmetic procedure, which in turn may require costly medical treatment. A patient's health-insurance provider may refuse to cover the costs incurred for this medical treatment if the complication is the result of a cosmetic operation that was not financed by it to start with. If interested, the surgeon or patient should clarify whether insurance cover for consequential damages is available for cosmetic operations to cover the potential monetary risk in case of medical complications ("follow-up costs insurance"). either the doctor can take out insurance for the patient, or patients themselves may take care of a subsequent cost insurance for cosmetic surgery. Physicians should inform patients about this option while explaining financial repercussions. Many patients find this reassuring.

24.11 Glasses

Not all patients are able to do without glasses and use contact lenses instead, although contact lenses are a better option for the postoperative period. Glasses may leave pressure marks on the skin if they are worn too early and for too long after the operation. The same also applies to sunglasses, protective laboratory goggles, skiing and diving goggles, etc. Glasses with light frames can be used after approximately 3 weeks, and initially only for a short period of about 15–30 minutes. The duration can be gradually prolonged if the glasses do not create pressure points.

24.12 Hair Washing, Showering

Patients should ensure that showering does not dislodge the nasal taping or aluminum splint postoperatively. It is best not to wash one's hair at all during the first 2 days after the procedure. An assistant can help with hair washing at least initially, with the patient's head tilted backward, while hairdressers can do this professionally.

If possible, shampoo or soap should not be applied to the surgical wounds at the nasal base, to avoid irritation and allow uncomplicated wound healing.

24.13 Homeopathic Remedies

Some patients believe in specific herbal remedies and are keen to take these to promote better wound healing and immunity. One should not advise against these alternative remedies, even though modern medicine has not confirmed that they have any effects. The preparations do not usually have any known adverse effects, and the patient may subjectively perceive a beneficial effect.

24

24.14 Inner Nose

Decongestant nasal sprays can be used during the first few days if swelling within the nose hinders breathing. They can be discontinued after a few days when no longer necessary. Decongestant sprays in the xylometazoline group in addition cause vascular constriction and prevent minor bleeding.

An oily nasal spray containing retinol and tocopherol, or oily herbal solutions (such as GeloSitin), which are often perceived as pleasant, are also used to moisturize the mucosa from about the second week onward.

Nasal irrigation with suitable mild saline solutions or specially designed products (e.g., Pari Montesol, etc.) may help cleanse the nasal cavities. However, the procedure should be carried out after the second or third week, as it requires manipulation of the nostrils, and only after the fourth week after wedge and sill resections.

If crusts and secretions in the nose lead to serious obstruction, nasal care through suctioning and/or instrumental cleaning needs to be done professionally by an experienced physician.

24.15 Outpatient/In-Patient

Many patients wish to have the procedure performed on an outpatient basis. This is possible in principle, especially if the patients do not live very far away and adequate care is available at home or in a hotel.

Others decide early on to stay one night in the hospital after the operation, in view of the likely condition after 3 hours of anesthesia with a freshly operated nose.

If organizationally feasible, it is sometimes useful in the case of a planned outpatient operation to give the patient the option of staying one night postoperatively in hospital, where a night nurse will be present all the time and a doctor can be called in relatively quickly – although this is only necessary extremely rarely.

24.16 Pain

The fear of pain is mentioned as an issue by many patients in the discussion before the operation. Fortunately, there is no need to be overly concerned about this. Most patients have no pain at all after the procedure. Occasionally, a few tablets of a mild pain reliever like cyclooxygenase inhibitors (e.g., ibuprofen) are given if needed. The surgical steps that cause pain are performed under anesthesia. Postoperatively, even the osteotomy lines no longer cause any pain, as long as they do not move.

Very rarely, patients later report a feeling of pressure and perhaps slight pain at the lines of the osteotomy, particularly if glasses are worn. Patience may be required over a longer period of time until these symptoms subside. A new spectacle frame that is lighter and has different contact points on the bridge of the nose may help.

On the other hand, if an operation on the nose is performed under local anesthesia, the surgeon must be aware of the sensitivity of the nasal skin, especially at the tip of the nose. Injections of local anesthetic therefore start first in the periphery – i.e., at the transition to the cheek – before slowly infiltrating the skin of the nose itself and finally the tip of the nose.

24.17 Payment

Advance payment is commonly requested for cosmetic surgery, the cost of which is not generally covered by health-insurance companies, but by the patients themselves. The surgeon may also be willing to draw up a payment plan in some cases. However, to remove the issue of finances from the doctor–patient relationship as much as possible, it may be advantageous to refer a patient who wishes to pay in installments to a company that professionally finances aesthetic procedures.

24.18 Physical Exertion

Even activities that may not be directly dangerous to the nose may have undesirable consequences due to an increase in blood pressure, with subsequent bleeding. Patients should therefore only take part in strenuous physical activity after 3–4 weeks.

24.19 Public Appearance

Patients who are in contact with clients, and public figures who have to appear in front of the camera or on television, etc., should not be reassured with an overly optimistic outlook about the timing of their next public appearance. When the operation is being planned, a period of 4–6 weeks off should be expected, even if the postoperative course is uneventful and might make a public appearance possible within 3 weeks after surgery.

24.20 Revision Surgery

The possibility that surgery may fail must be clearly explained to patients preoperatively and in writing, and they must be informed that cosmetic failure is the most significant complication of cosmetic rhinoplasty – even higher than the risk of functional disorders. The sequence of events in case of an undesirable outcome of the planned operation should be discussed with the patient before surgery – including revision surgery, even though that is extremely undesirable and also not highly probable statistically. Discussing possible blemishes in the result of the operation also opens up the possibility of allaying the patient's shyness about a possible revision operation at an early stage. It is essential not to make the revision operation sound like a disastrous situation, but rather a viable option to significantly improve on an outcome that may not be initially satisfactory in all respects. On the basis of extensive experience, one may safely point out that revision surgery often entails circumscribed, minor interventions that are nowhere near as comprehensive as the initial operation.

It must be made amply clear to the patient both preoperatively and postoperatively that any decision regarding possible revision cannot be arrived at before the ninth to twelfth postoperative months. At this point, patients are usually happy to note that they will not be charged the same amount as for the initial operation (see also section 24.10).

Despite detailed explanations, some patients panic very early after the operation, when the inevitable swelling does not yet allow a final assessment of the result and certain abnormalities seen in the mirror still diverge from the expected result.

The surgeon first has to explain the situation in a reassuring and empathetic manner in such cases, pointing out that a great deal will change for the better in the coming weeks and months. However, this may not be helpful in some instances, and patients may become prematurely preoccupied with the prospect of revision surgery at a most inappropriate time point.

Even if surgeons see disturbing abnormalities on the patient's nose that they would like to eliminate, they should not be tempted to carry out a hasty revision. The postoperative outcome can only be reliably assessed 9–12 months after surgery, once edema has subsided and wound healing is complete. Any revision surgery undertaken during this period would be considered premature and involves a risk of impaired wound healing due to incomplete restoration of blood circulation and tissue stability.

There is also another reason why revision surgery should be postponed: in the early postoperative period, it is only natural for patients to devote practically all their attention to the nose and the surgical result (possibly with supporting observation by their "best friend" or partner) and to be completely preoccupied with it. This changes over time as they get on with daily life. Patients and those around them notice gradual improvement in the nose, and the desire for revision surgery thus usually fades over time. It is therefore essential to help the patient come through an initial period of nervousness, uncertainty, and possible temporary dissatisfaction.

24.21 Sensory Disorders, Stiffness

Some patients find postoperative changes in sensation at the nasal tip annoying, as well as some stiffness in the tip, even if this has been explained preoperatively. Sensations occasionally take weeks or months to return to normal. It is rare for abnormal sensations to persist for years after the operation.

With regard to the strength of the anterior nose, it may be helpful to explain to the patient that this stability is important for keeping the nostrils open for breathing.

24.22 Sick Leave

If purely cosmetic surgery has been performed on the nose, then strictly speaking the postoperative state is not an illness. Surgeons and patients depend on the local regulations in their individual countries in relation to whether sick leave of an appropriate duration may be granted for concomitant functional surgery that is indicated on medical grounds (e.g., septoplasty, turbinate reduction, paranasal sinus surgery).

24.23 Skin Preparation

Pretreatment of the skin in patients with acne or rosacea, using appropriate dermatological agents, may be advisable before surgery (see Chapter 13). A rhinoplasty surgeon may not be specially trained in this field, and the patient can be advised to consult a dermatologist or a cosmetic institute if appropriate. The patient will continue to benefit from such therapeutic regimens for skin problems in the future, regardless of the planned rhinoplasty. Antibiotic and cortisone-containing ointments or gels (such as Jellin-Neomycin ointment) may be helpful for pretreatment of acute skin inflammation.

24.24 Sleeping Posture

Sleeping with the upper body raised by about 30° in the first week after the operation may be beneficial. This counters a nocturnal increase in facial edema, which is usually pronounced in the morning and then regresses during the day. Sleeping in the supine or lateral position is not prohibited; patients usually spontaneously avoid the unfavorable prone position in the immediate postoperative period.

24.25 Sports and Exercise

Simple sporting activities and exercise should only be gradually resumed after 2–3 weeks (e.g., jogging on flat ground, treadmill). Sports in which direct contact with the nose cannot be ruled out – e.g., ball sports such as tennis or soccer, contact sports, horseback riding, swimming, high diving, etc. – are better avoided for 8 weeks postoperatively.

Sports professionals engaged in these sporting activities who are unable to defer training for prolonged periods (e.g., professional soccer players, etc.) should wear customized face masks manufactured by an orthopedic shoemaker or by appropriate contacts at their club, which may allow them to train or play games relatively safely.

24.26 Stitches

The stitches at the columella incision are usually pulled around days 5–7 after surgery. If the suture lines from alar wedge and nostril sill resections are stable, these stitches are pulled simultaneously. If not, the latter are left in place for another 2–3 days.

24.27 Sun, Solarium

Patients are advised not to use a solarium and to avoid strong sunlight as much as possible for about 4–6 weeks after surgery, to protect the skin during the healing phase. Staying in the shade, using a peaked cap or similar, and applying sun creams with skin protection factor (SPF) 30 and higher are advisable.

Patients occasionally request surgery in the winter months, on the basis of information available from the Internet mentioning possible dangers of exposure to the sun. There is no truth in this, and it can be pointed out that the same operation is regularly performed in places like Australia, South America, and Africa, where exposure to sunlight plays a far greater role than in moderate climate zones.

24.28 Swelling, Hematomas

Patients must be informed preoperatively that considerable facial swelling may occur after surgery, although wide interindividual variations may be present; the postoperative course cannot be predicted beforehand.

Swelling can be expected to be most pronounced on the second and third postoperative days after piezosurgery, after which facial edema rapidly subsides. Postoperative edema and bluish-green facial hematomas are observed after hammer-and-chisel operations significantly more often than with piezoelectric techniques. The hematomas gravitate under the skin of the cheeks and neck within 1–2 weeks and then fade away. Edema takes longer to subside after the use of classic instruments than with piezoelectric devices.

24.29 Taping

About a week after surgery, the external aluminum splint and all tapes are removed from the nose, so that the skin will recover quickly. Patients sometimes ask if they will be receiving more taping of the nose beyond that period, as they may have picked up information from the Internet or another source. However, according to my experience, continued use of tapes brings no benefits or advantages. On the contrary, tapes should be removed as soon as possible to benefit skin recovery.

24.30 Work

Patients can generally start working on the computer or at a desk in the home office as early as 2–3 days after surgery. Returning to work depends to a great extent on the amount of physical stress associated with the specific job, and the patient must be advised accordingly.

Apart from that, it is important whether a patient is working in public or in direct contact with customers, or perhaps even as an actor on stage or in front of a camera. In general, the time point for returning to work may vary roughly between 5 days and 4 weeks after a rhinoplasty.

> ✔
>
> I give patients a leaflet with an overview of the most important information (▸ Fig. 24.1). However, this does not replace the additional recommendations that need to be given in the individual situation.

Bibliography

Yamasaki A, Warinner C, Lindsay R. Patient recovery and satisfaction with perioperative care after rhinoplasty. Facial Plast Surg Aesthet Med. 2022; 24(4):282–288

Index

Note: Page numbers set **bold** or *italic* indicate headings or figures, respectively.